Textbook of

Oral

Medicine and

Radiology

Textbook of
Oral
Medicine and
Radiology

Tapasya Karemore

MDS (Oral Medicine and Radiology), Fellow FAIMER

Associate Professor
Department of Oral Medicine and Radiology
VSPM's Dental College and Research Centre
Nagpur, Maharashtra

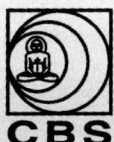

CBS

CBS Publishers & Distributors Pvt Ltd

New Delhi • Bengaluru • Chennai • Kochi • Kolkata • Mumbai
Hyderabad • Jharkhand • Nagpur • Patna • Pune • Uttarakhand

Textbook of
Oral
Medicine and
Radiology

ISBN: 978-93-90709-17-5

Copyright © Author and Publisher

First Edition: 2021

Published by Satish Kumar Jain and produced by Varun Jain for
CBS Publishers & Distributors Pvt Ltd
4819/XI Prahlad Street, 24 Ansari Road, Daryaganj, New Delhi 110 002, India
Ph: 011-23289259, 23266861, 23266867   Fax: 011-23243014
Website: www.cbspd.com   e-mail: delhi@cbspd.com; cbspubs@airtelmail.in

Corporate Office: 204 FIE, Industrial Area, Patparganj, Delhi 110 092, India
Ph: 011-49344934   Fax: 011-49344935   e-mail: publishing@cbspd.com; publicity@cbspd.com

Branches
- **Bengaluru:** Seema House 2975, 17th Cross, K.R. Road, Banasankari 2nd Stage, Bengaluru 560 070, Karnataka, India
  Ph: +91-80-26771678/79   Fax: +91-80-26771680   e-mail: bangalore@cbspd.com
- **Chennai:** 7, Subbaraya Street, Shenoy Nagar, Chennai 600 030, Tamil Nadu, India
  Ph: +91-44-26680620, 26681266   Fax: +91-44-42032115   e-mail: chennai@cbspd.com
- **Kochi:** 42/1325, 1326, Power House Road, Opposite KSEB, Power House, Ernakulum-682018, Kochi, Kerala, India
  Ph: +91-484-4059061-67   Fax: +91-484-4059065   e-mail: kochi@cbspd.com
- **Kolkata:** 6/B, Ground Floor, Rameswar Shaw Road, Kolkata-700 014 (West Bengal), India
  Ph: +91-33-22891126, 22891127, 22891128   e-mail: kolkata@cbspd.com
- **Mumbai:** PWD Shed, Gala No. 25/26, Ramchandra Bhatt Marg, Next JJ Hospital Gate No. 2
  Opp. Union Bank of India, Noorbaug, Mumbai-400009, Maharashtra, India
  Ph: +91-22-66661880/89   e-mail: mumbai@cbspd.com

Representatives
- **Hyderabad**   0-9885175004
- **Patna**   0-9334159340
- **Jharkhand**   0-9811541605
- **Pune**   0-9623451994
- **Nagpur**   0-9421945513
- **Uttarakhand**   0-9716462459

Printed at: Nutech Print Services, Faridabad, Haryana, India

to
all my beloved
students and dental professionals

Foreword

Oral medicine and radiology was started as a new speciality in India in the early 1970s, by starting MDS in Bangalore and Ahmedabad. Soon, the Dental Council of India made it a separate subject of study and examination for the BDS course in the final year. Before this era, textbooks used by the students were either on oral medicine or radiology, published from abroad. Towards the end of the last century, textbooks on oral medicine and radiology by Indian authors dealing with all topics mentioned in the curriculum and syllabus for BDS examination in the subject came into circulation. This book by the principal author Dr Tapasya Karemore and illustrious co-authors is the latest addition to the list.

The book is in two sections. All topics mentioned in the syllabus by the Dental Council of India are included in this textbook. The first section deals with the methods to learn oral diagnosis, clinical medicine, therapeutics and diagnostic tests. In the present century biotechnology has advanced very rapidly and, in most diseases, the final diagnosis is based on sophisticated molecular biological tests. Attempts made by the authors to include newer techniques in genomics and proteomics for diagnosis are applaudable.

The new cancer control programme (2017) of the Government of India includes screening of oral cancers at the primary health centre level. This programme has already been implemented in more than 100 districts. General medical practitioners and dental surgeons working in such programmes will find this book beneficial, as it contains several original, clinical photographs which would help them in diagnosing the same.

Newer areas of interest by the speciality like geriatrics, forensic medicine and physiotherapy in dentistry are added attractions.

Second section covers all the topics in oral radiology. The chapters on advanced imaging, soft tissue calcifications and ossifications as well as trauma teeth and jaws are novel and very useful.

In short, *Textbook of Oral Medicine and Radiology* principally authored by Dr Tapasya Karemore and the group of 31 brilliant specialists from India and abroad, is very comprehensive with all the topics as per the BDS syllabus and curriculum.

I wish the readers can take as much possible from this enriched resource.

07.07.2020

Babu Mathew
MDS (Oral Pathology, 1969)
MDS (Oral Medicine and Radiology, 1976)
President, Cancer Control Foundation of India
Ex-Professor, Community Oncology
The Regional Cancer Centre
Trivandrum, India
Former Principal/Dean/Research Director
Rajas Dental College, Vadakkangulam
Azeezia Dental College, Kollam and
PMS Dental College, Vattappara,
Trivandrum, India
Visiting Professor
University of Malmö, Sweden

Preface

Knowledge is power. Information is liberating. Education is the premise for progress..!
—Kofi Annan

Textbook of Oral Medicine and Radiology is a long cherished dream comes true for me as an author. I realize that it follows closely in the wake of several excellent textbooks in the subject. However, I sincerely felt that my knowledge, experience and wisdom gathered over the years of teaching and clinical practice can add value to what has already been written in this field.

I have tried to compile all concepts in the subject keeping in mind the needs of the undergraduate dental students towards learning the subject. One of the unique features of this textbook is the critical content validation from stalwarts having more than 20 years experience in the subject. Each chapter has undergone a comprehensive review procedure with strict adherence to the protocol till the final draft was found precise. Every topic covered has been kept abreast with updated knowledge and written in an 'easy to understand' format, along with special impetus to their clinical implications.

Another exclusive feature is, those topics that could be combined, to discuss and correlate clinical and radiologic characteristics, have been included as a separate section. As per the changing paradigms in the subject, a few more novel topics such as 'Role of Oral Physiotherapy', 'Commonly Practiced Diagnostic Tests' and 'Drugs in Oral Medicine' have also been incorporated in the book. All the clinical pictures and radiographs included in the book are original and flowcharts and schematic diagrams have been used wherever deemed necessary. As the principal author of the book, I wish to offer this work to the budding dental health professionals of the society. It is my honest attempt to help the students to inculcate the knowledge in oral medicine and radiology and build confidence in diagnosis and management of various oral and maxillofacial conditions.

I sincerely hope students and professionals enjoy reading it and benefit from it.

Tapasya Karemore

Acknowledgments

It was a pleasure to complete this work along with all the authors, who have contributed wholeheartedly towards the completion of this book. I would like to acknowledge the contribution of all the authors, out of which some were my teachers, colleagues and my students. I, therefore, consider this as a unique opportunity to have three generations working for the project together and so the knowledge and experience over a long period of time could be compiled together. I am deeply indebted to the reviewers of this book Dr Mukta Motwani, Dr Shirish Degwekar, Dr Deepak Samdani, Dr Ramhari Sathwane and Dr Ranjitkumar Patil who gave critical inputs and helped me to improve myself as an author and to refine the scientific content. I thank my colleagues in the department Dr Apeksha, Dr Anurag, Dr Smriti and Dr Apurva for their timely help and cooperation. I am also indebted to my students and postgraduates Dr Manjiri, Dr Shruti, Dr Adeeba, Dr Shreya, Dr Rajni, Dr Trushita and Dr Rutuja for taking efforts in collecting clinical pictures of the patients. Dr Adeeba Siddiqui needs special mention for her contribution to the radiography section of the book.

Heartfelt thanks to the best critics Dr Laxmikant Hedaoo, Dhwani Suchak, Simran Tahilyani, Mrunali Dahikar, Jeenal Manglani for being the student reviewers.

I also thank Dr Ranjitkumar Patil, Dr Vidya Lohe, Dr Ambika Gupta, Dr Harshkant Gharote, Dr Amit Parate, Dr Abhijeet Deoghare and Dr Silky Jasuja, Dr Saurabh Shrivastav, Dr Kriti Shrivastav, Dr Deepali Agrawal and Dr Vandana Singh for providing clinical images and radiographs apart from contributing to their own chapters as well.

I thank Dr Babu Mathew for his precious words as Foreword for this book and Dr Rahul Bhowate for penning down his feelings in the About the Author section.

My gratitude to CBS Publishers & Distributors Pvt. Ltd., especially Mr. YN Arjuna, for meticulous designing and compilation of my work. I greatly appreciate their uncompromising attitude towards quality of the production.

I express my sincere gratitude towards Dr Usha Radke, Dean and Dr Ramakrishna Shenoi, Vice Dean, VSPM's Dental College and Research Centre, Nagpur, for their continuous guidance and support.

I want to express my love and appreciation for my friends Dr Rajlakshmi Banerjee and Dr Saee Deshmukh for always being there to hold my hand and encourage me.

I thank my guide and mentor Dr Mukta Motwani for her tremendous positive influence on my professional development.

I heartily thank my parents, for believing in me and giving me the freedom to fulfill my dreams.

My beloved husband Dr Vaibhav has been by my side in all my endeavours as an integral part. Thanks in words cannot express my feelings for him. I am truly blessed.

It was heartening to see my sons Divit and Nivedit being always very supportive as such projects intrude a lot into family time. A big thanks to both of them.

Gratitude to the creator of this world 'God' for keeping me motivated enough throughout and blessed me with wonderful people around, to work harder!!

Tapasya Karemore

Esteemed Reviewers

Deepak Samdani
MDS
Former Professor and Head
Department of Oral Medicine
and Radiology
Dasmesh Institute of Research
and Dental Sciences, Faridkot
Punjab, India

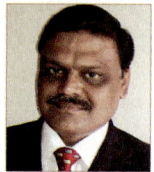

Ranjitkumar Patil
MDS
Vice Dean
Professor and Head
Department of Oral Medicine
and Radiology
Faculty of Dental Sciences
King George Medical University, Lucknow
Uttar Pradesh, India

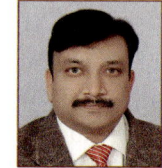

Mukta Motwani
MDS
Professor and Head
Department of Oral Medicine
and Radiology
VSPM's Dental College and
Research Centre
Digdoh Hills, Hingna
Nagpur
Maharashtra, India

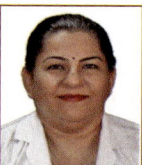

Shirish Degwekar
MDS
Former Professor and Head
Department of Oral Medicine
and Radiology
Datta Meghe Institute of
Medical Sciences
Sawangi (M), Wardha
Maharashtra, India

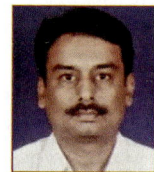

Ramhari Sathwane
MDS
Professor and Head
Department of Oral Medicine
and Radiology
SDK Dental College, Nagpur
Maharashtra, India

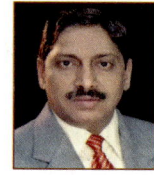

Contributors

Aarati Panchbhai
MDS PhD

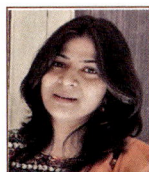

Professor
Department of Oral Medicine and
Radiology
Sharad Pawar Dental College
and Hospital,
DMIMS (Deemed to be University)
Sawangi (Meghe), Wardha
Maharashtra

Author: Diseases of Tongue, X-ray Film,
Intensifying Screen and Grid, Film Processing

Abhijeet Deoghare
MDS

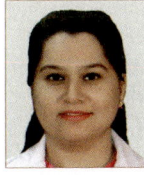

Professor and Head
Department of Oral Medicine
and Radiology
CDCRI, Rajnandgaon
Chhattisgarh

Author: Physiotherapy in Dentistry, and Soft Tissue
Calcifications and Ossification

Ambika Gupta
MDS

Senior Professor and Head
Department of Oral Medicine
and Radiology
Post Graduate Institute of
Dental Sciences
Rohtak

Author: Diseases of Bones Manifested in the Jaws

Amit R Parate
MDS

Associate Professor
Government Dental College
and Hospital
Aurangabad
Maharashtra

Author: Radiation, Safety and Protection

Anuraag B Choudhary
MDS

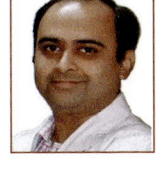

Assistant Professor
Department of Oral Medicine &
Radiology
VSPM's Dental College and
Research Centre, Nagpur

Author: Red Blood Cell Disorders—
Oral Manifestations and Dental Considerations

Apurva Mohite Khator
MDS

Assistant Professor
Department of Oral Medicine
and Radiology
VSPM's Dental College and
Research Centre, Nagpur

Author: Neuromuscular Disorders

Avinash Tejasvi ML
MDS

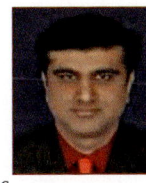

Professor
Department of Oral Medicine
and Radiology
Kamineni Institute of Dental Sciences
Telangana

Author: Intraoral Radiographic Techniques

Bhavana Sujanamulk
MDS

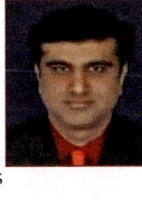

Reader
Department of Oral Medicine and
Radiology
Drs Sudha & Nageswara Rao
Siddhartha Institute of Dental Sciences
Vijayawada, Andhra Pradesh

Author: Temporomandibular Joint Diseases
and Radiation Biology

Chetana Ramesh Ratnaparkhi
MBBS MD (Radiodiagnosis)
Associate Professor
Department of Radiodiagnosis
NKP Salve Institute of Medical
Sciences and Lata Mangeshkar
Hopsital, Digdoh Hills, Hingna,
Nagpur
Author: Advance Imaging
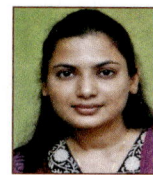

Nikhil Diwan
MDS PhD PGDEMS
Professor and PG Guide
MA Rangoonwala College of Dental
Sciences and Research Centre, Pune
Author: Benign Tumors of the Jaw
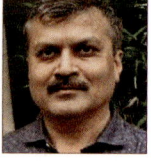

Harshkant P Gharote
MDS
Professor
Oral Medicine and Radiology
Oral Sciences Division
Dentistry Program
Batterjee Medical College, Jeddah, Saudi Arabia
Author: Projection Geometry, Trauma: Teeth and Jaws

Kanak Tripathi
MDS
Senior Lecturer
Department of Oral Medicine
and Radiology
Nanded Rural Dental College and
Research Center, Nanded
Co-author: Soft Tissue Calcification and Ossification

Keerthi G
MDS
Department of Oral Medicine
and Radiology
KLE Society's Institute of Dental
Sciences, Bengaluru
Author: Systemic Diseases and Dental
Considerations (Chapters 14–20)

Kshitij Bang
MDS (OMFS), FIBOMS FAOCMF
Associate Professor
VSPM's Dental College and
Research Centre, Nagpur
Author: Orofacial Pain
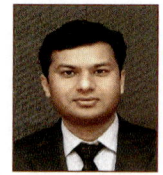

Mohit Gunwal
MDS
Assistant Professor
Department of Conservative Dentistry
VSPM's Dental College and
Research Centre, Nagpur
Author: Dental Caries
Co-author: Diseases of Pulp and
Periradicular Region
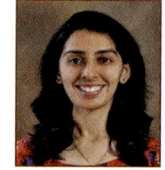
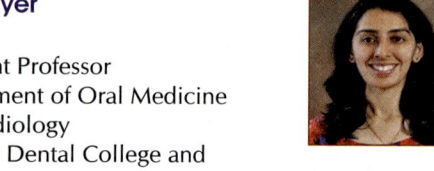

Neha Iyer
MDS
Assistant Professor
Department of Oral Medicine
and Radiology
VSPM's Dental College and
Research Centre, Nagpur
Author: Digital Imaging
Co-author: Extraoral Radiography
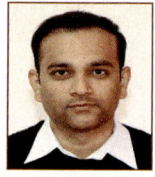

Pawan Motghare
MDS
Assistant Professor
Department of Oral Medicine and
Radiology
Government Dental College
Nagpur
Co-author: Radiation Physics
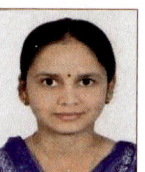

Priti Chawla
MDS
Associate Professor
SGRD Institute of Dental Sciences
and Research, Amritsar, Punjab
Author: Ulcerative Vesiculobullous
Lesions
Co-author: Oral Cancer and Radiologic
Considerations of Malignant Lesions
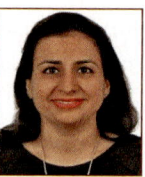

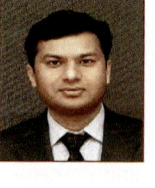

Priya Sahni
MDS
Professor and Head
Department of Dentistry
Ananta Institute of Medical Sciences
and Research Centre, Rajsamand
Rajasthan
Author: Red and White Lesions
Co-author: Clinical Investigations and Diagnostic Aids
in Oral Medcine: An Overview

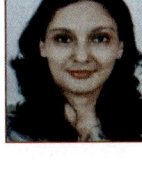

Raghavendra Byakodi
MDS
Professor
Department of Oral medicine
and Radiology
Vasantdada Patil Dental College and
Hospital
Kavalapur Sangli, Maharashtra
Author: Normal Anatomical Landmarks

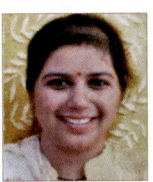

Rashmi Nivasrkar
MDS
Oral Medicine and Radiology
Co-author: Physiotherapy in
Dentistry

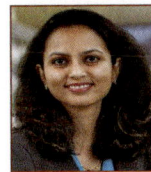

Rujuta Katkar
MDS MS Dipl. ABOMR
Associate Professor
Oral & Maxillofacial Radiology
Department of Comprehensive
Dentistry
University of Texas Health Science Center
San Antonio, 7703 Floyd Curl Drive
San Antonio, TX 78229
Author: Paranasal Sinus Diseases

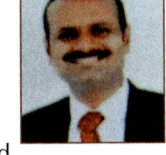

Samantha Thakur
BDS, MSc (FM)
Reader
Department of Oral Pathology and
Microbiology
MA Rangoonwala College of
Dental Sciences and Research Centre
Azam Campus, Pune
Author: Forensic Odontology

Silky Rajesh Punyani
MDS
Associate Professor
Department of Dentistry
Ananta Institute of Medical Sciences
and Research Centre, Rajsamand
Rajasthan
Author: Clinical Investigations and Diagnostic Aids
in Oral Medicine: An overview
Pigmented Lesions of Oral Cavity
Co-author: Red and White Lesions

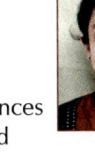

Smriti Golhar
MDS
Assistant Professor
Department of Oral Medicine
and Radiology
VSPM's Dental College and
Research Centre, Nagpur
Author: HIV Infection and Acquired Immune
Deficiency Syndrome (AIDS)

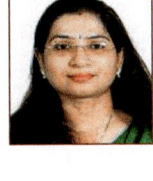

Sonam Khurana
MDS
Resident
Department of Oral and
Maxillofacial Radiology
University of Texas Health
San Antonio
Co-author: Paranasal Sinus Diseases

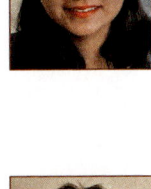

Sumanth Kumbargere Nagraj
MDS
Professor and Head
Department of Oral Medicine and
Radiology
Faculty of Dentistry
Melaka-Manipal Medical College
Bukit Baru, 75150, Melaka, Malaysia
Author: Dental Therapeutics and CBCT—
Principles and Applications in Dentistry

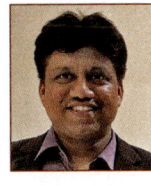

Suwarna Dangore-Khasbage
MDS
Professor
Department of Oral Medicine and
Radiology
Sharad Pawar Dental College
and Hospital, Sawangi (M), Wardha
Maharashtra
Author: Geriatric and Oral Health

Tapasya Karemore
MDS
Fellow FAIMER
Associate Professor
Department of Oral Medicine
and Radiology
VSPM's Dental College and Research Centre
Nagpur

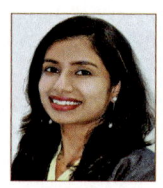

Author: History Taking and Diagnosis in
Oral Medicine, Oral Cancer and Radiologic
Considerations of Malignant Lesions,
Radiation Physics, Extraoral Imaging,
Panoramic Imaging, Periapical Pathologies

Co-author: Temporomandibular Joint Diseases and
Radiologic Considerations, Processing and Errors,
Radiologic Considerations in Periodontal Diseases

Vaibhav Karemore
MDS
Associate Professor
Department of Periodontia
Government Dental College, Nagpur

Author: Radiologic Considerations in
Periodontal Diseases

Vidya K Lohe
MDS
Professor and Head
Department of Oral Medicine and
Radiology
Sharad Pawar Dental College and
Hospital
Datta Meghe Institute of Medical Sciences
Sawangi (M), Wardha, Maharashtra

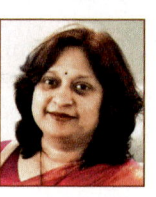

Author: Cyst of the Orofacial Regions

Vikram Khanna
MDS
Associate Professor
Department of Oral Medicine and
Radiology
Faculty of Dental Sciences
King George's Medical University
Lucknow, Uttar Pradesh

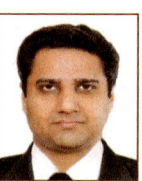

Author: Salivary Gland Disorders—Clinical and
Radiologic Considerations

Contents

Section I

Oral Medicine

Section II

Oral Radiology

Oral Medicine

Case History, Diagnosis and Systemic Considerations

Chapter 1

DEFINITION (AAOM)

Oral medicine is the specialty of dentistry that deals with the diagnosis and management of diseases that are non-surgical in nature, that may occur only in the oral cavity or may be an oral manifestation of systemic disease.

Oral cavity can reflect majority of systemic illness in children as well as adolescents. Oral health is integral factor of overall general health to which a clinician should be oriented while aiming at proper diagnosis and management.

Case history is defined as the data concerning an individual and his or her family and environment, including the individual's medical history that may be useful in analyzing and diagnosing his or her case or for instructional purposes. *(Grossman 13th Edition)*

History taking is an art, which a doctor learns over the years by repeated practice and experience. *(PJ Mehta)*

First interaction with the doctor can influence patient to answer every necessary leading question. It is advisable to consider patient's psyche as well, and not only the status of the disease.

IMPORTANCE OF HISTORY

* To aim at diagnosis
* To develop rapport with patient

* To know the psycho-social, economical, educational and health status of the patient so as to help in treatment planning.

Assessing patient's health, obtaining and evaluating history meticulously is mandatory for oral diagnostician. This method of history recording is divided into 4 major steps.

Steps:
1. Obtaining relevant information
2. Deriving provisional diagnosis
3. Carrying out necessary test to get final diagnosis
4. Formulating an accurate treatment plan.

Obtaining a patient's consent is another significant segment of case history taking.

A good case history should have the following information in a systematic manner.

a. **Demographic details:** This includes patient's name, age, sex, address, occupation, religion and marital status.
b. **Chief complaint:** This narrates about complaint with which patient has visited to doctor. These complaints should be recorded in chronological order along with duration.
c. **History of present illness:** This is related to complaints which patient had been dealing with, with all the symptoms right from initial days to present. Details of each symptom must be recorded separately. Associated symptoms must

3

be inquired and recorded. Similar illness in the past, duration and sequelae should be asked.

d. **Personal history:** It includes patient's appetite, diet, bowel and bladder habits, sleep cycle and associated habits of tobacco, kharra, betel nut, alcohol, snuff, khaini, smoking, etc.

e. **Family history:** The state of health of family members like, parents, grand-parents, siblings should be noted. That history may include chronic and serious illness.
   * Few diseases run in family, so family history is of significance when a clinician deals with patient, e.g. X-linked recessive diseases—hemophilia, G6PD deficiency
   * Autosomal dominant disorders—neurofibromatosis familial hyperlipidemias
   * Autosomal recessive disorder—sickle cell anemia, beta thalassemia

f. **Menstrual and obstetric history:** Menstrual history is important to know, as it can be co-related with hormonal cycle and pregnancy.

GENERAL EXAMINATION

Includes following details:

In general examination we observe whether patient is conscious, cooperative and well-oriented with time, place and person, along with it we examine all vital parameters.

1. Built
2. Body proportions
3. Nutrition
4. Decubitus
5. Clubbing
6. Cyanosis
7. Jaundice
8. Pallor
9. Lymphadenopathy
10. Edema
11. Skin, hair and nails, vertebral column
12. Temperature
13. Pulse
14. Blood pressure
15. Respiratory rate

1. **Built:** It is the skeletal structure in relation to age and sex compared to a normal person. Conditions where altered built can be observed are:
   * *Tall:* Gigantism, hyperpituitarism, Marfan's syndrome
   * *Shrot:* Genetic, malnutrition, skeletal deformities, renal diseases.

2. **Body proportions**
   * *In adults:* Upper segment is equal to the lower segment
   * *In infants:* Upper segment is greater than the lower segment.
   * Due to genetic disorders this ratio can be altered, e.g. Marfan's syndrome, Klinefelter's syndrome

3. **Nutrition:** Proteins, fats, carbohydrates, vitamins and minerals are important for nourishment of human body. Deficiency of any of the nutritional factor should be observed and mentioned in the history, e.g. iron deficiency can cause pallor, koilonychia, calcium can cause tetany.

4. **Decubitus:** It is posture of the patient which he adapts when lying in bed, e.g.
   * *Hemiplegia:* One side of patient is immobile
   * *Tetanus:* The patient has neck stiffness.
   * *Pneumonia:* The patient is uncomfortable on lying on the affected side.

5. **Clubbing:** It is bulbous enlargement of soft parts of the terminal phalanges with both transverse and longitudinal curving of the nails. This occurs due to interstitial edema and dilation of the arterioles and capillaries.
   * Conditions leading to clubbing are: Tuberculosis, infective endocarditis, Crohn's disease, myxedema, etc.
   * *Schamroth's sign:* When two fingers are held together with nails touching each other, a diamond-shaped space is seen, which is lost in case of clubbing.

× Hypoxia is considered as possible cause for causing clubbing

6. **Cyanosis:** It is bluish discoloration due to reduced hemoglobin in capillary blood

   × Types of cyanosis are central, peripheral and mixed.

   × Causes of cyanosis can be, congestive cardiac failure, chronic obstructive lung disease, exposure to high altitude or cold, etc.

   × *Cause of cyanosis:* When the amount of reduced hemoglobin exceeds 5 gm% in the capillaries, the blood appears dark, giving the tissue a bluish hue.

7. **Jaundice:** It is a symptom complex which is characterized by yellow discoloration of tissue and body fluids due to increase in the bile pigments. Jaundice can be positive in intra-corpuscular defects, extra-corpuscular defects, disturbance in bilirubin transport and hepatocellular diseases. Normal serum bilirubin: 1 mg% (total)

8. **Pallor:** Pallor is paleness of skin and mucous membrane due to circulating red blood cells or diminished blood supply. Causes of pallor can be anemia, shock and peripheral vascular disease.

9. **Lymphadenopathy:** It is an inflammatory or non-inflammatory enlargement of lymph nodes. There are various causes of lymphadenopathy like inflammatory diseases, neoplastic diseases, and neurological diseases. It can be categorized as generalized or regional lymphadenopathy. For oral and maxillo-facial infections regional lymph nodes are commonly enlarged or show changes.

10. **Edema:** It is a collection of fluid in the interstitial spaces or serous cavities. It may occur due to increased capillary permeability like, in acute inflammation, increased capillary pressure, e.g. cardiac failure or decreased osmotic pressure of the blood in hypoproteinemia. So, various cardiac, renal, hepatic endocrinal and nutritional disorders are responsible for edema.

11. **Vertebral column, skin, hair, nails.**

    × **Vertebral column** has no lateral curvature. It should be examined for any abnormality, angular deformity, swelling or tenderness.

    × Patient can be asked to bend forwards, backwards, and sideways to evaluate changes in vertebral column, which maybe a result of scoliosis, kyphosis, gibbus, lordosis.

    × **Skin** can be examined for its color, pigmentation, eruptions, macule, vesicle, hemorrhage. Types of skin are dry, moist, thick, thin, and pinched.

    To deal with history of **hair**, various details can be obtained as, falling of hair (typhoid), patent hair loss, loss of eyebrows or excessive growth (Cushing's syndrome).

    × **Nails** should be examined for shape, size, pallor and relation to nail bed. Conditions that affect nails are: anemia, tuberculosis, cyanosis or clubbing due to systemic diseases, hemorrhagic condition.

Vital Parameters

12. **Temperature:** Fever is associated with release of endogenous pyrogens which activate T cell and shows active host defense. It refers to body temperature mechanism of the viscera and tissue of the body. It can be best recorded by mercury thermometer and is recorded in axilla as a chair-side method but can also be recoded by keeping thermometer orally or rectally (kids).

    Normal range of temperature; 36°–37°C or 98°–99°F. Fever is an increase of more than 1°C or any rise above normal temperature.

    Probable causes of fever can be infections, neoplasms, vascular diseases, trauma, immunologic diseses, endocrinal diseases, metabolic diseases, etc.

13. **Pulse:** The normal pulse with regular intervals has normal range of 60–100/minute.

Pulse can be *anacrotic pulse, dicrotic pulse, pulsus bisferiens, pulsus parvus of tardus, pulsus alternans, pulsus paradoxus, thread pulse, and water hammer pulse.*

14. **Blood pressure:** BP is measured in terms of systolic and diastolic. Systolic BP is controlled by stroke volume of heart and stiffness of the arterial vessels, whereas diastolic BP is controlled by peripheral resistance.

   Variation in BP can be due to emotional alteration, exercise, meals, alcohol, tobacco, bladder distension, pain or temperature rise. Also circadian rhythms, age and face can influence BP.

   Measuring BP can aid in diagnosis of hypertension, hypotension, pulsus paradoxus, pulsus alternans, and aortic incompetence.

15. **Respiratory rate (RR):** Normal rate of respiration is 16–20/minute.
   * Increased RR (tachypnea) is evident in a few conditions like, exertion and excitement, fever, anorexia, and anemias while decreased RR (bradypnea) can be seen in poisoning like narcotic drugs and brain tumor.
   * Dyspnea is breathlessness, which can be seen with congestive cardiac failure, asthma, pneumonia, COPD.

BODY SYSTEMS: EVALUATION FOR SYMPTOMS (PAST MEDICAL HISTORY)

Obtaining accurate past medical history (PMH) is also important in history taking as it helps to identify oral manifestation of systemic disorders, in diagnosing and treating the condition and sometimes in handling relevant medico-legal issues.

* **Respiratory system:** Chest pain, wheezing, dyspnea, cough, hemoptysis.
* **CVS:** Chest pain, dyspnea, edema, claudication
* **GIT:** Appetite, dysphagia, nausea, vomiting, hematemesis, indigestion, pain, diarrhea, constipation, bloating, jaundice.
* **Genito-urinary:** Urinary frequency, dysuria, hematuria, nocturia, incontinence, discharge.
* **Endocrine:** Polyuria, polydypsia, pigmentation, temperature intolerance.
* **Hematologic:** Spontaneous gingival bleeding, long bleeding time, easy bruising, epistaxis.
* **Dermatologic:** Pruritus, rashes, pigmentation, eruptions, allergy.
* **Musculoskeletal (spasm of muscles of TMJ and accessory muscles of mastication):** Changes in range of motion of joint, joint swellings, joint deformities, pain of muscles or joint, joint sounds.
* **Lymphatic system:** Enlarged nodes, mobility.
* **ENT:** Oropharynx, nasopharynx, voice changes.

EXTRAORAL EXAMINATION

It includes examination of head, facial symmetry, TMJ, lymph nodes, ears, nose, eyes.

   Examination is carried out in a dental chair with the head completely rested or supported. This aids in accurate extraoral examination of the patient.

   This examination in dental office is restricted to the superficial tissues of the oral cavity, head and neck.

* **Facial symmetry:** This can guide towards uniformity of facial structures, bilaterally. It can be examined under two headings—symmetrical or asymmetrical.

   Face can be asymmetrical due to swelling, genetic disorder, trauma, etc.
* **TMJ:** Joint is examined for range of motion, swelling, pain of muscles, joint, palpation of muscles and joint or any other obvious abnormality (detail examination of TMJ is covered in chapter on TMJ diseases)
* **Ear, nose:** Examined for observable pathology, bleeding and pain.
* **Lips:** Lips are examined for presence of lip seal. Swelling, painful ulcer, gingival enlargement, etc. can alter competency of lips.

× **Eye:** Eyes are examined for intercanthus and eyeball distance, vision or other developmental abnormalities.

× **Neck (lymph nodes):** Regional lymph nodes are cervical group of lymph nodes (submental, submandibular, parotid, post-auricular, pre-auricular, occipital, and others are superficial, deep and anterior cervical nodes).

Nodes are examined under the headings of group of lymph nodes, mobility, side enlargement, dimension, tenderness, number, discharge, fixity to underlying structure, consistency and overlying skin.

Lymph node examination: For submandibular LN clinician stands behind the patient. With fixed neck, clinician uses tip of the first two fingers placing them medial to the body of mandible to palpate the nodes.

Cervical group of LN can be palpated anteriorly and posterior to the sterno-cleidomastoid (SCM) muscle. (By rotation of neck to opposite side, SCM becomes prominent which facilitates LN examination). There are many clinical conditions causing lymphadenopathy like local or systemic. Most common causes include infections of odontogenic origin, tuberculosis, malignancy, lymphomas or other non-specific lymphadenopathy, etc.

In acutely inflamed ulcers, the regional lymph nodes become enlarged, tender and show signs of acute lymphadenitis. Later on the nodules become soften to form an abscess.

In malignant ulcers, the nodes are stony hard and may be fixed to the neighboring structures in the later stages.

INTRAORAL EXAMINATION

Hard tissue and soft tissue examinations are covered in this section of history.

Hard tissue involves teeth while soft tissue includes all mucosae, tongue, gingiva, oropharynx, faucial pillars, uvula hard palate.

× **Lips:** Normal is pink, smooth and moist. It shows minor salivary glands.

× **Cheeks:** Moist and pink, Fordyce's granules, salivary gland opening (parotid)

× **Floor of mouth:** Lingual frenum, sublingual fold, sublingual carbuncle.

× **Tongue**
- *Dorsum:* Papilla present and median furrow.
- *Ventral surface:* Lingual frenum attached and varicosities
- *Movements*
- *Lateral borders*

× **Palate (soft/hard):** Minor salivary glands and their opening.

× **Gingiva**
- Coral pink in color.
- Firm and resilient in consistency.
- Stippling present with orange peel appearance.

× **Orifice of salivary ducts**
1. Parotid gland: Parotid duct
   - The duct opens into the mouth on the inner surface of cheek usually opposite to the maxillary 2nd molar.
2. Submandibular gland: Wharton's duct
   - It opens by narrow opening on the summit of a small papilla at the side of frenum on the tongue.
3. Sublingual gland: Bartholins's duct
   - The sublingual glands are drained by 8–20 excretory ducts known as duct of Rivinus.
   - Most of the remaining small sublingual ducts open into the floor of the mouth.

× Tonsillar pillar

× **Hard tissue:** Teeth
   Hypoplasia
   - Enamel hypoplasia
   - Dentin dysplasia
   - Fluorosis

× **Caries:** Initial/moderate/deep/pulp involvement

× Missing

× Filled

× Endodontically treated

× **Mobile**
  - Periodontitis
  - Pulpal infection
  - Trauma
  - Malignancy
  - Trauma from occlusion (TFO)
× Wasting disease
× **Over retained**
  - Ankylosis of tooth
  - Incomplete resorption of primary tooth
× **Supernumerary teeth**
  - Cleidocranial dysplasia
  - Familial adenomatous polyposis
  - Trichorhinophalangeal syndrome,
  - Type I: Rubinstein-Taybi syndrome
  - Nance-Horan syndrome
  - Opitz BBB/G syndrome
  - Oculofaciocardiodental syndrome
  - Autosomal dominant Robinow syndrome.
× Malposed
× Malformed
× Root stumps
× **Discolored/non-vital**
  - Trauma, physical/chemical injuries, caries, etc.
× **Fractured**
  - Trauma, malocclusion, dysplastic teeth, abrasion, erosion, etc.
× **Impacted**
  - Various syndromes are associated with impacted teeth which are either pathogenic or genetic (cleidocranial

TABLE 1.1: Causes of stains	
Extrinsic	*Intrinsic*
× Remnant of Nasmyth membrane × Poor oral hygiene × Existing restoration × Gingival bleeding × Plaque and calculus × Eating habits: Tea, coffee, stains, etc. × Tobacco chewing habit × Chromogenic bacteria × Mouthwashes: Chlorohexidine	× Hereditary disorders × Medication × Excess fluoride × High fever associated with early childhood illness and other types of trauma. × Stains located inside enamel and dentin.

dysplasia, Gardner's syndrome, Down syndrome, etc.)
× **Migration**
  - Pulpal or periodontal infections
  - Pathogenic cause like cyst, tumors, etc.
× Removable partial denture
× **Edentulous jaw:** Roots pieces, bone spicules, tori, etc.
× **Deposits:** Stains
  - Calculus
  - Plaque
× Periodontal status

Gingiva Examination

× Color, contour
× Consistency
× Bleeding on probing

TABLE 1.2: Clinical signs of pulpitis, periodontitis and gingivitis		
Signs of pulpitis	*Signs of periodontitis*	*Signs of gingivitis*
× No sensation to cold and hot temperature × Sharp shooting, piercing and lancinating pain (due to involvement of delta nerve fibres) or dull, boring, gnawing and excruciating (C-fibres). × Often localized to apex, with a fistulous tract. × Mobility of the tooth may or may not be present. × Often severe and difficult to localize. × Tooth may have large restoration. × Problem related to apex.	× Tooth sensitive to hot or cold stimuli. × Presence of periodontal pocket. × Presence of bleeding on probing. × Presence of recession × Mobility × Malodour × Teeth migration × Dull aching pain on mastication	× Tooth sensitive to hot or cold stimuli. × Presence of gingival pocket. × Presence of bleeding on probing × Reddish discoloration and swelling in the marginal gingival. × Increase in gingival crevicular fluid.

* Enlargement
* Recession
* Surface texture
* Interdental papillae
* Irritation from prosthesis or overhanging restoration.

Examination of Swelling (Extraoral)

Inspection

* Site, number	Edge
* Extent	Pulsation
* Shape	Overlying skin
* Surface texture	Surrounding tissue
* Color	Limitation of movement
	Sinus/fistula discharge

Palpation

All inspectory findings are confirmed by palpation
* Temperature
* Tenderness
* Consistency
* Fixity to underlying structure
* Translucency
* Compressibility
* Pulsatile
* Fixity to overlying structures
* Blanching effect

Examination of Swelling (Intraoral)

Intraoral Inspection

* Site
* Number
* Size
* Shape
* Surface texture
* Color
* Edge
* Number
* Pulsation
* Limitation of movement
* Surrounding tissue

Palpation

All the inspectory findings are confirmed on palpation.
* Temperature
* Tenderness
* Consistency
* Fixity to underlying structures
* Translucency
* Compressible
* Pulsatile
* Fixing to underlying tissue

ULCER EXAMINATION

Inspection

* Size, shape and color
* Number
* Site
* Edge (raised/sloping/punched out/undermined/rolled out/everted.)
* Floor
* Discharge
* Surrounding area

Palpation

* Tenderness
* Edge
* Base
* Depth
* Bleeding
* Relation to deeper structures
* Surrounding area

Intraoral Inspection

* Size and shape
* Number
* Position
* Edge

Provisional diagnosis: After detailed history taking and critical clinical examination, the signs and symptoms collected can guide to arrive at a diagnosis which is known as provisional diagnosis.

Differential diagnosis: Similar disorders, or diseases with overlapping features are rearranged as a list with most probable lesion ranked at the top and least probable at the bottom.

Chair Side Clinical Investigation

Vitality Test

- Thermal tests
- Electric pulp testing (EPT)
- Bite test
- Anesthesia testing
- Test cavity
- Laser-Doppler flowmetry
- Pulse oximetry
- Dual wavelength spectrophotometry
- **Thermal:** Heat, cold, electric pulp testing
- Aspiration

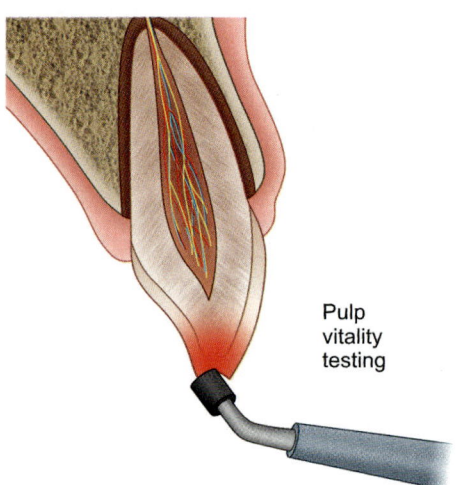

Pulp vitality testing

Fig. 1.1: Electronic pulp test

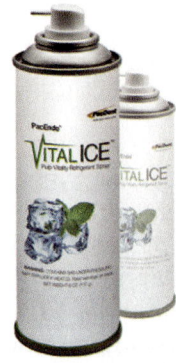

Fig. 1.2: The brand Vital Ice for cold test

Radiographic Investigations

This includes conventional (intraoral and extraoral) and advanced imaging modalities used to arrive at final diagnosis.

Conventional radiographic investigations: PA view or any other advanced imaging investigations include CT, MRI, VSG, scintigraphy, PET scan.

Laboratory investigations like routine hemogram, ESR, calcium, blood sugar, etc. are suggested related to the case to be diagnosed.

Special Investigations

1. **Blood test**
   - To detect any systemic disorder.
   - Total and differential count of WBC, hemoglobin, RBC count, ESR should be done.
2. **Examination of urine**
   - Particularly sugar estimation, to exclude diabetes, is important.
3. **Bacteriological examination of the discharge**
   - It is particularly important in inflamed and spreading ulcers.
   - This will not only give a clue as to the type of organism present in the ulcer, but also its sensitivity to a particular antibiotic.
4. **Biopsy**
   - Very important in malignant ulcers.
   - Biopsy is generally taken from edge of the ulcer, taking apportion of surrounding health tissue.
   - Biopsy material is then examined histologically to know the type of tumor, its invasiveness and whether differentiated or anaplastic.

Other tests include, scrape cytology, staining techniques and culture sensitivity tests.
- Final diagnosis
- Treatment plan
- Drugs/prescription
- Prognosis

Examination of Ulcer

An ulcer is a break in the continuity of the covering epithelium, skin or mucous membrane. It may either follow molecular death of the surface epithelium or its traumatic removal.

History

1. Mode of onset
2. Duration
3. Pain
4. Discharge
5. Associated disease

Local Examination

1. **On inspection**
   i. *Size and Shape*
      - *Oval:* Generally seen in tuberculous ulcers.
      - *Circular:* Seen in syphilitic ulcers.
      - *Irregular:* Seen in carcinomatous.
   ii. *Number*
      - *Multiple ulcers:* Herpetic ulcers
      - *Usually single:* Syphilitic and tuberculous ulcer
   iii. *Floor:* This is the exposed surface of the ulcer.
      - *Red granulation tissue:* Healing ulcer.
      - *Pale and smooth granulation tissue:* Slow healing ulcer.
      - *Watery granulation tissue:* Tubercular ulcer.
   iv. *Edge:* 5 common types of edges:
      a. Undermined edge is most commonly seen in tuberculous ulcer.
         - The overhanged skin is thin, friable, reddish blue and unhealthy.
      b. Punched out edge is most commonly seen in a gummatous ulcer or in a deep trophic ulcer.
         - The edge drops down at right angle to the skin surface as if it has been cut out with a punch.
      c. Sloping edge is mostly seen in healing traumatic or venous ulcers.
         - Every healing ulcer has a sloping edge, which is reddish purple in color and consists of new healthy epithelium.
      d. Raised and pearly-white beaded edge is a feature of rodent ulcer.
         - This type of edge develops in invasive cellular disease and becomes necrotic at the centre.
      e. Rolled out (everted) edge is a characteristic feature of squamous cell carcinoma.
   v. *Discharge:* The character of discharge and its amount should be noted.
      - *Scanty serous discharge:* Healing ulcer
      - *Purulent discharge:* Spreading inflamed ulcer
      - *Blood:* Malignancy.
   vi. *Surrounding area*
      - If the surrounding area of an ulcer is glossy, red and edematous, the ulcer is acutely inflamed.
      - All the findings of inspection are confirmed on palpation.
      a. *Tenderness*
         - *Exquisitely tender:* Acute inflamed ulcer
         - *Slightly tender:* Chronic ulcers like tuberculous
         - *Never tender:* Neoplastic
      b. *Edge and margin*
         - *Edge* is the area between the margin and the floor of the ulcer.
         - *Margin* is the junction between normal epithelium and ulcer, so it is the boundary of the ulcer.
      c. *Base:* It is on which the ulcer rests.
         - If an attempt is made to pick up the ulcer between the thumb and the index finger, the base will be felt.
         - *Slight indurations*: Chronic ulcer.
         - *Marked indurations*: Squamous cell.
      d. *Depth*
         - It can be recorded in mm.

× Trophic ulcers may be as deep to reach even the bone.
  e. *Bleeding*
    × Whether the ulcer bleeds to touch or not?
    × Commonly seen in malignant ulcer.
  f. *Relation with deeper structures.*
    × The ulcer is made to move over the deeper structures to know whether it is fixed to any of these structures.
    × Malignant ulcer is fixed to the deeper structure by infiltration.
  g. *Surrounding skin*
    × Increased temperature and tenderness of the surrounding skin indicates the ulcer to be of acute inflammatory origin.
    × Fixity to deeper structures indicates the malignant nature of the lesion.
vii. *Position*

EXAMINATION OF SWELLING

Definition

1. Swelling is an abnormal enlargement of a part of body, typically as a result of an accumulation of fluid
2. Swelling is a vague term which denotes any enlargement or protuberance in the body due to any cause.

1. Inspection

a. Site
  × Exterior angular dermoid: Lateral end of eyebrow
  × Meningocele: Back in midline
b. Size (in cm)
c. Shape
d. Surface
  × Smooth: Sebaceous cyst
  × Modular: Multinodular goiter
e. Skin
  × Pigmentation/ulceration/discharge
f. Surrounding area
  × Pigmentation/edema/discoloration
g. Others
  × Number
  × Color
  × Edges
  × Extent
  × Visible parameters

2. Palpation

a. Temperature
  × Increase in inflammation
b. Tenderness
  × Swelling related to nerves
c. Inspectory findings
  × Size, shape, surface
  × Edge and extent
  × Depth
d. Consistency
e. Fluctuations
  × Fluid or gas
  × Hydrocele

TABLE 1.3: Types of swellings				
Congenital	*Inflammatory*	*Traumatic*	*Neoplastic*	*Miscellaneous*
× Dermoid cyst × Hemangioma	× Abscess (pyogenic, pyemic, cold abscess) × Boil × Carbuncle × Erysipelas × Cellulitis	× Implantation dermoid	× Fibroma × Lipoma × Lymphangioma × Neurofibroma × Malignant (basal cell carcinoma, squamous cell carcinoma, malignant melanoma, sarcoma)	× Sebaceous cyst × Warts × Condyloma × Keloid/hypertrophic scar × Keratoacanthoma × Callosity/corn

f. Translucency (transmission of light through swelling)
   × Positive: Clear fluid and their transparent walls.
   × Negative: Wall thick, turbid liquid (blood or pus or lymph)
g. Reducibility: Can disappear completely and reappears by straining or coughing.
   × Hernia
   × Varicocele
h. Compressibility (swelling on pressure reduces in size, but only partially. It does not disappear completely).
   × Hemangiomas
i. Pulsatility
j. Fixity to skin
   × Fixed to skin cannot be lifted.
   × Skin moves over swelling.

3. Percussion

Not needed

4. Auscultation

Look for any bruit over pulsating swelling.
a. **Color**
   × Arterial haemangioma: Bright red
   × Venous haemangioma: Purple
   × Malignant melanoma: Black
   × Benign naevus: Black
   × Ranula: Bluish
b. **Skin overlying swelling**
   × Red and edematous: Inflammatory
   × Black punctum: Sebaceous cyst
   × Pigmentation: Moles, naevi
   × Scar
   × Ulcers

c. **Surface**
   × Smooth: Cystic swelling
   × Lobular: Lipoma
   × Nodular: Multinodular
   × Matted: Lymph nodes
   × Irregular: Carcinoma

d. **Edge**
   × Well-defined and irregular: Benign neoplasm
   × Well-defined and irregular: Neoplasm
   × Ill-defined and diffuse: Inflammatory swelling

e. **Consistency**
   × Soft: Lipoma
   × Cystic: Chronic abscess
   × Firm: Fibroma
   × Bony hard: Osteoma
   × Variable consistency: Malignancy

BIBLIOGRAPHY

1. Das S. A manual on clinical surgery. 4th edition Calcutta: S. Das; 1996.
2. Mehta P. Practical medicine. 16th edition Mumbai : National Book Depot; 2003.
3. Greenberg M and Glick M. Burket's Oral medicine diagnosis and treatment. 10th edition: BC Decker Inc; Elsevier; 2003
4. Greenberg M and Brightman V. Burket's Oral medicine diagnosis and treatment. 9th edition: Lippincott
5. Woud N and Goaz P. Differential diagnosis of oral and maxillofacial lesions. 5th edition: Elsevier; 2007.
   (www.ncbi.nlm.nih.gov/pubmed/27250821)

Clinical Investigations and Diagnostic Aids in Oral Medicine: An Overview

INTRODUCTION

Oral medicine as a speciality deals with a diagnosis and management of a vast variety of oral and systemic disorders that affect the oral cavity. Thorough recording of the patient's history, proper clinical examination remains the basis for arriving at a correct diagnosis and proper patient management. At the same time the importance of valid laboratory investigations and diagnostic aids cannot be undermined. It is of prime importance that the oral diagnostician be well aware of the relevant tests and investigations required when posed with a diagnostic challenge.

The pertinent laboratory investigations and diagnostic aids in oral medicine may broadly be classified under the following:

- Hematological investigations
- Biochemical investigations
- Histopathology and cytology
- Adjunct diagnostic aids for oral cancer and precancer
- Investigations for auto-immune disorders of the oral cavity
- Diagnostic microbiology
- Tests for allergy

HEMATOLOGICAL INVESTIGATIONS

Complete Blood Counts (CBC)

The basic test performed on the peripheral blood is the "Complete Blood Count" (CBC). It is one of the most informative investigations, expressing the health and disease status of the body. CBC is a comparatively inexpensive but powerful diagnostic tool in a variety of hematological and non-hematological disease conditions. It provides a myriad of valuable information about the blood and partly about the bone marrow. Over the past 3 decades, hematology analyzers have evolved by leaps and bounds, i.e. from semiautomated to fully automated ones.

The CBC is useful informative tool for various clinical situations like:

- Diagnosis of anemias (etiological and morphological types) and hemoglobino-pathies (thalassemia, sickle cell anemia, and hemolytic anemia)
- Nutritional deficiencies (iron, vitamin B_{12}, folic acid)
- Parasitic infections (malaria, filaria, leishmania)
- Thrombocytopenia [primary (due to nonproduction), secondary (due to

peripheral destruction) and bleeding disorders]
- Diagnosis of infections, leukocytosis, leukopenias, eosinophilia, monocytosis, lymphocytosis, etc.
- Hematopoietic malignancies like leukemias, various dysplasias like myelodysplastic syndrome, spillage of lymphoproliferative solid tumors, metastatic malignancies
- Diagnosis of effects of various drugs including chemotherapy and radiation therapy and effects of various toxins and chemicals.

Components

A complete blood count (CBC) is a series of tests used to evaluate the composition and concentration of the various cellular components of blood. It consists of the following tests:

- Red blood cell (RBC) count, white blood cell (WBC) count, and platelet count and parameters.
- Measurement of hemoglobin and calculation of hematocrit and red blood cell indices.
- White blood cells (WBC) total and differential count.
- Presence of parasites

Tests for bleeding and clotting disorders.
A range of screening and confirmatory tests are recommended for disorders affecting the coagulation pathway, broadly stated as bleeding and clotting disorders.

Table 2.1 shows the normal values for various blood component counts, hematological indices, and bleeding and clotting investigations and the conditions affecting them.

Sr. no.	Parameter	Normal value	Increased	Decreased
	TABLE 2.1: Normal values for various blood component counts, hematological indices, and bleeding and clotting investigations and the conditions affecting them			
1.	× Red blood cell count	× Male: 4.5 to 6.0 million/mm^3 × Female: 4.0 to 5.5 million/mm^3	× Polycythemia vera × Congenital heart disease × Anabolic steroids × Kidney tumors due to erythropoietin overproduction	× Anemia × Bone marrow depression × Leukaemia × Thalassemia × Erythropoietin deficiency due to chronic renal disease
2.	× Hemoglobin %	× Male: 13.5 to 17.5 g/dl × Female: 12 to 16 g/dl	× Same as above	× Same as above
3.	× Packed cell volume (hematocrit) × It gives the cell volume in a given quantity of blood	× Male: 41 to 53% × Female: 36 to 46%	× Dehydration × Low availability of oxygen (smoking, high altitude, pulmonary fibrosis) × Congenital heart diseases	× Anemia × Leukaemia
4.	× Mean corpuscular volume (MCV)	× 80–94 fl (femtolitres)/cell	× Macrocytic anemia	× Microcytic anemia

Contd.

TABLE 2.1: Normal values for various blood component counts, hematological indices, and bleeding and clotting investigations and the conditions affecting them (*Contd.*)

Sr. no.	Parameter	Normal value	Increased	Decreased
5.	⚹ Mean corpuscular hemoglobin (MCH)	⚹ 27–32 pg/cell	⚹ Macrocytic anemia	⚹ Microcytic anemia
6.	⚹ Mean corpuscular hemoglobin ⚹ Concentration (MCHC)	⚹ 31–37 gm/dl	⚹ Macrocytic anemia	⚹ Microcytic anemia
7.	Reticulocyte count	⚹ Infants at birth: 2–6% ⚹ Children up to 5 years: 0.2–5% ⚹ Adults: 0.2–2%	⚹ Iron supplementation ⚹ Megaloblastic anemia ⚹ Hemolytic anemia	⚹ Myelosclerosis ⚹ Aplastic anemia ⚹ Thalassemia ⚹ Erythroleukemia ⚹ Sideroblastic anemia
8.	Erythrocyte sedimentation rate ⚹ The rate at which red blood cells settle out when anticoagulated whole blood is allowed to stand ⚹ It is a non specific measure of inflammation	*Westergren's method* ⚹ Men under 50 years old: <15 mm/hr ⚹ Men over 50 years old: <20 mm/hr ⚹ Women under 50 years old: <20 mm/hr ⚹ Women over 50 years old: <30 mm/hr *Children* ⚹ Newborn: 0–2 mm/hr ⚹ Newborn to puberty: 3–13 mm/hr	⚹ Inflammation ⚹ Pregnancy ⚹ Anemia ⚹ Autoimmune disorders (such as rheumatoid arthritis and lupus) ⚹ Infections ⚹ Malignancies such as lymphoma and multiple myeloma	⚹ Polycythemia vera ⚹ Sickle cell disease ⚹ Congestive heart failure
9.	WBC	Total: 4000–11000/mm³ Differential: ⚹ Neutrophils: 35 to 73% ⚹ Lymphocytes: 23 to 33% ⚹ Monocytes: 2 to 6% ⚹ Eosinophils: 1 to 3% ⚹ Basophils: 0 to 1%	⚹ Infection ⚹ Inflammation ⚹ Tissue damage from burns ⚹ Myeloproliferative disorders ⚹ Acute or chronic leukaemia	⚹ Old age ⚹ Low immunity states—HIV infection ⚹ Autoimmune conditions ⚹ Bone marrow depression ⚹ Chemotherapy and radiotherapy ⚹ Malnutrition.
10.	Platelet count	150,000–400,000/ mm³	⚹ Essential thrombo-cythemia (due to bone marrow hyperactivity)	⚹ Leukemia ⚹ Aplastic anemia ⚹ Viral infections, such as hepatitis C or HIV

Contd.

TABLE 2.1: Normal values for various blood component counts, hematological indices, and bleeding and clotting investigations and the conditions affecting them (*Contd.*)

Sr. no.	Parameter	Normal value	Increased	Decreased
			✕ Reactive thrombo-cytosis (due to infection, anemia, malignancy, splenectomy)	✕ Drugs (heparin, quinine, chemo-therapeutic agents, sulfa containing antibiotics, anticonvulsants) ✕ Heavy alcohol consumption ✕ Pregnancy ✕ Auto-immune diseases—rheumatoid arthritis, lupus
11.	Bleeding time (the time taken to arrest bleeding after puncture is made on the skin surface allowing free flow of blood)	1 to 9 min (Ivy method)	*Hereditary causes* ✕ von Willebrand disease ✕ Glanzmann thrombasthenia ✕ Bernard-Soulier syndrome ✕ Connective tissue diseases *Acquired causes* ✕ Medications (NSAIDs, penicillins, TCA, anticoagulants) ✕ Vitamin C deficiency ✕ Alcohol intoxication ✕ Uraemia ✕ Liver failure ✕ Leukemias ✕ Myelodysplastic syndrome ✕ Amyloidosis ✕ Disseminated intravascular coagulations (DIC)	
12.	Clotting time: This is the time taken before a specimen of blood clots	4 to 9 min (Lee-White)	✕ Hemophilia ✕ Anticoagulant therapy ✕ Vitamin K deficiency ✕ DIC	

Contd.

TABLE 2.1: Normal values for various blood component counts, hematological indices, and bleeding and clotting investigations and the conditions affecting them (*Contd.*)

Sr. no.	Parameter	Normal value	Increased	Decreased
13.	Prothrombin time ✗ This is the time taken to clot citrated plasma sample in the presence of thromboplastin (tissue factor—TF) and calcium ions. ✗ It reflects the integrity of the extrinsic and common pathways of the coagulation system	✗ 9.5–13.5 seconds	✗ Warfarin use ✗ Vitamin K deficiency from malnutrition, biliary obstruction, malabsorption syndromes, or use of antibiotics ✗ Liver disease ✗ Deficiency of VII, X, II/prothrombin, V, or fibrinogen ✗ Disseminated intravascular coagulopathy (DIC) ✗ Fibrinogen abnormality ✗ Massive blood transfusion due to dilution of plasma clotting proteins ✗ Hypothermia	✗ Vitamin K supplementation ✗ Fresh frozen plasma transfusion
14.	International normalised ratio (INR) ✗ The INR was devised to standardize the result of the prothrombin time as the results may vary according to the analytical system used. ✗ The INR is typically used to monitor patients on warfarin or related oral anticoagulant therapy	✗ Normal individuals: 0.8–1.2 ✗ For people on warfarin therapy an INR of 2.0–3.0 is usually targeted.		

Contd.

TABLE 2.1: Normal values for various blood component counts, hematological indices, and bleeding and clotting investigations and the conditions affecting them (*Contd.*)

Sr. no.	Parameter	Normal value	Increased	Decreased
15.	✕ Activated partial thromboplastin time (APTT) ✕ The APTT is typically used to monitor heparin therapy	✕ 30–40 seconds (more than 70 seconds signifies spontaneous bleeding)	✕ Congenital deficiencies of intrinsic system clotting factors such as factors VIII, IX, XI, and XII, including hemophilia A and hemophilia B. ✕ von Willebrand's factor ✕ Hypofibrinogemia ✕ Liver cirrhosis ✕ Heparin therapy ✕ Vitamin K deficiency ✕ DIC ✕ SLE, rheumatoid arthritis due to circulating antibodies against coagulation factors	✕ Early stages of DIC; due to circulating procoagulants. ✕ Malignancies with metastasis ✕ Immediately after acute hemorrhage.

BIOCHEMICAL INVESTIGATIONS

One important aspect of oral medicine is the diagnosis and management of oral manifestations of systemic diseases. Hence, it is important for the oral physician to be aware of the biochemical investigations that help in diagnosis of systemic diseases. Biochemical investigations in oral medicine may broadly be subdivided into analysis of blood/serum, urine and saliva.

Blood and Serum Analysis

Blood and serum analysis is useful for assaying the levels of glucose, minerals, trace elements, vitamins, enzymes, proteins, lipid profile, hormones and antibodies. These tests need to be prescribed as indicated to rule out underlying systemic disease. Specific enzymes and parameters are defined for assessing kidney and liver functions, a complete description of which is beyond the scope of this textbook. Important tests and their values that have implications particularly in oral disorders are described in Table 2.2.

Urine Analysis

A urine analysis is a group of physical, chemical, and microscopic tests used to detect several substances in the urine, such as byproducts of normal and abnormal metabolism, cells, cellular fragments, and bacteria. It is indicated to diagnose and/or monitor several diseases and conditions, such as kidney disorders or urinary tract infections (UTIs) and metabolic disorders like diabetes mellitus. Table 2.3 summarizes the normal findings of a urine analysis and clinical implications.

TABLE 2.2: Important serum tests of relevance in oral medicine

S.no	Parameter	Normal range	Increased in	Decreased in
1.	Blood glucose	✗ Fasting: 72 to 99 mg/dl (4.0 to 5.4 mmol/L) ✗ Post-prandial: Up to 140 mg/dl (7.8 mmol/L) 2 hours after eating. ✗ Random: 79–160 mg/dl (4.4–8.9 mmol/L)	✗ Uncontrolled diabetes mellitus ✗ Acute stress ✗ Pancreatitis ✗ Drugs—corticosteroids, TCA ✗ Endocrinal causes: Acromegaly, Cushing's syndrome, hyperthyroidism ✗ Chronic renal failure	✗ Insulin overdose, insulinoma ✗ Adrenal insufficiency ✗ Drugs: Acetaminophen ✗ Endocrinal causes: Hypopituitarism, hypothyroidism ✗ Liver disease ✗ Starvation
2.	Serum calcium	✗ 8.5 to 10.5 mg/dl	✗ Hyperparathyroidism ✗ Bony metastasis ✗ Multiple myeloma ✗ Hypervitaminosis D ✗ Ectopic production of PTH-like substance ✗ Milk-alkali syndrome ✗ Sarcoidosis	✗ Hypoparathyroidism ✗ Osteomalacia ✗ Rickets ✗ Decreased intestinal absorption of calcium ✗ Renal insufficiency
3.	Serum phosphorus	✗ Adults: 3.0–4.5 mg/100 ml ✗ Children: 4.0–7.0 mg/100 ml	✗ Hypoparathyroidism ✗ Chronic renal disease ✗ Healing bone fracture ✗ Growth hormone excess ✗ Hypervitaminosis D	✗ Hyperparathyroidism ✗ Osteomalacia ✗ Rickets ✗ Antacid drugs
4.	Serum parathyroid hormone	✗ 10–65 ng/L	*Primary hyperparathyroidism* ✗ Pathology of parathyroid gland (adenoma, hyperplasia or malignancy) *Secondary hyper-parathyroidism* ✗ Vitamin D deficiency ✗ Renal failure *Tertiary hyperparathyroidism* ✗ Unregulated autonomously functioning parathyroid gland following longstanding secondary hyperparathyroidism	✗ Injury to the parathyroid glands during thyroid or neck surgery ✗ Radioactive iodine treatment for hyperthyroidism ✗ Very low magnesium level in the blood ✗ Autoimmune destruction ✗ DiGeorge syndrome ✗ Familial hypopara-thyroidism
5.	Serum alkaline phosphatase	✗ 1–4 Bodansky units ✗ 3–13 King Armstrong units	✗ Osteitis deformans (Paget's disease) ✗ Hyperparathyroidism ✗ Osteogenic sarcoma ✗ Infectious mononucleosis ✗ Metastatic bone tumor	✗ Hypophosphatasia ✗ Hypothyroidism ✗ Scurvy

Contd.

TABLE 2.2: Important serum tests of relevance in oral medicine (*Contd.*)

S.No	Parameter	Normal range	Increased in	Decreased in
		⨯ 30–110 IU	⨯ Granulomatous or infiltrative disease of liver	
6.	Serum acid phosphatase	⨯ 2 ng/ml	⨯ Osteopetrosis ⨯ Prostate gland pathologies	
7.	Serum iron	⨯ Males: 55–160 g/dl ⨯ Females: 40–155 g/dl	⨯ Hemochromatosis ⨯ Hemosiderosis caused by excessive iron intake (e.g., multiple transfusions, excess iron administration) ⨯ Hemolytic anemia ⨯ Pernicious anemia ⨯ Aplastic or hypoplastic anemia ⨯ Thalassemia	⨯ Iron deficiency anemia ⨯ Nephrotic syndrome (loss of iron-binding proteins) ⨯ Chronic renal failure ⨯ Active hematopoiesis ⨯ Malnutrition
8.	Thyroid profile T3, T4, TSH	⨯ TSH: 0.40–4.2 mIU/L ⨯ T4: 4.6–12 µg/dl ⨯ T3: 80–180 ng/dl	⨯ Congenital hypothyroidism ⨯ Primary hypothyroidism ⨯ TSH—secreting pituitary tumors (uncommon) ⨯ Pituitary resistance to thyroid hormone (uncommon) ⨯ Drugs: Dopamine antagonists, chlorpromazine, haloperidol, iodine-containing drugs ⨯ Amiodarone	⨯ Hyperthyroidism ⨯ Pituitary (secondary) hypothyroidism ⨯ Nonthyroid illness ⨯ Drugs: Exogenous thyroxine, glucocorticoids, dopamine, levodopa
9.	⨯ Antinuclear cytoplasmic antibodies (ANCA) ⨯ Perinuclear anti-neutrophil cytoplasmic antibodies (P-ANCA)		⨯ Rheumatoid arthritis ⨯ Ulcerative colitis ⨯ Glomerulonephritis ⨯ Vasculitis/polyangiitis	

Salivary Analysis

Saliva is a biofluid composed of water (99.5%), electrolytes (0.5%) and a number of organic compounds. The electrolytes found in saliva include sodium, potassium, calcium, magnesium, bicarbonate, and phosphates. The organic compounds present in saliva are immunoglobulins (IgA, IgG and IgM), proteins, enzymes, mucins, and nitrogenous products, such as urea and ammonia. Normal unstimulated salivary flow is 0.25–0.35 ml/min, whereas the stimulated salivary flow is 1–3 ml/min.

In addition to its normal constituents, a number of analytes that may be detectable are steroid hormones, cytokines and chemokines, growth factors, nucleic acids and certain drugs. Hence, salivary analysis that was earlier restricted to disorders affecting the salivary glands (xerostomia, Sjögren's syndrome, etc.) now encompasses

TABLE 2.3: Urinalysis normal findings and clinical implications

S. No.	Parameter	Normal finding	Clinical implication
1.	Color	Straw yellow to amber	⌗ Red/dark brown: Hemoglobinuria/ hematuria/porphyria ⌗ Bright yellow: Bilirubin ⌗ Green: Medications like amitriptyline, propofol ⌗ Orange: Pseudomonas infection
2.	pH	4.7 to 8.0 (mean, 6.3)	⌗ Very alkaline urine > 8: Strict vegetarian diet; diuretic/ alkali therapy; infection with a urea-splitting organism, such as *P. mirabilis*, vomiting ⌗ Acidic pH <4.5: Metabolic acidosis
3.	Volume	1500 ml/day	⌗ Less than 400 ml: Oliguria; in dehydration, kidney disease ⌗ Excess of 2000 ml: Polyuria; in diabetes mellitus and diabetes insipidus
4.	Specific gravity	1.016 to 1.022	⌗ It reflects the ability of kidney to concentrate the urine. ⌗ Increased in patients with diabetes mellitus and in individuals on multiple medications ⌗ Decreased in diabetes insipidus ⌗ Same as plasma in kidney failure.
5.	Glucose	Negative	⌗ Glycosuria is an indicator of diabetes mellitus; ⌗ When blood glucose levels rise above 160 mg/dl, glucose will be present in the urine.
6.	Protein	Negative	⌗ Presence indicates kidney disorder
7.	Ketones	Negative	⌗ Presence indicates: Type I diabetes mellitus, pregnancy, glycogen storage diseases
8.	Bilirubin	Negative	⌗ Presence indicates hepatic disease or hepatobiliary obstruction
9.	Blood	Negative	Presence of blood may be seen in: ⌗ Excessive red cell destruction ⌗ Glomerular disease ⌗ Kidney or urinary tract infection ⌗ Urinary tract injury or malignancy.
10.	Erythrocytes	0 to 2/ high-power field	⌗ Same as above (blood)
11.	Leucocytes/ Pus cells	0 to 5/ high-power field	⌗ Increased amount suggests urinary tract infection
12.	Leucocyte esterase	Negative	⌗ Presence indicates urinary tract infection
13.	Nitrite	Negative	⌗ A positive test for nitrite indicates the presence of bacteria including staphylococci, Proteus, Salmonella, Pseudomonas
14.	Urobilinogen	0–2 Ehrlich units	⌗ Increased in prehepatic jaundice ⌗ Hepatitis and hepatic necrosis
15.	Cellular casts and abnormal crystals	Absent on microscopic examination	⌗ Kidney disease

a wide range of conditions. It is useful for diagnosis and monitoring of patients with both oral and systemic diseases and drug monitoring as well. Saliva is biofluid that is easily collected, stored and is ideal for early detection of diseases as it contains specific soluble biological markers. Thus, contemporary salivary diagnostics has gained profound importance in the diagnosis of oral squamous cell carcinoma, understanding the pathogenesis of dental caries and periodontitis as well as the diagnosis of fungal and viral diseases of the oral cavity.

HISTOPATHOLOGICAL INVESTIGATIONS

Oral Biopsy

The phrase "biopsy" originates from the Greek terms *bios* (life) and *opsis* (vision): Vision of life. Biopsy is the removal of a tissue sample from a living body with the objective of providing the pathologist with a representative, viable specimen for histopathologic interpretation and diagnosis. Biopsies are an important diagnostic tool for the diagnosis of lesions ranging from simple periapical lesions to malignancies.

Indications for Oral Biopsy

- Any lesion that persists for more than 2 weeks with no obvious etiologic basis.
- Any inflammatory lesion that does not respond to the treatment even after 2 weeks.
- Clinical suspicion of malignancy, such as an enlarging mass, hyperkeratotic lesion with areas of erythema, chronic ulceration, tissue friability, induration on palpation or persistence of mucosal changes despite removal of local irritants.
- New or enlarging pigmented lesions, especially those with an irregular border and nonhomogenous coloration.
- Clinically benign or reactive (e.g. pyogenic granuloma, mucocele osseous lumps or fibrous hyperplasia interfering with oral function) may be excised for esthetic or functional reasons.
- Anesthesia or paresthesia and pain associated with lesions of unclear etiology.
- Lichen planus, mucous membrane pemphigoid, pemphigus vulgaris and other immune-mediated disorders may be biopsied for definitive diagnosis.
- Labial, buccal, or lingual muscles showing interstitial lesions.

Contraindications for Biopsy

- Vascular lesion—caution must be exercised in the biopsy of any lesion with red, purple or blue coloration or with blanching or pulsation on palpation.
- When acute, virulent, pyogenic infection is present.

Caution and Concerns

- Location of the lesion in an esthetic region (e.g. vermilion border of the lip), referral to a specialist should be considered in such cases.
- Oral sites, such as the floor of the mouth, may be challenging to access, difficult to provide hemostasis and risks damage to anatomic structures (e.g. submandibular duct).
- Obtain medical clearance the case of medically compromised patients, including those with severe or poorly controlled systemic diseases such as coronary artery disease, renal or hepatic impairment, and various endocrinopathies immune-compromised states and patients with significant risk of hemorrhage due to underlying bleeding diatheses.
- Patients undergoing bisphosphonate therapy or radiotherapy may be predisposed to osteonecrosis if the biopsy procedure exposes bone.

Types of Oral Biopsies

Scalpel Biopsy

Depending on the technique employed, biopsies can be classified as *incisional or excisional*.

The incisional technique involves the removal of a representative portion of the target lesion and of a part of healthy tissue. Such an approach is indicated in the case of suspected malignancy or precancerous lesions and lesions greater than 2 cm in size.

An excisional biopsy in turn involves total removal of the lesion, with slight peripheral and in-depth safety margins. It is indicated in lesions, less than 2 cm in diameter. Such biopsies play a diagnostic and therapeutic role, since complete removal of the lesion is carried out, ensuring the inclusion of a peripheral margin of normal tissue.

Punch Biopsy

The punch biopsy technique is an alternative to the traditional incisional biopsy. Essentially the punch comprises a circular blade attached to a plastic handle (Fig. 2.1). Diameters of two to ten millimetres are available. This removes a core of tissue the base of which can be simply and atraumatically released using curved scissors. Alternatively, the specimen can be lifted from the mucosal surface and the base undermined with a scalpel. The resultant wound may not require suturing if using the smaller diameter punches.

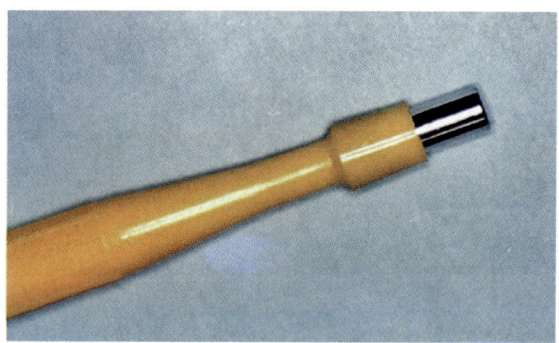

Fig. 2.1: An oral biopsy punch

Other Methods

× Surgical tissue removal by cautery or a high-frequency cutting knife
× Soft tissue laser

An elliptical incision is preferred as it is easier to suture (Fig. 2.2).

Frozen Section Biopsy

It is performed while surgery for a malignant lesion is in progress to get an immediate histological report. It is done to ascertain if the entire lesion has been removed. The tissue obtained from the lesion is kept in deep freezer. The frozen tissue is sectioned, stained, studied and report immediately. In this type of biopsy slides cannot be preserved for future reference.

Exfoliative Cytology

Surface cells from the epithelium are constantly being exfoliated and these can

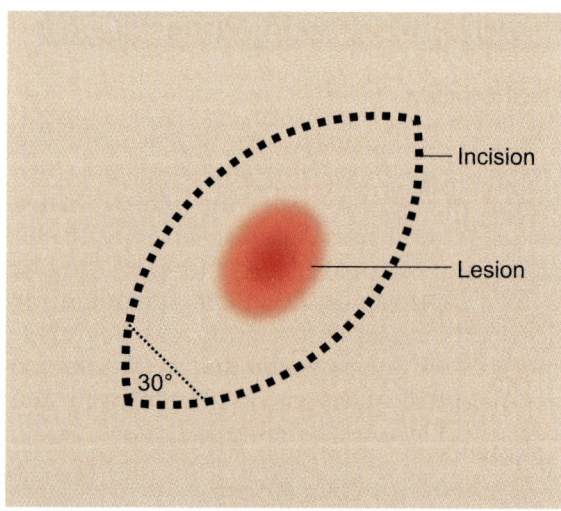

Fig. 2.2: An elliptical biopsy incision (*Image Source*: http://img.medscapestatic.com/pi/meds/ckb/80/10280tn.jpg)

be collected by scraping of the surface epithelium and examined microscopically.

Exfoliative cytology is the study of cells which exfoliate or abrade from the body surfaces. When the epithelium becomes seat of any pathological condition, the cells may lose their cohesiveness, and cells in the deeper layer may shed along with the superficial cells. These exfoliated cells as well as cells which are scrapped off by means of specific instruments, can be studied quantitatively or qualitatively. Considerable interest has developed in the use of exfoliative oral cytology for the diagnosis of oral mucosal lesions. It is a quick, simple, painless and bloodless procedure.

Indications

* This technique is of utmost value in evaluation of suspected malignancies. (a Papanicolaou stained smear is used generally for this purpose).
* Follow-up detection of recurrent carcinoma in previously treated cases.
* In the diagnosis of certain specific cells in diseases like herpes simplex infection, herpes zoster, pemphigus vulgaris, benign familial pemphigus, keratosis follicularis, hereditary benign intraepithelial dyskeratosis, white sponge nevus, and pernicious and sickle cell anemia.
* Also, studies have been done to determine antioxidant levels and gender determination from exfoliated cells, recently.

Procedure

* The surface of oral lesion is cleaned of debris and mucus.
* The mucosa is stretched and the scraper (metal spatula, moistened tongue blade, cytobrush) is placed on the lesion, pressed firmly and the surface is scraped until a visible quantity of material is collected.
* The collected material is transferred onto a microscopic slide, spread evenly and fixed in a mixture of alcohol and ether before the specimen dries.
* The smear is then stained and examined under the microscope.

Interpretation

The cytologic smear will usually be reported by the cytologist as falling into one of five classes:

* **Class I (normal):** Indicates that only normal cells were observed
* **Class II (atypical):** Indicates the presence of minor atypia but no evidence of malignant changes
* **Class III (indeterminate):** This is an in between cytology that separates cancer from noncancer diagnosis. The cells display wider atypia that may be suggestive of cancer, but they are not clear-cut and may represent precancerous lesions or carcinoma *in situ*. Biopsy is recommended.
* **Class IV (suggestive of cancer):** A few cells with malignant characteristics or many cells with borderline characteristics. Biopsy is mandatory.
* **Class V (positive for cancer):** Cells that are obviously malignant. Biopsy is mandatory.

Aspiration/Fine Needle Aspiration Cytology

This is the procedure whereby small amount of tissue/cells/fluid (in case of cystic lesions) are aspirated from a lesion with the help of a small bore (usually 22 gauge) needle.

Advantages

* It is a safe, economical, outpatient procedure that does not require anesthesia.
* Less traumatic than the conventional biopsy.
* Results can be obtained within an hour
* The procedure is easier to repeat.

Disadvantages

* Not suitable in many non-neoplastic conditions where detailed examination of tissue architecture is necessary for the diagnosis.
* The procedure may produce complications, e.g. bleeding, infection, seeding of tumor cells.

Indications

* Cystic lesions
* Clinically suspicious lymph nodes
* Evaluation of salivary gland tumors.

Procedure

The skin/mucosa above the area is sterilised with an antiseptic solution. A needle of very fine diameter 22–25 gauges on a syringe

TABLE 2.4: Enlists the type of aspirate that may be found in some oral lesions

S. No.	Lesion	Aspirate characteristics
1.	Radicular cyst	Straw color fluid; it may appear shimmering due to the presence of cholesterol crystals; total protein content between 5 and 11 g/dl
2.	Dentigerous cyst	Straw colored fluid; the total protein content in the dentigerous cyst is usually 4–8 g/100 ml
3.	Odontogenic keratocyst	Dirty white cheesy material with Keratin squames; Total protein content is <5 gm/100 ml; the ratio of soluble protein to total protein content is lower than that in serum
4.	Mucocele/ranula	Mucous aspirate
5.	Anuerysmal bone cyst	Blood tinged sero-sanguinous fluid/no aspirate
6.	Dermoid cyst	Thick sebaceous material
7.	Stafne's cyst	Empty cavity
8.	Solid tumor mass	No aspirate
9.	Unicystic ameloblastoma	Amber colored fluid
10.	Salivary gland tumors	Lesional tissue/fluid

is passed into the swelling. The plunger is withdrawn slowly in stages thus aspirating the fluid/tissue material from the lesion. The needle is withdrawn and the aspirate is spread on a glass slide, fixed, stained and studied (in case of tissue aspirate) or examined for its physical characteristics and chemical analysis (in case of cystic fluid) (Table 2.4).

IMMUNOHISTOCHEMISTRY

Immunohistochemistry is a histopathological technique that involves the application of monoclonal or polyclonal antibodies to determine the tissue distribution of an antigen of interest in health and disease. It is widely used for diagnosis of cancers and tumors because specific tumor antigens are expressed *de novo* or up-regulated in certain cancers.

Principle

IHC requires the availability of tissue sections that are incubated with an appropriate antibody. The site of antibody binding is visualized under an ordinary or fluorescent microscope by a marker such as fluorescent dye, enzyme, radioactive element, or colloidal gold, which is directly linked to the primary antibody or to an appropriate secondary antibody.

Advantages

- It affords a significant advantage in the diagnosis of difficult and equivocal tumors.
- Immunohistochemistry has also provided insight into tumor histopathogenesis. Predictable tumor expression of many of the same antigens (a macromolecular protein or polysaccharide that can bind to an antibody molecule) as their cells of origin or normal tissue counterparts validate the principle of tumor classification by immunohistochemistry.
- Application of immunohistochemistry in distinguishing undifferentiated oral neoplasms of different origins was achieved through the detection of tumor antigens using known antibodies. Thus, immunohistochemistry is important in diagnosis, investigation, and determining the behavior and pathogenesis of oral tumors (Table 2.5).

TABLE 2.5: Describes the tissue specific general IHC markers

S. No.	Markers	Diagnostic applications
1.	Cytokeratins	Epithelial tumors
2.	Vimentin	Mesenchymal tumors
3.	Desmin	Muscle tumors, muscle lesions
4.	S-100 protein	Nerves, Schwann cells, chondrocytes, melanocytes, Langerhans cells, APUD cells
5.	Neuron-specific enolase	Melanoma, neuroendocrine tumors, neuroblastoma, Wilms' tumors.

ADJUNCT DIAGNOSTIC AIDS FOR ORAL CANCER AND PRECANCER

Brush Biopsy

This technique is an advanced variation of the exfoliative cytology.

- The oral brush biopsy, also known as "oral CDx brush test system" (Fig. 2.3), consists of a method of collecting a trans-epithelial sample of cells from a mucosal lesion with representation of the superficial, intermediate and parabasal/basal layers of the epithelium.

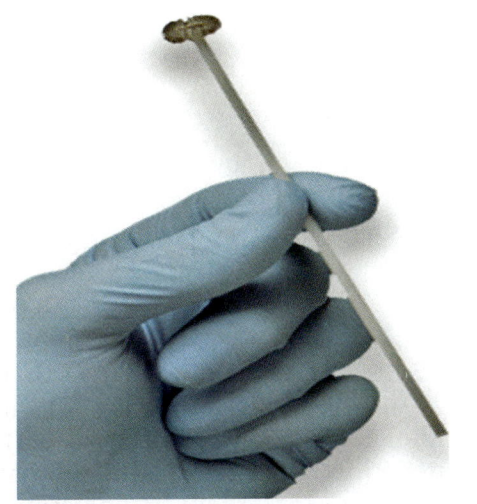

Fig. 2.3: Oral CDx brush (image source www.cdxdiagnostics.com)

- This test was specifically designed for lesions with low-risk clinical features.
- A specially designed brush is used for epithelial cell collection. Samples are fixed onto a glass slide, stained with a modified Papanicolaou test and analyzed microscopically via a computer-based imaging system.
- Results are reported as "positive" or "atypical" when cellular morphology is highly suspicious for epithelial dysplasia or carcinoma or when abnormal epithelial changes are of uncertain diagnostic significance respectively. Results are defined as negative when no abnormalities can be found. The test is considered an intermediate diagnostic step as a scalpel biopsy must follow when an abnormal result is reported (atypical or positive).
- Current data show that Oral CDx's cytologic test is highly sensitive and specific in detecting dysplastic changes in high-risk mucosal lesions.

Vital Staining

Supravital staining has long been used as an adjunct in the early diagnosis of malignant lesions. The technique has been applied in the oral setting for over 30 years by means of the dye toluidine blue. Apart from toluidine blue, other stains such as methylene blue (MB), Lugol's iodine, and acetic acid have also been tried in the diagnosis of cancerous lesions.

Toluidine Blue Staining

TB was first used by Richart in 1963 to stain uterine cervical carcinoma *in situ* and dysplasia.

Properties

TB chemically is referred to as *tolonium chloride*. It is an acidophilic dye of the thiazine group that selectively stains acidic tissue components, including deoxyribonucleic acid (DNA) and ribonucleic acid (RNA). It has the staining property of metachromasia, which is due to the presence of repetitive phosphate groups in the nucleic acids and is dependent on temperature and the pH. The recommended pH is 6.0–7.0. The temperature should not exceed 30°C above which the metachromatic property diminishes in strength. The TB solution can be prepared in the laboratory or it is also available commercially as ready to use kit, which consists of three component systems. One component is 1% TB solution and the other two are the pre- and post-rinse solutions consisting of 1% acetic acid.

Principle

- The dye attaches to phosphate bonds and the extent of binding depends on the amount of DNA, which is related to number and size of nuclei present in the superficial layers.
- Its use *in vivo* is based on the fact that dysplastic and anaplastic cells contain quantitatively more nucleic acids than normal tissues, shows loss of cell cohesion and increased mitosis.
- In addition, malignant epithelium may contain wider intracellular canals; a factor that enhances penetration of the dye.
- It stains to the depth of 2–10 cell layers, and hence just reflects only the epithelial changes, the invasion into the underlying connective tissue, or the changes in the submucosa cannot be appreciated.

TECHNIQUE OF STAINING

TB can be used in two forms. It is either applied to the site of the lesion with a cotton applicator or it is used as mouth rinse. The procedure of staining is as follows:
- Oral examination
- Rinsing the mouth twice with water for 20 s to remove the debris
- Application of 1% acetic acid for 20 s to remove any ropey saliva
- Application of 1% TB solution for 20 s either with cotton swab when a mucosal

lesion is seen or given as a rinse when no obvious lesion is detected
- Application of 1% acetic acid to reduce the extent of mechanically retained stain
- Rinsing oral cavity with water
- Oral examination and recording of the stained areas.

Interpretation

A dark blue (royal or navy) stain of either the entire lesion or a portion of it is considered as positive stain, lack of color absorption by the lesion as negative stain, and light or pale blue staining as doubtful. These cases are usually due to mechanical surface retention or inadequate removal of the stain. False positive dye retention may occur in inflammatory and ulcerative lesions, but false negative retention is uncommon.

Advantages

- TB staining is a simple, quick, noninvasive, and highly cost effective procedure.
- It is used as an adjunctive aid in the detection of premalignant and malignant lesions.
- In selecting biopsy site and in the screening of second primaries of the oral cavity
- And multicentric tumors.
- In obtaining the marginal control of carcinoma, and during the follow-up of treated lesions.

Lugol's Iodine

Lugol's iodine is a solution of elemental iodine. Lugol's solution consists of iodine and potassium iodide.

Principle

- The basic principle with iodine staining is its affinity for carbohydrates and starch in the tissues.
- As the malignancy is associated with reduction in the glycogen content of the tissues, the malignant tissue remains unstained and on the contrary, the normal epithelium gets stained brown or black.

- This selective staining delineates the inflammatory and carcinomatous epithelium from the normal epithelium.
- Iodine infiltrates and reacts with the glycogen mainly in the upper superficial layer of the nonkeratinized epithelium.
- Glycogen content is inversely related to the degree of keratosis, suggesting a role of glycogen in keratinization. Throughout the oral mucosa, the content of glycogen varies with the type of keratinization of the mucosa. This may limit the use of Lugol's iodine in keratinized lesions and in such case its uptake should be assessed carefully.
- This technique also cannot be used for the detection of subepithelial infiltrating tumors.

Double Staining

- Studies have been done wherein a few authors have used combination of two dyes to aid in the assessment of oral malignant diseases.
- The combination of toluidine blue and Lugol's iodine has been used.
- TB will stain the abnormal epithelium, whereas Lugol's solution binds to glycogen present in the normal epithelium.
   Other stains used for vital tissue staining are methylene blue and acetic acid.

Chemiluminescence (ViziLite)

This technique involves the use of a chemiluminescent light that is shone inside the mouth to detect areas that may harbour premalignant and malignant changes. Under this light the abnormal tissue glows differently from the normal tissue thus demarcating it.

Components of the ViziLite system (Fig. 2.4)
1. ViziLite rinse (1% acetic acid solution)
2. ViziLite capsule (chemiluminescent light stick)
3. ViziLite retractor (sheath and handle)

Principle

- Normal epithelium absorbs ViziLite and appears dark, whereas abnormal

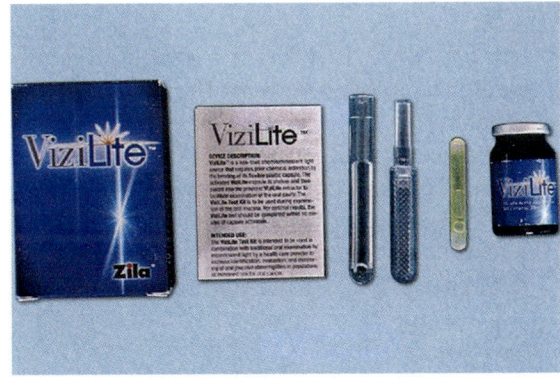

Fig. 2.4: The ViziLite kit [Image available via license: CC BY-NC-SA 3.0]

epithelium reflects ViziLite and appears white.
- As a cell becomes more dysplastic, nucleus becomes larger compared with the neighbouring normal cells. The enlarged nucleus reflects light and thus appears white.

Fluorescence (VELScope: Visually Enhanced Lesion Scope)

The VELscope® System (Fig. 2.5) is a revolutionary hand-held device that provides the oral health care professionals, an easy-to-use adjunctive mucosal examination system for the early detection of abnormal tissue. It can also aid the surgeon to identify diseased tissue around a clinically apparent lesion and thus help in determining the appropriate margin for surgical excision.

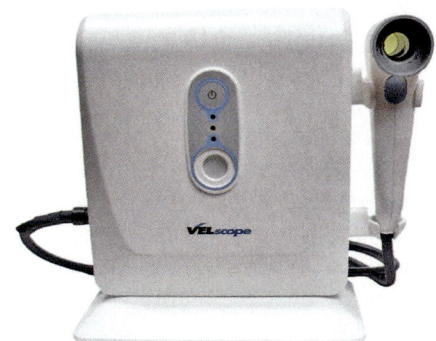

Fig. 2.5: The VELscope [*Image source* https://ledapteryx.com]

Principle

- It is based on the direct visualization of tissue fluorescence and the changes in fluorescence that occur when abnormalities are present.
- The VELscope® System Handpiece emits a safe blue light into the oral cavity, which excites the tissue from the surface of the epithelium to the basement membrane and into the stroma beneath, causing it to fluoresce.
- The clinician is then able to immediately view the different fluorescence responses to help differentiate between normal and abnormal tissue
- Under examination with the VELscope® System, abnormal tissue typically appears as an irregular, dark area that stands out against the otherwise normal, green fluorescence pattern of surrounding healthy tissue.

Investigations for Autoimmune Disorders of the Oral Cavity

Immunofluorescence is an immuno-histochemical method used to demonstrate the presence of antigen and antibodies in the tissues or serum. It is an auxiliary diagnostic tool for the autoimmune bullous and inflammatory disorders. It detects the *in situ* and circulating immune deposits that are involved in the pathogenesis of immunobullous diseases.

Fluorescence is the property of absorbing light rays of one particular wavelength and emitting rays with a different wavelength. Fluorescent dyes show up brightly under ultraviolet light as they convert ultraviolet light into visible light. In 1941 Coons and Kaplan showed that these fluorescent dyes can be conjugated with antibodies and they are called labeled antibodies. These labeled antibodies can be used to locate and identify antigens in the tissues.

The most commonly used fluorochromes are:
- Fluorescein isothiocyanate (FITC) which produces apple-green color
- Tetramethylrhodamine isothiocyanate with a red color of fluorescence
- Phycoerythrin which also shows red fluorescence.

2 basic types of IF technique

- **Direct IF (DIF):** DIF is the earliest form of immunohistochemistry. In this direct technique, the antigen is reacted directly with a fluorescein-conjugated antibody specific for the material sought within the tissue. Patients tissue biopsy is used (Table 2.6).
- **Indirect IF (IIF):** Indirect IF (IIF) is a two-step serological technique for detecting the circulating antibodies in the body fluids. It uses serial dilution of patients serum applied to the section of suitable tissue substrate.[1] Conjugated antihuman IgG is then applied to localize the autoantibodies from the patient's serum that are bound in the tissue substrate. Patients serum is used.

Nikolsky's Sign

The Nikolsky's sign is a well-described clinical sign seen in some vesiculobullous disorders which manifest as dislodgement of intact superficial epidermis by a shearing force. The pathophysiology associated with Nikolsky's sign is the acantholysis[8], i.e. loss of coherence between epidermal cells due to the breakdown of their intercellular bridges. It is characteristically seen in intraepidermal bullous disorders; whereas in subepidermal VB diseases, the sign is generally absent.

Elicitation of the Nikolsky's Sign

When a tangential pressure is applied on apparently normal skin/mucosa, or on peri-lesional skin/mucosa or on affected skin/mucosa with the thumb or finger, the resulting is a shearing force dislodges the upper layers of epidermis from the lower epidermis resulting in formation of new blister.

TABLE 2.6: Direct immunofluorescence appearance of some vesiculobullous lesions

Disease	Antigenic self-protein, autoantibody and location in direct immunofluorescence
Pemphigus vulgaris	✕ Antibodies are formed against desmoglein 3 and 1, the intercellular cementing substance, resulting in the formation of intra-epithelial blisters (Fig. 2.6). ✕ DIF shows intercellular deposits of IgG and C3, the latter are predominantly located in the lower layers of the epithelium. Chicken wire, fish net appearance (Fig. 2.6A)
Paraneoplastic pemphigus	✕ Autoantibodies target desmoglein 3, desmoplakins and basement membrane zone [BMZ] antigens. ✕ DIF shows similar pattern to that of PV, along with linear, intercellular and intraepithelial deposition of IgG in the basement membrane. ✕ One way to differentiate PNP from PV is to perform IIF.
Bullous pemphigoid	✕ Antibodies are formed against BP 180 and 230 ✕ Deposition of C3, IgG or both at the BMZ. ✕ Deposition of C3 with significantly higher intensity than IgG strongly favors the pemphigoid group of diseases (Fig. 2.6B)
Cicatricial pemphigoid	✕ Antibodies are formed against BP 180 and laminin V ✕ Linear deposits of C3, IgG, and IgA at the dermal epidermal junction, "shore line appearance" (Fig. 2.6C)
Epidermolysis bullosa acquisita	✕ Antibodies are formed against type VII collagen ✕ Deposition of IgG, IgA and lesser amounts of C3 at the basement membrane zone
Linear IgA disease	✕ Antibodies are formed against desmoglein 3, desmocolin 1 and 2 ✕ Linear IgA deposits in the basement membrane.
Dermatitis herpetiformis	✕ Antibodies are formed against tissue transglutaminase ✕ Granular deposition of IgA and C3 in the papillary dermis and along the BMZ is diagnostic of dermatitis herpetiformis ✕ Deposition of IgG or IgM or both is less frequent and less intense (Fig. 2.6D)
Erythema multiforme	✕ Antibodies are formed against desmoplakins ✕ Granular deposits of IgG, C3, IgM and fibrinogen around dermal vessels and at the dermal-epidermal junction
Systemic lupus erythematosus	✕ Anti-nuclear antibodies are formed ✕ Deposits of IgG, C3, IgM at the basement membrane zone and around blood vessels; "positive lupus band test" (Fig. 2.6E)

Applications of the Nikolsky's Sign

Nikolsky's sign is also useful in differentiating various blistering diseases. It is usually positive in intraepidermal blistering disease, while in subepidermal blistering disease such as bullous pemphigoid, the sign is usually absent. Nikolsky's sign is positive in pemphigus vulgaris, pemphigus foliaceous, chronic erythema multiforme, epidermolysis bullosa acquisita, Stevens-Johnson syndrome, toxic epidermal necrolysis.

It is of prognostic significance also in the treatment of pemphigus vulgaris as the sign is positive in the active phase and becomes negative with response to the immunosuppressive therapy.

DIAGNOSTIC MICROBIOLOGY

Infectious diseases of the oral cavity may be bacterial, viral or fungal in origin. The most common means of bacterial isolation and identification is culture of an appropriate bacterial specimen (pus, exudate, sputum or blood). Other methods of bacterial identification include methods like phage

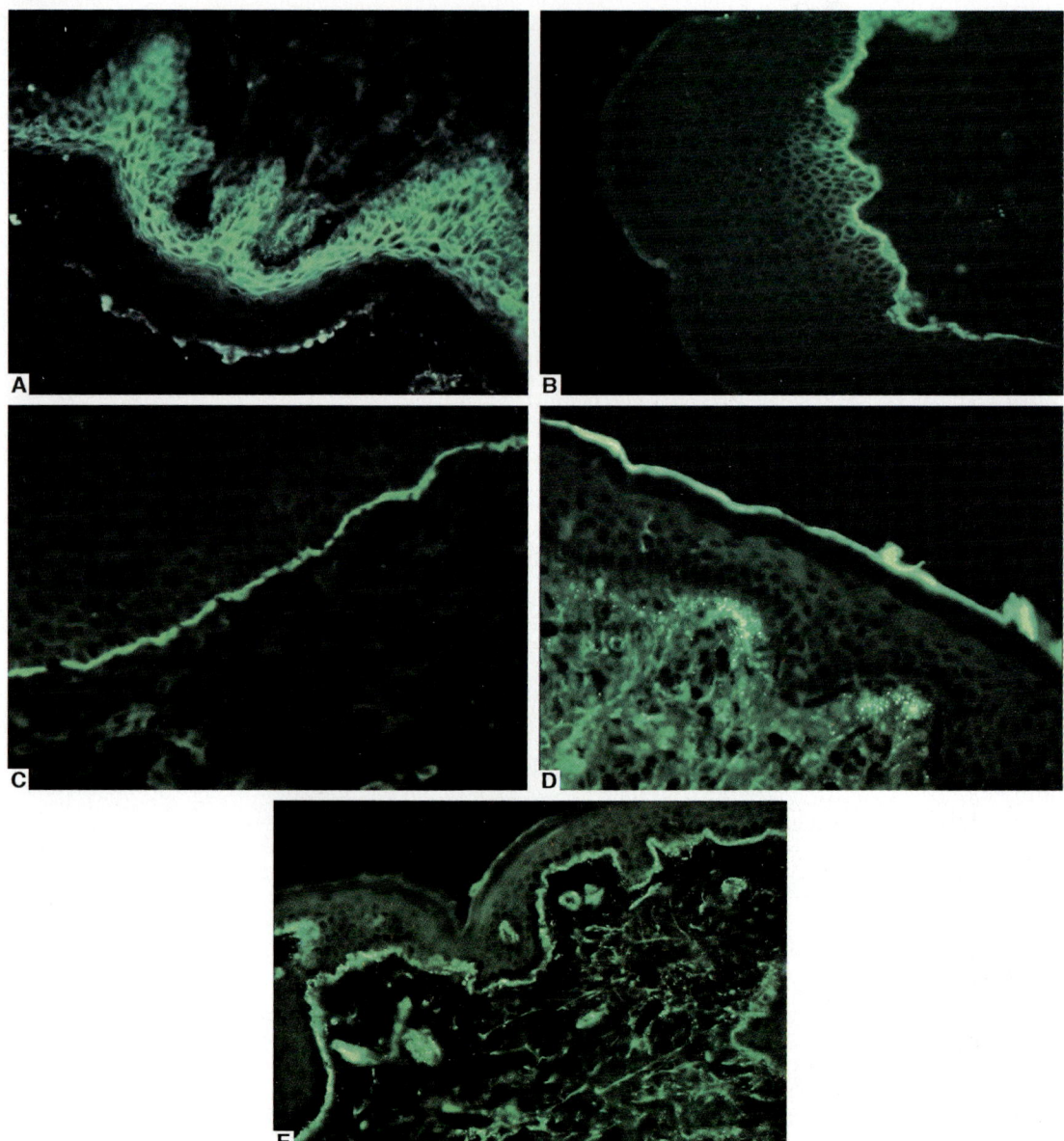

Fig. 2.6: Direct immunofluorescence patterns in: (A) Pemphigus vulgaris; "fishnet appearance"; (B) Bullous pemphigoid; (C) Cicatricial pemphigoid 'shore-line appearance'; (D) Dermatitis herpetiformis; (E) SLE 'positive lupus band' [*Image source:* http://www.ijdvl.com/text.asp?2012/78/6/677/102355]

typing, bacterial PCR, and identification of antibodies to bacteria (ELISA, precipitation assays, etc).

Most oral infections are of a mixed nature, so both aerobic and anaerobic cultures may be necessary.

Table 2.7 delineates the commonly used culture media for infections that may affect the oral cavity.

Table 2.8 shows the recommended tests for bacterial infections that may have oral manifestations.

Fungal Infections

Candidiasis is the most common fungal infection of the oral cavity.

Laboratory Investigations for Candida

- Potassium hydroxide (KOH) wet mount for direct demonstration of fungal hyphae under microscope.
- Periodic acid–Schiff (PAS) stain and methenamine silver stain
- Fungal culture with Sabouraud's dextrose agar, corn meal agar

- **Serology:** Serum (1,3) β-D-glucan and mannan detection assays (these are fungal cell wall components).

Viral Infections

Herpes simplex viruses (1 and 2), human papillomaviruses (HPV) and human immunodeficiency virus (HIV) are the common viruses implicated in viral diseases of the oral cavity (Table 2.9).

TABLE 2.7: Commonly used culture media for infections that may affect the oral cavity

S. No.	Culture media	Organism
1.	Nutrient agar (1 to 2% agar)	Basal media in microbiology Supports the growth of all non-fastidious organisms
2.	Blood agar	Staphylococcal and streptococcal infections
3.	Robertson's cooked meat broth	Anaerobic culture
4.	MM10 sucrose blood agar	Ideal medium for normal and disease-associated dental plaques
5.	Lowenstein-Jensen medium	Selective media for isolation of *Mycobacterium tuberculosis* from sputum and other samples
6.	Mannitol salt agar	Selective and indicator media for *S. aureus*
7.	Polymyxin B, neomycin, fusidic acid media (PNF)	Selective media for *S. pyogenes* (or β-hemolytic Streptococcus)
8.	Mueller-Hinton agar	Performing antimicrobial susceptibility for bacteria

TABLE 2.8: Recommended tests for bacterial infections that may have oral manifestations

S. no.	Infection	Tests
1.	Tuberculosis	- Mantoux tuberculin skin test - Acid-fast bacilli (AFB) smear and culture - PCR for *M. tuberculosis* specific DNA - Interferon gamma release assay
2.	Syphilis	*Screening:* - Venereal Disease Research Laboratory (VDRL) test, - Rapid plasma reagin (RPR). *Confirmatory:* - Fluorescent treponemal antibody-absorption (FTA-ABS), microhemagglutination assay-*T. pallidum* (MHA-TP), - *T. pallidum* particle agglutination (TPPA) test
3.	Leprosy	- Acid-fast bacilli (AFB) smear and culture - Serologic assay to detect phenolic glycolipid-1 (specific for *M. leprae*)
4.	Actinomycosis	- Examination of "sulphur granules" - Anaerobic culture

TABLE 2.9: Various tests recommended for the laboratory diagnosis of these conditions

S. No.	Virus	Diseases	Diagnosis
1.	HSV 1 and 2	⚹ Acute herpetic gingivostomatitis ⚹ Herpetic labialis and whitlow	⚹ Viral isolation in tissue culture ⚹ Tzanck smear ⚹ Detection of viral DNA by polymerase chain reaction (PCR) ⚹ Direct fluorescent antibody staining ⚹ Serum antibody titres.
2.	Epstein-Barr virus	⚹ Infectious mononucleosis	⚹ Paul-Bunnel test ⚹ Monospot test
3.	HIV 1 and 2	⚹ HIV infection and AIDS	⚹ Screening: ELISA to detect antibodies to the virus ⚹ Confirmatory: Western blot ⚹ Antigen detection assay: Done for p24 antigen (for early testing) ⚹ CD4 + counts—for disease surveillance ⚹ Viral load assessment by PCR—therapeutic monitoring.

ALLERGY TESTING

A possible allergic reaction to a drug or dental medicament is a significant cause of concern for the dentist. An anaphylactic shock is a severe kind of allergic reaction that could be potentially life-threatening, that could be encountered in a dental setting. Allergies include hypersensitivity reactions could be immediate or delayed.

1. Skin Tests

Useful for both immediate and delayed hypersensitivity reactions.

Skin tests for allergy include:

Intradermal injection: The test involves injection of a small amount of the suspected allergen into the superficial layer of the dermis with a fine bore needle (26 or 27 gauge). The amount of quantity injected is approximately 0.05 ml or the amount that causes a visible weal. The preferred sites for intradermal injection are the flexor aspect of forearm or the back. A control (e.g. normal saline) must also be injected at a comparable site. After about 20 minutes the area is examined for a reaction at the site. A typical reaction looks like a small hive with swelling and redness. Examples are tuberculin test, sensitivity testing for Xylocaine. Resuscitation equipment and 1 in 1000 epinephrine should be available in case of any untoward allergic reaction.

Prick test: This is a modification of the intradermal injection. A small amount of test solution is placed on the skin and a shallow prick is made through it with a sharp needle. Care should be taken to avoid inducing any bleeding. The size of the visible flare is measured after 15 to 20 minutes. The concentration of prick test solutions is higher than those used for intradermal testing.

Patch test (epicutaneous test): Patch tests are used to detect contact allergy of the delayed hypersensitivity type. It involves applying patches with test substances in small chambers or discs to a person's back. The patches are secured with hypoallergenic tapes. They are usually read at 48–72 hours and again at 1 week. A positive patch test reaction will produce an area of active dermatitis, which is itchy, in the area of application.

2. Serum Tests

These tests require a small sample of blood (about 5 ml) from which the serum is obtained. The different serum assays used for allergy testing include:

1. **Histamine release assay:** For immediate hypersensitivity reactions
2. Assay for the concentration of IgE antibodies against a specific allergern
3. **Lymphocyte proliferation and lympho-kine production assay:** For delayed hypersensitivity reaction.

Frequently asked questions
1. Pathergy test
2. Biopsy
3. Nikolsky sign
4. Toluidine blue staining

BIBLIOGRAPHY

1. Kamal AH, Tefferi A, Pruthi RK. How to interpret and pursue an abnormal prothrombin time, activated partial thromboplastin time, and bleeding time in adults? *Mayo Clin Proc.* 2007 Jul. 82(7):864–73. [Medline]
2. McPherson RA, Matthew R. Pincus MR. Henry's Clinical Diagnosis and Management by Laboratory Methods. 22nd ed. Philadelphia: Elsevier Saunders; 2011. 254–5.
3. Hayward CP. Diagnostic approach to platelet function disorders. Transfus Apher Sci. 2008 Feb. 38(1):65–76. [Medline].
4. Schafer A. Hemorrhagic disorders: Approach to the patient with bleeding and thrombosis. Goldman L, Ausiello D, eds. Cecil Medicine. 23rd ed. Saunders Elsevier: Philadelphia, Pa; 2007. 178.
5. Kamal AH, Tefferi A, Pruthi RK. How to interpret and pursue an abnormal prothrombin time, activated partial thromboplastin time, and bleeding time in adults. Mayo Clin Proc. 2007 Jul. 82(7):864–73. [Medline].
6. Levy JH, Szlam F, Wolberg AS, Winkler A. Clinical Use of the Activated Partial Thromboplastin Time and Prothrombin Time for Screening: A Review of the Literature and Current Guidelines for Testing. Clin Lab Med. 2014 Sep. 34(3):453–477. [Medline].
7. Goldstein DA. Serum Calcium. In: Walker HK, Hall WD, Hurst JW, editors. Clinical Methods: The History, Physical, and Laboratory Examinations. 3rd edition. Boston: Butterworths; 1990. Chapter 143. Available from: https://www.ncbi.nlm.nih.gov/books/NBK250/
8. Seshadri D, Kumaran MS, Kanwar AJ. Acantholysis revisited: Back to basics. Indian J Dermatol Venereol Leprol 2013;79:120–6
9. Malamud D. Saliva as a diagnostic fluid. Dent Clin North Am. 2011;55(1):159–178. doi:10.1016/j.cden.2010.08.004
10. Humphrey SP, Williamson RT. A review of saliva: Normal composition, flow, and function. The Journal of Prosthetic Dentistry. 2001; 85:162–169.
11. Fedele S. Diagnostic aids in the screening of oral cancer. *Head Neck Oncol.* 2009;1:5. Published 2009 Jan 30. doi:10.1186/1758–3284–1–5.
12. Nithya SJ, Sankarnarayanan R, Hemalatha VT, Sarumathi T. Immunofluorescence in oral lesions. *J Oral Maxillofac Pathol.* 2017;21(3):402–406. doi:10.4103/jomfp.JOMFP_207_17
13. Melrose RJ, Handlers JP, Kerpel S, Summerlin DJ, Tomich CJ, American Academy of Oral and Maxillofacial Pathology. The use of biopsy in dental practice. The position of the American Academy of Oral and Maxillofacial Pathology. Gen Dent. 2007;55(5):457–61.
14. Mashberg A, Samit A. Early diagnosis of asymptomatic oral and oropharyngeal squamous cancers.*CA Cancer J Clin.* 1995;45(6):328–51.
15. Driemel O, Kunkel M, Hullmann M, von Eggeling F, Müller-Richter U, Kosmehl H, et al. Diagnosis of oral squamous cell carcinoma and its precursor lesions. *J Dtsch Dermatol Ges.* 2007;5(12):1095–100.
16. Patton LL, Epstein JB, Kerr AR. Adjunctive techniques for oral cancer examination and lesion diagnosis: a systematic review of the literature. *J Am Dent Assoc.* 2008 Jul. 139(7):896–905; quiz 993–4. [Medline].
17. Avon SL, Klieb HB. Oral soft tissue biopsy: an overview. *J Can Dent Assoc.* 2012. 78:c75. [Medline].
18. Hunasgi S, Koneru A, Manvikar V, Amrutha R, Reddy KMP. Oral biopsy in general dental practice. J Adv Clin Res Insights 2017;4:162–165.
19. Oliver RJ, Sloan P, Pemberton MN. Oral biopsies: methods and applications. British Dental Journal, 2004;196:329–333.
20. Sudheendra US, Sreeshyla HS, Shashidara R. Vital tissue staining in the diagnosis of oral precancer and cancer: Stains, technique,

utility, and reliability. Clin Cancer Investig J 2014;3:141–5.

21. Duraiyan J, Govindarajan R, Kaliyappan K, Palanisamy M. Applications of immuno-histochemistry. J Pharm Bioallied Sci. 2012;4(Suppl 2):S307–S309. doi:10.4103/0975–7406.100281

22. Patil DB, Tekale PD, Patil HA, Padgavankar PH. Emerging applications of immunohistochemistry in head and neck pathology. J Dent Allied Sci 2016;5:89–94.

23. Gupta LK, Singhi M K. Tzanck smear: A useful diagnostic tool. Indian J Dermatol Venereol Leprol 2005;71:295–9.

24. Rastogi V, Sharma R, Misra SR, Yadav L. Diagnostic procedures for autoimmune vesiculobullous diseases: A review. J Oral Maxillofac Pathol. 2014;18(3):390–397. doi:10.4103/0973–029X.151324

25. Chhabra S, Minz RW, Saikia B. Immunofluorescence in dermatology. Indian J Dermatol Venereol Leprol 2012;78:677–91

26. Soni AG. Nikolsky's sign: A clinical method to evaluate damage at epidermal-dermal junction. J Indian Acad Oral Med Radiol 2018;30:68–72.

27. Syed SA, Loesche WJ. Efficiency of various growth media in recovering oral bacterial flora from human dental plaque. *Appl Microbiol.* 1973;26(4):459–465.

28. Epidemiology, clinical presentation, and antibody response to primary infection with herpes simplex virus type 1 and type 2 in young women. Clin Infect Dis. 2013 Feb. 56 (3):344–51.

29. Qaseem A, Snow V, Shekelle P, Hopkins R Jr, Owens DK. Screening for HIV in health care settings: a guidance statement from the American College of Physicians and HIV Medicine Association. Ann Intern Med. 2009 Jan 20. 150(2):125–31.

30. Scully C. *"Oral and Maxillofacial Medicine"*. 3rd edition. London. Churchill Livingstone. 2013.

31. Burket. Greenberg MS, Glick M, Ship J (ed). Burket's oral medicine: diagnosis and treatment. 11th edition. 2008. Hamilton, Ont: BC Decker.

32. Centers for Disease Control and Prevention. Sexually Transmitted Disease Surveillance 2007 Supplement, Syphilis Surveillance Report. Centers for Disease Control and Prevention. Available at http://www.cdc.gov/std/Syphilis2007/. Accessed 2nd June 2019.

33. The World Health Organization. Diagnosis of Leprosy. Leprosy Elimination. Available at http://www.who.int/lep/diagnosis/en/. Accessed: 2nd June 2019.

Dental Therapeutics

The scope of this chapter is limited to the clinical practice of dentistry and does not cover alternative medicines. The dosages and drug preparations described in this chapter are based on the Indian Standard Pharmacopeia (ISP). The reader is cautioned to use the information provided based on their diagnosis and sound pharmacological knowledge. Drug interactions and adverse effects should be considered before prescribing any medications.

GENERAL PRINCIPLES OF DENTAL THERAPEUTICS

A budding dentist usually ponders if he/she is eligible to prescribe all those drugs which was taught in the graduate course. Indeed, the author of this chapter has been asked the same query by many colleagues and students. It should be understood that the subject of pharmacology has been taught and tested in the course of BDS programme which makes a dentist eligible to prescribe drugs with certain exceptions. Diseases which are not in the scope of dentistry should not be treated by a dentist alone.

How to prescribe?
Any prescription has to follow the basic principles taught in the subject of pharmacology (Fig. 3.1). Both written and electronic prescriptions need to be signed by

the licensed dentist with his official stamp. However, prescriptions through social media, text messages or telephonic conversations, commonly known as e-pharmacy is better to be avoided. The Drugs Controller General of India (DCGI) has banned the sale of medicines through e-pharmacies on 30th December, 2015[1].

What are over-the-counter medications?
Some of the medications commonly used for oral care are available as over-the-counter (OTC) medications and do not need any prescriptions. NSAIDs like paracetamol and ibuprofen, toothpastes, mouthwashes containing chlorhexidine or chlorine dioxide are a few examples for the OTC products.

Are there any legal issues in drug prescription?
Yes. Any authorized prescription is a legal document and can be used as a piece of evidence by the law of the land. It is a good practice to maintain copies of prescriptions in the patient records. Prescriptions for sedatives, hypnotic agents and opioid analgesics should be for short duration only. If necessary, new prescriptions are issued. These precautionary measures are to safeguard patient's health and avoid any misuse of prescriptions.

Prescriptions are valid from the date of issue to the number of days the drug is prescribed. No prescription can be reused and loses its legal validity if done so.

Faculty of dentistry, Xxxxxxxxxxxxxxxxxxxxxxxxxx
xxxxxxxxxxxxxxxxxxxxxxxxxxx

Mr. Yyyyyyy **Folder number:** 899898 **OPD number:** XYZGHKIL	**Diagnosis:** Periapical abscess **Age:** 27 yrs

R_X

1. Caps Amoxycillin 500 mg x tid for 5 days
   (to be taken 30 minutes after food only)

2. Tab Ibuprofen 400 mg sos—maximum one tablet per 8 hours
   (to be taken 30 minutes after food only)

Dr. XYZ
Annual practice registration number: 12345678
Date:

Fig. 3.1: Model prescription

Self-prescription is not a valid prescription and does not have any legal validity. It is not illegal to self-prescribe (including immediate family members) most of the medications (except for controlled drugs). However, such practices should be avoided.

Are there any cultural and religious issues related to drug prescriptions?
A dental practitioner should develop the cultural competence so that the values and beliefs of patients are taken into consideration during a drug prescription. Halal drugs, medications containing animal products, IV fluid administration during religious fasting are a few common issues that needs to be understood by the reader.

Should we prescribe trade name or generic name of the drug?
According to the circular of Medical Council of India (2017)[2] 'every physician should, as far as possible, prescribe drugs with generic names legibly and preferably in capital letters and he/she shall ensure that there is a rational prescription and use of drugs'.

The circular also states the provision for disciplinary action against defaulters.

Antibiotics

Any chemical produced by microbial organisms used against other microbial organisms are known as antibiotics and can be an antibacterial or antifungal drug. For the sake of convenience, in this chapter we have used antibiotic terminology for antibacterial and antifungal is used separately.

General guidelines for antibiotic prescription:
- Antibiotics is always a prescribed drug
- Complete dosage of antibiotic should be prescribed
- Start with an extended spectrum antibiotic and if therapeutic target is not achieved, should not hesitate to advise culture and sensitivity and followed by a narrow spectrum antibiotic.
- Seldom, antibiotics are prescribed for longer duration (>10 days) in the field of dentistry.

- Prophylactic antibiotics should be based on the standard guidelines rather than any speculation of infection without a clinical evidence.
- Local delivery of antibiotics should be restricted to periodontal treatment procedures and special cases like a dry socket.
- A standard drug duration of 5, 7 or 10-day regimen should be followed and should be based on the clinical judgement.
- Antibiotics are always combined with dental treatment procedures like RCT or extraction or curettage.

Dentoalveolar Infections

Majority of the dentoalveolar infections can be controlled using extended spectrum penicillin like amoxicillin and ampicillin[3]. 30% of these infections are caused by resistant strains to penicillin. Clavulanic acid in combination with amoxicillin is preferred in such cases.

To avoid development of antibiotic resistance to these drugs, a 3-day regimen has been advised[4]. However, the authors believe in the traditional school of thought, i.e. first 3 days of antibiotics are to kill the bacteria and next 2 days to kill the spores, thus making it a minimum of 5 days of prescription.

The traditional amoxicillin piggy backed with metronidazole can increase the effectiveness in treating dentoalveolar infections to 99%[5].

Periodontal and Pericoronal Infections

Periodontal infections are anaerobic infections or mixed infections and thus to be treated with combination drugs like amoxicillin and metronidazole or drugs which are excreted in gingival crevicular fluid like doxycycline.

As a guidance, Table 3.1 gives an overview of antibiotics for common dentoalveolar and periodontal infections.

Cephalosporin group of drugs and ciprofloxacin are commonly not advised in dental infections. However, such prescriptions are valid when supported with culture and sensitivity reports.

Osteomyelitis

Amoxicillin and clavulanic acid combination with metronidazole for 2–3 weeks, or ciprofloxacin combined with clindamycin in penicillin allergic patients are usually advised in jaw osteomyelitis patients. Newer antibiotics like linezolid are good for

TABLE 3.1: An overview of antibiotics for common dentoalveolar and periodontal infections

Infection	Antibiotic	Cost	Comments
Localised, no penicillin allergy	- Amoxicillin 500 to 750 mg *tid* for 5 days	- Economical	- Good compliance
Localised, allergic to penicllin	- Clindamycin 300 mg, *bid* for 5 days	- Expensive	- Avoid in patients with h/o colitis
	- Doxycycline 100 mg *bid* on first day and *od* for 4 days	- Economical	- No interference with food
Spreading, no penicillin allergy	- Augmentin 625 mg *bid* for 5 to 7 days	- Expensive	- Causes diarrhea
Spreading, allergic to penicillin	- Azithromycin, 500 mg *bid* for 5 to 7 days	- Expensive	- For patients with history of diarrhea after taking antibiotics
Alternative drugs	- Metronidazole 400 mg *tid* for 5 days	- Economical	- Should be used with amoxycillin, no alcohol, side effect like colitis

methicillin-resistant strains and vancomycin for nosocomial infections.

Common adverse events related to antibiotics:
A 5 days course of antibiotics such as amoxicillin and augmentin can sometimes result in diarrhea. A prior information of such a possibility should be provided to patients. This is a transient adverse effect which can be treated with probiotic tablets containing *Lactobacillus acidophilus*. Agents like metronidazole, tinidazole and ornidazole can result in metallic taste, xerostomia and fixed drug eruptions. These agents are also known for their 'disulfiram like' effect and hence a warning to avoid alcoholic drinks should be printed in the prescription. Tetracycline and ciprofloxacin should be avoided in pregnant patients and children less than 12 years.

Antifungals

Commonly used topical antifungal agents are clotrimazole, nystatin and miconazole. Resistant infections and deep fungal infections are treated with systemic antifungals like fluconazole, ketoconazole and amphotericin-B.

In denture stomatitis patients, topical antifungal agents are to be applied both on the lesion and on the denture-tissue surface. Topical antifungals are also used as first line of treatment for non-scrapable white lesions. Table 3.2 describes the commonly used topical and systemic antifungal agents.

Antiviral Agents

In this section we have described antiviral agents commonly used for orofacial viral infections. Antiretroviral drugs are not in the scope of this chapter.

Antiviral agents prescribed in a dental office are acyclovir, famciclovir and penciclovir for herpetic infections. Table 3.3 describes the various conditions and the dosage of antiviral agents used.

Nonsteroidal Anti-inflammatory Drugs (NSAIDs)

Unlike antibiotics, there is no rigid course for NSAID prescription. These drugs are always given 'as and when needed (*SOS*)'. However, appropriate drug should be chosen based on the severity or duration of pain. Table 3.4

TABLE 3.2: Commonly used topical and systemic antifungal agents

Infection	Antifungal agent	Dosage	Adverse reactions
Denture stomatitis, angular cheilitis and non-scrapable white lesions	⚹ Clotrimazole ⚹ Nystatin	⚹ 10 mg lozenges five times/day for two weeks or 1% solution *tid*/day topical for 2–4 weeks ⚹ 100,000 units qid/day topical for two weeks	⚹ Erythema, stinging, irritation ⚹ Nonspecific myalgia, bronchospasm, tachycardia
Resistant oral candidiasis	⚹ Fluconazole ⚹ Ketoconazole ⚹ Amphotericin-B oral suspension	⚹ 50 to 150 mg/day for two weeks ⚹ 200 to 400 mg/day for 2 weeks ⚹ 1 ml of 100 mg/ml oral suspension or 10 mg lozenges or 100–200 mg tablets *qid*	⚹ Diarrhea, flatulence, taste disturbance ⚹ Adrenal insufficiency, GI disturbances, photophobia are seen ⚹ Local irritation, pruritus and skin rash
Deep fungal infections like blastomycosis, cryptococcosis and rhinosporidiosis	⚹ Amphotericin-B	⚹ 250 µg/kg/day up to 1 mg/kg/day	⚹ Pain at injection site, renal toxicity, peripheral neuropathy

TABLE 3.3: Various conditions and the dosage of antiviral agents used

Condition	Antiviral agent	Dosage
Primary herpes simplex	Acyclovir	200 mg five time/day for 10 days
Recurrent herpes labialis	Acyclovir cream Penciclovir cream	5% five time/day for 1–2 weeks 1% five time/day for 2 weeks
Recurrent herpes simplex	Acyclovir	400 mg bid/day for 5–10 days
Herpes zoster	Acyclovir Famciclovir	800 mg five times/day for 10 days or IV 5 mg/kg 8 hourly 500 mg tid for 7 days
Prophylaxis of herpes simplex in immunocompromised patients	Acyclovir	200–400 mg qid/day for 1–2 weeks

TABLE 3.4: Appropriate choice of NSAIDs for dental practice

Condition	NSAID	Cost	Comments
Dentoalveolar infection with swelling and fever	Paracetamol 650 mg	Economical	✗ Not safe in patients with liver disorders. ✗ Preferred drug in children, pregnant patients and asthmatics
Dental extraction	Diclofenac sodium 50 mg Ibuprofen 400 mg	Economical	✗ Can cause gastric irritation
TMJ pain	COX-2 inhibitors like valedicoxib 10 mg or etoricoxib 60 mg	Expensive	✗ Not indicated in patients with liver impairment
Dental infections with fever in children	Mefenamic acid 250 mg	Economical	✗ Not indicated in asthmatic patients

describes the appropriate choice of NSAIDs for dental practice.

It should be noted that there is no therapeutic advantage of using COX-2 inhibitors to treat acute dental pain compared to Ibuprofen[6].

Opioid Analgesics

Indications for opioid analgesics in the field of dentistry is limited. Chronic pain in head and neck cancer patients, facial trauma and patients undergoing minor oral surgery might need these drugs. However, the addiction possibility, misuse of drug and side effects related to opioids need to be taken care in such cases.

Opioid analgesics are contraindicated in patients with cardiac problems, head injury and hypotension. They are not safe to be prescribed in pregnancy, children and teenagers.

Commonly prescribed drugs are tramadol, buprenorphine, pethidine, fentanyl, codeine and pentazocine (Table 3.5). Readers should update themselves with the regulations related to these drugs before any prescriptions are given.

Sedatives and Hypnotics

Alprazolam, barbiturates, clonazepam, diazepam and midazolam are the commonly used sedatives and hypnotics. Alprazolam is used in stress-related disorders leading to chronic orofacial pain. Clonazepam and diazepam are used as central muscles

TABLE 3.5: Commonly prescribed drugs

Type of opioid analgesic	Dosage	Indications	Adverse reactions
Tramadol	50 to 100 mg	Acute and chronic pain	Dizziness, vomiting and fatigue
Buprenorphine	200 to 400 mcg sublingual	Moderate to severe pain Medication assisted treatment	CNS depression, hallucinations and vertigo
Pethidine	50 to 150 mg IV	Moderate to severe acute pain	Hallucinations, dependence
Fentanyl	100 µg sublingual	Chronic pain	Bronchoconstriction, hypotension
Codeine	15 to 60 mg	Mild to moderate pain	Miosis, anorexia, confusion
Pentazocine	25 mg	Mild to moderate pain	Urinary retention and disorientation

relaxants. Topical clonazepam is used in burning mouth syndrome cases. Midazolam is used as a preoperative sedative agent for treating pediatric dental patients.

These group of drugs should be prescribed for short duration and related adverse effects should be informed to the patients.

Instructions to be given to patients on sedatives or hypnotics:

1. Follow the recommended dose.
2. Your medications can induce drowsiness. Please take such medications only before bed and do not drive/work after ingestion of such medications.
3. After taking these medications, do not work with fire, electric appliances and sharps.
4. These medications might cause dry mouth which is a temporary side effect.
5. Do not re-use the prescription.
6. Dispose remnant medications.
7. Keep the medications away from children.

Muscle Relaxants

Central muscle relaxants are more commonly used compared to peripheral ones. These drugs are mainly used for TMDs along with NSAIDs. Chlorzoxazone, orphenadrine, tizanidine, baclofen and thiocolchicoside are commonly used oral muscle relaxants. Other than these drugs, sedative agents like clonazepam and diazepam can be used as muscle relaxants.

We have not covered parenteral muscle relaxants in this section as it is not in the scope of this book. Table 3.6 describes the dosage, indications and key adverse reactions of these drugs.

TABLE 3.6 Dosage, indications and key adverse reactions of these drugs

Type of muscle relaxant	Dosage	Indications	Adverse reactions
Baclofen	5 to 10 mg	Severe chronic spasticity	Dry mouth, taste alterations, dizziness
Chlorzoxazone	250 mg	Painful muscle spasm	Altered liver function test, drowsiness
Orphenadrine	100 mg	Muscle spasm	CNS depression, tachycardia, euphoria, increased intraocular pressure
Thiocolchicoside	4 to 8 mg	Muscle spasm	Photosensitivity reactions
Tizanidine	2 mg	Spasticity and painful muscle spasm	Drowsiness, fatigue, dizziness, insomnia

Corticosteroids

In this textbook, corticosteroid is used as an equivalent terminology to glucocorticoid. We have not covered anabolic steroids and mineralocorticoids in this chapter.

In the field of dentistry, short and medium acting steroids are more commonly used compared to long-acting steroids. Table 3.7 shows the classification of corticosteroids with examples.

TABLE 3.7: Classification of corticosteroids with examples

Types	Examples
Short-acting (8–12 hours)	Hydrocortisone, cortisone
Medium-acting (12–36 hours)	Prednisolone, prednisone, methyl-prednisone, triamcinolone
Long-acting (36–72 hours)	Betamethasone, dexamethasone, deflazacort

Other than these, some of the glucocorticoids are used as topical agents only and belong to short-acting category. For example, budesonide, beclomethasone, clobetasone, fluticasone and mometasone.

In the field of dentistry, majority of corticosteroid prescriptions are topical. Corticosteroids are available in market as ointment, cream, paste and gel. It is advisable to use either gel or cream due to the presence of saliva in oral cavity. Because of saliva, ointment may not get absorbed through oral mucosa.

It should be noted by the reader that we seldom have the luxury of getting a topical corticosteroid manufactured for intraoral usage. Thus, we have to depend on the preparations marketed for skin lesions. Such topical preparations have warnings mentioned on the package prohibiting intraoral or intraocular usage. These warnings can panic a patient who has been advised to use the same intra orally. It is a good practice to explain these issues to the patients and take their consent or prescribe specific intraoral usage agents like Kenacort® with Orabase®.

Topical agents have the advantage of lesser systemic effects and lesser adverse event rate. However, there are many limitations which should not be overlooked. Challenges like standardized dispensing of steroid gel, consumption of food or fluids diluting the effect of the drug, unpleasant taste and flavor, messy application methods and difficulty in applying to posterior oral cavity can influence the overall drug effectiveness.

To handle lesions on the posterior parts of the oral cavity, topical prednisolone solution used as mouth rinse is comparatively more acceptable to patients in author's experience, except for its bitter taste. Local drug delivery systems like mucosal patch have yielded promising results[7].

Table 3.8 shows the WHO classification of topical corticosteroids[8].

TABLE 3.8 WHO classification of topical corticosteroids

Types	Examples
Ultra high potency	Clobetasol proprionate cream 0.05%
High potency	Flucinonide gel 0.05%
Moderate potency	Triamcinolone acetonide cream 0.1%
Low potency	Hydrocortisone acetate 1%

Systemic corticosteroids are prescribed either in the form of oral tablets or intralesional injections. Most commonly prescribed oral tablets are either prednisolone or prednisone. It is advisable to restrict the prescription of oral tablets up to 30 mg per day in any dental practice due to associated complications and the possible immunosuppression. Cases which need higher dosage should be managed as an inpatient or internal medicine specialist consultation would be needed.

Systemic steroids dosages prescribed in dose of >20 mg/day and/or >3 weeks are usually tapered gradually to allow the adrenal glands to resume their normal function. For patients under systemic steroid therapy presenting with oral infections, steroid dosage should be increased to combat the stress. It should be noted that despite steroid being an immunosuppressive agent, it is not withdrawn in cases of infection[9]. However, antibiotics and local treatment procedures to combat infection should be done simultaneously.

Intralesional corticosteroids are used specifically for managing trismus in oral submucous fibrosis cases, major aphthae, TMJ osteoarthritis, long-standing mucocele and large central giant cell granulomas. Complications such as local infection, scarring secondary to injections are not uncommon in such cases.

Pulse therapy is a special type of corticosteroid administration in conditions like erythema multiforme in which infusions of methylprednisolone is given in dose of 20–30 mg/kg to a maximum of 500 mg over 2–3 hours on consecutive days.

Prophylactic corticosteroids are used in 3rd molar surgery, edema reduction in trauma cases before open reduction of fractures and in pre-prosthetic surgeries. Although there are some conflicting effects, there is current evidence for such usage in 3rd molar surgery[10].

Occlusive therapy using custom trays are used to localize topical steroid medications on the gingival tissues in cases of desquamative gingivitis. Systemic complications like increase in blood glucose levels can be seen in such cases, which is unusual with conventional topical application of corticosteroids.

Other clinical scenarios where corticosteroids are used with varying success rates are to manage postoperative edema and pain, pulp capping agent, cavity liner, dry socket, Bell's palsy, Melkersson-Rosenthal syndrome, infectious mononucleosis and Behçet's syndrome.

Immune Modulators

Immune modulators can be immunosuppressors or immunoactivators. Although, corticosteroids are potent immunosuppressors, in this section we will limit the discussion to non-steroidal drugs.

Immune suppressors are usually prescribed in autoimmune disorders and have grave clinical implications as the recipient is vulnerable for opportunistic infections. It is best practice to discuss such therapies with an internal medicine specialist beforehand and necessary follow-ups and prophylactic measures should be considered.

Agents such as azathioprine, cyclosporine, methotrexate, sirolimus, tacrolimus and thalidomide are documented in the dental literature for management of autoimmune disorders affecting oral cavity. Oral PUVA therapy is combination of oral psoralen tablets with UV-type A rays for management of resistant type of oral lichen planus.

Some of these immune suppressors are also otherwise known as 'disease modifying anti-rheumatoid drugs (DMARDs)'. Nonbiologic DMARDs are hydroxychloroquine, sulfasalazine, minocycline, methotrexate and leflunomide[11]. Biologic DMARDs are etanercept, adalimumab, infliximab, certolizumab pegol, and golimumab which are related to tumor necrosis factors[11].

Immune activators like levamisole, interferons, interleukin-2, BCG injections and thalidomide have been used in management of aphthous ulcers, oral submucous fibrosis, oral premalignant and malignant lesions. However, there is a clear lack of evidence to ascertain the clinical advocacy of these drugs in these oral disorders.

Dentifrices

Two types of dentifrices are used for dental care, viz. antiplaque or anti-decay toothpaste and desensitizing toothpaste.

Antiplaque toothpastes, if fluoridated, have to declare the fluoride concentration on the label[12] and can range from 1000 to 1500 ppm. The maximum fluoride content in the toothpaste varies between countries. There are non-OTC high fluoride concentration toothpastes available in some countries. However, the recently published Cochrane review suggests that there is no evidence to choose toothpastes containing fluorides more than 1500 ppm[13].

Non-fluoridated toothpastes are available for both adults and children in India. As toothpastes with higher fluoride content can increase the risk of enamel defects because of fluorosis in children, some countries have restricted the usage of fluoridated toothpastes up to certain age. There is moderate-certainty evidence that 1500 ppm fluoride toothpaste reduces caries increment compared to non-fluoride toothpaste in primary dentition of young children[13]. Readers are advised to further read the American Academy of Pediatric Dentistry recommendations to make decisions related to the use of fluoride toothpaste[14].

Commonly used desensitizing toothpastes in India contain potassium nitrate, sodium fluoride, strontium ion or arginine bicarbonate. These toothpastes should be used for longer duration to see clinical benefits and should be applied with finger and wait for a few minutes before brushing. As these desensitizing agents cannot be combined with the common detergent used in toothpastes (sodium lauryl sulphate), there is comparative lack of freshness and foaming with these toothpastes.

Sodium lauryl sulphate, a detergent and foaming agent, presents in toothpastes can cause recurrent aphthous stomatitis in some individuals. Such patients can be prescribed toothpastes which contain alternative detergents such as non-ionic polyethylene glycol ethers of stearic acid[15].

Mouthwashes

Mouthwashes are antiseptic solutions used after brushing. Whereas, a mouthrinse is used before brushing to freshen the breath. However, these two terminologies are used synonymously in majority of the literature. In this chapter, we have used the terminology 'mouthwash' which includes both mouthwash and mouthrinse.

Antiseptic mouthwashes contain different agents like 0.12% chlorhexidine gluconate, 0.2% chlorhexidine gluconate, hydrogen peroxide, cetyl peridium chloride, chlorine dioxide, povidine-iodine, benzethonium chloride, essential oils or alcohol either as a stand-alone content or in combination. These mouthwashes are used for 1–2 weeks to establish any therapeutic effect. However, there are no evidence-based guidelines for the prescription duration.

Fluoride mouthwashes are used for its anti-cariogenic effect. These mouthwashes are prescribed to patients with high caries risk and post-orthodontic de-bonding cases.

Anodyne mouthwashes are used to reduce burning sensation or pain due to oral ulcers in patients undergoing cancer treatment. These mouthwashes contain benzydamine 0.15% or ketamine or morphine sulphate 2% or doxepin 0.5% and have shown promising results in pain reduction. Mouthwashes containing local anesthetic agents such as lignocaine and benzocaine are usually combined with diphenhydramine and magnesium aluminum hydroxide and dispensed as 'magic solution'. Antacid solutions can be used effectively to control pain or burning sensation in such patients. As a cleansing and debriding mouthwash, carbamide peroxide (10–15%), hydrogen peroxide (3%), or sodium bicarbonate solutions are used with varying success rates in aphthous ulcer patients. Antihistamine syrups such as Benadryl® are successfully used to manage allergic stomatitis.

Miscellaneous Drugs

Topical Agents

Amlexanox 5%, a potent inhibitor of inflammatory mediators, in the form of oral paste is used for aphthous ulcers to reduce pain and healing time. Hyaluronic acid is used topically in cases of oral ulcers including aphthous. 25% podophyllin resin is used to treat oral hairy leukoplakia along with antiviral medications. Preparations containing choline salicylate are regularly used in managing oral ulcers, inflamed mucosa and teething pain.

In cases of xerostomia, artificial saliva or oral humectants such as Biotene® gel or gels containing aloe vera can be prescribed. Systemic drugs (parasympathomimetic drugs) like pilocarpine, cevimeline, anetholetrithione have severe adverse effects and should be weighed over benefit before prescribing.

In case of leukoplakia, topical vitamin A preparations like retinoic acid, tretinoin, isotretinoin are used if no dysplasia is found in the biopsy reports. In case of dysplasia, topical bleomycin 1% cream is recommended.

Systemic Agents

It is recommended to prescribe H2 blockers like ranitidine or cimetidine or proton-pump inhibitors like pantoprazole or lansoprazole to reduce the gastric irritation along with long-term prescriptions of NSAIDs.

In cases of allergic manifestations, antihistamines such as cetirizine hydrochloride or diphenhydramine can be prescribed. However, in cases of type I anaphylactic reaction, IM administration of hydrocortisone is preferred drug of choice.

Neuralgias can be managed with carbamazepine, oxycarbazepine, phenytoin sodium, gabapentin or baclofen as first-line of treatment. These drugs can be given in combinations depending on the tolerance of the patient.

In potentially malignant conditions as oral submucous fibrosis, antioxidants like beta carotene, vitamin C, vitamin E, lycopene, manganese, selenium are prescribed as chemo-preventive agents. Intralesional injections of antioxidants, especially placental extracts are traditionally used along with local anesthetics and steroids.

Other than these medications, there are disease-specific agents like obtundants, mummifying agents, disclosing agents, denture cleansers, bleaching agents and cauterization solutions. These are explained in detail in the specialty textbooks and hence not covered in this chapter.

Pediatric Dose Calculation

An example is shown here:

A parent brought a 5-year-old boy, who was weighing 17 kilograms to the dental clinic who had pain in his decayed upper front teeth. He was examined and was diagnosed with acute periapical abscess in #51, #61. Prescribe appropriate drugs in the standard format.

In this case, the pediatric drug dose can be calculated either using Young's formula or Clark's rule.

Young's formula: Adult dose × Age / Age + 12 = Child's dose

500 mg × 5 / 5 + 12 = 147 mg

Clark's rule: Adult dose × Weight (in pounds) / 150 = Child's dose

500 × (17 x 2.2*) / 150 = 125 mg

> **Note:** Amoxycillin syrup is sold in the concentration of 125 mg/5 ml. So, the dosage of amoxicillin in this case will be ~5 ml (125 mg).
>
> Similarly, Ibuprofen syrup is sold in the concentration of 100 mg/5 ml. So, the dosage of ibuprofen in this case will be ~6 ml (125 mg)
>
> *1 kilogram = 2.2 pounds (In Clark's rule, body weight of the child has to be in pounds).

BIBLIOGRAPHY

1. Priyanka VP, Ashok BK (2016) E-pharmacies Regulation in India: Bringing New Dimensions to Pharma Sector. Pharmaceut Reg Affairs 5:175. doi: 10.4172/2167–7689.1000175
2. Medical Council of India: Circular on Generic Medicine. 2017. [accessed on May 6, 2019]. Available from: https://old.mciindia.org/circulars/Public-Notice-Generic-Drugs-21.04.2017.pdf
3. Fouad AF. Systemic Antibiotics in Endodontic Infections. In: Fouad AF, editor. Endodontic

Microbiology. Second ed.: Wiley-Blackwell; 2017: 269–85.

4. AAE Guidance on the Use of Systemic Antibiotics in Endodontics (2017). [accessed on May 6, 2019]. Available from: https://www.aae.org/specialty/wp-content/uploads/sites/2/2017/06/aae_systemic-antibiotics.pdf

5. Baumgartner JC, Xia T. Antibiotic susceptibility of bacteria associated with endodontic abscesses. J Endod. 2003 Jan;29(1):44–7. PubMed PMID: 12540219.

6. Huber MA, Terezhalmy GT. The use of COX-2 inhibitors for acute dental pain: A second look. J Am Dent Assoc. 2006 Apr;137(4):480–7. Review. PubMed PMID:16637477.

7. Sumanth KN, Ongole R, Rimal J. Efficacy of Dexamethasone Mucosal Patch for Oral Submucous Fibrosis (OSMF): A Pilot Study. Int Poster J Dent Oral Med 2010, Vol 12 No 2, Poster 484.

8. WHO model prescribing information: Drugs used in skin diseases, Classification of topical corticosteroids, Geneva: World Health Organisation; 1997; 117–8 [accessed on 7th May 2019]. Available at https://apps.who.int/medicinedocs/en/d/Jh2918e/32.html].

9. Tripathi, KD (2011) Essentials of Pharmacology for Dentistry. 2nd Edition. Jaypee Brothers Medical Publishers, New Delhi.

10. Ngeow WC, Lim D. Do Corticosteroids Still Have a Role in the Management of Third Molar Surgery? Adv Ther. 2016;33(7):1105–39. doi: 10.1007/s12325–016–0357-y. Epub 2016 Jun 10. PubMed PMID: 27287853.

11. Cohen S, Cannella A. Patient education. Disease modifying anti-rheumatoid drugs (DMARDs): Beyond basics. [accessed on 7th May 2019]. Available at https://www.uptodate.com/contents/disease-modifying-antirheumatic-drugs-dmards-beyond-the-basics

12. India cosmetics regulation. [accessed on 7th May 2019]. Available at https://cosmetic.chemlinked.com/countrypage/india-cosmetics-regulation

13. Walsh T, Worthington HV, Glenny AM, Appelbe P, Marinho VC, Shi X. Fluoride toothpastes of different concentrations for preventing dental caries in children and adolescents. Cochrane Database Syst Rev. 2010 Jan 20;(1):CD007868. doi: 10.1002/14651858.CD007868.pub2. Review. Update in: Cochrane Database Syst Rev. 2019 Mar 04;3:CD007868. PubMed PMID: 20091655.

14. Fluoride therapy. Recommendations: Best practices. American Academy of Pediatric Dentistry Reference Manual. 2017;20(6):250–3. [accessed on 8th May 2019]. Available at https://www.aapd.org/research/oral-health-policies--recommendations/fluoride-therapy/

15. Sälzer S, Rosema NA, Martin EC, Slot DE, Timmer CJ, Dörfer CE, van der Weijden GA. The effectiveness of dentifrices without and with sodium lauryl sulfate on plaque, gingivitis and gingival abrasion--a randomized clinical trial. Clin Oral Investig. 2016;20(3):443–50. doi: 10.1007/s00784–015–1535-z. Epub 2015 Aug 22. PubMed PMID: 26293981.

Physiotherapy in Dentistry

INTRODUCTION

Physiotherapy, a treatment in orofacial dysfunction, is considered to be an estranged abstract to dentist as well as people. This novel method is an important adjunctive therapy used in dentistry based on the traditions of orthopedics concerned with the management and rehabilitation of the patient. Postoperative physiotherapy is essential for the prevention or management of temporomandibular joint hypermobility or ankylosis. People with muscle weakness of mouth may benefit from facial strengthening exercises. Various oral motor exercises may be used as an aid in the management of Bell's palsy, trismus, oral submucous fibrosis. This non-invasive, reversible, and cost effective therapeutic modality is a major part of the comprehensive management of patients with orofacial disorders. The concept of physiotherapy goes way back to immemorial times of Hippocrates, deemed as the great Father of Medicine, who acknowledged that movement of body parts promotes good blood circulation necessary for a patient's recovery.

DEFINITION

World Confederation for Physical Therapy (WCPT) defines physical therapy as "Physical medicine and rehabilitation specialty that remediates impairments and promotes mobility, function and quality of life through examination, diagnosis, prognosis and physical intervention using mechanical force and movements".

—Oxford Textbook of Palliative Medicine

Treatment modalities of physiotherapy are broadly classified into:

- **Physical therapy:** Massage, deep tissue massage, trigger point therapy, spray and stretch, physical activity.
- **Electrotherapy:** Transcutaneous electric nerve stimulation (TENS), electronic galvanic stimulation (EGS), electro-accupuncture, diathermy, ultrasonography, lasers, iontophoresis.
- **Thermal therapy:** Hot packs, ice pack.

PHYSICAL THERAPY

Physical therapy refers to light physical activities that help in the release of endorphins for a sense of physical mental and social well-being. It stimulates muscle spindles for contraction and Golgi tendons for stretching, to maintain the normality of tissues.

Massage

It is mechanical manipulation of tissue with rhythmical pressure. Massage reduces pain and restores the proper length and flexibility of the muscles. It stimulates parasympathetic activity which in turn reduces stress and anxiety. Deep massage assists in mobilizing tissues, increasing blood flow to the area, and eliminating trigger points. It is most effective when it follows 10–15 minutes of preparation of the tissues with deep moist heat which tends to relax the muscle tissue, decreasing pain. Commonly used in cases of masticatory muscle pain.

Spray and Stretch Technique

Vapocoolants ethyl chloride or fluoromethane spray prior to stretching the muscles provides a temporary anesthesia effect to the muscles, so a more intense stretch can be achieved without pain. Sudden cold and the tactile stimulation provided by the vapocoolant spray, inhibit the pain and the reflex motor, and autonomic responses in the central nervous system. When the pain stimuli subside or suppress, an effective relaxation takes place that allows the gently stretching and lengthening of the muscle. The muscle is stretched and vapocoolant is applied in parallel sweeps in one direction till pain reference area. Commonly used in cases of masticatory muscle pain.

Physical Activity

Physical activity can be achieved by:

I. Soft Tissue Mobilisation

It is accomplished by superficial and deep massage which helps in mobilizing the tissues, increase blood flow to the area, and eliminate trigger points. Soft tissue therapy (STT) is the assessment, treatment, and management of soft tissue injury, pain, and dysfunction primarily of the neuromusculoskeletal system.

II. Joint Mobilisation

Distraction is accomplished by placing the thumb in the patient's mouth over the lower second molar area on the side to be distracted. With the cranium stabilized with the other hand, a downward force is applied on the molar with the thumb as the rest of the same hand pulls up on the anterior portion of the mandible. It is not indicated in inflammatory joint disorder. It inhibits pain, reduces muscle spasm and improves range of motion.

III. Muscle Conditioning

There are exercises that can help restore normal function and range of movement of the orofacial musculature. Four types of exercises can be instituted:

a. **Mobilization exercise:** Mobilizing the temporomandibular joints, the exercise aims to improve flexibility and extensibility of muscles, muscle fascia, tendons, and ligaments of masticatory muscles, as well as the facial muscles around the mouth so as to result in pain relief.
   - *Passive muscle stretching:* Instruct the patient to slowly and deliberately open the mouth until the pain is felt. While observing in a mirror patient is encouraged to open on a straight opening pathway.
   - *Assisted muscle stretching:* It is used when there is a need to regain muscle length. Instruct the patient to apply stretching force gently and intermittently to the elevator muscle with the fingers. If pain is elicited, then the force should be decreased or the exercise is stopped completely.

b. **Muscle-strengthening exercise (resistance exercises):** The patient is instructed to place the fist under the chin and open the mouth gently against the resistance. These exercises are repeated 10 times each session, six sessions a day. If they elicit pain, they should be discontinued. It is used to strengthen the power of targeted muscles.

c. **Coordination exercise:** Open-close or lateral movements of the mandible are effective to obtain coordination of muscle activity in masticatory muscles. It improves imbalanced muscle activity of painful muscles by repetitive alternate movements and thus relieve the muscle pain.

d. **Postural training:** In temporomandibular disorder (TMD) patients with muscle pain who also have a forward head posture, training the patient to keep the head in a more normal relationship with the shoulders may be helpful in reducing the TMD symptoms. Postural exercise includes head posture correction, correction of mandibular position including tongue postural exercise, and myofascial release.

Exercise for Facial Musculature

- **Facial-strengthening exercises:** Wide open the lips, puckering of the lips and moving from one side to the other, smiling by showing the teeth and gums, tightly closing the lips, puffing of cheeks 'O' exercise.
- **Tongue exercises:** Straight tongue the stretch, side tongue stretch, up and down stretch, by sliding the tongue along the outside of the teeth and gums, making circles in the mouth, pushing the tongue against the inside of the cheek, etc.

Tongue Exercises

Employed in cases of temporomandibular joint disorders, clicking related intracapsular

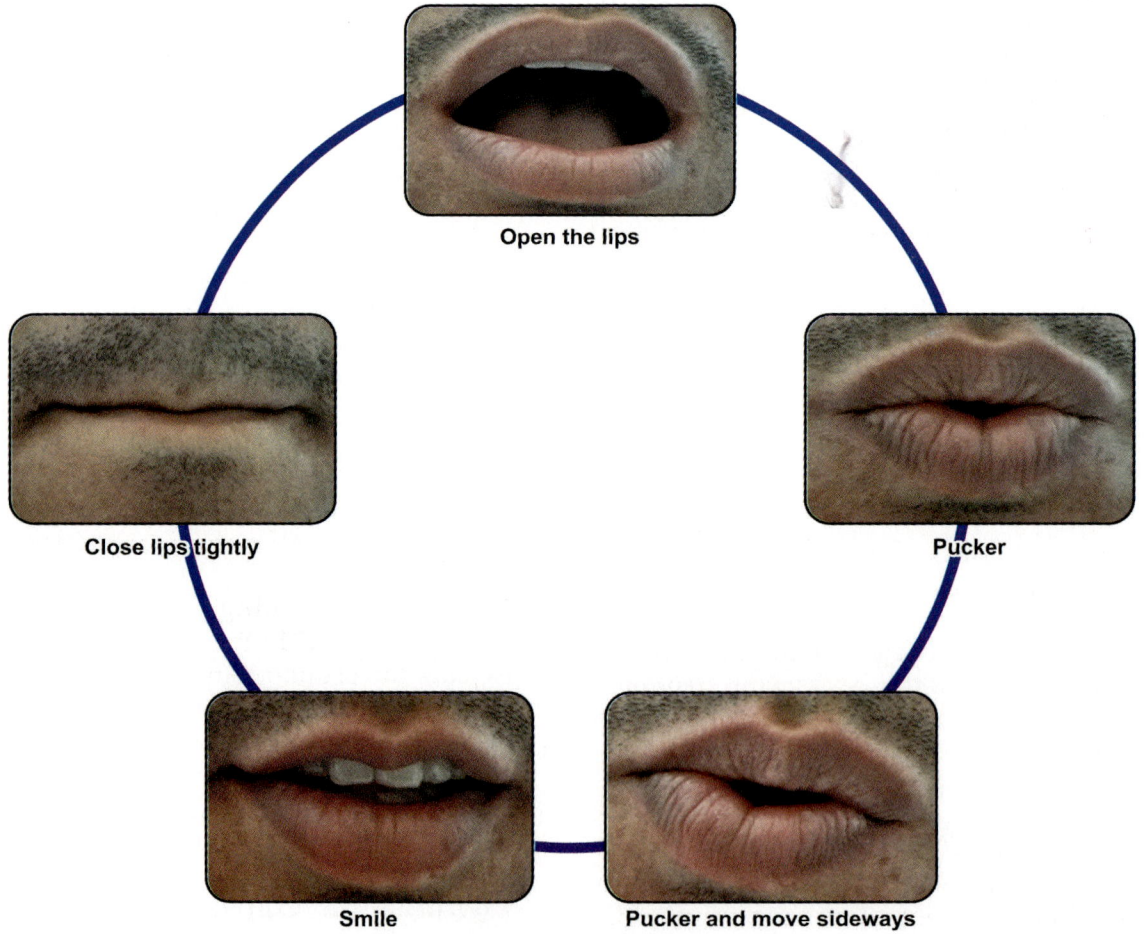

Open the lips

Close lips tightly

Pucker

Smile

Pucker and move sideways

Fig. 4.1: Lip exercises

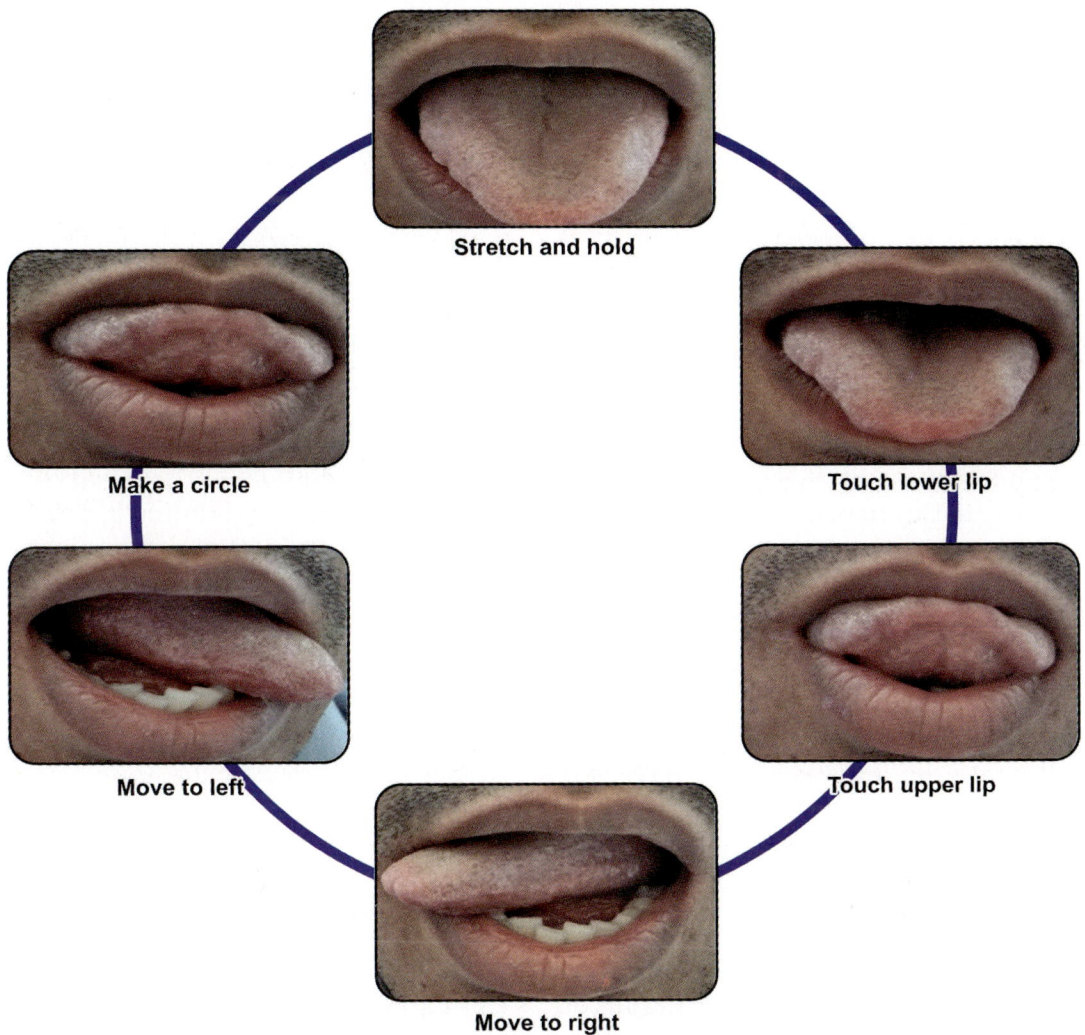

Fig. 4.2: Tongue exercises

joint disorder, acute lock, trauma-induced joint pain, chronic closed lock, capsulitis, hypermobility, hypomobility and oral submucous fibrosis.

Electrotherapy creates an electric field to stimulate or alter healing process, resulting in pain relief and tissue regeneration.

× **Transcutaneous electrical nerve stimulation:** It utilizes a high frequency (50–100 Hz), but very low intensity electric current which stimulates the nociceptive A-beta cutaneous afferents that activate the descending pain-inhibitory mechanism. It is perceived as a tingling or vibratory sensation with phasic muscle/no phasic muscle contraction. It is useful in acute pain, chronic intractable pain, trigeminal neuralgia, peripheral nerve injuries, myofascial pain dysfunction syndrome, post-TMJ surgery and causalgia.

Contraindications listed by manufacturers include pregnancy, infection, malignancy, and pacemaker.

Serious adverse events are rare although skin irritation and contact dermatitis beneath electrodes are erupt.

× **Electrogalvanic stimulation therapy:** A rhythmic electrical impulse of high-voltage, low-amperage is applied to the muscle, creating repeated involuntary contractions and relaxations resulting in the break-up of the muscle spasm as well as increases the blood flow to the muscles. Commonly employed in cases of masticatory muscle pain and post-TMJ surgery cases.

× **Electroacupuncture:** Acupuncture involves the insertion of small, solid needles, stainless steel needles that uses the body's own anti-nociceptive system to decrease the levels of pain felt. Stimulation of acupuncture points appears to cause the release of endorphins which effectively block the transmission of noxious impulses and thus reduce the sensation of pain. Electroaccupuncture requires a current of sufficient intensity to cause pain and muscle contraction. Used in cases of Bell's palsy, masticatory muscle pain, and temporomandibular joint disorders.

× **Diathermy:** Uses short wave (wavelength 3–30 m, frequency 10–100 MHz) or microwave (wavelength 0.001–1 m, frequency 300 MHz–300 GHz) electro-magnetic radiation to produce heat within body tissue through conversion. Results in selective heating of epithelial connective tissue that results in physiofibrinolysis. Commonly employed in cases of oral submucous fibrosis.

× **Ultrasonography:** Use physiotherapy in the form of penetrating heat to increase the blood flow in deep tissues and increases the flexibility and extensibility of connective tissue. The frequency range of therapeutic ultrasound is 0.75 to 3.3 MHz. Used in cases of oral submucous fibrosis, TMDs, and masticatory muscle pain.

× **Cold laser:** LASER (Light Amplification by Stimulated Emission of Radiation) is monochromatic, coherent and highly directional light. Low level lasers with red and near-infrared wavelength reduce the transmission of neurotransmitters resulting in decreased stimulation and thus reducing the pain. Act on trigger points by reducing the vascularity and thus diminishing the number of trigger points. Used in masticatory muscle pain and temporomandibular disorders.

× **Iontophoresis:** Local anesthetics and anti-inflammatory agents are placed in a pad and the pad is placed on the desired tissue area. Then a low electrical current is passed through the pad that drives the medication into the tissue. Scientific studies suggested iontophoresis can deliver dexamethasone between 8 and 17 m deep and long duration application of 3 hours via low current is more effective. Employed for TMDs and intracapsular joint disorders.

THERMOTHERAPIES

× **Humans** are warm blooded and their tissues are affected by the application of heat or cold.

× **Superficial mild heat** is used in thermo-therapy to increase circulation, soft tissue extensibility, enhance healing, control pain, metabolic, neuromuscular, and hemodynamic activity.

× **Cold application** reduces pain and body temperature, anesthetize an area, control hemorrhage, and growth of bacteria and reduce inflammation.

× **Thermotherapy:** A hot, moist towel is applied over the symptomatic area for 20 minutes, two to three times a day at tolerant temperature. Heat causes vasodi-lation, increased circulation to the area, and reduces symptoms.

× **Coolant therapy:** Ice is directly applied to the affected area and is moved in a circular motion without pressure on the tissues for a period of 5–7 minutes. When numbness begins, ice should be removed. Types of cryotherapy include cold packs (–12°F), ice packs vapor coolant (cools at 5°C at 2 cm depth), chemical gel packs, vapocoolant spray, controlled cold compression units, and cold water immersion.

- **Alternate fomentation:** Studies suggest that superficial heat and cold application have similar positive effects in relieving pain because of similar action. Cold therapy has a rapid analgesic effect, reduces acute inflammation and prevents edema in acute injury, whereas thermal therapy increases tissue extensibility thus causing relaxation. Alternate hot and cold fomentation, results in accelerated local circulation and stimulate healing. During the warming period in between applications, it increases the blood flow. Stimulation of cutaneous nerve fibers occur which in turn shuts down the smaller pain (C) fibers. Used in cases of muscle and joint stiffness. Cryotherapy should precede thermal therapy.
- Employed in cases of temporomandibular joint disorders, clicking related intra-capsular joint disorder, acute trauma induced joint pain, chronic closed lock, capsulitis, hypermobility, hypomobility, and masticatory muscle spasm.

Summary

Applications in orofacial conditions:
- Temporomandibular joint disorders
- Intracapsular joint disorders (clicking and clicking-related jaw incoordination as a result of disc displacement)
- Intracapsular joint disorders (trauma-induced acute pain, chronic closed lock, capsulitis and arthritic change)
- Masticatory muscle pain
- Hypermobility and hypomobility
- Post-orthognathic surgery
- Post-TMJ surgery
- Oral submucous fibrosis
- Bell's palsy

BIBLIOGRAPHY

1. Sodhi A, Nair PK, Hegde S. Physiotherapy: Key to the kinetics of orofacial musculature. J Indian Acad Oral Med Radiol 2014; 26:419–24.
2. Steve Heinrich P.T. (1991) The Role of Physical Therapy in Craniofacial Pain Disorders: An Adjunct to Dental Pain Management.
3. Pain Disorders: An Adjunct to Dental Pain Management, CRANIO®, 9:1, 71–75.
4. Agrawal A, Keluskar V. Role of physiotherapy in treatment of certain Orofacial disorders. Biosci Biotech Res Comm. 2010, 3(1): 7–13.
5. Kumar SP, Jim A. Physical therapy in palliative care: From symptom control to quality of life: A critical review. Indian J Palliat Care 2010;16:138–46.
6. Panga SS, Sekhar R, Sekhar GR, Tupii S. Diagnosis and Treatment Modalities for Temporomandibular Disorders (Part II). Int J Prostho Resto Dent 2011;1(3):192–5.
7. Gloth M, Matesi M. Physical therapy and exercise in pain management. Clin Ger Med. 2001; 17(3):525–35.
8. Shimada A, Ishigaki S, Matsuka Y, Komiyama O, Torisu T, Oono Y, Sasaki K. Effects of exercise therapy on painful temporomandibular disorders. J Oral Rehab. 2019; 46(5): 475–81.
9. Shaffer SM, Brismee JM, Sizer PS, Courtney CA. Temporomandibular disorders. Part 2: conservative management. Journal Manual and Manipulative Therapy 2014; 22(1): 13–23.

Ulcerative Vesiculobullous Lesions

TERMINOLOGIES

1. **Ulcer:** A defect in the epithelium; it is well-circumscribed depressed lesion over which epidermal layers have been lost with molecular necrosis. It is also described as break in the continuity of epithelium due to molecular necrosis, e.g. aphthous ulcer, traumatic ulcer, herpetic ulcer.
2. **Macule:** Well-circumscribed, flat lesions that are noticeable because of their change from normal skin color. May be red due to the presence of vascular lesions or inflammation, or pigmented due to presence of melanin, hemosiderin, drugs, e.g. hemangioma, oral melanotic melanoma.
3. **Papule:** Solid lesions, raised above the skin surface that are smaller than 1 cm diameter, e.g. erythema multiforme, rubella, lupus erythematosus, papules of pseudomembranous candidiasis.
4. **Plaque:** Solid raised lesions that are over 1 cm in diameter; they are larger papules, e.g. leukoplakia.
5. **Vesicle:** Raised fluid-filled lesions containing clear fluid with diameter less than 1 cm, e.g. pemphigus, erythema multiforme.
6. **Bulla:** Elevated blister-like lesions containing clear fluid that are over 1 cm in diameter, e.g. pemphigus.
7. **Nodule:** These lesions are present deep in the dermis and the epidermis can be easily move over them. They protrude above the skin or mucosa, e.g. lipoma.
8. **Pustule:** Raised lesions containing purulent material.
9. **Erosion:** Moist red lesions often caused by the rupture of vesicles or bullae as well as trauma, e.g. oral lichen planus.
10. **Purpura:** Reddish to purplish discolorations caused by leakage of blood and varies in size from 0.4 to 0.9 cm which do not blanch on pressure.

The oral mucosa is thin and friable leading to rapid rupture of vesicles and bullae forming ulcers and erosions. A patient presenting with ulcerative or vesiculobullous lesions should be asked the following important questions:

1. **Since when:** Duration (acute/chronic)
2. **How many:** Number (single/multiple)
3. **Recurrent or first time:** Primary or recurrent
4. Presence of fever or systemic complaints, joint pains
5. History of eye, genital or skin lesions

CLASSIFICATION

1. Classification of Vesiculobullous Lesions (Fig. 5.1)

i. **The patient with acute multiple lesions**
   × Herpesvirus infection

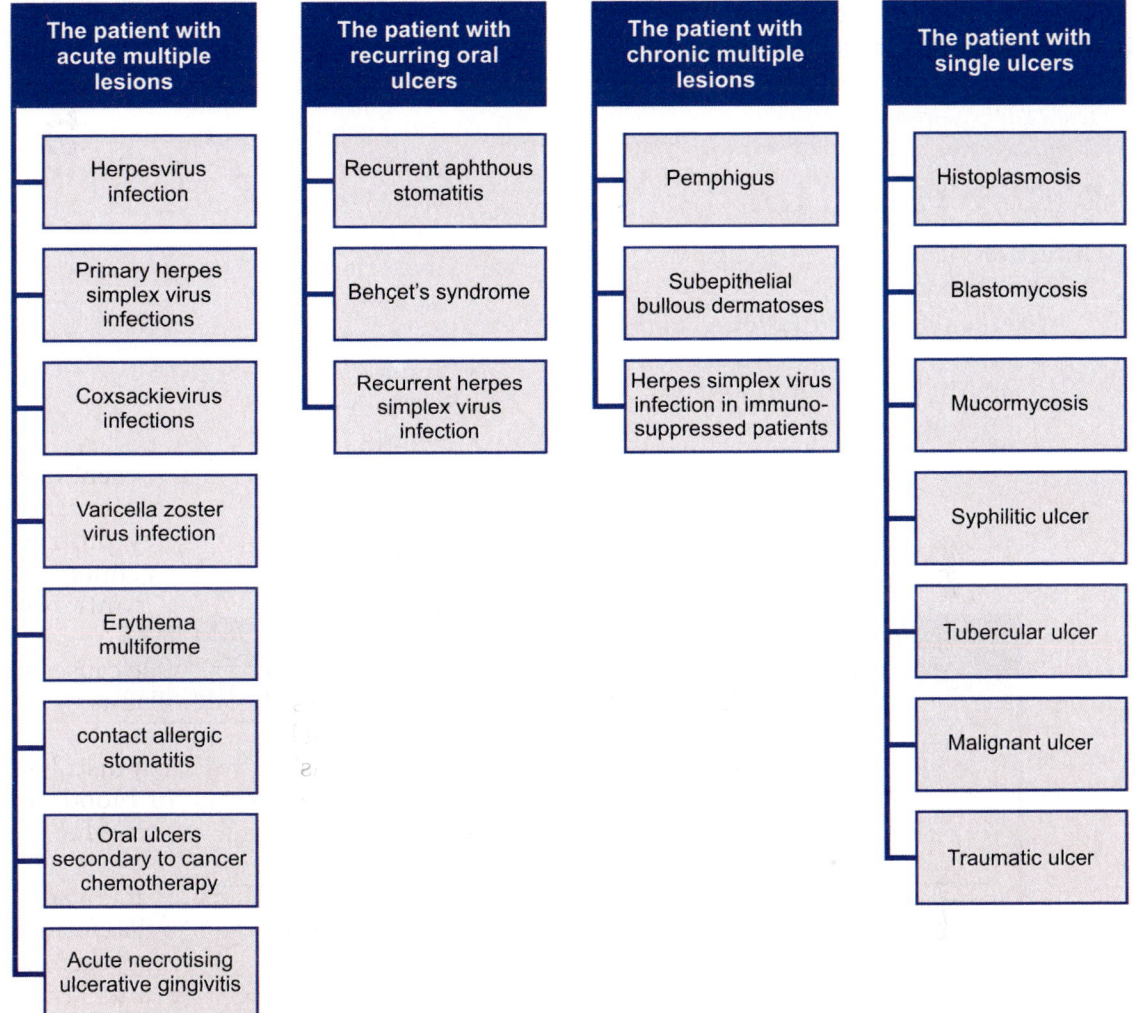

Fig. 5.1: Classification of vesiculobullous lesions based on clinical presentation

- Primary herpes simplex virus infections
- Coxsackievirus infections
- Varicella zoster virus infection
- Erythema multiforme
- Contact allergic stomatitis
- Oral ulcers secondary to cancer chemotherapy
- Acute necrotising ulcerative gingivitis

ii. **The patient with recurring oral ulcers**
- Recurrent aphthous stomatitis
- Behçet's syndrome
- Recurrent herpes simplex virus infection

iii. **The patient with chronic multiple lesions**
- Pemphigus
- Sub-epithelial bullous dermatoses
- Herpes simplex virus infection in immunosuppressed patients

iv. **The patient with single ulcers**
- Histoplasmosis
- Blastomycosis
- Mucormycosis
- Syphilitic ulcer
- Tubercular ulcer
- Malignant ulcer
- Traumatic ulcer

2. Classification of Ulcerative, Vesiculo-bullous Lesions based on Etiology

1. **Traumatic**
   - Mechanical irritation
   - Chemical irritants
   - Thermal burns
   - Radiation burns
2. **Infections**
   A. *Viral infection*
   - Herpes simplex infection
   - Herpes zoster
   - Hand-foot-and-mouth disease
   - Herpangina
   - Measles
   - Infectious mononucleosis
   - HIV-AIDS

   B. *Bacterial infection*
   - Syphilis
   - Tuberculosis
   - ANUG
   - Gonorrhea
   - Leprosy
   - Actinomycosis
   - Noma
   - Scarlet fever
   - Diphtheria

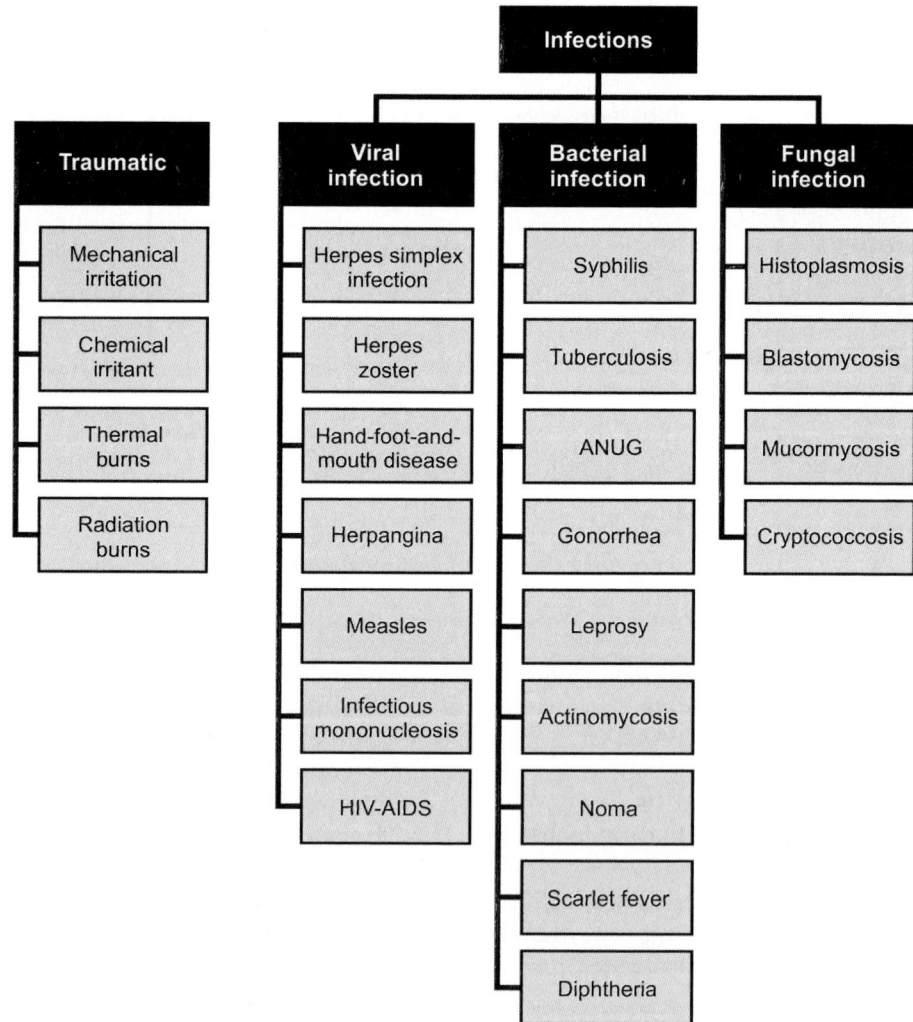

Fig. 5.2: Classification of ulcerative, vesiculobullous lesion based on etiology

C. *Fungal infections*
  - Histoplasmosis
  - Blastomycosis
  - Mucormycosis
  - Cryptococcosis
3. **Neoplasms**
  - Squamous cell carcinoma
  - Malignant melanoma
  - Non-Hodgkin's lymphoma
4. **Systemic disorders**
   Blood disorders
  - Agranulocytosis
  - Leukemia
  - Aplastic anemia
5. **Nutritional deficiency**
  - Scurvy
  - Riboflavin deficiency
  - Inflammatory bowel disease

6. **Conditions associated with immunologic dysfunction**
  - Aphthous ulcers
  - Behçet's syndrome
  - Reiter's syndrome
  - Erythema multiforme
  - Lupus erythematosus
  - Drug reactions
  - Contact allergic stomatitis
  - Wegener's granulomatosis
  - Chronic granulomatous disease
  - Cyclic neutropenia
A. **Intraepithelial vesicles:** The lesion is formed within the epithelium
  - *Acantholytic vesicles:* This is because of the breakdown of specialized attachments called the desmosomes, e.g. pemphigus

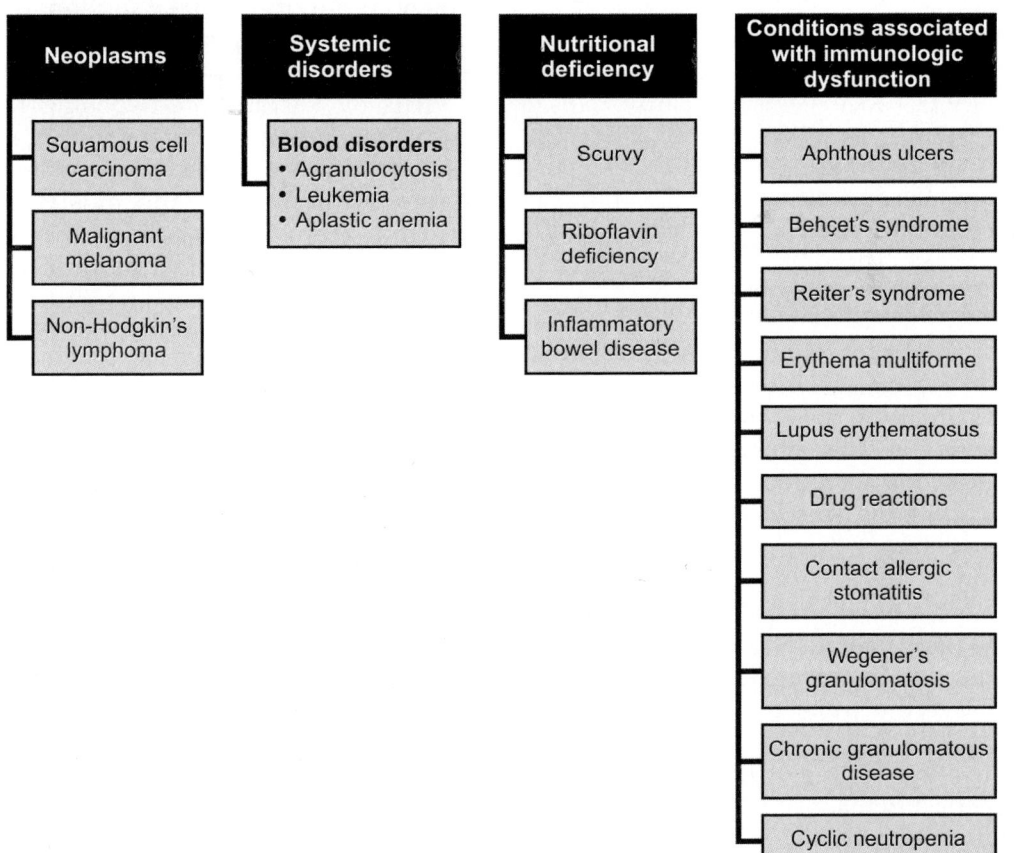

Fig. 5.3: Classification based on various conditions

* *Non-acantholytic vesicles:* It is usually seen in viral infections because of the death or the rupture of the group of cells
B. **Sub-epithelial vesicles:** Lesions formed between the epithelium and the lamina propria, e.g.
   * Erythema multiforme
   * Pemphigoid
   * Epidermolysis bullosa

Acute Multiple Vesiculobullous Lesions

Human herpesvirus infection: Seven types of herpesvirus are known to be pathogenic for humans, with six of them linked to head and neck region.

The Herpesviridae family of viruses contain nine different viruses that are pathogenic in humans. These are:

1. Herpes simplex virus 1
2. Herpes simplex virus 2
3. Varicella zoster virus
4. Cytomegalovirus
5. Human herpesvirus 6
6. Human herpesvirus 7
7. Human herpesvirus 8
8. Simian herpesvirus
9. Epstein-Barr virus

HERPESVIRUS INFECTION

HSV-1 causes infections above the waist and HSV-2 causes infections below the waist. Primary herpes infection is acquired by inoculation of the mucosa, skin and eyes with infected secretions. The virus then travels along the sensory nerve to establish a chronic latent infection in the sensory ganglion.

Two types of HSV: HSV-1 and HSV-2.

HSV-1 affects oral, facial and ocular areas. The pharynx, intraoral sites, lips, eyes and skin above the waist are involved. It can cause:

* Acute herpetic gingivostomatitis
* Herpetic eczema
* Keratoconjunctivitis
* Meningoencephalitis
* Herpes labialis

HSV-2 involves genitalia and skin below the waist. It can cause genital herpes.

Predisposing Factors

* Sunlight
* Trauma
* Menstruation
* Fever
* Immunosuppression
* Decompression of the trigeminal nerve
* Irritation by dental instruments.

Clinical Features

It manifests in two forms: Primary infection and recurrent/recrudescent form

1. **Primary HSV/primary herpetic gingi-vostomatitis**

   Primary infection may be manifested only by a few and mostly the individuals experience a subclinical state. HSV exhibits latency in the trigeminal ganglion, nodosa ganglion of vagus nerve, dorsal root ganglia, sympathetic ganglia and brain. Reactivation of virus by various predisposing factors causes secondary or recurrent infection. The newborn are protected by placentally transferred antibodies and mostly affects children from 6 months to 6 years. Generalized prodromal symptoms like fever, malaise, irritability, headache and cervical lymphadenopathy are mostly accompanied with the infection.

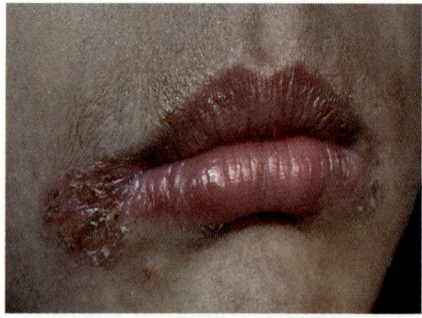

Fig. 5.4: Primary herpes clinical presentation

The vesicles tend to appear in clusters on skin, vermilion border of lips and keratinized oral tissues like palate and gingiva. Thin-walled vesicles (*drops of dew appearance*)

TABLE 5.1: Types of HHV

Type of human herpesvirus (HHV)	Primary infection	Recrudescent lesions in healthy hosts	Recrudescent lesions in Immunocompromised hosts
Herpes simplex virus 1 (HHV-1)	Gingivostomatitis, kerato-conjunctivitis, genital and skin lesions	Herpes labialis ("cold sores" "fever blisters"), intraoral ulcers, kerato-conjunctivitis, genital and skin lesions	Ulcers at any mucocutaneous site, usually large and persistent; disseminated infection
Herpes simplex virus 2 (HHV-2)	Genital and skin lesions, gingivostomatitis, kerato-conjunctivitis, neonatal infections, aseptic meningitis	Genital and skin lesions, gingivosto-matitis, aseptic meningitis	Ulcers at any mucocutaneous site, usually large and persistent; disseminated infection
Varicella-zoster virus (HHV-3)	Varicella (chickenpox)	Zoster (shingles)	Disseminated infection
Cytomegalovirus (HHV-4)	Infectious mononucleosis, hepatitis, congenital disease		Retinitis, gastroenteritis hepatitis, severe oral ulcers
Epstein-Barr virus (HHV-5)	Infectious mononucleosis like hepatitis, encephalitis		Hairy leukoplakia, lympho-proliferative disorders, mucocutaneous ulcers
HHV-6	Roseola infantum (affects children below 3 years), exanthema subitum, otitis media, encephalitis		Fever, bone marrow suppression
HHV-7	Roseola infantum		
HHV-8	Infectious mononucleosis like febrile exanthema		Kaposi sarcoma, lympho-proliferative disorders, bone marrow suppression

affecting any part of the oral mucosa, rupture to form painful, smooth, round, shallow, symmetrical and small ulcers

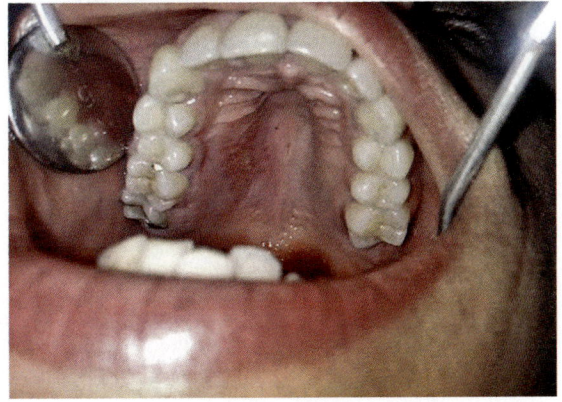

Fig. 5.5: Intraoral herpes infection

with surrounding tissue tags (*moon crater appearance*). The ulcers heal without scarring in 1 to 2 weeks. There is erythematous involvement of marginal gingiva which is characteristic of herpes infection. It may be associated with pharyngitis and there is cervical lymphadenopathy.

2. **Secondary or recurrent herpes simplex infection**

Predisposing factors cause reactivation of virus and the patient experiences prodromal symptoms of tingling, burning or pain at the site. Clusters of vesicles form, which often go unreported by the patient, since they soon rupture and coalesce to form large ulcers. Vesicular lesions mostly occur only on the lips and are referred as recurrent herpes labialis (RHL). Sometimes *clusters of smooth, round, shallow, symmetrical ulcers along with marginal gingivitis* occur mostly on keratinized mucosa (gingival and hard palate) and is described as recurrent intraoral herpes infection [RIOH].

Recurrent lesions in immunocompromised patients like HIV/malignancy are very severe and large. Infection of the thumbs or fingers may occur in health professionals during treatment of infected patients or as a result of self-inoculation in children with orofacial herpes and is called *herpetic whitlow*. Recurrences on the digits may result in paresthesia and permanent scarring.

Primary cutaneous herpetic infection in areas of previous epithelial damage is called *herpes gladiatorum or scrumpox.*

Diagnosis

Clinical examination is most commonly the diagnostic feature of the lesion caused by HSV.

1. **Cytology:** HSV can be identified from the scrapings from the base of the lesions smeared on to the glass slides. These can be stained with Wright's Giemsa (Tzanck test) or Papanicolau staining to demonstrate the characteristic multinucleated giant cells or intranuclear inclusions of herpesvirus.
2. **HSV isolation** by cell culture is the gold standard test for the diagnosis for HSV-1 infections since it grows readily in tissue culture. The advantage of a culture is that it has high sensitivity and specificity and allows for amplification of virions subtyping and testing for sensitivity to antiviral drugs.
   Disadvantage: It needs specialized equipment, is expensive, and may take upto several days for final result.
3. **Recently PCR (polymerase chain reaction)** from swabs has been shown to detect HSV antigen.
4. **Recurrent infection** is associated with rise in IgG antibody titre in acute sera but a fourfold rise is seen in only 5% patients.

Management

RHL is usually self-limiting. Treatment is directed at promoting lesion healing and providing palliation. Adequate food and fluid intake should be ensured. Patients should restrict contact with active lesions to prevent spread and should avoid contact with children. Topical anesthetic agents like dyclonine hydrochloride 0.5 to 1% as oral rinse provides palliation. NSAIDs like ibuprofen can be given for fever.

Antivirals can be given for severe lesions. Topical acyclovir in cream or suspension in a rinse and swallow technique. Systemically acyclovir can be given as 200 mg five times daily in very severe lesions, as in severe immunosuppression.

Penciclovir cream 1% during prodromal stage prodrome and then every 2 hours.

Differential Diagnosis

- **Hand-foot-and-mouth disease:** Hands, feet and oral.
- **Herpangina:** Oropharyngeal and soft palate involvement. It affects children in

TABLE 5.2: Differential features of HSV and EM	
HSV	*EM*
SSSR	LIDB
Prodromal symptoms Period: 2 to 8 days	Fever may sometimes accompany No prodromal symptoms
Fever before	Sudden acute explosive onset
Age: Older	Age: Younger <50 years
Etiology: Viral	Hypersensitivity reaction
Marginal gingivitis	No gingival involvement Lips prominently involved
Cervical lympha-denopathy: +nt	−1 nt
No target/bull's eye lesion	Target/bull's eye lesion
Rx: Antiviral steroids are contraindicated	Rx: Steroids

late summer and early monsoon season on soft palate and facial area with fever and malaise.

TABLE 5.3: Differential features of HSV and HZV

HSV	HZV
Lesions do not heal by scarring	Scarring +nt
No osteonecrosis	In severe—osteonecrosis
HSV: 1° and 2° – RHL and RIOH	VZ: 1° Chickenpox and HZ
Bilateral	Unilateral
Prodromal symptoms; fever, malaise	Prodromal symptoms shooting pain, burning paraesthesia and tenderness along the nerve area—C_3, T_5, L_1, L_2
No pain only tingling	No h/o fever
Cytology: Tzanck cells	Non-specific cytology
Rx: Acyclovir 200 mg 5 times a day	Rx: Acyclovir 800 mg 5 times a day

TABLE 5.4: Differential features of HSV and herpangina

HSV	Herpangina
Severe	Mild
Non-epidemic	Epidemic
Anterior portion of mouth especially gingiva	Posterior portion
Gingivitis	No gingivitis
Larger SSSR	Smaller lesions Macule, papule, vesicles, ulcers
DNA virus	RNA virus
HSV	A4 coxsackie
Cytology shows multi-nucleated Tzanck cells	Absence of multi-nucleated giant cells
Rx: Specific antiviral for HSV	Self-limiting and supportive Rx.

- **Aphthous stomatitis:** No stomatitis, no general systemic symptoms and lesions are less numerous and more oftenly found in adults.

- **Bullous lichen planus:** It is painful condition characterized by large blister on tongue and cheek which rupture and undergo ulceration.
- Erythema multiforme
- Acute necrotizing gingivostomatitis
- Thermal burns
- CMV infection

COXSACKIE VIRUS

Coxsackie virus is a RNA virus and causes following infections
1. Herpangina
2. Hand-foot-and-mouth disease
3. Acute lymphonodular pharyngitis

Herpangina

It is caused by coxsackie group of virus with type 1 through 6, 8, 10, 16 and 22. Herpangina is derived from herpes and angina.

Herpes: Vesicular eruptions and angina: Inflammation of throat.

Infection occurs through ingestion, direct contact, or through droplet spread and multiple cases in a single household are common. It occurs in epidemic with highest frequency from June to October.

Clinical Features

Majorly affected are young children aged 3 to 10 years, and adults are only occasionally affected. Herpangina is chiefly a summer disease, and many children may actually harbor the virus at this time without exhibiting clinical manifestation of the disease. The incubation period is 2–10 days.

Generalized symptoms: Mild and of short duration. It begins with sore throat, cough, rhinorrhea, low-grade fever, headache, sometimes vomiting, prostration, and abdominal pain.

Oral Manifestations

The first oral symptoms of herpangina are sore throat and pain on swallowing. Commonly occur on the anterior faucial pillars and sometimes on the hard and soft palates, posterior pharyngeal wall, buccal mucosa and tongue. Small vesicles form and persist for short duration which rupture to form crops of ulcers with a gray base and inflamed periphery. The ulcers less painful, although dysphagia may occur.

Symptoms resolve within a few days. Ulcers generally heal within 7–10 days.

Recurrence: Children have been affected several times in one season by infection with different strains of coxsackie virus. A permanent immunity to the infecting strain usually develops rapidly and most adults have neutralizing antibodies against numerous strains.

Laboratory Findings

1. Viral isolation

Differential Diagnosis

1. Herpangina and primary HSV

Treatment

No treatment is necessary, since the disease usually appears to be self-limiting and presents with a few complications.

Hand-Foot-and-Mouth Disease

Hand-foot-and-mouth disease is an epidemic infection, caused by the enterovirus coxsackie A16 and has been reported to be cause less frequently by types A5 and A6, and occasionally even by B2, B6 or enterovirus 71. Despite the similarity in names, it bears no relationship to hand-foot-and-mouth disease, another viral disease with an animal vector.

Clinical Features

It primarily affects young children between age of 6 months and 5 years. It is characterized by the appearance of maculopapular, exanthematous, and vesicular lesions of the skin, particularly involving the hands, feet, legs, arms, and occasionally the buttocks. There is anorexia, low-grade fever and sometimes lymphadenopathy, diarrhea and vomiting.

Oral Manifestations

The oral lesions are usually located on hard palate, tongue and buccal mucosa and sometimes involving the lips, gingival, pharynx and the tonsils. The patient complains of sore mouth with difficulty to eat. This is due to small, multiple vesicular and ulcerative oral lesions that are more numerous than seen in herpangina. The tongue may also become red and edematous.

Laboratory Findings

Intracytoplasmic viral inclusions can sometimes be demonstrated in vesicular scrapings of the lesions. Viral isolates may usually be obtained from vesicular fluid itself. There is rise in acute or convalescent serum antibody titre to coxsackie A16.

Differential Diagnosis

- **Herpetic gingivostomatitis:** Entire oral cavity is affected. No hand and feet involvement.
- **Varicella zoster infection:** Segmental distribution along the anatomical location of nerve (unilateral lesions)
- **Herpangina:** Affect children mostly in late summer and early monsoon and lesions are common on soft palate and facial area with fever and malaise.
- **Allergic stomatitis:** Sudden appearance, no prodromal symptoms with itching and noticeable erythema.
- **Chickenpox:** In addition to intraoral changes, polymorphic exanthematous lesions on the entire body and severe lesions.

Measles (Rubeola, Morbilli)

It is an acute, contagious, dermotropic viral infection, primarily affecting children, and occurring many times in epidemic form.

It is caused by paramyxovirus 'which' belongs to the family paramyxoviridae, which is an RNA virus.

Transmission

Spread of disease occurs by direct contact with a person or by droplet infection, the portal of entry being the respiratory tract.

Epidemiology

It is contagious from first or second day even before the onset of serious illness or appearance of rash.

It is transmitted mainly through respiratory secretions and also through direct contact of droplets.

The incubation period is generally from 8–12 days. It is mainly transmitted in large families, crowded homes and slums.

It is a self-limiting disease in healthy immune competent children, but morbidity and mortality is high in malnourished and immunocompromised individuals.

Pathogenesis

Upon invasion of respiratory epithelium it reaches reticuloendothelial system through blood stream and thereby infects skin, respiratory tract, and other organs.

The invasion of T-lymphocytes and increased levels of suppressive cytokines leads to transient suppression of cellular immunity. Monocyte is mainly infected.

Symptoms show mainly due to the infection of the entire respiratory epithelia and the secondary infection with bacteria.

Viremia develops, but specific antibodies are not developed before the onset of rash. Cellular immunity plays a major role in host defense against measles.

Clinical Features

- **Incubation period:** It is 8 to 10 days.
- **Symptoms:** It is characterized by the onset of fever, malaise, cough, conjunctivitis, photophobia, lacrimation, and eruptive lesions of the skin and oral mucosa.
- **Skin:** It usually begins on the face, in the hair line and behind the ears, and spreads to the neck, chest, back and the extremities. These appear as tiny red macules or papules which enlarge and coalesce to form blotchy, discolored, irregular lesions which blanch upon pressure and gradually fade away in four to five days with a fine desquamation.

Oral Manifestations

Oral lesions are prodromal, frequently occurring two to three days before the cutaneous rash, and are pathognomonic of this disease.

- **Site:** The most common site is on buccal mucosa.
- **Koplik's spot:** Intraoral lesions are called Koplik's spots and occur in 97% of cases. Immune reaction to the virus in the endothelial cells of dermal capillaries plays a role in the development of spots. The spots disappear after the onset of rash.
- **Appearance:** They are small, irregularly shaped flecks which appear as bluish white specks surrounded by bright red margins. These macular lesions increase in number rapidly and coalesce to form small patches. Palatal and pharyngeal petechiae as well as generalized inflammation, congestion, swelling and focal ulceration of the gingival, palate and throat may also occur.

Complications

Measles is a disease which lowers the general body resistance and for this reason often leads to complications.

- Bronchial pneumonia
- Encephalitis
- Otitis media
- Noma

In addition, measles has an immunosuppressive effect through impairment of cell-mediated immunity, so delay in wound healing. It may also cause induction of remission of leukemia and Hodgkin's disease. The disease is rarely fatal except in the case of secondary complications.

Differential Diagnosis

- **Smallpox:** High fever, monoform exanthema.

* **Chickenpox:** Typical exanthema that follows the intraoral lesion. The diagnosis can be established microscopically (blister swab) and virologically.

Control Measures

Measles vaccines are available as single or in combination (MMR).

In Asian countries 'typically' in India, the Edmonton Zagrd (EZ strain) 5 ml of vaccine is given subcutaneously. Studies have suggested the age for vaccination as nine months. A second dose should be given in the form of MMR at 15–18 months for adequate immunity.

Management

* The patient should be isolated, if possible.
* Antiviral drug
* Vitamin A should be given.

Varicella Zoster Virus Infections

Varicella zoster virus (VZV) is responsible for 2 major clinical infections:
1. Chickenpox (Varicella) and
2. Herpes zoster (Shingles / Zona)

Primary infection: 'Chickenpox' is a generalized primary infection that occurs the first time an individual contacts the virus and is accompanied with fever and malaise. It generally occurs in first two decades of life. Lesions begin on trunk and spread centrifugally. It is characterized by intensely pruritic maculopapular rash followed by vesicles which are described as '*Dew Drops on Rose Petals*'. The vesicles turn into scab and crust in 7–10 days.

After the primary disease is healed, VZV becomes latent in the dorsal root ganglia of cranial nerves. There is involvement of C3, T5, L1, L2. The varicella zoster virus may get reactivated due to: Stress, trauma, malignancy, radiotherapy, chemotherapy, immunosuppressive therapy or underlying malignancy.

Herpes zoster virus infection: Herpes zoster is an acute infectious viral disease of extremely painful and incapacitating nature. It is characterized by inflammation of the dorsal root ganglion. It is associated with vesicular eruptions of skin and mucous membrane of the area supplied by the affected sensory nerve. Transmission is through respiratory route.

Clinical Features

It affects adults and there is no sex predilection. Prodromal period of 2 to 4 days in which shooting pain, paraesthesia, burning and tenderness appear along the course of affected nerve. The reason for shooting pain is occurrence of active ganglionitis with resultant neuronal necrosis and severe neuralgia. The pain is present in the area supplied by the affected nerve (dermatome). There may be altered sensation of hypoesthesia or hyperesthesia. Nerves commonly affected are C3, T5, L1, L2 and first division of trigeminal nerve. It may affect motor nerves also. Zoster ophthalmicus results when ophthalmic branch of trigeminal nerve is involved and can lead to acute retinal necrosis.

Unilateral vesicles on an erythematous base appear in clusters, chiefly along the course of nerve and giving picture of a single dermatome involvement. This is called '*zosteriform*' pattern. Thoracic and lumbar dermatome are most commonly involved followed by craniofacial area. Lesions do not cross midline and heal by crustation. *Zoster sine eruptione or zoster sine herpete* is the zoster infection without the appearance of dermatological lesion, making diagnosis difficult. Cutaneous zoster infection of the side of tip of nose is termed *Hutchinson sign*:

*Syndrome associated: **Ramsay Hunt syndrome*** [triad of ipsilateral facial paralysis, ear pain and vesicles on face and ear, loss of taste sensation is typical presentation]. There is involvement of geniculate ganglion of facial nerve.

Oral Manifestations

Varicella zoster virus causing herpes zoster involving 2nd and 3rd divisions of trigeminal nerve leads to oral manifestation. Involvement of 2nd division leads to lesion of midface and upper lip and involvement of 3rd division leads to lesion of lower face and lower lip. It may be found on buccal mucosa, tongue, uvula, pharynx and larynx. Presence of pain, burning, tenderness usually on the palate on one side. After a few days of pain, intact vesicles appear (*drops of dew on rose petals*) which soon rupture leaving tissue tags (*moon crater appearance*) to leave areas of erosion.

HZ has been associated with dental anomalies and severe scarring of the facial skin when trigeminal HZ occurs during tooth formation. Pulpal necrosis and internal root resorption have also been related to HZ. Necrosis of the underlying bone and exfoliation of teeth may be seen in immunocompromised patients. In immunocompromised patients the disease is more severe and last for about three weeks.

Complication

1. **Post-herpetic neuralgia:** Pain of herpes zoster may continue for weeks to months, even after the lesions have healed. The pain that lingers on for more than 120 days even after lesions have healed is called post-herpetic neuralgia. It usually occurs in elderly persons due to inflammation, fibrosis and scarring of the nerve and may cause severe pain which is sharp, stabbing, burning or gnawing in nature.
2. **Tooth extirpation** associated with osteonecrosis.
3. **Involvement** of ophthalamic division leads to corneal scarring and sometimes blindness.
4. **Immunocompromised patient** may experience atypical involvement of multiple dermatome, retinitis, encephalitis and even sometimes bilateral lesions.

Diagnosis and Investigations

1. **Clinical diagnosis:** *Unilateral* lesions along the distribution of the nerve will give clue to the diagnosis.
2. **Cytology:** A simple smear stained with a standard laboratory stain would reveal the presence of multinucleated epithelial cells, it is a rapid method of evaluation.
3. **Fluorescent antibody** stained smears using fluorescein monoclonal antibodies: More reliable than routine cytology.
4. **Viral isolation in tissue culture:** More expensive and results take days rather than hours. It is *the best way to confirm the diagnosis.*
5. **PCR:** Used to detect viral antigen. *Expensive and highly sensitive.*

Treatment

- **Antiviral drugs:** Systemic acyclovir 800 mg 5 times daily / famciclovir (500 mg 3 times daily) for 7 days and topical acyclovir application 5 times daily. Antiviral drugs should be started within 72 hours of onset of infection.
- **Symptomatic treatment:** Antipyretics along with antipruritics (diphenhydramine), aspirin especially in children with viral infection may be associated with development of Reye syndrome causing liver damage.
- To prevent post-herpetic neuralgia prednisone 40 to 60 mg daily for 1 to 2 weeks may be given.
- Gabapentin, topical anesthetics, topical capsaicin 0.025% 4 times a day for treatment of post-herpetic neuralgia.
- Steroid injection can be given in a patient with age more than 60 years, for the treatment of post herpetic neuralgia.
- Antidepressants like amitriptyline, other tricyclic antidepressant and opioid analgesics have been used to minimize painful sequelae of this infection for post-herpetic neuralgia.
- Sympathetic nerve block and chemical and surgical neurolysis for post-herpetic neuralgia.

× Botulinium toxin also been suggested for post-herpetic neuralgia.

Differential Diagnosis

1. **Herpes simplex infection:** Patient will have history of generalized prodromal symptoms (fever, headache, malaise, nausea, vomiting) that precede the lesions by 1 or 2 days. Lesions may not be unilateral (Fig. 5.6)
2. **Herpangina:** Acute infection, posterior part of oral cavity is affected and occur in seasonal epidemics.
3. **Hand-foot-and-mouth disease:** Oral lesions accompanied with maculopapular and vesicular lesions on hand and foot.
4. **Erythema multiforme:** Local lesions and systemic symptoms appear together.
5. **Pemphigus and pemphigoid:** Chronic lesions and do not present unilaterally.

ERYTHEMA MULTIFORME

It is an acute inflammatory mucocutaneous disease that can occur in both the genders at any age. It causes a variety of lesions, hence the name *multiforme*. Initiated either by deposition of immune complexes in the superficial microvasculature of skin and mucosa or cell-mediated immunity.

Etiology and Predisposing Factors

It is immunologically mediated disease in which there is deposition of immune complexes in the blood vessels of skin and oral mucosa. It is hypersensitivity reaction to infectious agents or medications.

× **Infections** (mainly HSV and sometimes tuberculosis, histoplasmosis mycoplasma pneumoniae).

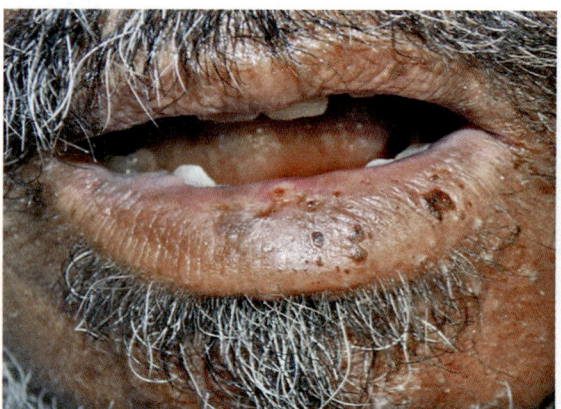
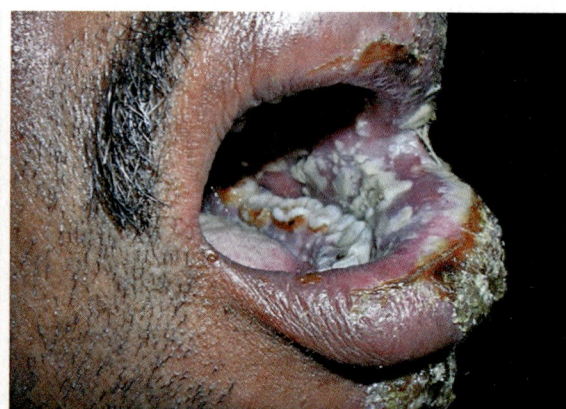
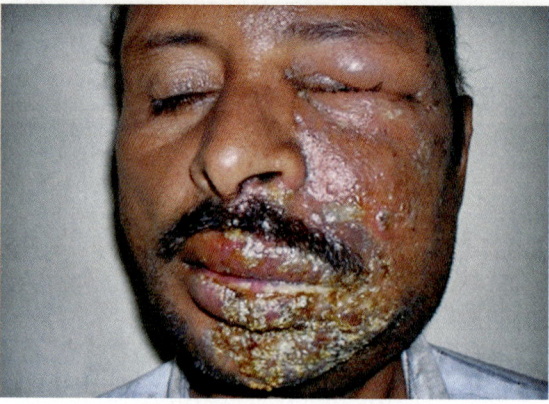

Fig. 5.6: Herpes zoster

× **Drugs** (Barbiturates and sulfonamides, phenytoin, carbamazepine, penicillin, anticonvulsants oxicam NSAIDs and allopurinols).

× **Other factors:** Malignancy, vaccination, autoimmune disease, radiotherapy and ultraviolet light.

Immunologic attack by CD8+ cytotoxic effector cells on the 'HSV' expressing keratinocytes. The CD8+ cells induce apoptosis of these keratinocytes causing necrosis in lesions. There may be history of recurrent episodes (in the spring and autumn). Recurrent erythema multiforme (EM) is preceeded with recurrent HSV infection.

Clinical Features

Mostly occurs in young adults (30–40 years) and affects both sexes equally. There may be prodromal symptoms if associated with HSV. There may be a prodrome of fever, malaise, headache, sore throat, rhinorrhea, and cough. These symptoms suggest a viral (especially respiratory tract) infection.

It is characterized by sudden, acute, explosive onset. Skin lesions appear rapidly over a few days and begin as red macules that become papular, starting primarily in the hands moving centripetally towards the trunk area. There are erythematous discrete macules/papules or occasional vesicles and bullae in the skin and oral cavity. It appears as concentric zones with a central blister surrounded by a ring of pale edematous area and another concentric ring of erythematous halo. This lesion appears *as target, iris or bull's eye.*

PART OF ORAL MANIFESTATIONS

Oral Manifestations

The oral lesions are large ulcers, which are irregular in shape and deep and thus they often bleed. There may be blood tinged saliva. The oral lesions heal without scar formation. It is not characterized by *lymphadenopathy.* **The oral lesions start as bullae on an erythematous base, but intact bullae are rarely seen by the clinician because they break rapidly into irregular ulcers.** There is characteristic *hemorrhagic crusting* of the vermillion borders *of the lips* it is most common in the lips and gingival involvement is rare. In fully blown clinical cases, lips are extensively eroded and large portions of the oral mucosa are denuded of epithelium.

There is difficulty in eating, swallowing and drooling of blood tinged saliva, within 2 or 3 days lateral lesions begin to crust, healing occurs in 2 weeks.

Types

EM is classified as

× **EM minor** if there is less than 10% skin involvement and there is minimal to no mucous membrane involvement, whereas

× **EM major** has more extensive but still characteristic skin involvement with mucous membrane affected.

× Historically, the fulminant forms of erythema multiforme were labelled as *Steven Johnson Symdrome and Toxic Epidermal Necrolysis* (TEN/Lyell's disease).

SJS is a less severe variant of TENs and separate clinically and etiopathogenetically from EM. Although all three are hypersensitivity reactions and give rise to oral bullae, erosions, ulcers and crusted lips , the skin lesions of SJS and TENs are different from EM. They are more severe and tend to arise on the chest rather than the extremities on erythematous and purpuric macules; these lesions are called "atypical targets".

Clinical Features

EM is characterized by

× Sudden acute explosive onset.
× Large, irregular deep ulcers with bleeding.
× Characteristic iris/bull's eye lesion.
× Involvement of vermillion border of lip with crustation.
× There may be history of preceding HSV infection

Histopathlogically, most of the lesion is localized in the epidermis presumably this being the site where the drug or its metabolites are bound, with less inflammation in the dermis. The primary cytokine involved is tumor necrosis factor-alpha. There is lymphocytic infiltration in epidermal dermal junction, necrosis of basal keratinocytes and degeneration of basal cell layer.

Differential Diagnosis

The differential diagnosis includes:
* Herpes simplex (Refer to Table 5.5 in HSV)
* Pemphigus vulgaris.
* Benign mucous membrane pemphigoid.
* Bullous lichen planus.
* Recurrent aphthous ulcers

Treatment

* **Mild:** Topical anesthetic mouthwashes, topical steroids and soft/liquid diet.
* **Moderate to severe:** 30–50 mg/day of prednisolone for several days which is then tapered.
* **Recurrent cases:** Dapsone, azathioprine, levamisole or thalidomide.

Pemphigus	EM
Large, irregular ulcers, but no bleeding present	Large, irregular deep and bleeding
No prodromal symptoms	Fever may sometimes accompany (no prodromal symptoms) Sudden acute explosive onset
Age: Older	Age: Younger <50 years
Etiology: Auto-immune	Hypersensitivity reaction (drug/HSV)
No bloody lip crustation	Lips are extensively eroded and large portions of the oral mucosa are denuded of epithelium. Lips show bloody crustation
Chronic	Acute
No target/ bull's eye lesion	Target/ bull's eye lesion
Rx: Steroids to be given for long duration	Rx: Steroids for short duration

TABLE 5.5: Differential features of HSV and EM

HSV	EM
SSSR	LIDB
Prodromal symptoms (Period: 2 to 8 days) Fever before	Fever may sometimes accompany (no prodromal symptoms) Sudden acute explosive onset
Age: Older	Age: Younger <50 years
Etiology: Viral	Hypersensitivity reaction
Marginal gingivitis	No gingival involvement Lips prominently involved
Cervical lymphadenopathy: +nt	–nt
No target/bull's eye lesion	Target/bull's eye lesion
Rx: Antivirals Steroids are contraindicated	Rx: Steroids

TABLE 5.6: Differential features of pemphigoid and EM

Pemphigoid	EM
Large irregular ulcers, but no bleeding present	LIDB
Prodromal symptoms absent Chronically present	Fever may sometimes accompany (no prodromal symptoms) Sudden acute explosive onset
Age: Older	Age: Younger <50 years
Etiology: Autoimmune	Hypersensitivity reaction
Desquamative gingivitis present	No gingival involvement Lips prominently involved
No target/ bull's eye lesion	Target/bull's eye lesion
Rx: Steroids are for long term	Rx: Steroids are for short duration

TABLE 5.7: Differential features of RAS and EM

RAS	EM
× SSSR (smooth, round, shallow, symmetrical)	× LIDB (large, irregular, deep and bleeding)
× Acute but recurrent	× Sudden acute explosive onset
× Age: Older	× Age: Younger <50 years
× Etiology: Autoimmune, hematological, etc.	× Hypersensitivity reaction to a drug or HSV
× No lip crustations present	× Lips prominently involved
× No target/ bull's eye lesion	× Target/bull's eye lesion
× Rx: Steroids are for short term	× Rx: Steroids are for short duration

Antiviral drugs (acyclovir) in HSV associated EM patients.

× Hydroxychloroquine, mycophenolate-mofetil, azathioprine, colchicines, methotrexate, and intravenous immunoglobulin are the other drugs which can be given.

ALLERGIC STOMATITIS

Also known as allergic contact stomatitis, or allergic contact gingivostomatitis. It is basically a type IV delayed hypersensitivity reaction that occurs in susceptible atopic individuals when allergens penetrate skin or mucosa or it is described as an inflammatory reaction of the oral mucosa by contact with irritants or allergens.

Pathogenesis

× Allergens which may be different for different individuals combine with

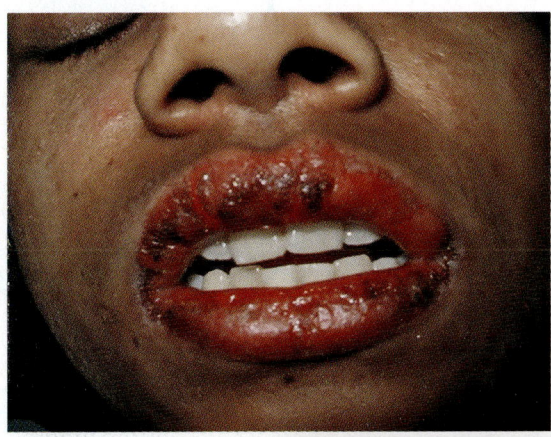
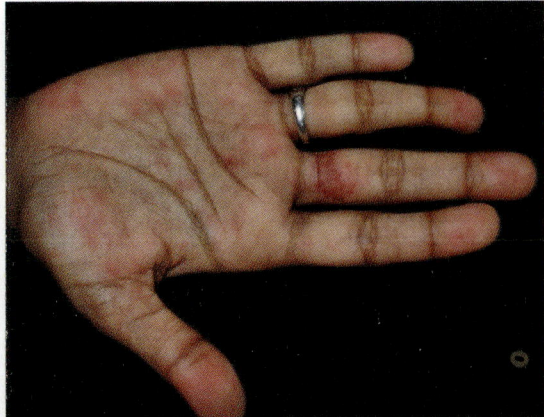
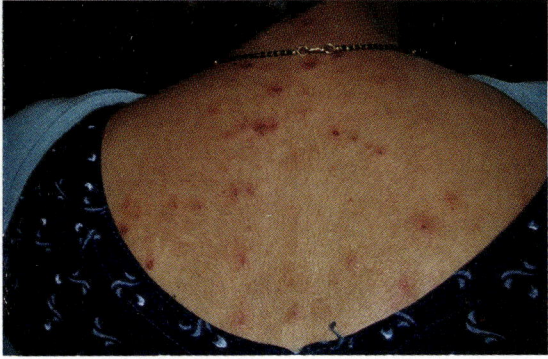

Fig. 5.7: Healed iris lesions

epithelial derived proteins forming haptens which bind with Langerhans cells in the mucosa, which in turn present the antigen on their surface to T lymphocytes, sensitizing them to that antigen and causing to produce many specific clones. The second time that specific antigen is encountered an inflammatory reaction is triggered at that site of exposure.

- Most common allergens that may cause allergic stomatitis in some individuals include:
  - Cinnamaldehyde, balsam of Peru, peppermint, mercury, gold, pyrophosphates, zinc citrate, free acrylic monomer, and nickel, fluoride and sodium lauryl sulfate.
- These allergens may originate from many sources, including various foods and drinks, chewing gums, toothpaste, mouthwash, dental floss, dental fillings, dentures, orthodontic bands or wires and many other sources.

Allergic oral reactions to systemic drugs are termed stomatitis medicamentosa and those to topical agents like toothpaste, acrylic resin, strongly flavoured foods, cosmetics and topical medications and chemicals are termed stomatitis venenata.

Clinical Features

Clinically it may be characterized by:
- Erythematous plaques
- Vesiculation
- Ulceration and/or hyperkeratosis
- Pain, burning sensation or itchiness

Oral hypersensitivity reaction may be of various forms:
1. Acute ulcer in erythema multiforme
2. Lichenoid drug reaction, a variant of allergic contact stomatitis, brought about by direct contact with the oral mucosa of certain metals in dental restorations.
3. Fixed drug eruptions
4. Plasma cell gingivitis and stomatitis
5. Angioedema of lips
6. Oral allergy syndrome without swelling.

- The features of allergic contact stomatitis are neither clinically nor histopathologically specific, so the diagnosis is usually presumptive and can only be confirmed by resolution of the inflammation after withdrawal or removal of suspected causative allergen.
- When allergic contact stomatitis is suspected but an allergen cannot be identified, *patch testing* is necessary.

Differential Diagnosis

Plasma cell gingivitis resembles desquamative gingivitis in pemphigoid and lichen planus and chronic granulomatous gingivitis.

Allergic contact stomatitis resembles chronic atrophic candidiasis

Treatment

- In persistent cases, topical corticosteroids are treatment of choice.
- For severe cases and extensive lesions, systemic corticosteroid and systemic antihistamines may be indicated.

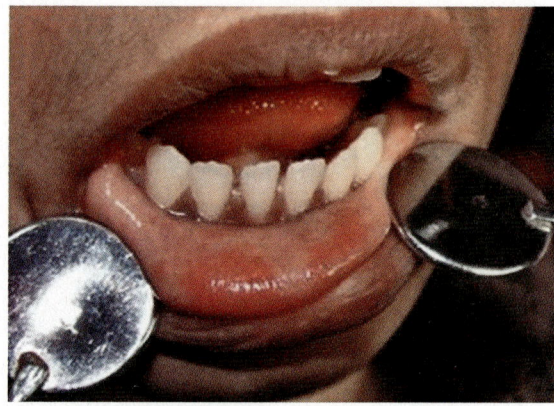

Fig. 5.8: Healed lesions of EM

ACUTE NECROTIZING ULCERATIVE GINGIVITIS

- Vincent's infection, trench mouth, acute ulceromembranous gingivitis, phagedenic gingivitis, fusospirochetal gingivitis.
- It is an acute, ulcerative lesion of gingiva and periodontal tissues. It was also called trench mouth since it was very frequent

among soldiers living in trenches during World War I.

Etiology and Pathogensis

Plaut and Vincent were the first who reported that ANUG is caused by specific bacteria like fusiform bacilli and spirochetes. Other microbes include Treponema species, *Prevotella intermedia, Fusobacteria nucleatum, Peptostreptococcus micros* and *Porphyromonas gingivalis Selenomonas* species, and *Campylobacter*. The tissue destruction is most probably result of production of endotoxins or immunological activation and subsequent destruction of gingiva and adjacent tissue.

It has strong association with immune suppression (AIDS), debilitation, smoking, stress, poor oral hygiene and diabetes.

Clinical Findings

ANUG may not be associated with fever and malaise, although lymphadenopathy may be present.

Oral Manifestations

It has rapid and acute onset. The gingiva is tender, erythematous and there is presence of pseudomembrane. The patient may experience excessive salivation, metallic taste, malodor, gingival bleeding. It rapidly develops into extremely painful and erythematous gingiva with scattered punched out crater like ulcerations, usually on the interdental papilla. Linear gingival erythema.

When ANUG progresses to involve mucogingival junction, it is called necrotising ulcerative periodontitis it may be characterized by sloughing of oral mucosa followed by sequestration of exposed necrotic bone. Necrotising ulcerative stomatitis may also accompany the lesions on gingiva.

Complications

If there is underlying systemic illness, NUG and NUP can spread rapidly from the gingiva to the periodontium and into the soft tissues, giving rise to cancrum oris, noma, or orofacial gangrene. The overlying skin becomes discolored, and perforation of the skin ensues. The orofacial lesions are cone shaped, with the base of the cone within the oral cavity and the tip at the skin aspect.

Fusobacterium necrophorum is likely to play an important role in the progression of NUP to cancrum oris because this organism produces toxins, leading to extensive tissue destruction. Noma is generally accompanied by fluctuating fever, marked anemia, high white cell count, general debilitation, and a recent history of some other systemic illness, such as measles.

Lab Findings

Secretions from the gingival sulcus grow mixed flora but in particular will be culture positive for *Treponema* species, *Prevotella intermedia, Fusobacterium nucleatum*, it may be appropriate to test the patient for HIV or other immunosuppressive conditions, such as blood dyscrasia.

Differential Diagnosis

- **Primary herpetic gingivitis:** It is a viral infection caused by herpes simplex virus.
- **Desquamated gingivitides** (cicatricial pemphigoid, pemhigus vulgaris, lichen planus) no acute course, no bad breath, whitish changes and skin symptoms.
- **Neutropenic ulcers** in patients on cancer chemotherapy may appear similar, leading to extensive ulceration and necrosis of the marginal gingiva and other mucosal surfaces.
- **Chronic periodontitis**

Management

- **First visit:** Instruct the patient to rinse with 3% of hydrogen peroxide H_2O_2 with equal volume of warm water every 2 hrs.
- **Antibiotics:** Amoxycillin 500 mg 6 hrly for 10 days if allergic, erythromycin 400 mg 6 hrly for 10 days and metronidazole 400 mg BD for 7 days.

- Ultra super soft toothbrush with bland dentifrice twice daily.
- **NSAIDs:** Ibuprofen SOS as required for pain relief.
- No scaling and root planing is to be done on 1st visit. Patient is called after 2 days.
- **2nd visit:** Once the acutely painful episodes have resolved, scaling and root planing to completely remove all residual plaque and calculus are indicated. Supragingival scaling is done
- Re-evaluation of patient.
- Patient is called after 5 days.
- **3rd visit:** Plaque control measures—3% H_2O_2 stopped.
- 0.12% chlorhexidine twice a day for 2–3 weeks.
- Scaling and root planing is repeated if required.
- Copious amount of fluid consumption
- Gingivoplasty and periodontal surgery may be necessary to correct gingival and periodontal defects.

B. Recurrent Oral Ulcers

The following present with recurrent ulcer:
1. Recurrent aphthous stomatitis
2. Behçet syndrome
3. Recurrent HSV infection
4. Recurrent oral EM

RECURRENT APHTHOUS STOMATITIS/ CANKER SORES

The term aphthous was given by Hippocrates and was first described by von Mikulicz and Kümmell in 1888. Recurrent aphthous stomatitis (RAS) is a common disorder characterized by recurring ulcers confined to the oral mucosa in patients with no other systemic disorder. It affects 20% of the general population.

Classification:

Lehner has classified it as follows:

Etiology: The major factors include:
1. *Genetic factors:* Genetic factor is considered as the main cause. Patients with RAS have HLA B$_{12}$, DR2, DR7, CW7 and B5.

2. *Immunological abnormalities:* Humoral and cell-mediated immunity. Research has suggested a relationship between RAS and lymphotoxicity, antibody-dependent cell-mediated cytotoxicity defects in lymphocyte cell subpopulation, and alteration in CD4 to CD8 lymphocyte ratio. There is exaggerated cell-mediated immune response resulting in ulceration of mucosa.
3. Hematological deficiency of iron, folate, vit. B$_1$, B$_{12}$
4. *Bacterial cause:* Allergy to *Helicobacter pylori*

Predisposing factors: Stress, anxiety, local trauma, food allergies and menstrual cycle, upper respiratory infections, food allergy. Aphthous like ulcer may be seen in celiac disease.

Clinical Features

They have been classified according to the clinical manifestations.

1. **Recurrent aphthous minor:** Also called Mikulicz ulcer. Most common disease and referred as canker sores. <1 cm, lasting 7–14 days, no scarring
2. **RA major:** Most severe form. Also called Sutton's disease, periadenitis mucosa necrotica recurrens, more than 1 cm, lasting for weeks, often with scarring.
3. **Recurrent herpetiform ulcerations:** Has clusters of ulcerations resembling herpetic lesions. <1 cm, >10 ulcers present continuously

Most common in 2nd decade of life. It is characterized by burning sensation, erythema, generalized edema of oral cavity, with no evidence of lymphadenopathy.

Oral Manifestations

The lesion begins at the oral mucosa with prodromal burning or a sensation of a papule in mucosa 1 to 2 hours before the ulcer develops. During initial period there's localized erythemataus, within hours, a small white papule forms, ulcerates and gradually enlarges over the next 48–72 hours.

TABLE 5.8: Types of RAS

Characteristics	Major	Minor	Herpetiform
Sex incidence	Females more than males	Females more than males	Females more than males
Age of onset	After puberty	Childhood or adolescence	Adulthood
Areas involved	Mostly labial mucosa, soft palate, lips, tongue, faces	Buccal and labial mucosa, tongue, soft palate, pharynx (mucosa not bound to periosteum)	Non-keratinized movable mucosa
Number of ulcers per episode	1–10	1–5	Many, may even be 100 (may coalesce to form large irregular ulcers)
Size of each ulcer	1–3 cm (large)	3–10 mm (small)	1–3 mm (tiny)
Ulcer duration	2–6 weeks	7–14 days	7–10 days
Rate of recurrence	May be in waves lasting 20 years or more	Episodes per month to one year	Remissions short
Ulcer healing	Scar formation	No scarring	No scarring
Pain	Present	May be severe	May be severe
Prodormal symptoms	Localised itching, burning sensation	Burning, itching, stinging	----------

The lesions are round, symmetrical, shallow, without tissue tags and develop mostly on non-keratinized mucosa like labial and buccal mucosa and tongue. In most severe cases, the ulcers become confluent, and are extremely painful, interfering with speech and eating. Patients experience multiple ulcer over several episodes in a year.

RA major: Develop ulcers that are deep and larger than 1 cm in diameter. Lesions last for weeks to months.

Lab Findings

Lab tests should be done when RAS becomes severe or occurs at the age past 40 years.

With other signs and symptoms
1. Investigations for systemic diseases.
2. Hematological tests for reduced levels of vit. B_{12}, Se. iron, folate, ferritin
3. Biopsy only to differentiate from diseases like Crohn's, sarcoidosis, etc.
4. CD4 counts in immunodeficients

Differential Diagnosis

1. Viral stomatitis, herpetic stomatitis is associated with prodromal symptom of fever, malaise, lymphadenopathy and commonly affects the keratinized mucosa like gingiva and palate.
2. Erythema multiforme
3. Chronic multiple lesions, e.g. pemphigus, pemphigoid: Lesions remain in the same site from week to months in contrast to RAS in which lesions heal and reoccur at a different site.
4. Lupus erythematosus
5. Traumatic ulcers
6. Herpangina
7. Erosive lichen planus

Management

1. Protective emollient such as orabase to promote healing
2. Topical anaesthetics such as benzocaine or lidocaine (for minor lesions) to provide pain relief.

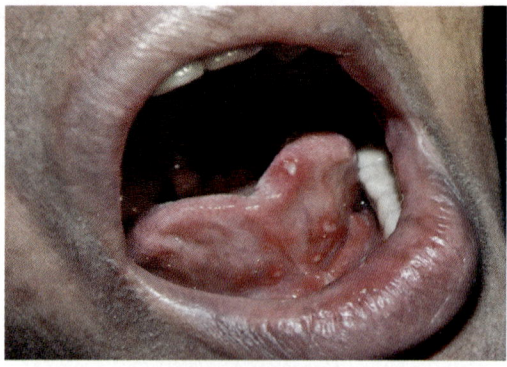

Fig. 5.9: RAS

3. High potency topical steroids such as clobetasol, betamethasone, fluocinonide placed directly over the lesion (shortens the healing time and reduces the size of the ulcer).
4. Amlexanox paste, topical doxycycline, tetracycline can be used with a guaze over a lesion in larger-sized ulcers.
5. Thalidomide, though 1st being the drug of choice, has to be given very cautiously due to its prominent side effects such as phocomelia, teratogenicity, gastrointestinal complaints, DVT.
6. Levamisole has also been found useful to manage the disease.
7. Pentoxyfylline has also been tried in management of aphthous stomatitis.

BEHÇET'S DISEASE (BEHÇET'S SYNDROME)

Behçet's disease (BD) is a multisystem disorder with many possible manifestations. It was first described by Turkish dermatologist Hulusi Behçet. It is also known as Silk route disease and is known to involve areas around Mediterranean sea.

Behçet's disease (BD) presents with triad of symptoms including recurring oral ulcers, recurring genital ulcers, and eye involvement. BD is more severe in younger patients and patients with eye and GI involvement.

Etiology and Pathogenesis

BD is a systemic vasculitis characterized by hyperactivity of neutrophils with enhanced chemotaxis and elevated pro-inflammatory cytokines IL-8 and IL-17, with TNF-α playing a major role in the pathogenesis. The HLA-B51 genotype is most frequently linked to BD, especially in patients with severe forms of the disease in Asia.

Clinical Manifestations

The highest incidence of BD is in young adults around 25 to 40 years of age.

Oral involvement followed by genital lesions and eye involvement (uveitis, retinal vasculitis, vascular occlusion, optic atrophy, and conjunctivitis) mainly comprises the BD. Blindness is a common complication of the disease. Skin lesions resembling erythema nodosum or large pustular lesions occur in patients with BD. It is common for patients with BD to have a cutaneous hyperreactivity to intracutaneous injection or a needlestick **(pathergy).**

BD causes red and swollen joints as in rheumatoid arthritis, but with involvement of small joints.

- In some patients, central nervous system involvements causing brainstem syndrome, involvement of the cranial nerves and neurologic degeneration.
- Other reported signs of BD include thrombophlebitis, intestinal ulceration, venous thrombosis, and renal, cardiac, and pulmonary disease.
- Both pulmonary involvement and cardiac involvement are believed to be secondary to vasculitis.
- BD in children, which most frequently presents between the ages of 9 and 10 years, has similar manifestations to the adult form of the disease, but oral ulcers are a more common presenting sign in children, whereas uveitis is less common.
- It is characterized by mouth and genital ulcers with inflamed cartilage and is associated with relapsing polychondritis (MAGIC syndrome).

Oral Findings

The most common site of involvement of BD is the oral mucosa with recurrent oral aphthous ulcers. Some patients may have large, scarring lesions of major RAS. Lesions may appear anywhere on the oral or pharyngeal mucosa.

Differential Diagnosis

The following diagnostic criteria based on a point system where 4 or more points is strongly associated with BD: Oral, ocular, and genital lesions score 2 points each, while skin lesions, and neurologic and vascular manifestations score 1 point each. Positive pathergy test is an optional test but also scores 1 if positive.

BD is a clinical diagnosis based upon the criteria described above. Laboratory tests are used to rule out other diseases, such as connective tissue (e.g. lupus erythematosus) and hematologic diseases causing severe neutropenia.

Management

Prednisolone, azathioprine and other immunosuppressive drugs have been shown to reduce ocular disease as well as oral and genital involvement.

Pentoxifylline, which has fewer side effects than immunosuppressive drugs or systemic steroids, has also been reported to be effective. Dapsone, colchicine, and thalidomide have also been used effectively to treat mucosal lesions of BD.

Therapy with monoclonal antibodies such as infliximab and etanercept are playing an increasing role in therapy of BD particularly in patients who do not respond to anti-inflammatory and immunosuppressive drugs.

CHRONIC ULCERATIVE LESIONS

These lesions are present in the patients from weeks to months and are usually misdiagnosed as recurrent ulcerative lesions. Careful history will reveal that the patient has new lesions which heal and recur at a different site. However, the chronic lesions are present at the same site from weeks to months. The following lesions are included in the list of chronic ulcerative lesions.

1. Pemphigus vulgaris
2. Bullous and cicatricial pemphigoid
3. Erosive oral lichen planus
4. Herpes simplex infection in immuno-compromised patients.

Pemphigus

It is an autoimmune disease. Derived from Greek word 'pemphix' means bubble or blister.

Etiology

Autoimmune: Unknown triggering mechanism predispose genes to form auto-antibodies.

It occurs more commonly in Ashkenazi Jews in whom a strong genetic association is present with HLA-DR4 and DQ8 haplotypes. In pemphigus there are antibodies against desmoglein 1 and 3 which are adhesion molecules in the epithelium of skin and oral mucosa respectively resulting in acantholysis and intraepithelial bulla formation. PV has been reported coexisting with other autoimmune diseases, particularly myasthenia gravis and thymoma, lymphoma.

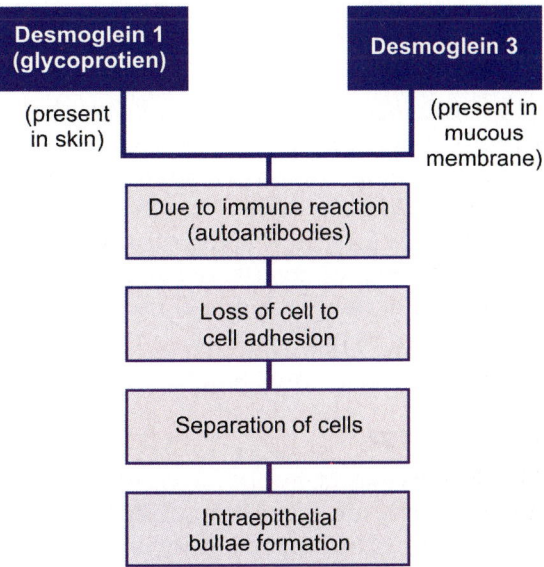

Fig. 5.10: Pathogenesis of pemphigus vulgaris

Drugs like penicillin, phenylbutazone, d-penicillamine and captopril are associated with drug-induced pemphigus.

Pemphigus foliaceous and erythematous affect desmoglein 1, hence there are no oral lesions in these forms.

Pemphigus foliaceous has blisters in superficial granular cell layer, whereas in pemphigus vulgaris it is present deep but above basal cell layer.

Clinical Features

Age: 50 to 60 years

Gender predilection: Male = Female
The subsets of pemphigus include:
- Pemphigus vulgaris
- Pemphigus vegetans (variant of pemphigus vulgaris)
- Pemphigus foliaceous
- Pemphigus erythematosus (variant of foliaceous)
- Paraneoplastic pemphigus
- Drug-related pemphigus

Sites: Oral mucosa and other mucosa involved are those of conjunctiva, cervix, urethra, penis, anus, pharyngeal, laryngeal and esophageal mucosa.

Pemphigus vulgaris has a classical thin-walled bulla which rapidly breaks to form ulcers and continue to extend which eventually leave denuded areas of skin. The bullae soon rupture to form large irregular asymmetric ulcers. Most of the lesions develop very slowly taking weeks to months.: 'Nikolsky sign' is the characteristic sign of disease in which application of lateral pressure on unaffected area results in formation of new lesion and it occurs due to pulling of upper layers of skin from basal layer.

Oral Findings

Oral lesions may be the first sign of the disease and may precede skin lesions. Initially, there is formation of bullae on non-inflammed base which breaks rapidly and there is formation of shallow irregular ulcers.

Thin epithelium layer peels away in irregular pattern and leaves denuded base which continue to extend covering large area. The lesion usually starts on buccal mucosa, gingiva and palate. The average time from the disease onset to diagnosis may often take over five months, and coexisting candidiasis may mask the typical clinical picture of the pemphigus lesions.

Differential Diagnosis

Recurrent aphthous stomatitis: Lesion is severe but heal and recur, but in pemphigus lesion continues to extend, is not round and symmetrical like RAS but is shallow and irregular.

Erythema multiforme: It has an acute sudden explosive onset in contrast to pemphigus which is chronic in onset.
- Mucous membrane pemphigoid
- Erosive lichen planus

Lab Findings

Biopsy: Best on intact vesicles and bullae in <24 hours and is taken from advancing edge of lesion.

Positive Nikolsky's sign

Direct immunofluorescence: Presence of IgG in combination with C3, IgA, IgM in epithelium of lesion or clinically normal epithelium of lesion.

Indirect immunofluorescent (iif) antibody tests performed on a patient's serum are helpful in distinguishing PV from pemphigoid.

An enzyme-linked immunosorbent assay (ELISA) can distinguish anti-DSG1 antibodies from anti-DSG3 in serum samples. The ELISA test results combined with results from direct and IIF are the most accurate method to confirm a diagnosis of PV.

For the **Ashboe-Hansen sign**, lateral pressure on the edge of a blister may spread the blister into clinically unaffected skin.

Management

It varies according to the severity of disease and rate of progression of disease.

- High dose corticosteroids 1–2 mg/kg/day
- The most commonly used adjuvants are immunosuppressive drugs such as mycophenolate mofetil, azathioprine, cyclophosphamide, and cyclophosphamide pulse therapy.
- When disease is under control, adjunct therapy like immunosuppressants are given to decrease the steroid dose as it causes serious complications.
- But studies show that there is no benefit of adding immunosuppressants to it as it increases the risk of malignancy and blood dyscrasias.
- If patient is having only oral involvement, low dose of prednisolone (topical+systemic) is given for short period.
- Other therapies like parentral gold therapy and dapsone is beneficial.
- May be treated with IV immunoglobulins, extracorporeal photophoresis or plasma exchange.
- Rituximab is presently being used and evaluated as a first line treatment although some studies demonstrated a high rate of infection.

Pemphigus Vegetans

- Uncommon variant of pemphigus vulgaris
- Benign variant because patient has ability to heal denuded areas. It has 2 types:
  - Neumann type (flaccid bullae and erosions)
  - Hallopeau type (pustules)
  - Neumann type is more common, whereas Hallopeau type is less aggressive and has verrucous hyperkeratotic lesions
- Both heal by hyperplastic granulation tissue.

Oral Findings

Gingival lesions may be lace like ulcer with purulent surface on red base or have granular or cobblestone appearance.

Characteristic feature is 'cerebriform tongue' with pattern of sulci and gyri on dorsum of tongue.

Lab Findings

Biopsy: Suprabasilar acantholysis, hyperkeratosis, pseudoepitheliomatous hyperplasia.

Immunofluorescence: Same as pemphigus vulgaris.

Management

Same as pemphigus vulgaris. Pemphigus foliaceus (superficial pemphigus, fogo selvagem).

Paraneoplastic Pemphigus (PNPP)

PNPP is a severe blistering disease, that is, a multiorgan disease associated with an underlying neoplasm, most frequently non-Hodgkin lymphoma, chronic lymphocytic leukemia, or thymoma.

This condition is also referred to as paraneoplastic autoimmune multiorgan syndrome because of the involvement of other systems such as the lungs in particular, and the variable skin findings, namely pemphigus, pemphigoid, EM-like, graft-vs-host disease-like and lichen planus-like.

The damage to the epithelium in PNPP is due to antibodies to desmogleins, plakins and an α-macroglobulin-like-protein.

Pathogenesis

Autoimmune reaction + cell-mediated cytotoxicity with epithelium cells.

Clinical Findings

Age: 7 to 76 years mean age of 60 years

Gender predilection: Male = Female
- Severe blisters and erosions of mucous membrane and skin.
- Has rapid onset and has severe oral and conjunctival lesions.
- The lesions resemble lichen planus, erythema multiforme, inflammatory lesion of drug reaction.
- It may involve respiratory epithelium.

* Nasal ulcers may cause epistaxis.
* In severe cases, the lesions may mimic TEN and often also involve the respiratory epithelium. Unlike EM or TEN, the lesions of PNPP continue to progress over weeks to months.

Oral Manifestations

Common sites are lips, tongue, soft palate, labial, buccal and lingual mucosae.

Lesions are large inflammed, necrotic erosions and are very painful.

The eruptions assume wide variety of morphology like morbilliforme, urticarial, bullous or erythema multiforme like lesions.

Erosions and crustations on vermillion border of lips are typical and is similar to Stevens-Johnson keratinocyte necrosis and acantholyis.

PEMPHIGOID

Pemphigoid is an **autoimmune disease** caused by malfunction of the immune system and results in skin rashes and blistering. It is the most common subepithelial blistering disease and occurs in older adults above 60 years of age.

Etiology

It is an autoimmune disease. Autoantibodies are directed against basement membrane proteins leading to a subepithelial split and subsequent vesicle formation.

Types of pemphigoid:
1. **Cicatricial pemphigoid:** This subepithelial blistering results in ulceration which then undergo scarring.
2. **Bullous pemphigoid**

Cicatricial Pemphigoid

It is an autoimmune disease in which the autoantibodies are directed against one or more components of basement membrane. In this antibodies are directed against basement membrane proteins, causing a subepithelial split resulting in vesicle formation. Antibodies to lamina lucida portion of the basement membrane are present, but antibodies to lamina densa may be sometimes the primary site of involvement. Drugs such as clonidine, d-penicillamine, and l-dopa have been reported as triggers for mucous membrane pemphigoid.

Clinical Features

It is seen in age group of 50–60 years with female predilection. Sites involved are skin, oral, nasal, laryngeal and conjunctival mucosa. Oral mucosa followed by conjunctival mucosa are the most common sites of involvement. Conjunctival involvement leads to scarring and adhesions developing between bulbar and palpebral conjunctiva called symblepharon. **Ocular** lesion includes subconjunctival fibrosis in which the conjunctiva is inflamed and eroded and when it attempts to heal, **scarring occurs** which close the opening of lacrimal glands leading to absence of tears which cause the eyes to become dry and cornea produce keratin causing blindness.

Laryngeal involvement causes pain, hoarseness, difficulty in breathing and may lead to death due to asphyxiation.

Esophageal involvement may cause dysphagia, which can lead to debilitation and death.

Skin lesions and genital involvement are also present.

Oral Manifestations

Oral mucosa is involved in more than 80% of cases. Oral lesions begin as **vesicle/bullae** which rupture to form large superficial **ulcerated** area which are **painful** and persist for weeks or months and heals **without scaring.** Gingival lesions are also found.

Desquamative gingivitis is the most common manifestation and may be the only manifestation of the disease appearing bright red.

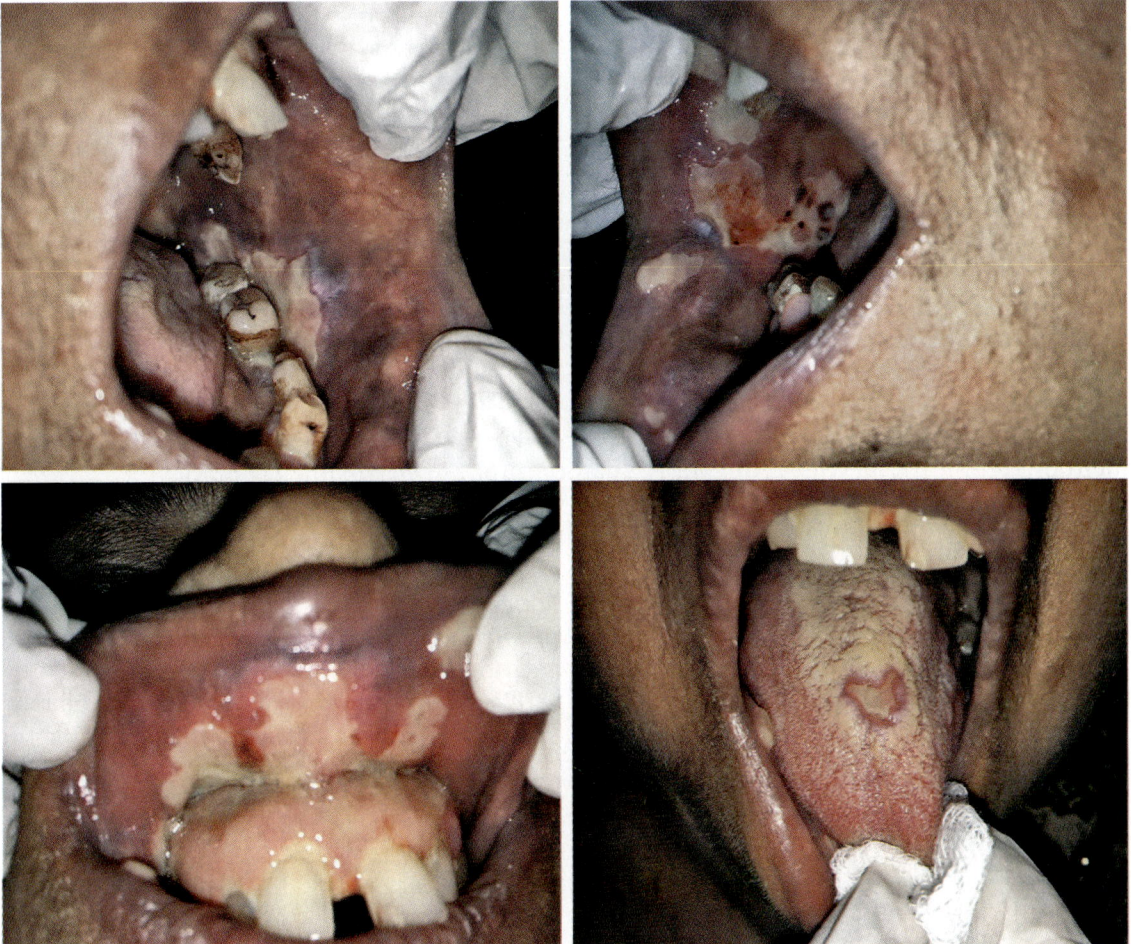

Fig. 5.11: Oral clinical presentation of pemphigus vulgaris

Diagnosis

- × **Biopsy** is taken for both routine and immunofluorescent study.
- × **Histopathology** shows sub-basilar cleavage.
- × **Direct immunofluorescent** technique is excellent for distinguishing cicatricial pemphigoid from pemphigus, it demonstrates positive fluorescence for immunoglobulin and complement in the basement membrane zone in 50–80% of patients. Only 10% patients demonstrate positive *indirect immunofluorescence* for circulating antibasement membrane zone antibodies.

- × Using the salt-split skin technique, immunoreactants usually localize to the roof of the split.

Treatment

Topical steroids, intralesional steroids
- × Depends on severity of symptoms, lesions confined to oral mucosa are treated by systemic corticosteroids.
- × Desquamative gingivitis can often be managed with topical steroids in a soft dental splint that covers the gingiva.
- × When topical or intralesional therapy is not successful, use of a tetracycline, such as doxycycline or minocycline is often helpful

in controlling desquamative gingivitis and other oral lesions.

- When there are severe oral lesions, conjunctival or laryngeal involvement dapsone therapy is recommended as the next choice. Before prescribing it, patient should be tested for G6PD deficiency as it is known to cause hemolysis.

Dapsone is also known to cause hypersensitivity syndrome, idiosyncratic disorder characterized by fever.

Immunosuppressive drugs such as cyclophosphamide, particularly when there is risk of blindness from conjunctival involvement or significant laryngeal or esophageal damage can be used.

Bullous Pemphigoid

It is the most common autoimmune subepithelial blistering condition.

Etiology

Autoantibodies are directed against components of basement membrane. Antigens are referred to as BP antigens, BP 180 and BP 230. The BP antigens are found in lamina lucida regions of basement membrane on the hemidesmosomes of basal epithelial cells. It is seen to be reported with diseases like multiple sclerosis and malignancy, drug therapy like diuretics. This damage to basement membrane results in subepithelial vesicle formation.

Clinical Features

It is seen in old age of about 60–80 years and no sex predilection is seen. The characteristic skin lesion of BP is a tense blister on an inflamed base which ruptures after several days resulting in crust formation which heals without scarring. These lesions are accompanied by pruritis and urticarial plaques involving the scalp, abdomen, extremities, axilla, and groin.

Oral Manifestations

Oral lesions are uncommon which begin as bullae and rupture to form large shallow ulcer. These lesions are less painful and do not involve the mucosa extensively, as in pemphigus. Gingival lesions consist of generalized edema, inflammation and desquamation with localized areas of discrete vesicle formation. Desquamative gingivitis has also been reported as the most common oral manifestation of BP, and the gingival lesions may be the only site of oral involvement. Recurrence is more common in BP than mucous membrane pemphigoid.

Diagnosis

- **Biopsy** is done in early stages when clinical differences are not apparent.
- **Histology** shows subepithelial bulla formation.
- **Indirect immunofluorescent** antibody testing demonstrate circulating IgG antibody against basement membrane antigen.
- **Direct immunofluorescent** is more reliable. The salt-split skin test is particularly useful in distinguishing BP from EBA that has IgG antibodies localized to the dermal side of the salt-split skin (floor of the blister).
- **ELISA:** Circulating autoantibodies against pemphigoid antigens BP 180 and BP 230 can be detected in serum samples using ELISA and are useful in both diagnosis and monitoring disease activity.

Differential Diagnosis

- **Erosive form of lichen planus:** The erosive areas and ulcers are surrounded by Wickham's striae.
- **PV:** Unlike the bullae in bullous pemphigoid does not extend at the periphery. The lesions of BP are less painful and do not involve the mucosa as extensively, as in pemphigus. The lesions of BP are shallow as compared to pemphigus. Intact vesicles are rarely seen in pemphigus in contrast to pemphigoid, as they rupture soon because of its intraepithelial location.
- **Subepithelial bullous dermatoses:** MMP, unlike ocular pemphigoid, rarely results in scarring.

Treatment

Topical steroids—clobetasol, betamethasone

TABLE 5.9: Differential features of pemphigus and pemphigoid	
Pemphigus	Pemphigoid
4 types: P. vulgaris, P. foliaceous, P. vegetans, P. erythematosus	2 types: Cicatriacial pemphigoid, bullous pemphigoid
Intraepithelial bullae formation (antibodies are formed against desmoglein 1 and 3)	Sub-epithelial bullae formation (antibodies to lamina lucida portion of the basement membrane are present)
Oral lesions precede the skin lesions. There is no involvement of conjunctiva	Oral mucosa followed by conjunctival mucosa are the most common sites of involvement. Laryngeal and esophageal, genital involvement has also been seen.
	Desquamative gingivitis is the most common manifestation
Has thin-walled bullae which rupture easily	Has thick-walled bullae which are intact for a period of time compared to pemphigus
Nikolsky sign is positive	Nikolsky sign is not seen
In direct immuno-fluorescence: Presence of IgG in combination with C3, IgA , IgM in epithelium of lesion or clinically normal epithelium of lesion.	In direct immuno-fluorescence: Positive fluorescence for immunoglobulin and complement in the basement membrane is seen
	Circulating autoantibodies against pemphigoid antigens, BP 180 and BP 230 can be detected in serum samples for bullous pemphigoid

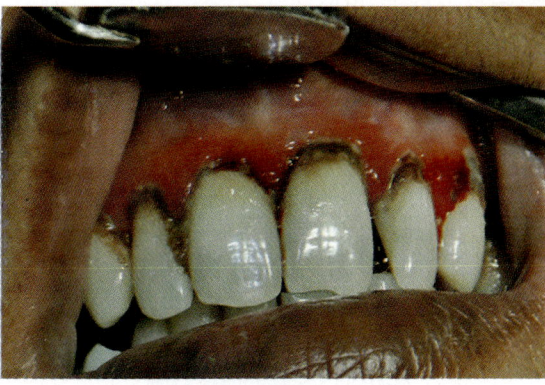

Fig. 5.12: Desquamative gingivitis in patient with pemphigoid

Systemic corticosteroid is usually necessary with lower dose and for short period of time. They may be combined with azathioprine, cyclophosphamide, mycophenolate, or rituximab.

Patients with moderate levels of disease may minimize the use of systemic steroids by the use of dapsone or tetracycline, doxycycline, or minocycline, which may be combined with niacinamide.

ORAL LICHEN PLANUS

Oral lichen planus (OLP) is a common mucocutaneous disease and is thought to affect 0.5–1% of the world's population.

The condition can affect either the skin or mucosa or both.

OLP is considered to be a premalignant condition. Patients with OLP are predisposed to develop oral carcinomas. Ulcerative lesions are suspected to be associated with malignant transformation.

Etiology

× Exact etiology is not known.
× The immune system has a primary role in the development of this disease (immunologically mediated disease).
× Other factors
  ▪ Stress
  ▪ Anxiety

- An association between OLP and hepatitis C virus (HCV). But no comprehensive explanation has been provided regarding this association.

Pathogenesis

Autoreactive T-lymphocytes may be of primary importance for the development of OLP.

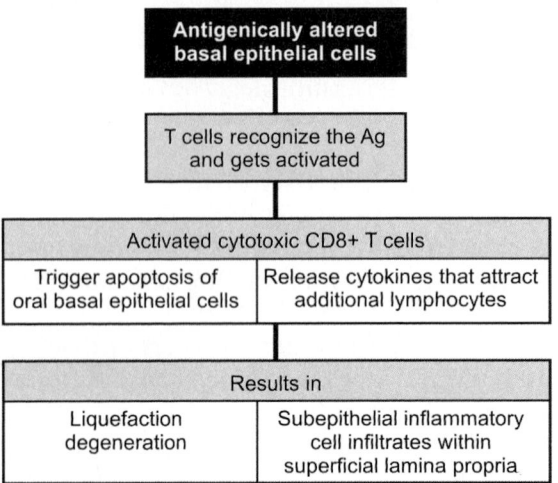

Epidemiology

- **Prevalence:** 0.5 – 2.2%
- **Gender:** More common in women than men.
- **Age:** Approximately 55 years

Clinical Manifestations

- Cutaneous lesions in approximately 15% of patients with OLP.
- Skin lesions are classically described as of pruritic, papular, polygonal, plaque, purple. They may be erythematous to violaceous papules that are flat topped.
- **Predilection sites:** Trunk and flexor surfaces of arms and legs. The patient reports relief following intense scratching of the lesions, but trauma may aggravate the disease, which is referred to as a Koebner phenomenon. Lichen planus involving genital mucosa, esophageal mucosa and nails have been reported.

Oral Manifestations and Clinical Classification

- Reticular
- Papular
- Plaque-like
- Bullous
- Erythematous
- Ulcerative/erosive

When mild degree of inflammation is present, it stimulates the epithelium to produce hyperkeratosis, whereas more intense inflammation leads to deterioration of epithelium leading to atrophic, erosive and ulcerative forms of lichen planus.

1. **Reticular form:**
   - Characterized by fine white lines or Wickham's striae and striae may show annular patterns. Found in all regions of the oral mucosa, most frequently observed bilaterally in the buccal mucosa.
   - It may be asymptomatic.
   - Reticular OLP can sometimes be observed at the vermilion border

2. **Papular type**
   - Initial phase of the disease
   - Characterized by small white dots, which in most occasions intermingle with the reticular form.

3. **Plaque type**
   - Homogenous well-demarcated white plaque that occurs in conjunction with striae. It resembles homogenous leukoplakia.
   - It usually presents on dorsum of tongue and patient may experience a feeling of roughness.

4. **Bullous form:** It is usually rare and appears as bullous structures surrounded by a reticular network.

5. **Erythematous OLP**
   - Characterized by a homogenous red area and striae are frequently seen at the periphery of the lesion.
   - Lesions may occur on attached gingiva without any papules or striae and presents as a desquamative gingivitis.

6. **Ulcerative lesions**
   - Most disabling form of OLP in which erythematous zone is surrounded by white striae.
   - Patients complain of severe burning sensations and discomfort on food intake.

Diagnosis

Pathognomonic Wickham's striae help to establish a correct clinical diagnosis. Desquamative gingivitis, plaque-like, erythematous, bullous, or ulcerative forms may exist together with the Wickham's striae.

Biopsy required for an accurate diagnosis of erythematous type of OLP .

Histopathology

1. Areas of hyperparakeratosis or hyper-orthokeratosis, often with a thickening of the granular cell layer and a saw: toothed appearance to the rete pegs.
2. "Liquefaction degeneration" or necrosis of the basal cell layer.
3. An eosinophilic band seen just beneath the basement membrane, containing fibrin covering the lamina propria.
4. A dense subepithelial band-shaped infiltrate of lymphocytes and macrophages is also characteristic of the disease.

Management

- Since the etiology behind OLP is unknown, thus all the treatment strategies are aiming at reducing or eliminating symptoms.
- Topical steroids like triamcinolone acetonide 0.1% ointment and clobetasol can be used as the primary therapeutic choice for symptomatic OLP. Topical steroids are used as a mouth rinses or a gel. It can be used by "swish and spit out" method. Apply the drug 2 or 3 times a day during 3 weeks followed by tapering during the following 9 weeks until a maintenance dose of 2 to 3 times a week is reached. When potent topical steroids are used, a fungal infection may emerge, and a parallel treatment with antifungal drugs may be necessary when the number of applications exceeds once a day and antifungal treatment itself may result in significant improvement of symptoms and clinical features. For desquamative gingivitis, steroid gels in prefabricated plastic trays may be used for 30 minutes at each application to increase the concentration of steroids in the gingival tissue.
- Several other topical drugs including calcineurin inhibitors like topical tacrolimus 0.1% ointment, topical cyclosporine and retinoids form the second line of treatment.
- Systemic steroids are used to control symptoms from recalcitrant lesions. 1 mg/kg daily for 7 days followed by a reduction of 10 mg each subsequent day.
- Since half of OLP lesions exhibit candidal infection, antifungal treatment may be used before treatment with steroids. Oral hygiene should be optimized prior to the beginning of steroid treatment.
- Retinoids, levamisole, dapsone, mycophenolate mofetil, cyclosporine, low dose heparin (enoxaprin), efalizumab are other treatment modalities which can be given in recalcitrant cases of oral lichen planus.
- Ultraviolet phototherapy, PUVA, photodynamic therapy and lasers are the non-pharmacological methods for treatment of oral licen planus.
- Relapses are common, and the general approach should be to use steroids at the lowest level to keep the patient free of symptoms.

Differential Diagnosis

1. Lichenoid contact reactions
2. Lichenoid reactions of graft-versus-host disease (GVHD)
3. Oral lichenoid drug eruptions
4. Discoid lupus erythematosus (DLE)
5. Systemic lupus erythematosus (SLE)
6. Homogenous oral leukoplakia (d/d of plaque-type)
7. Mucous membrane pemphigoid (d/d of erythematous type)

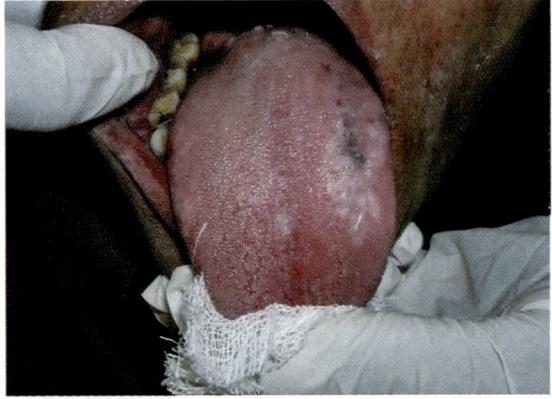

Fig. 5.13: Lichen planus involving tongue

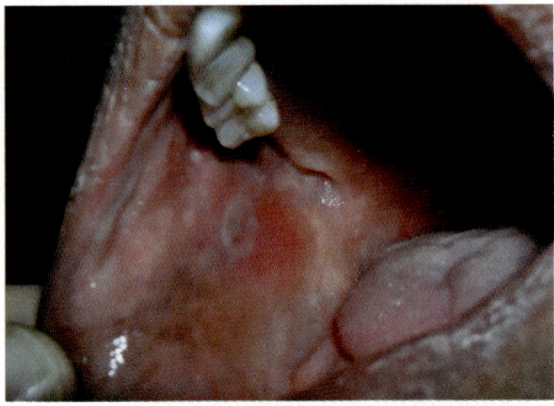

Fig. 5.15: Discoid lichen planus

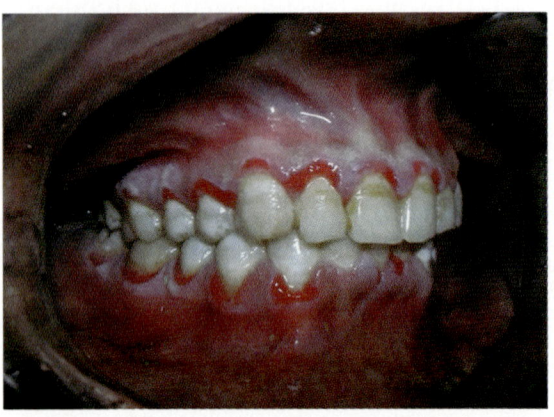

Fig. 5.14: Lichen planus involving gingiva

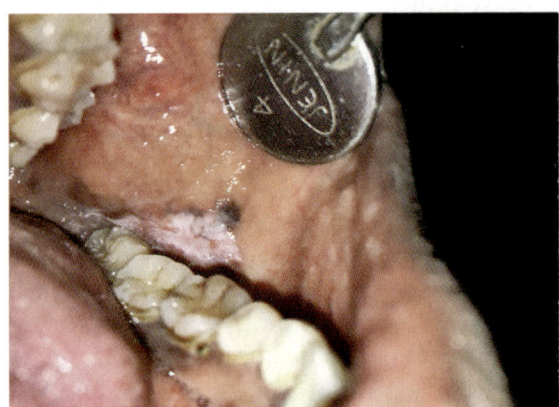

Fig. 5.16: Plaque type lichen planus

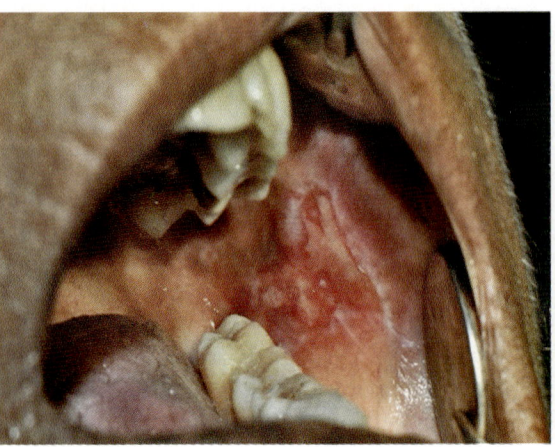

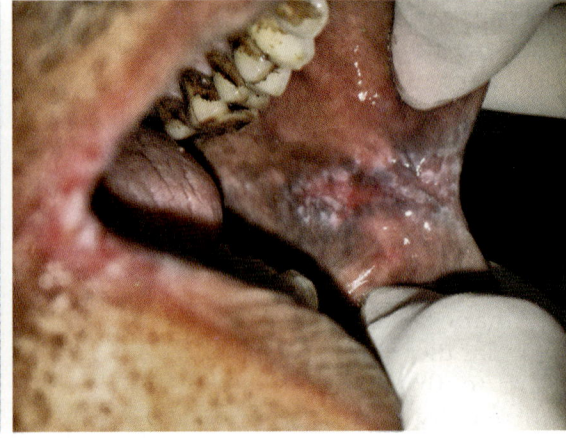

Fig. 5.17: Erosive lichen planus

SINGLE ULCERS

Traumatic Ulcers

Most common cause of single ulcers is due to trauma. It is a frequently encountered ulcerative lesion of mouth.

Causes

- **Direct physical/mechanical:** Acute bite injuries, sharp tooth (most common cause), ill-fitting prosthesis, overzealous toothbrushing, oral piercing.
- **Thermal:** Electrical burns, burns on palate from ingesting hot foods and beverages, reverse smoking, hot instrument (iatrogenic)
- **Chemical:** Placing noxious and caustic substances directly on mucosa such as silver nitrate, phenol, acetylsalicylic acid. Sucking on or chewing medications formulated to be swallowed (such as aspirin or oral bisphosphonates) may also lead to severe oral ulcers. Prolonged contact of methacrylate monomer on the mucosa may also lead to necrosis of the mucosa.
- A positive history about inciting agent helps in confirmation of etiologic agent.

Clinical Features

It can occur in persons of any age, with equal frequency in both the sexes. Appearance depends on the site of injury, the nature and severity of trauma and the degree of secondary infection present. It may persist for a few days and may last for weeks. May be crater-like, generally the result of repetitive trauma over a prolonged period, thereby preventing healing.

Oral Findings

Traumatic ulcer usually present as single, irregular ulcer in proximity of the offending sharp tooth or clasp of dental prosthesis and usually present on lateral borders of tongue. It may persist from many days to weeks. The ulcer may conform to the shape of etiologic agent and may be surrounded by a whitish keratotic area. Sometimes, trauma from natal teeth may present with ulcer in the sublingual area of neonates. These are described **as Riga-Fede's ulcer**.

Electrical burns in particular are caused by high heat, are generally fairly extensive, involve the lips, and are generally seen in young children and toddlers.

Burns from hot foods and beverages are generally small and localized to the hard palatal mucosa or lips and are usually seen in teenagers and adults, usually presents as an area of tenderness and erythema that develops into ulcers within hours of the injury.

Differential Diagnosis

A positive history about inciting agent will help to confirm the diagnosis.

- **Tubercular ulcer:** Undermined flabby borders, usually painless.
- **Primary syphilic lesion:** Painless indurated edema and lymph swelling.
- **Dystrophic ulcer:** Rare ulceration caused by deficient blood supply due to local anesthesia.
- **Malignant ulcer**
- **Recurrent intraoral** herpes infection of palate may resemble thermal burn.

Lab Findings

- Culture may be needed if the areas do not heal well or if suppuration develops, suggesting a secondary bacterial infection.
- A biopsy should be performed if the ulcer does not heal within a few weeks.

Management

- Pain control can be achieved with topical anesthetics (such as viscous lidocaine). Topical steroids or intra-lesional steroid injections may be useful.
- Electrical burns are deep and more extensive, and healing results in scarring and contracture.
- Smaller lesions caused by less severe thermal or chemical injury heal on their own once the irritant is removed.

* Antibiotics may be necessary to prevent a secondary infection.
* Chlorhexidine mouthwash or topical local anesthetics to relieve symptoms of pain.

ULCERS CAUSED BY FUNGAL INFECTIONS

Fungal infections are common and a variety of environmental and physiological conditions can contribute to development of fungal infections. Inhalation of fungal spores or localized colonization of the skin may initiate persistent infections; therefore, fungal infections often start in the lungs or on the skin. Fungal infections are usually confined to the subcutaneous tissues, but in rare cases they become systemic and produce life-threatening disease. Individuals with weakened immune systems, with HIV/AIDS, under steroid treatments, chemotherapy and uncontrolled diabetes tend to develop fungal infections.

Histoplasmosis

It is caused by fungus *Histoplasma capsulatum*, a dimorphic fungus. Primary infection which is mild, from inhaling dust contaminated with droppings, cause pulmonary disease that heals to leave fibrosis and calcification similar to TB. It occurs in immunocompromised states and may be the first sign of AIDS.

Oral Manifestations

Oral involvement is usually secondary to pulmonary involvement. It begins as an area of erythema that becomes a papule and eventually a painful, indurated, granulomatous ulcer appearing on palate, gingiva or tongue. It often resembles squamous cell carcinoma. It is accompanied with cervical lymphadenopathy.

Lab Diagnosis

A rapid diagnosis may be made with the use of a smear of the lesion stained with methenamine silver or a biopsy of the lesion stained with periodic acid–Schiff or methenamine silver, which will reveal the presence of the fungi within granulomas. Cultures should be performed on a portion of tissue removed during the biopsy. Diagnosis of disseminated histoplasmosis occurs by antigen detection via enzyme immunoassay in serum and urine, antibody detection via immmunodiffusion, identification of histoplasma DNA via various PCR techniques.

Differential Diagnosis

Ulcers present for weeks or months may represent other lesions of infectious etiology like deep fungal infections, tuberculous ulcer, traumatic ulcerative granuloma, squamous cell carcinoma, lymphoma, or other malignancy.

Management

* Intravenous amphotericin B
* Itraconazole in AIDS patient
* Systemic ketoconazole for 6 to 12 months in immunocompetent individuals

Blastomycosis

It is caused by blastomyces dermatitidis. Inhalation causes primary pulmonary infection that is acute self-limiting and remains asymptomatic, in some cases it is normal inhabitant of soil so it is more commonly associated with farmers and construction workers. And is not commonly associated with HIV infection.

The skin lesions (usually on exposed surfaces) start as subcutaneous nodules, slowly progressing to well-circumscribed indurated ulcers. If the infection goes untreated, the signs and symptoms may mimic TB and include dyspnea, weight loss, and production of blood-tinged sputum.

Oral Manifestations

Oral lesions are rarely the primary site of infection. Oral lesions are non-specific, painless, verrucous ulcer with indurated borders and is often mistaken for squamous cell carcinoma. Other oral lesions include hard nodules and radiolucent jaw lesions.

Diagnosis

PCR, antibody identification through enzyme immunoassay, biopsy, and culture on Sabouraud agar.

Management

* Itraconazole therapy is used to manage mild cases of blastomycosis. More advanced cases infections are treated with amphotericin B
* Ketoconazole
* Fluconazole

Mucormycosis (Phycomycosis, Zygomycosis)

It causes opportunistic infections in debilitated patients, patients with decreased host resistance, those with poorly controlled diabetes or hematologic malignancies, post-solid-organ transplantation cancer chemotherapy or immunosuppressive drug therapy. It may occur as a pulmonary, gastrointestinal, or rhinocerebral infection.

Clinical Features

The two most common forms of mucormycosis are pulmonary/sinus and cutaneous. In pulmonary/sinus mucormycosis, spores are inhaled from the environment. It is characterized by arterial invasion and a fulminant course, frequently resulting in death. The hallmark of infection is the formation of emboli with resulting necrosis of involved tissue.

Oral Findings

The most common signs are ulceration of palate, which results from necrosis due to invasion of palatal vessels. Lesions are large and deep, causing denudation of underlying bone. Ulcers have been reported on gingiva, lip and alveolar ridge. More advanced disease with ulcer and palatal perforation may lead to invasion of maxillary sinus and involvement of brain.

Lab Diagnosis

* Biopsy for culture and direct examination must be performed. The histopathology shows necrosis and nonseptate hyphae, which are best demonstrated by a periodic acid–Schiff stain or the methenamine silver stain
* PCR

Management

* Control the predisposing factors such as diabetes.
* Surgical debridement of infected area.
* Systemic administration of amphotericin B

Tuberculous Ulcer

Tuberculosis is an infectious granulomatous disease caused by acid-fast bacilli *Mycobacterium tuberculosis*. Although, oral manifestations of tuberculosis has a rare occurrence, but it has been considered to account for 0.1–5% of all the TB infections. These lesions are usually secondarily inoculated with infected sputum or due to haematogenous spread. Nowadays, oral manifestations are re-appearing as a consequence of the outbreak and emergence of drug-resistant TB. Dental identification of the tuberculosis lesions have the potential of serving as an important aid in the first line of control for this dangerous and often fatal disease.

The following symptoms are common: Chronic cough, moderate fever, night sweats, fatigue, decreased appetite, and weight loss.

Oral Manifestations

Lesions may occur in the oral tissues and the neck lymph nodes. The latter is termed scrofula.

Tongue is the most commonly affected followed by palate, lips, buccal mucosa, and gingiva. It may be preceded by an **opalescent vesicle or nodule**, a result of caseation necrosis which breaks down into an ulcer which is usually superficial or deep and painful. Tubercular ulcers are generally oval in shape but their coalescence may give an irregular crescentic border. The edge of the ulcer is **undermined** with minimum induration. It tends to be increased slowly in size. The disease spreads in and destroys the subcutaneous tissue faster than it destroys the skin. The overhanging skin is thin, friable, reddish blue and unhealthy. The mucosa is **inflamed** and **oedematous.**

Base: The base of ulcer is pale with scanty granulation tissue.

Floor: The floor of the ulcer is watery / apple jelly appearance.

Differential Diagnosis of Tubercular Ulcer of Oral Cavity

- **Syphilitic ulcer:** Primary lesion is harder and spirochetes are found.
- **Traumatic ulcer:** Short duration and history of trauma.
- **Sarcoidosis:** Tuberculin test negative, the granuloma of sarcoidosis are of non-necrotizing type.
- **Lupus erythematosus:** Histology, causative agent tests negative, skin changes.
- **Leukaemia:** Immature WBCs, prolonged bleeding and clotting time.

Laboratory Diagnosis

The diagnosis of latent disease is initiated by performing a tuberculin skin test (TST) on the forearm with purified protein derivative, a mycobacterial antigen. If a red welt forms within 72 hours, the patient is considered to have been exposed to *M. tuberculosis*. A chest radiograph often reveals pulmonary involvement. Confirmation of active TB involves collecting patient sputum to look for the infecting organism.

Treatment

The patient diagnosed with a latent TB infection is typically treated with one of the following regimens from four to nine months: Isoniazid, isoniazid plus rifapentine, or rifampicin.

Malignant Ulcers

Ulcer can be defined as break in the continuity of the covering epithelium of the skin or mucous membrane. Malignant ulcers include squamous cell carcinoma, basal cell carcinoma, malignant melanoma.

Etiology

- Smokeless tobacco and alcohol
- Genetic changes
- Immunosuppressed patient
- Exposure to UV light
- Chemical and physical irritants, viruses, and hormonal effects

Clinical Features

- Male predominance
- Age above 60 years
- Site = Lower lip, anterior floor of the mouth, lateral borders of the tongue.
- Appearance = Red, white or mixed red-white lesions, change in surface texture, presence of mass or ulcerations
- Ulcers are irregular, indurated with raised everted edges. It may be accompanied with a proliferative growth.
- Superficial and deep lymph nodes affected, enlarged and firm to hard on palpation. There may be pain, discomfort and trismus accompanied with the ulcer.

Differential Diagnosis

- Major aphthous ulcers
- Long standing ulcers in herpes
- Basal cell carcinoma
- Primary syphilitic lesion
- Verrucous carcinoma

Treatment

Surgery and radiation

Syphilitic Ulcers

It is also called lues, caused by *Treponema pallidum*. There are three stages of infection in syphilis and sometimes may develop at the site of inoculation in the oral cavity.

Etiology

× Sexual contact
× Maternal transmission

Primary Syphilis

× **Site:** Most frequently on genitalia, lip, tongue, nostrils and to some extent gingiva and tonsillar area.
× The lesion is called chancre which is highly infectious. The chancre is painless, necrotic, covered with grayish white membrane, and may be painful due to secondary infection. The ulcers are characterized by rolled out borders and lymphadenopathy.

Secondary Syphilis

Commences six weeks after primary syphilis
× **Site:** Tongue, soft palate, cheek, tonsils, buccal mucosa
× **Appearance:** Slightly raised, greyish white, glistening patches on mucous membrane called 'mucous patches'. The mucous patch presents as thickened whitish plaques with necrosis and sloughing. The lesions are accompanied with fever, lymphadenopathy, weight loss.
× **Snail track ulcers:** Mucous patches coalesce to form snail track ulcers. The leions in secondary syphilis are described as interstitial glossitis or leutic glossitis. These lesions constitute a premalignant condition.
　Patients with syphilis who are not treated in the secondary stage will develop tertiary syphilis which can cause complications including paralysis and dementia.

Tertiary Syphilis

Site: The lesion in tertiary syphilis is called gumma. It most commonly affects hard palate, soft palate, lips and tongue. Gumma manifests as painless, firm nodular mass with deep, punched out borders.
　Gumma begins as small, pale, raised area of mucosa that ulcerate and rapidly progress to large zone of necrosis and denudation of bone in case of palate and may lead to oro-nasal fistula.

Congenital Syphilis

It is characterized by:

Hutchinson's incisors: Screw driver shaped incisors and mulberry molars. In late congenital syphilis, over two years of age, a number of complications develop including Hutchinson's notched incisors, mulberry-shaped molar teeth, corneal keratitis, deafness, frontal bossing, saddle nose, hard palate defects, and swollen joints.

Diagnosis

1. Darkfield microscopy to identify organisms from lesion
2. *Antibody to Treponema:* The more specific fluorescent treponemal antibody absorption test.
3. Venereal disease research laboratory (VDRL) test

Differential Diagnosis

× **Primary syphilis**
　▪ Ruptured vesicles of herpes simplex
　▪ Traumatic ulcer
× **Secondary syphilis**
　▪ Aphthous ulcers
　▪ Erythema multiforme
　▪ Lichen planus
　▪ Malignant ulcer
　▪ Tuberculous ulcer

Treatment

× Antibiotics

Cytomegalovirus Infection

CMV causes an infectious mononucleosis like disease especially in the immuno-compromised patient such as HIV, organ transplant. CMV remains latent in connective tissue cell and causes vascular inflammation. It is associated with mild fever, lymphadenopathy and splenomegaly. It results in CMV retinitis and CMV enteritis in HIV patients.

Oral Manifestations

In immunocompromised patient CMV is known to cause single large ulcer and rarely multiple which are painful and last for weeks to months.

Differential Diagnosis

* Tuberculous ulcer
* Ulcer caused by fungal infection
* Malignant ulcer
* Traumatic ulcerative granuloma

Treatment

Topical anaesthetics and antiviral drugs

FREQUENTLY ASKED QUESTIONS

1. Write clinical features, differential diagnosis and management of the following:
   a. Herpes simplex
   b. Herpes zoster
   c. Recurrent aphthous ulcers
   d. Pemphigus
   e. Erythema multiforme
2. Define macule, papule, vesicle, bullae

BIBLIOGRAPHY

1. Glick M. Burket's oral medicine. 12th edition Shelton, USA: Peoples Medical Publishing House; 2015.
2. Venkataraman BK. Diagnostic oral medicine 1st edition: Wolters Kluwer; 2013.
3. Woud N. Goaz P. Differential diagnosis of oral and maxillofacial lesions. 5th edition Elsevier; 2007.
4. Greenberg M. Glick M. Burket's Oral medicine diagnosis and treatment. 10th edition: BC Decker Inc; Elsevier; 2003
5. Greenberg M. Brightman V. Burket's Oral medicine diagnosis and treatment. 9th edition: Lippincott 1997.
6. Nair GR, Naidu GS, Jain S, Nagi R, Makkad RS, Jha A. Clinical effectiveness of aloe vera in the management of oral mucosal diseases— A systematic review. J Clin Diagn Res. 2016 Aug;10(8):Ze01–7
7. Misra N, Maiti D, Misra P, Singh AK. 940 nm diode laser therapy in management of recurrent aphthous ulcer. BMJ Case Rep. 2013 Apr 17;2013
8. Preeti L, Mangesh K, Rajkumar K, Karthik R. Recurrent Aphthous Stomatitis. J Oral Maxillofac Pathol 2011 Sep; 15(3):252–6
9. Ahluwalia J, Han A, Kusari A, Eishenfield Lf. Recurrent herpes labialis in the pediatric population: Prevalence, therapeutic studies, and associated complications. Pediatr Dermatol 2019 Sep 9.
10. Rutnin S, Chanprapaph K. Vesiculobullous diseases in relation to lupus erythematosus. Clin Cosmet Investing Dermatol 2019 Sep 4; 12:653–667.
11. Yanovsky Rl, Mcleod M, Ahmed AR. Treatment of pemphigus vulgaris: Part 2 - Emerging Therapies. Expert Rev Clin Immunol. 2019 Oct 2. doi: 10.1080/1744666X.2020.1672539.
12. Stamatis Gregoriou, Ourania Efthymiou, Christina Stefanaki, and Dimitris Rigopoulos. Management of pemphigus vulgaris: Challenges and solutions. Clin Cosmet Investig Dermatol. 2015; 8: 521–527.
13. Wim Opstelten, Just Eekhof, Arie Knuistingh Neven, Theo Verheji. Treatment Of Herpes Zoster. Can Fam Physician. 2008 Mar; 54(3): 373–377.

Red and White Lesions

The oral cavity is a complex anatomical space delimited by structures of different nature and functions. The oral mucosa covering the different oral structures and areas has a different role and may be affected by a plethora of pathologic conditions of variable etiology and significance. Oral soft tissue lesions result from histologic changes occurring at a molecular and microscopic level that affect the oral epithelium and the underlying connective tissue. These changes may lead to a color change of the mucosa, causing red and/or white appearing lesions of the oral cavity.

A white appearance of the oral mucosa may be caused by a variety of factors including an increased production of keratin (hyperkeratosis), an abnormal, benign thickening of stratum spinosum (acanthosis), intracellular and extracellular accumulation of fluid in the epithelium, necrosis of the oral epithelium or microbes, particularly fungi, that produce a whitish pseudomembranous appearance. A red lesion of the oral mucosa may develop as a result of atrophic epithelium, characterized by a reduction in the number of epithelial cells or increased vascularization.

Classification

The red and white appearing lesions on the oral mucosa have a multifactorial etiology. Based on the underlying pathology and etiology, these lesions may be classified as

1. **Potentially malignant disorders**
   - Oral leukoplakia
   - Erythroplakia
   - Actinic cheilitis (cheilosis)
   - Actinic keratosis
   - Oral submucous fibrosis.

2. **Immunologically mediated diseases**
   - Oral lichen planus
   - Drug-induced lichenoid reactions
   - Lichenoid reactions of graft-versus-host disease.
   - Lupus erythematosus.

3. **Infectious disease**
   - Oral candidiasis
   - Hairy leukoplakia

4. **Allergic reactions**
   - Lichenoid contact reactions
   - Reactions to dentifrice and chlorhexidine

5. **Toxic reactions**
   - Reactions to smokeless tobacco
   - Smokers palate.

6. **Reactions to mechanical trauma**
   - Morsicatio
   - Frictional keratosis

7. Others
- Benign migratory glossitis
- Leukoedema
- White sponge nevus
- Pachyonychia congenita
- Dyskeratosis congenita

POTENTIALLY MALIGNANT ORAL DISORDERS

Oral cancer is one of the most common malignancies in southeast Asia, accounting for 30–40% of all malignancies in India. The survey burden of cancer and their variations across Indian states showed that cancer of the oral cavity and lip accounts for 7.2% cases and was identified as a leading cause of death. SEER data has demonstrated an increase in the incidence of tongue cancer in young individuals (age less than 40 years) from 3–6% over time. The complex association between poverty, education, reduced access to treatment, low prioritization of the disease and the specific cultural and social habits are the main reasons for increased incidence of oral cancer in the Indian population.

Many oral malignancies develop from the premalignant disorders affecting the oral cavity including leukoplakia, erythroplakia, lichen planus, etc. Early detection of premalignant lesions can improve the prognosis and is well proved as an effective aid in disease prevention. The prevalence of potentially malignant disorders varies by geographic location and population ranging from 1 to 5% despite all limitations. Most affected patients are middle aged or elderly men but trends have shifted and men:women ratio has reduced considerably with time. This trend is thought to be the reflection of general acceptance of habits of smoking and drinking by both the sexes. Most commonly affected sites in general are the buccal mucosa, lower gingiva, tongue, floor of the mouth.

In 1978, WHO classified precancer into precancerous lesions and precancerous conditions.

- A precancerous lesion is a morphologically altered tissue in which oral cancer is more likely to occur than its apparently normal counterpart.
- A precancerous condition is a generalized state associated with a significantly increased risk of cancer.

The current Working Group of WHO in its latest monograph (2005) did not favour the subdividing of the precancer to lesions and conditions and the consensus view was to refer to all clinical presentations that carry a risk of cancer under the term 'potentially malignant disorders' to reflect their widespread anatomical distribution.

A proposed definition for potentially malignant oral disorder is:

"It is a group of disorders of varying aetiologies, usually tobacco; characterized by mutagen-associated, spontaneous or hereditary alterations or mutations in the genetic material of oral epithelial cells with or without clinical and histomorphological alterations that may lead to oral squamous cell carcinoma transformation".The suggested definition depicts the molecular nature of the oral potentially malignant disorders along with the possible presence and absence of clinical and histomorphological alterations.

Oral Leukoplakia

Definition

In 1978, WHO defined oral leukoplakia as"A white patch or plaque that cannot be characterised clinically or pathologically as any other disease." The term leukoplakia is unrelated to presence or absence of epithelial dysplasia.In a monograph by WHO (1977) the phrase any other definable disease was replaced by other "definable lesion". No clarification was provided for this change. In 2005, WHO changed the definition of oral leukoplakia to "A white plaque of questionable risk having excluded other known diseases or disorders that carry no increased risk for cancer". Leukoplakia has been considered a potentially malignant or precancerous disease and not a lesion since it is well known that cancer development not only occurs in or close to a leukoplakic patch but can also occur at any other site of the oral cavity. A combination of 1978 and 2005 WHO definition has led to the following text:

"A predominantly white patch or plaque that cannot be characterized clinically or pathologically as any other disorder. Oral leukoplakia carries an increased risk of cancer development either in or close to the area of leukoplakia or elsewhere in the oral cavity or the head and neck region."

The diagnosis of leukoplakia mainly denotes that the mucosa is irritated by mechanical, chemical, or galvanic means and the mucosa is trying to adapt to the noxious stimuli by undergoing hyperkeratinisation of its surface.

Classification

Traditionally, two major clinical types of oral leukoplakia (OL) are recognized: Homogenous and Non-homogenous. Figure 6.1 illustrates a simple classification of leukoplakia.

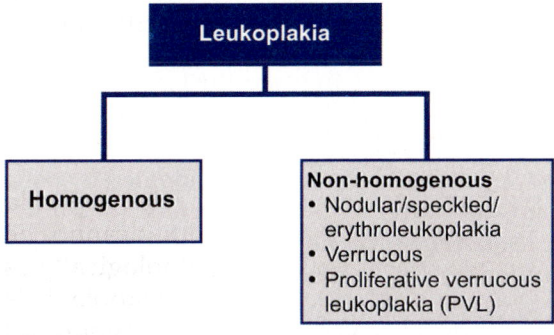

Fig. 6.1: A simple classification of leukoplakia

The homogenous type is characterized by a thin, flat, and homogenous whitish appearance giving the lesion a cracked mud appearance.

The non-homogenous type consists of:
- *Nodular/speckled:* Red and white (erythroplakia)
- *Verrucous*
- *Proliferative verrucous leukoplakia (PVL):* This was introduced by Hansen et al. It may start as simple keratosis at one end to invasive carcinoma at the other.

Epidemiology: Almost all leukoplakias in India occur in tobacco users. A definitive dose—response between leukoplakia and various forms of tobacco use has been demonstrated particularly as smoking.

Etiology

The etiology of oral leukoplakia is multifactorial.

1. **Tobacco:** The habit of tobacco smoking/chewing is associated with leukoplakia. There is a dose response relationship between oral leukoplakia and tobacco. It has been observed that reducing or cessation of tobacco use may result in the regression or disappearance of oral leukoplakia. The smokeless tobacco habit often leads to a clinically distinctive white plaque called "tobacco pouch keratosis" which is not a true oral leukoplakia.

2. **Alcohol:** Alcohol along with tobacco does have a synergistic effect in oral leukoplakia as in cancer. People excessively using mouthrinses with an alcohol content greater than 25% may have greyish buccal mucosal plaques but not true leukoplakia.

3. **Sanguinaria:** Toothpastes or mouthrinses containing sanguinaria may lead to the development of true oral leukoplakia. Sanguinaria associated oral leukoplakia are located in maxillary vestibule or on the alveolar mucosa of the maxilla. The lesions may persist even after the cessation of the use of product.

4. **Ultraviolet rays:** UV rays are causative factor for oral leukoplakia of lower lip vermillion. Immunocompromised persons, especially transplant patients, are prone to the development of leukoplakia and squamous cell carcinoma of lower lip vermillion.

5. **Candida:** Candida can colonize the superficial epithelial layers of the oral mucosa often producing a thick granular

plaque with a mixed white and red color. The term 'candidal leukoplakia or hyperplastic candidiasis' has been used to describe such lesions and biopsy may show hyperplastic histopathological changes. It is not known whether Candida produces dysplasia or secondarily infects altered epithelium. There is reduction or disappearance of these lesions after the use of antifungal therapy.

6. **Human papillomavirus (HPV):** HPV subtypes 16 and 18 have been identified in some oral leukoplakias. HPV 16 has been shown to induce dysplasia like changes in normally differentiating squamous epithelium, particularly with exophytic verrucous leukoplakia.

7. **Trauma:** Several keratotic lesions which were until recently considered as variants of oral leukoplakia are now considered as precancer. *Nicotine stomatitis* is a generalized white palatal hyperkeratotic response to heat generated by tobacco smoking (pipe smoking) rather than a response to carcinogens within smoke. *Frictional keratosis* is a chronic mechanical irritation that can produce a white lesion similar to true oral leukoplakia. Such a lesion can be reversed after elimination of the trauma. Traumatic lesions such as linea alba, morsacatio, toothbrush and gingival abrasion along with denture trauma or masticatory keratosis should be differentiated from groups of precancer.

8. **Nutritional deficiency:** It has been observed that serum levels of vitamins A, B_{12}, C, beta carotene and folic acid significantly decrease in Indian patients of leukoplakia.

Clinical Features

The onset of oral leukoplakia usually starts after the age of 30 years. However, younger age groups between 20 and 30 years have also been reported. Peak incidence is above the age of 50 years. The gender distribution in India is strong male predominance, however other studies have reported 1:1 male to female ratio in the Western world.

Leukoplakias are most commonly encountered on the buccal mucosa, gingiva, floor of the mouth, tongue, lip vermillion. Almost 90% of cases on the tongue, floor of the mouth or lip vermillion will show dysplasia or carcinoma. Early or mild leukoplakias are thin, greyish white plaques, somewhat translucent in appearance, fissured or wrinkled and may disappear on discontinuation of smoking or continue unchanged. These may later become thick and distinctly white appearance, leathery on palpation and fissures may deepen and become numerous. At this stage, the lesions are often called *homogenous leukoplakia*. These may remain regress or disappear, few may become severe develop surface irregularities and are called verrucous or verruciform leukoplakia.

Speckled leukoplakia/erythroleukoplakia/ nodular leukoplakia is a non-homogeneous type of leukoplakia. Speckled leukoplakia (SL) according to WHO, is a leukoplakia with a mix of white and red plaque lesions. It is a form of leukoplakia that is rarely found with very aggressive high risk for transformation into malignancy, and also considered as precursor lesion for squamous cell carcinoma. Clinically the lesion appears in the form of plaque/whitish nodules that have a granular surface against a reddish background. SL is often accompanied by pain and discomfort.

Verrucous leukoplakia appears as an adherent white plaque that has numerous papillary projections on its surface.

A high-risk aggressive form of leukoplakia, *proliferative verrucous leukoplakia (PVL)* is characterised by the development of multiple keratotic plaques with roughened surface projections. The multiple plaques of PVL tend to slowly spread and involve other oral mucosal sites. Gingiva is frequently involved with spread to the other sites as well. The PVL lesions begin as simple, flat hyperkeratosis that are indistinguishable from ordinary leukoplakia. PVL exhibits persistent growth, becoming exophytic and verrucous in nature.These lesions have a strong female predilection (1:4) and minimal association with tobacco use and mostly associated with human papilloma virus. The lesions rarely regress despite therapy.

Severe leukoplakia lesions may become invasive and scattered patches of redness called erythroleukoplakia or speckled leukoplakia. The red areas usually represent sites where epithelial cells are so immature or atrophic that they lose their ability to produce keratin and hence intermixed red and white areas are seen. These lesions frequently represent advanced dysplasia on biopsy.

Diagnostic Procedures

Clinical examination with directed conventional biopsy remains the best means of assessing oral leukoplakia. Biopsy should be taken from the site of symptoms if present or site of redness or induration for the confirmatory diagnosis. Diagnostic methods other than histological examination like supra-vital staining or cytologic listing (brush biopsy) have their limitations when dealing with oral leukoplakia.

Histopathologic Features

Microscopically, leukoplakia is characterized by a thickened surface keratin layer described as hyperkeratosis. The keratin layer may consist of parakeratin (hyperparakeratosis) or orthokeratin (hyperorthokeratosis) or a combination of both. There is thickening of spinous cell layer (acanthosis). Some lesions may show surface hyperkeratosis but may demonstrate atrophy or thinning of underlying epithelium. Subadjacent connective tissue may show variable number of chronic inflammatory cells.

Verrucous leukoplakia has papillary or pointed surface projections, varying keratin thickness and broad blunted rete ridges.

PVL shows a variable microscopic appearance depending on the stage of the lesions. Early PVL appears as a hyperkeratotic lesion with time, the lesion becomes papillary, exophytic, verrucous hyperplasia. In later stages, the papillary proliferation exhibits downgrowth into the epithelium with broad, blunt rete ridges invasion into underlying CT. This stage is similar to verrucous carcinoma. Furthermore, the invading epithelium becomes less differentiated transforming into a full-fledged squamous cell carcinoma (SCC). Due to variable clinical and microscopic appearance, careful correlation of findings is required.

Most leukoplakia lesions demonstrate no dysplasia on biopsy.

Dysplasia

A loss in the uniformity and architectural pattern of the individual cells is termed dysplasia. The dysplastic features typically begin at the basilar or suprabasilar areas of the epithelium and may go on to involve the entire thickness of the epithelium. The dysplastic features include architectural features and cytologic features.

Architectural Features

* Asymmetric epithelial stratification
* An increased number of mitotic figures
* Dyskeratosis
* Drop-shaped rete pegs
* Loss of polarity of basal cells
* Basal cell hyperplasia or anaplasia

Cytologic Features

* Cellular and nuclear pleomorphism
* Increased nuclear cytoplasmic ratio
* Prominent nucleoli
* Hyperchromatism

These dysplastic features could be mild, moderate, or severe depending on restriction of features to lower one-third to two-thirds and more than two-thirds of the epithelium respectively.

Carcinoma in situ is the term applied when the entire thickness of epithelium is involved in which the dysplasia extends from the basal layer to the overlying mucosa without invading the underlying connective tissue.

The risk for malignant transformation of oral leukoplakia includes
- Female gender
- Long standing oral leukoplakia
- Oral leukoplakia in non-smokers (idiopathic)
- Location on tongue, floor of the mouth
- Size greater than 200 mm
- Non-homogenous type with presence of Candida infection
- Presence of epithelial dysplasia

Differential Diagnosis

Table 6.1 enumerates the list of lesions affecting the oral mucosa that must be considered in the differential diagnosis of oral leukoplakia and their differentiating points.

TABLE 6.1: Differential diagnosis of oral leukoplakia and their differentiating points

Lichen planus (LP)	✗ Typical lacy white lesions; ✗ "Wickham's striae" are seen possible presence of concurrent skin lesions ✗ Plaque-like LP lesions are also associated with reticular areas at periphery ✗ LP is commoner in females as opposed to leukoplakia ✗ Biopsy of the lesion helps in making a definitive diagnosis in case of multiple lesions/co-existing lesions
Leukoedema	✗ Occurs bilaterally on the buccal mucosa ✗ Disappears on stretching ✗ Appears as a faint milky opalescence as opposed to the definite white appearance of the leukoplakia
Cheek-biting lesion/ *Morsicaio buccarum*	✗ Buccal mucosa takes on a roughened, whitish lesion with a ragged, eroded surface. ✗ Careful questioning of the patient usually elicits the cause and promotes the proper diagnosis.
Smokeless tobacco lesion	✗ Lesion often has a more wrinkled pattern and is easily identified by its location in the vestibule and history of tobacco chewing use
Lupus erythematosus	✗ Leukoplakia-like intra-oral lesions are seen in DLE ✗ Lesions are frequently bilateral ✗ Classic oral lesion in DLE has a central atrophic area with small white dots and a slightly elevated border zone of irradiating white striae. ✗ Concurrent skin lesions and work-up for lupus help to distinguish
Hyperplastic candidiasis	✗ Occurs as a result of chronic infection of *C. albicans*. ✗ It may be difficult to identify whether the lesion is a primary candidal lesion or a secondarily infected leukoplakia. ✗ Multiple lesions favour the diagnosis of candidiasis.
Hairy leukoplakia	✗ Occurs usually on the lateral or ventral surfaces of the tongue in HIV-positive patients. ✗ Associated features of HIV infection are present ✗ HIV testing and biopsy of the lesion are helpful in making a definitive diagnosis
Electro-galvanic reactions	✗ They are keratotic plaque-like lesions similar to leukoplakia that arise due to a microgalvanic current from dissimilar metal restorations on the adjacent mucosa ✗ Lesions disappear when the different metal restorations are replaced or when the teeth are extracted.
White sponge nevus	✗ Familial pattern ✗ Widespread folded white lesions develop in childhood as opposed to leukoplakia that occurs in older individuals

Contd.

Treatment

When diagnosed with leukoplakia, the clinician should try to eliminate the possible cause either by stoppage of habit or removal of mechanical irritation. The treatment options for leukoplakia may be broadly subdivided into non-surgical treatment and surgical treatment.

Non-surgical Management

1. The use of beta-carotene in a dose of 60 mg/day for 12 months has been proven to have an effective response in preventing dysplasia in OL.
2. Retinoids are derivative compounds of natural vitamin A (retinol). Both systemic and topical therapies with vitamin A derivatives have been documented.

   Systemic-13-cis retinoic acid: A decrease in the size of oral leukoplakia was reported in patients who were provided systemic (1–2 mg/kg per day) for 3 months. However, systemic vitamin A therapy is associated with significant dose dependant toxicity including skin rash, dryness and bleeding of the nasal mucosa, conjunctivitis, oral mucositis, cheilitis, hypertriglyceridemia, and teratogenic effects.

   Topical vitamin A: Topical therapy has the potential advantages of high local dose with low systemic exposure, limiting the risk of systemic side effects.

   * 0.05% tretinoin gel applied topically 4 times per day has been proved to show complete clinical remission in some cases.
   * Topical 0.1% 13-*cis* retinoic acid (isotretinoin) gel 3 times is also effective in reducing the size of the lesion. Isotretinoin oral lozenges containing 1–5 mg 13-*cis* retinoic acid has been reported to have a similar effect.
3. Lycopene, an antioxidant, protects cells against damage and plays a protective role against progression of dysplasia by inhibiting tumor cell proliferation. 8 mg of lycopene in daily dose is an effective treatment.
4. Topical bleomycin, a cytotoxic antibiotic, has been used in the treatment of OL in dosages of 0.5%/day for 12 to 15 days.
5. Fenretinide (4-HPR) or N-(4-hydroxyphenyl) retinamide is a vitamin A analogue that has also been used in the chemoprevention of oral leukoplakia. 4 HPR has been used in both topical and systemic forms. Systemic use of 4-HPR with 200 mg/day for 3 months has been reported to produce partial clinical resolution of existing lesions.
6. **Photodynamic therapy:** The principle of this therapy is to produce photochemical reaction by using photosensitizer drugs, oxygen and visible light to eradicate the lesion. Drugs like photofrin, 5-aminolevulinic acid (ALA), verteporfin, Foscan have been used.
7. **Cryotherapy:** This method locally destroys the lesional tissues by freezing *in situ*. It has several advantages like bloodless treatment, a very low incidence of secondary infection and a relative lack of scarring and pain. Oral leukoplakia can be treated by direct application of CO_2 snow or liquid nitrogen by spray.

Surgical Treatment

1. In case of moderate to severe dysplasia surgical excision is the treatment of choice. The lesions on the ventral and lateral borders of the tongue, floor of the mouth, soft palate and oropharynx should be completely excised. Close surveillance and follow-up are mandatory for all lesions. Surgical removal is the treatment of choice for PVL.
2. **Laser surgery:** The use of carbon dioxide, Nd:YAG and KTP lasers has been suggested for the vaporization or excision of oral leukoplakia. Their precision allows a conservative and site-specific, minimally invasive surgery with sterilization of the surgical area and minimal intraoperative hemorrhage, with less postoperative swelling and pain with minimal scarring.

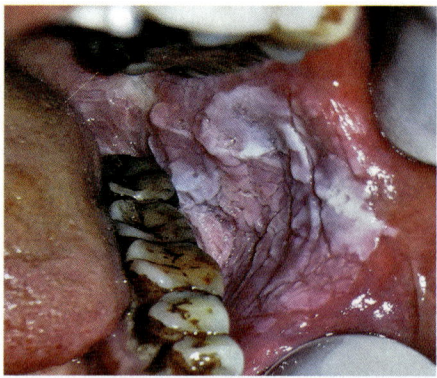

Fig. 6.2: Intra-oral photograph showing white patch, with cracked mud appearance on the left buccal mucosa, suggestive of homogenous leukoplakia

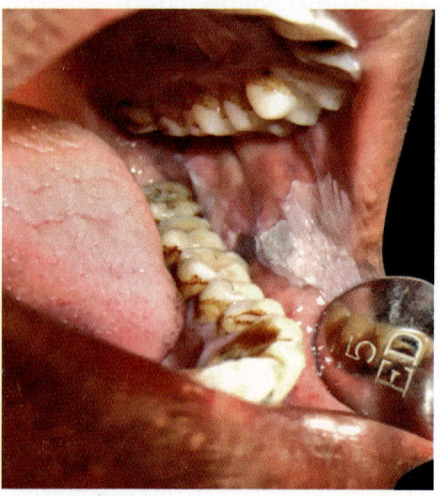

Fig. 6.3: Homogenous leukoplakia of lower left commissure and buccal mucosa

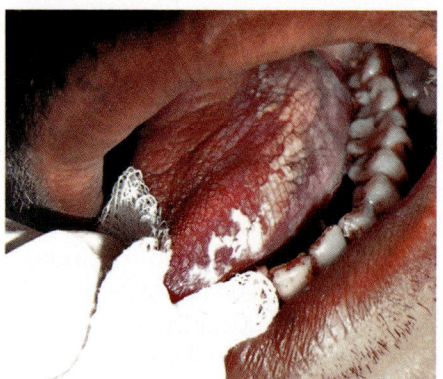

Fig. 6.4: Homogenous leukoplakia on the left lateral border of tongue

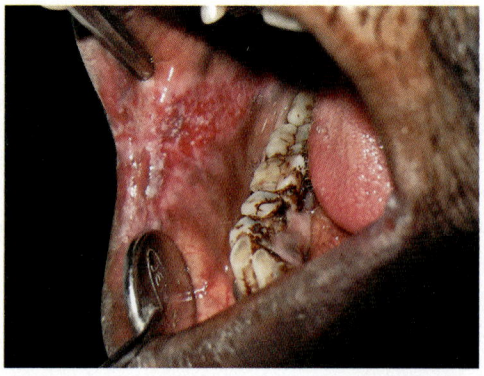

Fig. 6.5: Speckled/nodular leukoplakia lesion present on the right buccal mucosa, note the intermingled red and white clinical components and severe staining on the teeth due to heavy tobacco use

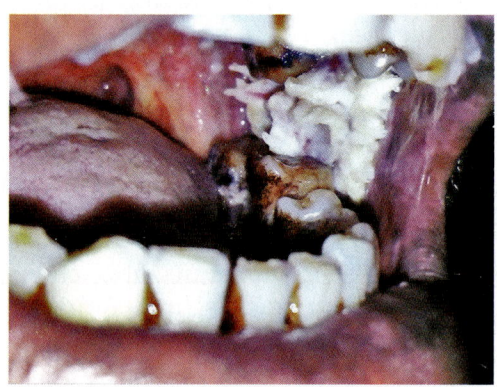

Fig. 6.6: Verrucous leukoplakia with minute projections imparting a warty, "cauliflower" like appearance

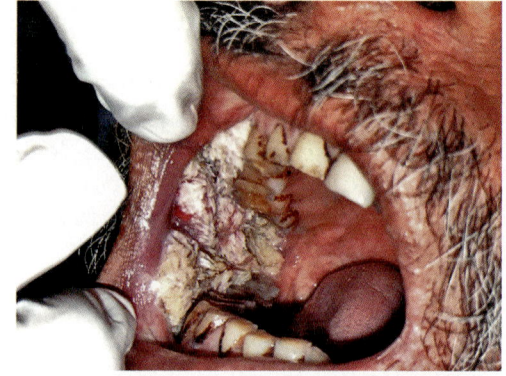

Fig. 6.7: An extensive PVL lesion on the right buccal mucosa and buccal vestibule

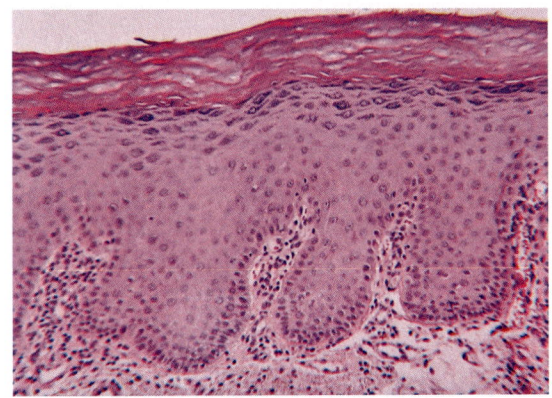

Fig. 6.8: Photomicrograph of an oral leukoplakia. H and E stained section

Erythroplakia (Erythroplasia of Queyrat)

The term erythroplakia is defined as "a red patch that cannot be clinically and pathologically diagnosed as any other condition." Queyrat used the term "erythroplasia" to describe a precancerous red lesion that develops on the penis. Almost all true erythroplakias demonstrate significant epithelial dysplasia, carcinoma *in situ* or invasive SCC. These may occur in conjunction with leukoplakia and has been found with a large proportion of early invasive oral carcinomas.

Clinical Features

Erythroplakia has no sex predilection but most cases are reported in the sixth and seventh decades. The etiology is by and large similar to that of squamous cell carcinoma. The floor of the mouth, tongue and soft palate are the most common sites of involvement and multiple lesions may be present. The altered mucosa appears as a well-demarcated erythematous macule or plaque with a soft velvety texture. It is usually asymptomatic and may be associated with adjacent leukoplakia.

Diagnosis

On histopathologic examination, the epithelium shows lack of keratin production and is often atrophic but it may be hyperplastic. This allows the underlying microvasculature to show through, thereby imparting the red color. The epithelium by far shows dysplastic changes, carcinoma *in situ* or invasive SCC. The underlying connective tissue often demonstrates chronic inflammation. Differentiation of erythroplakia from malignant change can be done by using toluidine blue applied topically or through an oral rinse.

Differential diagnosis: Non-specific mucositis, candidiasis, erosive lichen planus, or vascular lesion may mimic erythroplakia and biopsy is often required.

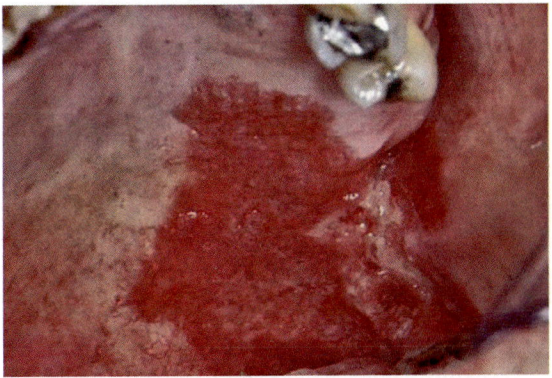

Fig. 6.9: Erythroplakia appearing as a well-demarcated red patch on the left side of the hard and soft palate

Treatment

Red lesions of the floor of the mouth and ventral or lateral tongue should be biopsied. For lesions in other locations, source of irritation, if identified should be removed, then biopsy should be performed if the lesions fail to regress after 2 weeks. As with leukoplakia the treatment of erythroplakia is guided by definitive diagnosis obtained by biopsy. Recurrence and multifocal oral mucosal involvement are common with erythroleukoplakia, hence long-term follow-up is suggested for treated patients.

Actinic Cheilitis (Cheilosis)

This is a premalignant alteration of the lower lip vermillion that results from long-term exposure to UV light or sunlight with compromised immunity.

Clinical Features

It occurs in older males more than 45 years. MF is 10:1 in some studies. The earliest change includes atrophy of the lower lip vermillion border, characterized by smooth surface and blotchy pale areas. As the lesion progresses it becomes rough, scaly and thicken resembling leukoplakia. Further, focal ulceration may develop at more than one sites finally proceeding to SCC.

Histopathology

There is an atrophic stratified squamous epithelium with marked keratin production. Varying degrees of dysplasia may be encountered.

Differential Diagnosis

Cheilocandidiasis, lip chapping, traumatic ulcer.

Treatment

Carbon dioxide or erbium: YAG laser ablation, photodynamic theory, chemoexfoliation or chemical peel with trichloroacetic acid is done. Long-term follow-up is necessary.

Actinic Keratosis (Solar Keratosis)

This is a premalignant lesion caused by cumulative ultraviolet radiation to sun exposed skin, particularly in fair-skinned people.

Etiopathogenesis

UV light exposure can produce mutations in the p53 tumor suppressor gene. Mutations in the telomerase gene represent delayed apoptosis. Apart from UV light, other potential risk factors include immunosuppression, arsenic exposure, genetic abnormalities like albinism, xeroderma pigmentosum, Cockayne syndrome, Bloom syndrome, Rothmund-Thomson syndrome.

Clinical Features

This is found in older individuals, above 40 years of age. The head, neck, face, scalp of bald-headed men, forearm, dorsum of the hands are the most common sites of occurrence. The lesions are irregular, scaly plaque which vary in color from normal to white, grey, brown superimposed an erythematic background. The lesion may be as small as 7 mm and may reach a size of 2 cm, with minimal elevation above the surface of the skin. Occasional lesions may produce so much keratin that a 'horn' may be seen arising from the central area.

Diagnosis

Histopathologically, there is hyperparakeratosis and acanthosis of epithelium. Tear drop rete ridges of the epithelium with mild epithelial dysplasia are noted. When full thickness dysplasia is noted, then it is termed **Bowenoid actinic keratosis**. Suprabasilar acantholysis with melanosis and lichenoid inflammatory infiltrate is seen. The dermis exhibits band of sun damaged collagen and elastic fibres (solar elastosis) appearing as pale basophilic area. There is increase in elastic fibres seen in this band and thickness may increase with increased exposure to actinic rays.

Differential Diagnosis

Seborrheic keratosis, skin lesions of DLE, Bowen's disease.

Treatment

The lesion is either surgically removed or destroyed by liquid nitrogen cryotherapy, curettage, electrodessication due to its precancerous nature. It is observed that 10% actinic keratosis will progress to SCC over a period of approximately 2 years.

Oral Submucous Fibrosis (OSF)

OSF is a chronic progressive, scarring disease that predominantly affects the south Asians. First described by Schwartz (1952) as "atropia idiopathica mucosa oris" and was later described by Joshi (1953) in Mumbai, who predesignated the condition as oral submucous fibrosis.

In 1966, Pindborg defined OSMF as an insidious chronic disease affecting any part of the oral cavity and sometimes the pharynx. It is associated with juxtaepithelial inflammatory reaction followed by fibroelastic changes in the lamina propria layer, along with epithelial atrophy which leads to rigidity of the oral mucosa, proceeding to trismus and difficulty in mouth opening.

Other terms such as juxtaepithelial fibrosis, idiopathic scleroderma of mouth, idiopathic palatal fibrosis, sclerosing stomatitis and diffuse OSMF have also been used. It can occur at any age but most commonly it is seen in young adults (2nd–4th decade). Onset of disease is insidious and is often 2–5 years duration. It is more prevalent in southeast Asian and Indian subcontinent. The prevalence rate in India is 0.2–0.5%. The increased prevalence is due to increased use and popularity of commercial products prepared from areca nut and tobacco products like gutkha, paan masala, flavoured supari, etc. The malignant transformation rate of OSMF is almost 7.6%.

Etiopathogenesis

It is multifactorial in origin with main etiological factors being areca nut, capsaicin in chillies, micronutrient deficiencies of iron, zinc, essential vitamins like vitamin A and B_{12}. Autoimmune etiological basis with demonstration of autoantibodies against specific HLA antigens has also been suggested.

Areca nut chewing: Areca nut (betel nut) chewing is one of the most common causes of OSMF. It contains tannins, alkaloids such as arecoline, arecadine, guanacine, guacoline. Arecaidine is an active metabolite in fibroblast stimulation and proliferation, thereby inducing collagen synthesis. With addition of slaked lime, Ca (OH) to areca as seen in Indian subcontinent, causes hydrolysis of arecoline to arecadine making it available in the oral environment. Tannin reduces the collagen degradation by inhibiting collagenase. OSMF is a combined effect of tannins and arecoline which causes excessive production of collagen and reduced degradation.

Lime is a major component of betel quid preparation which alters the oral environment to severely alkaline. Under pH more than 9.5, areca nut releases reactive oxygen species (ROS) and areca phenols (tannins and catechins) undergo auto-oxidation to release superoxide radicals and hydrogen peroxide. Also transition metal ions Cu^{2+}, Fe^{2+}, Fe^{3+}, promote reactive oxygen species (ROS) production by interacting with areca nut constituents. These ROS are capable of formation of mutated cells during replication.

Copper: Areca nut releases copper after chewing which is brought directly in contact with mucosal epithelial cells for prolonged period of time. Uptake of Cu^{2+} ions, by cells is a non-energy, non-enzyme dependent diffusion. Copper causes upregulation of enzyme lysyl oxidase which plays a crucial role in cross-linking of collagen and elastin molecules.

Nutritional deficiency: Deficiency of iron, vitamin B complex, minerals and malnutrition are the promoting factors that disturb the repair of inflamed oral mucosa, thus leading to deranged healing and resultant scarring and fibrosis. The resulting atrophic mucosa is more susceptible to the effects of chillies, betel nuts and other irritants causing burning sensation.

Genetics and immunology: The genes COL1A2, COL3A1, COL6A1, COL6A3 have been linked in the progression of disease. There is polymorphism for gene coding for TNF-α which inhibits collagen phagocytosis. Patients with OSMF have increased frequency of HLA-A10, HLA-B7 and HLAD3. There is increase in autoantibodies directed towards the gastric parietal cells, thyroid gland, anti-nuclear antibodies and anti-smooth muscle antibodies in OSMF. Humoral immunity may also play a role with increased serum levels of IgG and IgA. Serum-derived antibodies provide a basis for increase in the mucosal permeability and thereby accentuating the existing pathologic condition. A viral origin (HPV, HSV) is also linked with OSMF as decreased immune response is mediated by viral antigens and associated transformation of epithelium.

Various grading/staging classification systems have been documented by various authors in the past, which involves clinical classification, histopathological classification or their combination. A combination of clinical and histopathological classification by Khanna and Andrade is the most referred classification. A newer classification by Passi D et al (2017) includes all the parameters and components of OSMF along with treatment and prognosis. None of the previous classifications includes these features in a single classification. The main drawback of this classification is that it is lengthy and complex to read.

Clinical Features

Early stage: The prodromal symptoms include burning sensation in the mouth when consuming spicy food, appearance of vesicles especially on the palate, labial and buccal mucosa, melanosis, excessive salivation, defective gustatory sensation and dryness of the mouth (xerostomia). There are periods of exacerbation manifested by appearance of vesicles on cheek and palate for 3 months to 1 year. Petechiae are observed in about 22% of OSF cases mostly on the tongue followed by labial and buccal mucosa and soft palate. Submucosal fibres can be palpated with pain in the areas, the mucosa develops blotchy, marble-like pallor. Buccal mucosa, retromolar area, soft palate are the most commonly affected sites.

Advanced stage: As the disease progresses buccal mucosa and lips are affected symmetrically with fibrous bands in buccal mucosa running in the vertical direction. Circular bands can be felt around entire rimaorris (mouth orifice) and more marked around lower lip. There is impairment of tongue movement with significant atrophy of the tongue papillae. The density of deposition of the fibrous bands varies from a slight whitish area on the soft palate to a dense fibrosis causing fixation, shortening and deviation of the uvula and soft palate. The faucial pillars may also show slight to dense fibrosis extending deep into the pillars and causing strangulation of the tonsils. The fibrosis around pterygomandibular raphe, causes varying degrees of difficulty in the mouth opening. Sometimes fibrosis spreads to the pharynx and down to the piriform fossae. Leukoplakia on the surface of the buccal mucosae may be noted. With progressing fibrosis mouth opening reduces, inability to whistle or blow and difficulty in swallowing may be noted. When the fibrosis involves nasopharynx, there is referred pain in the ear and a nasal voice.

Histopathology

Epithelial changes include hyperplasia (early) and atrophy (advanced) changes, associated with an increased tendency for keratinizing metaplasia. Association with parakeratotic leukoplakia and atrophic epithelial changes predisposes OSF to malignancy.

Subepithelial changes

On the basis of H and E stained sections, OSF can be grouped into four clearly definable stages.

Very early, early, moderately advanced and advanced

The criteria depend on:
- Presence or absence of oedema
- Physical state of mucosal collagen
- Overall fibroblastic response
- State of blood vessel
- Predominant cell type in the inflammatory exudate

Vascular response due to inflammation has been noted in OSMF. Normal, dilated and constricted blood vessels can be seen in combination in the same section. The narrowing of smaller vessels appears first in upper mucosa and with the advancing stage involves larger, deeper vessels. Persistent dilation has been noted in moderately advanced and advanced cases. In earlier stages, mast cells predominate which fall to fewer numbers at a later stage. The inflammatory cells are mainly lymphocytes and plasma cells. In the advanced stage, submucosal connective tissue shows extremely dense and avascular collagenous tissue, variable numbers of chronic inflammatory cells. Epithelial dysplasia without carcinoma may be evident in large number of biopsy tissues (10–15%) with frank carcinoma in at least 5% cases. The excessive fibrosis in the submucosa seems to occur earlier than atrophic changes in the epithelium.

Investigations and Blood Chemistry

There is increased ESR, anemia and eosinophilia, increased gamma globulins, reduction in serum iron, and increase in total iron binding capacity. A significant alteration in the serum copper and zinc ratio is also reported.

Differential Diagnosis

× *Oral manifestations of scleroderma:* Scleroderma can be distinguished by other cutaneous, systemic, and characteristic laboratory findings.
× Subjective symptoms of burning sensation of the oral mucosa may be confused with those caused by oral lichen planus and anemia as the latter are also associated with atrophic oral mucosa.
× Other causes of trismus including TMJ dysfunction, tetanus and localised infection are easily distinguishable by proper history and examination.

Management

The management of oral submucous fibrosis depends on the degree of clinical involvement. If the disease is detected at a very early stage, cessation of the areca nut/tobacco chewing habit along with cessation of smoking, alcohol and restriction of hot and spicy food are sufficient. Moderate-to-severe oral submucous fibrosis is irreversible.

Medical Management

1. *Nutritional supplement and antioxidants:* Lycopene is a tomato extract and one of the most potent carotenoid antioxidants. Lycopene capsules in a daily dose of 8–16 mg have been proven to have a beneficial effect in reducing the OSF associated symptoms and in preventing the disease progress. As an antioxidant it has the highest singlet oxygen quenching capacity with high capability of quenching other free radicals. Lycopene also exerts an anti-inflammatory effect as well as inhibits abnormal fibroblast proliferation in OSF.

2. *Steroids:* Steroids suppress inflammatory reactions, thereby preventing fibrosis by decreasing fibroblastic proliferation and deposition of collagen. Topical applications triamcinolone acetonide 0.1% (kenacort) and betamethasone—0.5% (betnesol) have been reported to reduce the symptoms of burning sensation. Alternatively, injections of dexamethasone 1.5 ml, with hyaluronidase 1500 IU and 0.5 ml lignocaine HCl injected intralesionally biweekly for 4–6 weeks has also been tried and has been reported to produce a definite reduction in burning sensation, blanching of oral mucosa and marginal improvement in mouth opening.

3. *Placental extract:* Placental extract contains growth factors and anti-inflammatory agents and also has antiplatelet activity. It has biogenic stimulator action and is used on the basis of tissue therapy method. It stimulates metabolism, increases the vascularity and promotes regeneration and recovery of the tissue, upon implantation into the body. Submucosal injection of Placentrex (2 ml) are given alone/ in conjunction with intralesional steroids.

4. *Interferon gamma:* IFN-gamma is a known antifibrotic cytokine. IFN-gamma, through its effect of altering collagen synthesis, appears to be a key factor to the treatment of patients with oral submucous fibrosis, and intralesional injections of the cytokine may have a significant therapeutic effect on oral submucous fibrosis.

5. *Peripheral vasodilators:* Vasodilators like pentoxifylline and oral isoxsuprine have vasodilating properties and help in increasing the hampered mucosal vascularity in OSF. Pentoxifylline also suppresses leucocyte function and alters fibroblast physiology and stimulates fibrinolysis. Pentoxifylline in a dose of 400 mg 3 times daily, as coated, sustained release tablets have been used as an adjunct therapy in the management of oral submucous fibrosis.

6. *Herbal extracts:* Several herbal compounds including curcumin (found in turmeric), aloe vera and spirulina have been shown to possess antioxidant and anti-inflammatory properties and have accorded significant relief in subjective symptoms of OSF.

Surgical management

1. *Surgical excision:*
   × Surgical treatment of OSF by excision of the fibrous bands followed by inter-position of local flaps/graft material have been documented in severe cases of OSF.
   × The commonly used extra-oral and intra-oral flaps include the nasolabial flap, temporalis fascia flap, buccal pad of fat, tongue flap, palatal island flap.
   × Grafting materials used are split skin grafts (SSG), collagen membranes and artificial dermis for the mucomuscular defects in the surgical management of OSMF.
   × Adjunctive temporalis muscle myotomy and coroinoidectomy has also been used to maintain the mouth opening achieved.

2. *Laser surgery:* ErCr:YSGG laser and carbon dioxide laser fibrotomy under local anesthesia is a minimally invasive, cost effective, chairside procedure and an useful adjunct in management of moderate OSMF.

3. *Cryosurgery:* Cryosurgery is an efficient method for tissue destruction by means of freezing. It has been used in the management of various oral lesions like the oral submucous fibrosis, oral leukoplakia, pyogenic granuloma, actinic cheilitis, vascular lesions, mucocele, keratoacanthoma, etc.
   × *Advantages:* Absence of bleeding, minimal pain, low incidence of infection, economical and relatively safe in patients with a pacemaker, the elderly, and those with coagulopathies. Useful in cases of multiple and extensive lesions and areas of difficult surgical access.
   × *Procedure:* Cryosurgery is performed using N_2O refrigerant gas and cryoprobe. After placing the cryoprobe over the lesion coolant gas is allowed to flow through the channels in the metal tip of the cryoprobe for duration of about 7 s after which lesion is allowed to thaw to complete one freeze thaw cycle. The hypothermia produced by this procedure resulted in ice crystal formation leading to destruction of the tissue.

Adjuvant modalities

1. *Diathermy:* Diathermy is a selective deep heating therapy. Both shortwave and microwave diathermy have been tried as adjuvant treatment modalities in OSF. Heat therapy acts by fibrinolysis of bands. Microwave diathermy selectively heats only juxtaepithelial connective tissue further limiting the area to be treated. Thus, it is easy to apply with minimum discomfort. A proposed regimen advocates the use of microwave diathermy every day for 20 min at each

site of lesion by means of 20–25 watts of energy to create comfortable warmth.

2. *Ultrasound:* Therapeutic ultrasound is an effective adjuvant along with combination therapy in patients of OSMF. Therapeutic effects obtained by ultrasonic energy are due to increased vascular and fluid circulation, increase in cell permeability, and increase in pain threshold and a break in pain cycle.

3. *Physiotherapy:* This includes muscle stretching exercises and heat therapy. They are helpful in preventing any further reduction in mouth opening.

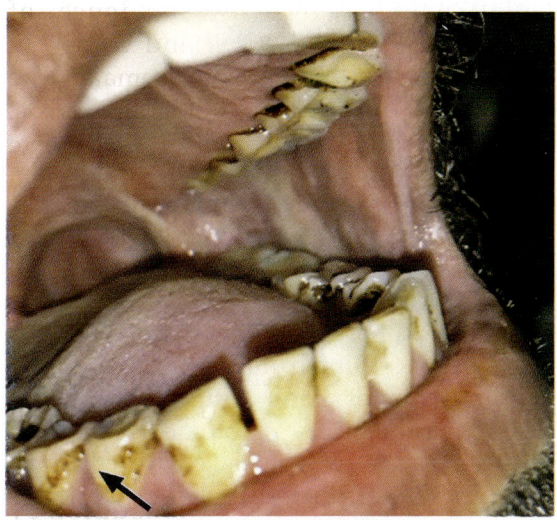

Fig. 6.10: Blanched, marble-like appearance seen on the buccal mucosa in OSF

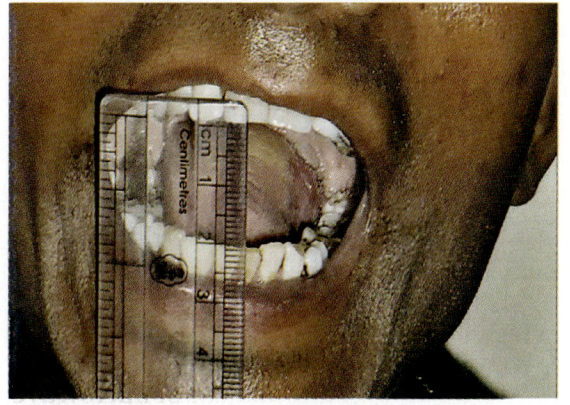

Fig. 6.11: Restricted mouth opening in OSF

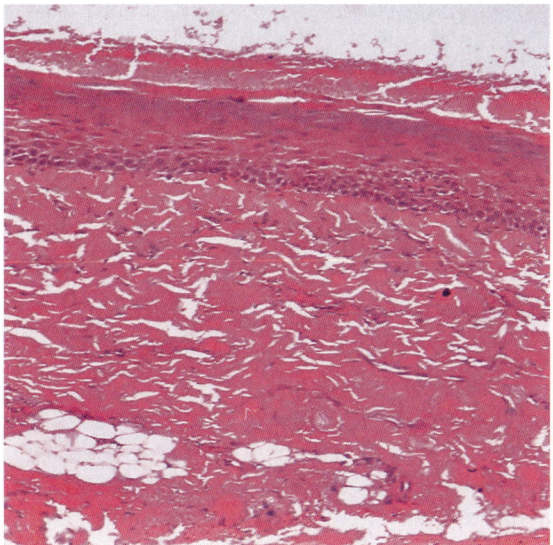

Fig. 6.12: Photomicrograph of H and E stained section showing atrophic epithelium with loss of rete ridges and hyalinization of connective tissue

IMMUNOLOGICALLY MEDIATED DISEASES

Oral Lichen Planus (OLP)

Lichen planus is a chronic mucocutaneous disorder of the stratified squamous epithelium that affects oral and genital membranes skin, nails and scalp. OLP is the mucous counterpart of cutaneous Lichen planus. It is derived from the Greek word *lichen* means tree moss and Latin word *planus* means flat.

History

The disease was first presented by the English physician Erasmus Wilson in 1866. He considered it to be the same disease described by Hebra previously as Lichen ruler. In 1892, Kaposi reported clinical variant of the disease, lichen rubber pemphigoid. In 1895, Wickham noted the characteristic reticulate white lines on surface of lichen planus papules, recognized as Wickham's striae. Darriel is credited with the first formal histopathological description.

Epidemiology

Different prevalence figures have been reported for OLP and vary from 0.5 to 2.2%. The proportion of women affected is higher with age range between 30 and 60 years. OLP occurs more frequently than cutaneous forms and tends to be more persistent and resistant to treatment.

Etiology

The exact etiology is unknown. Some of the factors associated with it are

* **Genetic background:** Familial cases are seen in association with HLA-A3, A11, A26, A28, B3, B5, B7, B8 DR1 and DRW9 have been noted. There is increase in HLA-DRW9 and Te 22 antigens in the Chinese population
* **Dental materials:** Silver amalgam, gold, cobalt, chromium, palladium, cadmium, have been identified as the triggering elements for OLP. Epoxy resins (composites) restorations and prolonged denture usage can also lead to OLP lesions.
* **Drugs:** Lichenoid like reactions may be triggered by systemic drugs, including NSAIDs, beta blockers, sulfonylureas, some anti-malarial ACE inhibitors.
* **Infectious agents:** OLP has been found to be associated with various viral agents such as HPV, EBV, HHV-6 and HIV virus. Epidemiological evidenced worldwide strongly suggest HCV as an etiological factor in OLP. Hepatitis C virus has been reported in the epithelial cells from the mucosa by rt-PCR or *in situ* hybridization. HCV specific CD4 and CD8 lymphocytes were reported in the subepithelial band. These suggest role of HCV in oral lichen planus.
* **Autoimmunity:** Autoreactive T lymphocytes may be of importance in the development of OLP. These cells cannot discriminate between the inherent molecules of the body and the foreign antigens. It may be associated with other autoimmune disorders such as primary biliary cirrhosis, chronic hepatitis, myasthenia gravis and thymoma. Bowel diseases showing concomitant OLP include celiac disease, ulcerative colitis and Crohn's disease.
* **Food allergies:** Food additives such as cinnamon have been found to be associated with OLP.
* **Stress:** Anxiety and stress have revealed the role of psychologic stress in the etiology of OLP
* **Trauma:** Could be a mechanism by which other etiological factors exert their effect.
* **Diabetes and hypertension** have been associated with OLP—'Greenspan syndrome'
* **Malignant neoplasm:** Lichen planus has been observed on the skin or mucosae of patients affected with breast cancer and metastatic adenocarcinoma.

Pathogenesis

OLP is a T-cell mediated autoimmune disease in which the auto-cytotoxic CD8+ T cells trigger the apoptosis of the basal cells of the oral epithelium. The CD+ lesional T cells may recognize an antigen associated with major histocompatibility complex (MHC) class I on keratinocytes. After antigen recognition and activation, CD8+ cytotoxic T Cells may trigger, basal cell apoptosis. Activated CD+T cells and keratinocytes release cytokines that attract additional lymphocytes into the developing lesion, thereby causing a vicious cycle.

Clinical Features

The cutaneous lesions of LP are characterized by 5 Ps—purple, polygonal, pruritic, papules and plaques. Initially evident cutaneous lesion is usually a discrete, flat topped papule that is 3 to 15 mm in diameter coalesce and form larger plaque. Initially, the lesions may appear red but eventually they take on reddish purple or violaceous hue. The centre of the papule may be slightly umbilicated and is surface is covered by characteristic, very fine, greyish white lines, called Wickham's striae. The lesions are seen more on the flexor surfaces of the limbs, inner aspects of knees and thighs and the trunk. The primary symptoms are severe pruritis. The severity of pruritis varies, some patients may report scalp, genital or nailbed involvement.

Oral Manifestations

The oral manifestations are different from that on the skin and is characterised by bilaterally symmetrical lesions consisting of radiating, white, grey, velvety, thread-like papules in a linear, annular or retiform pattern forming lacy reticular patches, rings and streaks. A tiny elevated white dot is present at the intersection of white lines known as striae of Wickham. Most commonly seen on the buccal mucosa, tongue, lips, gingiva, floor of the mouth palate and may appear weeks or months before appearance of cutaneous lesions. The oral lesions produce no significant symptoms, although patients may complain of burning sensation in the involved areas.

The oral lesions can have a clinically varied presentation (Fig. 6.13).

- **Reticular:** This is the most common clinical form and presents with fine, asymptomatic intertwined lace-like pattern called Wickham's striae in a bilateral symmetric form involving posterior aspect of buccal mucosa.
- **Atrophic:** Appears as smooth, red, poorly defined areas, often with peripheral striae evident on gingiva of postmenopausal women.
- **Ulcerative:** Vesicular or bulla formation may be seen which rupture and erode resulting into frankly ulcerated lesions, irregular in size and shape appears as raw, painful, areas. Despite the erosion of the mucosa, the characteristic radiating striae may be noted on the periphery, of the individual lesions.
- **Plaque-like:** Hypertrophic form appearing as well circumscribed, elevated white lesions resembling leukoplakia mainly on the buccal mucosa and tongue.
- **Papular:** This is a rarely observed form. It presents with small white papules with fine striae in its periphery.

Diagnosis: The history, typical oral lesions, skin and nail involvement are sufficient for clinical diagnosis. A biopsy is recommended to differentiate from the other lesions.

Histopathology

The histopathological findings include hyper para or orthokeratosis with the thickening of granular layer, acanthosis with intercellular edema of spinous layer in some instances or atrophic epithelium where the rete pegs may be shortened pointed giving a characteristic saw-tooth appearance of rete pegs. Band like subepithelial infiltrate consisting of T-cells and histiocytes, increased numbers of intraepithelial T-cells, degenerating basal keratinocytes that form, civatte (hyaline, cytoid) bodies which appear as homogenous eosinophilic globules. Degeneration of basal keratinocytes and disruptions of anchoring fibrils of epithelial basement membrane and basal keratinocytes weakens the epithelium connective tissue interface. As a result, a histologic cleft (Max-Joseph space) may form blisters that can be seen on the oral mucosa. Direct immunofluorescence studies on the oral lichen antibody planus have shown that the antifibrinogenic antibody reacts with the lesions and exhibits strap positive fluorescence that outlines basement membrane zone and numerous irregular extensions into superficial lamina propria.

Differential diagnosis: Lichenoid reactions, oral lesions of graft-versus-host disease (GVHD), leukoplakia, may be confused with reticular and plaque-like varieties. Erosive forms may mimic atrophic candidiasis, pemphigus, cicatricial pemphigoid, and erythema multiforme.

Malignant transformation: The potential of malignant transformation remains small, i.e. 0.3–3.8%. Most of the reported cases have been confined to erosive and atrophic forms.

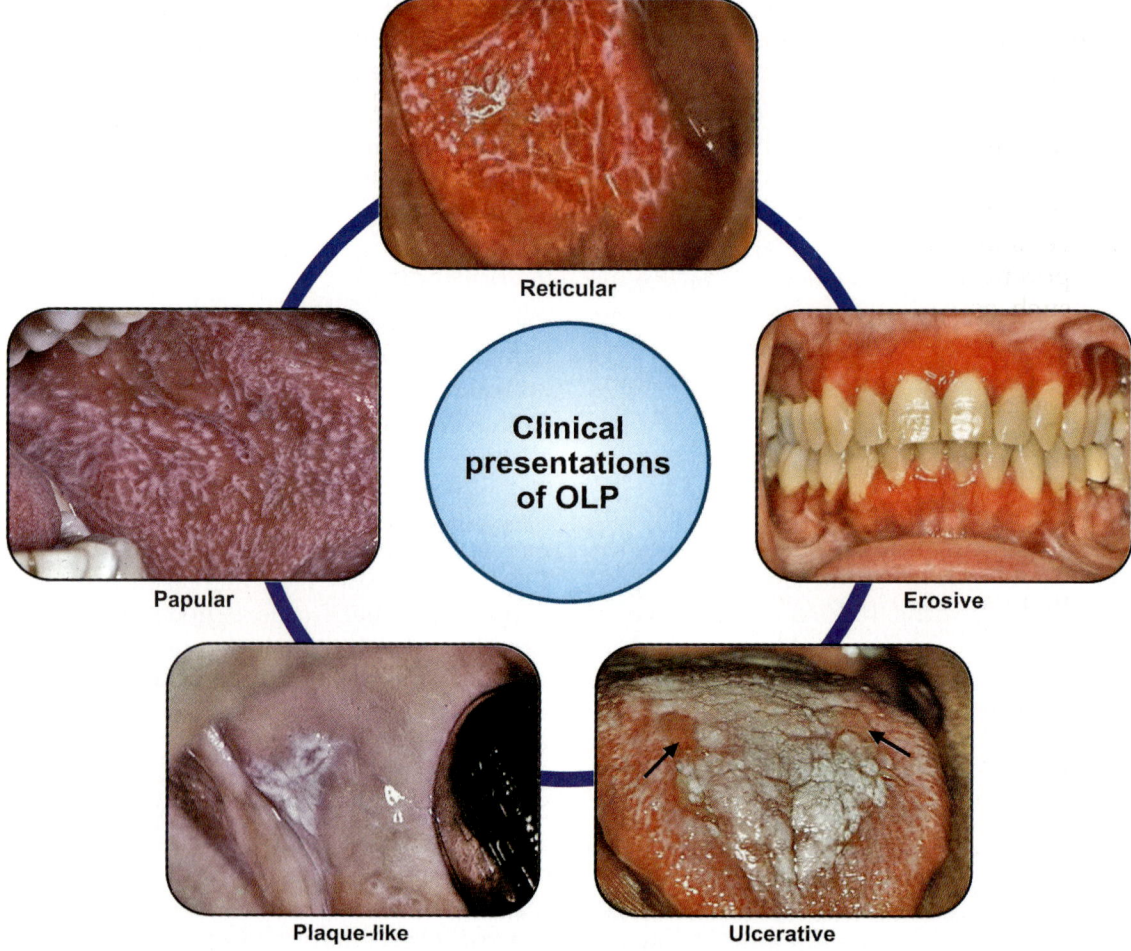

Fig. 6.13: The varied clinical appearances of oral lichen planus

Treatment: The primary aims of oral lichen planus therapy are the resolution of painful symptoms and oral mucosal lesions, the reduction of the risk of oral cancer, and the maintenance of good oral hygiene. In patients with recurrent disease, prolongation of the symptom-free intervals is another management goal. No treatment for oral lichen planus is definitely curative.

General Guidelines

* Eliminate all local exacerbating factors including sharp teeth, broken restorations or prostheses that are likely to cause physical trauma to areas of erythema or erosion.
* Thorough scaling of the teeth to remove calculus deposits.
* Removal and replacement of any dental restoration/drug identified as possible etiological factor for the lesion.
* General measure to reduce stress-like mediation and relaxation training.
* Patient education regarding the potentially malignant nature of the disease.
* Advise complete cessation of tobacco and alcohol consumption and advise a diet rich in fresh fruits and vegetables.

Medicinal Management

1. **Corticosteroids:** Corticosteroids have been the mainstay of management of

OLP. Corticosteroids act by reducing inflammation and immune reponse.

Topical therapy

- Topical midpotency corticosteroids such as triamcinolone acetonide (0.1%), high-potent corticosteroids such as fluocinonide acetonide, disodium betamethasone phosphate, and super-potent halogenated corticosteroids such as clobetasol (0.05%) are used based on the severity of the lesion. The greatest limitation in using topical corticosteroids is their lack of adherence to the mucosa for a sufficient length of time.
- Small and accessible erosive lesions located on the gingiva and palate can be treated by the application of the drug in an adherent paste with the help of a custom tray. This allows for accurate control over the contact time and ensures that the entire lesional surface is exposed to the drugs.
- Patients with extensive OLP lesions may be precribed high-potent and superpotent corticosteroids mouthwashes and intralesional injections.
- Long-term use of topical steroid can lead to the development of secondary candidiasis which necessitates antifungal therapy.

Systemic therapy

- Systemic corticosteroids are reserved for recalcitrant erosive OLP lesions where topical approaches have failed.
- Systemic prednisolone is the drug of choice, but should be used at the lowest possible dosage for the shortest duration. One milligram per kilogram daily for 7 days has been suggested, followed by a reduction of 10 mg each subsequent day. A maintenance dose with topical steroids may be commenced during the tapering of the systemic steroids.

2. **Immunomodulatory agents:** Calcineurin inhibitors

- *Cyclosporine:* Cyclosporine inhibits lymphokine production and interleukin release, leading to a reduced function of effector T-cells. It is used as a mouth-rinse or topically with adhesive bases in OLP. However, the drug is expensive and should be reserved for highly recalcitrant cases of OLP. It is known to cause dose-related gum hyperplasia which reduces when the drug is withdrawn. Systemically administered cyclosporin has been used in a dose of 150 mg, twice a day in cases of severe recalcitrant erosive lichen planus. Topically, cyclosporine oral solution (100 mg/ml) as a "swish and spit" medication, 3 times daily, each rinse cycle lasting for 5 min has also been tried.
- *Tacrolimus:* Tacrolimus is a macrolide immunosuppressant. It is 10–100 times as potent as cyclosporine and it has a greater capacity to penetrate the mucosa. It has been successfully used in recalcitrant OLP cases. The immunosuppressive action of tacrolimus is similar to that of cyclosporine. Burning sensation is a common side effect. A potential risk of development of carcinoma from its prolonged use is documented. Hence, its use is recommended for short periods of time. 0.1% ointment is used.
- *Pimecrolimus* has significant antiinfla-mmatory activity and immunomodu-latory capabilities with low systemic immunosuppressive potential. 1% topical cream of pimecrolimus has been successfully used as treatment for OLP.

Retinoids: Topical retinoids such as tretinoin, isotretinoin and fenretinide, with their immunomodulating properties, have been reported to be effective in OLP. Their use should be weighed against their significant side effects like cheilitis, elevation of serum liver enzymes and triglyceride levels and teratogenicity. Doses for these agents are same as used for the treatment of leukoplakia.

Dapsone: It is an antibacterial agent traditionally used in the treatment of leprosy. It is effective in the treatment of lichen planus due to its anti-inflammatory action and inhibition of mast cell activity. Dapsone 100 mg per day for 3 months has been reported to produce a significant improvement in the burning sensation and reduction in size of the erosive areas with minimal side effects (Fig. 6.14).

Others: Mycophenolate mofetil [MMF] (oral administration: Capsules containing 250 mg of MMF, tablets containing 500 mg of MMF, and as a powder for oral suspension, which when constituted contains 200 mg / ml MMF). **Efalizumab** (a monoclonal antibody, once a week as a sub-cutaneous injection)

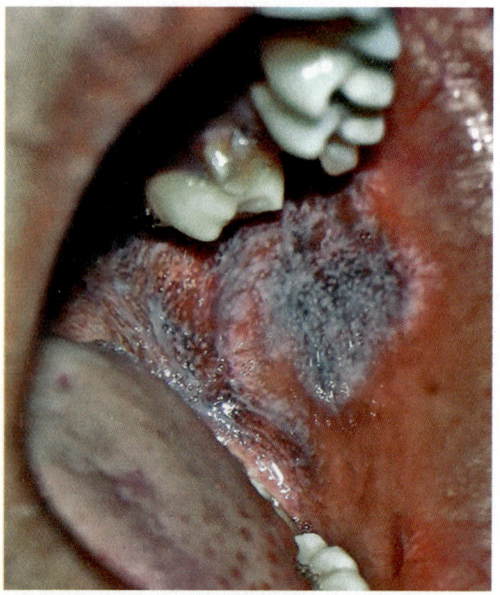

Fig. 6.14: Papular lichen planus with reticular form at the periphery and areas of hyperpigmentation

Non-pharmacological Modalities

PUVA therapy: PUVA (psoralen and ultra-violet A therapy) uses photochemotherapy with 8-methoxypsoralen and long wave ultraviolet light (PUVA). Psoralens are plant derive compounds that make skin temporarily sensitive to UV radiation. Methoxy psoralen is given orally 0.6 mg / kg, 2 hours before of UV irradiation, intraorally

in the affected sites. It has been successfully used in the treatment of severe cases of OLP. Disadvantages of this therapy include nausea and dizziness secondary to psoralen and photosensitivity for up to 24 hours.

Photodynamic therapy: Photodynamic therapy (PDT) is a technique that uses a photosensitizing compound like methylene blue which is activated by laser light of specific wavelengths, to produce oxidizers, which cause cellular damage. PDT is found to have immunomodulatory effects and induces apoptosis in the hyperproliferating inflammatory cells present in lichen planus.

Laser therapy: 980 nm diode laser, CO_2 laser, pulsed diode laser using 904 nm pulsed infrared rays have been tried in the treatment of oral lichen planus. All types of laser destroy the superficial epithelium by protein denaturation. A deeper penetrating beam like the diode laser destroys the underlying connective tissue with the inflammatory component along the epithelium (Fig. 6.15).

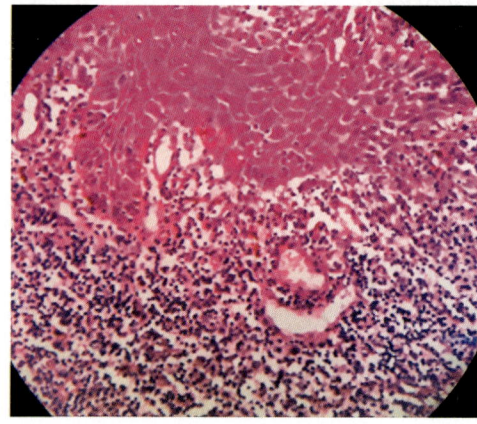

Fig. 6.15: Photomicrograph of lichen planus: H and E stained section

Drug-induced Lichenoid Reactions

Etiopathogenesis

Drug-induced lichenoid reactions are essentially delayed hypersensitivity type of reactions. It has been hypothesized that drugs or their metabolites act as hapten triggers for the lichenoid reaction. Some of the examples of drugs that cause drug-induced lichenoid reactions are penicillin, gold and sulphonamides. It has been postulated that drug-induced lichenoid reactions may result from poor drug metabolism because of genetic variation of the major cytochrome P-450 enzymes.

Clinical Features

The drug-induced lichenoid reactions are predominantly unilateral in appearance and with an ulcerative reaction pattern along with lesions appearing clinically similar to oral lichen planus.

Diagnosis

Drug-induced lichenoid reactions often pose diagnostic challenge as the condition may be associated with a large number of drugs (Table 6.2). However, diagnosis is easier if a new drug is recently started. Drug-induced lichenoid reactions often may not develop for several months after a new drug is started and may take weeks or months to disappear after withdrawal.

Differential diagnosis: Oral lichen planus, oral lichenoid contact reactions. Careful history and clinical examination help distinguish the drug-induced lesions.

Management

Discontinuation of the drug and topical steroid application are sufficient to treat drug-induced lichenoid reactions. Patient should be educated and made aware about the drug causing the lesion for the prevention of future drug-induced lichenoid reactions.

Graft-versus-host Disease

Etiopathogenesis

This disease occurs mainly in the recipients of allogenic bone marrow transplants for patients suffering from disease of blood or bone marrow. The donor supplies haematopoietic stem cells obtained from bone marrow, peripheral blood or umbilical cord blood. However, to provide the

TABLE 6.2: Drugs implicated to cause oral lichenoid reactions

Drugs known to cause lichenoid reaction	
ACE inhibitors	Mercury (amalgam)
Allopurinol	Metformin
Amiphenazole	Methyldopa
Antimalarials	Metronidazole
Barbiturates	Niridazole
BCG vaccine	NSAIDs
Captopril	Oral contraceptives
Carbamazepine	Oxpronolol
Carbimazole	Para-aminosalicylate
Chloral hydrate	Penicillamine
Chloroquine	Penicillins
Chlorpropamide	Phenindione
Cholera vaccine	Phenothiazines
Cinnarizine	Phenylbutazones
Clofibrate	Phenytoin
Colchicine	Piroxicam
Dapsone	Practolol
Dipyridamole	Prazosin
Ethionamide	Procainamide
Flunarizine	Propranolol
Gaunoclor	Propylthiouracil
Gold	Protease inhibitors
Griseofulvin	Prothionamide
Hepatitis B vaccine	Quinidine
Hydroxychloroquine	Quinine
Interferon	Rifampicin
Ketoconazole	Rituximab
Labetalol	Streptomycin
Levamisole	Sulfonamide
Lincomycin	Tetracycline
Lithium	Tocainide
Lorazepam	Tolbutamide
Mepacrine	Triprolidine

transplant, an HLA-matched donor must be found. Unfortunately, this HLA match is not always exact and despite the use of immunosuppressive drugs such as prednisolone, methotrexate, cyclosporin, the graft is recognized as foreign and the cells start attacking what they perceive as a foreign body and the condition which results is graft-versus-host disease (GVHD).

Clinical Features

The symptoms could be acute and chronic depending on milder disease in patients with better HLA match and age of the individual.

Acute GVHD: It is observed within first few weeks or first 100 days after transplant particularly in bone marrow transplant patients. The skin lesions may range from mild rash to severe sloughing resembling toxic epidermal necrolysis. The associated symptoms are fever, nausea, vomiting, diarrhoea, abdominal pain and liver dysfunction.

Chronic GVHD: It may represent previously diagnosed case of acute GVHD or appear after days. This forms mimics variety of autoimmune condition such as systemic lupus erythematosus, Sjögren's syndrome, primary biliary cirrhosis. Skin lesions may mimic lichen planus or systemic sclerosis.

Oral Manifestations

The lesions appear as a reticular network of white striae resembling OLP. Diffuse pattern of pinpoint white papules is also seen. Burning sensation of oral mucosa is often present along with candidiasis. Atrophy of oral mucosa may be seen. Ulcerations are seen related to chemotherapeutic conditioning and neutropenic state. Ulcers often develop during first 2 weeks of transplant. If they persist longer than 2 weeks than acute GVHD should be considered and differentiated from intra-oral herpes virus or bacterial infection. Xerostomia is a common complaint along with the development of small, superficial mucoceles on palate indicating destruction of salivary gland tissue by immunologic response.

Diagnosis

The diagnosis of GVHD may be difficult because of varied manifestations. However, oral lesions have a highly predictive index in presence of GVHD.

Differential diagnosis: Since oral GVHD may manifest as lichenoid, erosive or ulcerative lesions, these reactions may mimic lichen planus, drug-induced reactions and contact allergies.

Management

Primary strategy of dealing with GVHD is to reduce or prevent its occurrence. Careful HLA matching is performed and patient is given prophylactic immunosuppressive and immune modulating therapy with the combination of prednisone, cyclosporin or tacrolimus. If GVHD develops, then mycophenolate mofetil or azathioprine may be added. Topical steroids may facilitate healing of focal oral ulcerations and OLP like lesions. Use of PUVA therapy, i.e psoralen and UVA has shown to improve these lesions. In case of dentulous patients with xerostomia topical fluorides may be used to prevent xerostomia related caries. Salivary flow can be enhanced by using pilocarpine hydrochloride or cevimeline hydrochloride. Patient's oral health status may be evaluated before transplant to remove potential source of infection. In general, some degree of GVHD often develops after allogenic bone marrow transplant. Prognosis depends on disease progress and control.

Lupus Erythematosus

Etiopathogenesis

Lupus erythematosus (LE) is an immunologically mediated condition. Environmental factors include sun exposure, drugs, chemical substances and hormones which aggravate the disease. Genetic predisposition with elevated risk for siblings in monozygotic twins has been supported.

It has the following clinical subtypes:

- **Systemic lupus erythematosus (SLE):** SLE is a serious multisystem disease with a variety of cutaneous and oral manifestations. There is an increase in the activity of B-lymphocytes in conjunction with abnormal function of T-lymphocytes. There is an interplay between genetic and environmental factors in development of SLE.
- **Chronic cutaneous LE (CCLE):** It primarily affects skin and oral mucosa. This has fairly good prognosis.
- **Subacute cutaneous LE (SCLE):** It is a third form of disease which is intermediate between those of SLE and CCE.

Clinical Features

SLE: Women are affected 8–10 times more frequently than men. The average age is 31 years. In 40–50% of affected patients, a characteristic rash, having the pattern of a butterfly, develops over the malar area and nose typically sparing the nasolabial folds. Sunlight often worsens the lesions. Kidneys are affected in 40–50% of cases. The complications may ultimately lead to kidney failure. Cardiac involvement with pericarditis being the common complication. There are warty vegetations affecting heart valves in 50% of cases (Libman-Sacks endocarditis). Oral lesions predispose as lichenoid areas on buccal mucosa, gingiva and palate. Involvement of the vermillion border of lip is also seen. Varying degrees of ulceration, pain, erythema and hyperparakeratosis may be present. Xerostomia, candidiasis, periodontal disease, dysgeusia have also been described. Diagnosis can be confirmed by American Rheumatism Association and these include both clinical and laboratory findings (Table 6.3).

Chronic cutaneous lupus erythematosus (CCLE)—discoid lupus erythematosus (DLE): The skin lesions begin as scaly erythematous patches that are frequently

TABLE 6.3: American College of Rheumatology Criteria for systemic lupus erythematosus

1. Malar rash
2. Discoid lesions
3. Photosensitivity
4. Presence of oral ulcers
5. Nonerosive arthritis of two joints or more
6. Serositis
7. Renal disorder
8. Neurologic disorder (seizures or psychosis)
9. Hematologic disorder (hemolytic anemia, leukopenia, lymphopenia, or thrombocytopenia)
10. Immunologic disorder (anti-DNA, anti-SM, or antiphospholipid antibodies).

distributed on sun exposed skin in head and neck area. The lesions are exacerbated by sunlight. The lesions may heal with time, only to appear in another area. The healing results in cutaneous atrophy with scarring and hypopigmentation of the resolving area. Oral lesions of DLE are similar to erosive lichen planus and seldom occur without skin lesions. An ulcerated or atrophic, erythematous central zone surrounded by white fine, radiating striae characterizes oral lesion of DLE. Sometimes the central zone may show stippling of white dots. The ulcerative oral lesions may be painful.

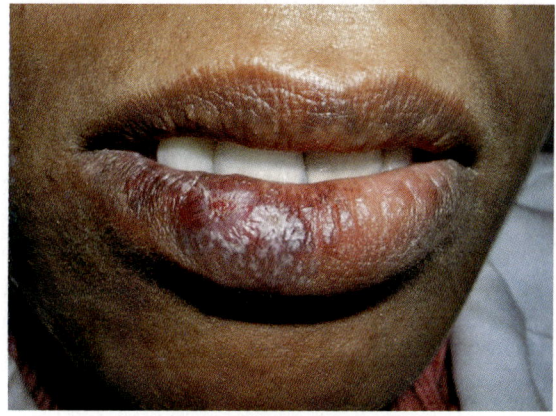

Fig. 6.16: DLE lesion involving lower lip

Subacute cutaneous LE: SCLE may be triggered by anyone of a variety of medications (Table 6.4). It is usually seen in the patients with arthritis or musculoskeletal problems. The skin lesions predominate in the sun-exposed areas.

TABLE 6.4: Drugs causing lupus erythematosus-like eruptions

Medications implicated in lupus erythematosus-like eruptions	
⁎ Carbamazepine	⁎ Etanercept
⁎ Chlorpromazine	⁎ Ethosuximide
⁎ Gold	⁎ Hydantoins
⁎ Griseofulvin	⁎ Hydralazine
⁎ Infliximab	⁎ Lithium
⁎ Isoniazid	⁎ Methyldopa
⁎ Penicillamine	⁎ Procainamide
⁎ Primidone	⁎ Quinidine
⁎ Reserpine	⁎ Thiouracil
⁎ Streptomycin	⁎ Trimethadione

Diagnosis

Histopathology

Skin lesions: There is presence of hyper-parakeratosis, with keratin plugging in hair follicles. In all forms of LE, degeneration of the basal cell layer is observed and underlying connective tissue shows patchy to dense aggregates of chronic inflammatory cells. Deeper areas of connective tissue show chronic inflammatory cells surrounding small blood vessels.

Oral lesions: The oral lesions typically mimic oral lichen planus. However, the two conditions can be distinguished by the presence of patchy deposits of PAS deposits materials in the basement membrane zone, subepithelial edema and a more diffuse, deep inflammatory infiltrate often in a perivascular orientation. Differentiation of LE from OLP is best seen by immunofluorescence studies.

Direct immunofluorescence: It shows the deposition of one or more immunoreactants (IgM, IgG or C3) in a shaggy or a granular band at the basement membrane zone. Evaluation of the serum obtained from the patients with SLE have antibodies against multiple nuclear antigens (ANA). Antibodies directed against the double-stranded DNA are noted. Also, antibodies against Sm, a protein that is complexed with small nuclear RNA is very specific for SLE.

Differential diagnosis
- **SLE:** The differential diagnosis for SLE includes sunburn, photosensitivity, rash caused by vitamin deficiency (pellagra), discoid lupus erythematosus, seborrheic dermatitis, dermatomyositis, and drug eruptions.
- **DLE:** The differential diagnosis for DLE includes seborrheic dermatitis, psoriasis, superficial basal cell carcinoma and systemic lupus erythematosus.

Treatment

To obtain relief from oral symptoms, topical steroids may be tried. Immunosuppressive drugs used to treat LE may precipitate opportunistic fungal and viral infections. Oral ulcerations may also occur due to frequent use of NSAIDs. Oral lesions may regress spontaneously but can also persist for months or even years. Table 6.4 delineates the various topical agents used in the treatment of SLE (Table 6.5).

TABLE 6.5: Topical treatment options for oral lesions or lupus erythematosus

	Directions for use
Topical steroids	
1. 0.05% fluocinonide gel	⁎ Place on affected areas twice a day for 2 weeks
2. 0.05% clobetasol gel	⁎ Place on affected areas twice a day for 2 weeks
3. Dexamethasone elixir (0.5 mg/ml)	
4. Triamcinolone acetonide 5 mg/ml	⁎ Swish and spit 10 ml 4 times a day for 2 weeks
	⁎ Intralesional injection

Contd.

TABLE 6.5: Topical treatment options for oral lesions or lupus erythematosus *(Contd.)*

	Directions for use
Topical antifungals 1. 10 mg clotrimazole troches 2. Nystatin suspension (100,000 U/ml)	× Dissolve in mouth, 5 times a day for 10 days × Swish and spit 5 ml 4 times a day for 10 days
Chlorhexidine rinse (0.12%)	Swish and spit 10 ml 2 times a day, until lesions resolve

INFECTIOUS DISEASE

1. Oral Candidiasis

Candidiasis is caused by yeast-like fungus *Candida albicans*. This is one of the commonest oral infections. *C. albicans* are one of the components of the normal oral microflora. There are many types of *Candida* species seen in the oral cavity. These include *C. albicans, C. glabrata, C. krusei, C. guilliermondii, C. parapsilosis, C. pseudotropicalis, C. stellatoidea, C. tropicalis*. Candida exists harmlessly in mucous membranes such as eyes, ears, nose, mouth, sinuses, skin, GIT, vagina, etc. It is a beneficial flora, however, if an imbalance of normal flora occurs, it can cause overgrowth of *Candida albicans*. The organism is present in two forms, a trait known as dimorphism. The yeast form is innocuous but hyphae form is associated with the invasion of host tissue. There exists a complex host and organism interaction; Candida infection may range from mild, superficial mucosal involvement to fatal disseminated disease in immunocompromised patients.

Etiology

Pathogen: Infection with *C. albicans* is associated with certain pathogenic variables. Adhesion of fungi to the epithelium is an important step in initiation of infection. This is promoted by certain fungal cell wall components like mannose, C3d receptors, mannoproteins, and saccharine other factors include persistence within the epithelial cells, endotoxins, induction of tumor necrosis factor and proteinases. Phenotypic switching from one morphological form to other depending upon environment has been implicated.

Host Factors

Local
× Impaired salivary gland function leading to xerostomia may predispose to candidiasis.
× Antimicrobial proteins in the saliva such as lactoferrin, sialoperoxidase, lysozyme, histidine-rich polypeptides and especially anti-Candida antibodies prevent overgrowth of Candida.
× Drugs such as inhaled steroids may alter the environment by possibly suppressing cellular immunity and phagocytosis. The local mucosal immunity reverts back to normal on discontinuation of inhaled steroids.
× Dentures predispose to infection with Candida in elderly people wearing full upper dentures. Dentures provide environment with low oxygen, low pH and an anaerobic environment, reduced salivary flow under dentures.
× Other factors include oral cancer and leukoplakias and high carbohydrate diet.

Systemic Factors
× Extremes of life predispose to infection due to reduced immunity. Drugs such as broad-spectrum antibiotics, immunosuppressive drugs, anti-neoplastic agents alter the oral flora, disrupting the mucosal surface and altering the character of the saliva.
× Other factors include smoking, diabetes, Cushing's syndrome, immunosuppressive conditions such as HIV, malignancies, leukaemia, nutritional deficiencies, vitamin B have been implicated.

Classification

The disease is classified as:

Primary oral candidiasis—Group I

- ✗ Acute
  - Pseudomembranous
  - Erythematous
- ✗ Chronic
  - Hyperplastic
  - Pseudomembranous
  - Erythematous
- ✗ Keratinized primary lesions super infected with Candida
  - Leukoplakia, lichen planus, lupus erythematosus
- ✗ Candida associated lesions
  - Angular cheilitis
  - Denture stomatitis
  - Median rhomboid glossitis

Secondary oral candidiasis—Group II: Oral manifestations of systemic mucocutaneous as a result of diseases such as thymic aplasia and candidiasis endocrinopathy syndrome.

PRIMARY CANDIDIASIS

The clinical manifestations of clinically important forms of primary candidiasis are described below.

◈ Acute Candidiasis

☛ Acute Pseudomembranous Candidiasis (Thrush)

This form is characterized by the presence of adherent white plaques that resemble cottage cheese or curdled milk on the oral mucosa. Sites frequently involved are the tongue, buccal mucosa, labial mucosa, palate. The white mass is composed of entangled hyphae, yeasts and desquamated epithelial cell debris. Scraping them with tongue blade or rubbing them off with a dry gauze sponge can remove these plaques leaving an underlying erythematous area.

This may be seen in patients on long-term, broad-spectrum antibiotics or by impairment of patients' immune system as in HIV infection or leukemic patients. Infants may also be affected due to underdeveloped immunity. Symptoms may be mild causing burning sensation or an unpleasant taste in the mouth described as salty or bitter. The oral surfaces frequently involved include labial and buccal mucosa, tongue, hard and soft palate and oropharynx. The involvement of both oral and oesophageal mucosa is prevalent in AIDS patients. The symptoms of the acute form are rather mild and the patients may complain only of slight tingling sensation or foul taste, whereas the chronic forms may involve the oesophageal mucosa leading to dysphagia and chest pains.

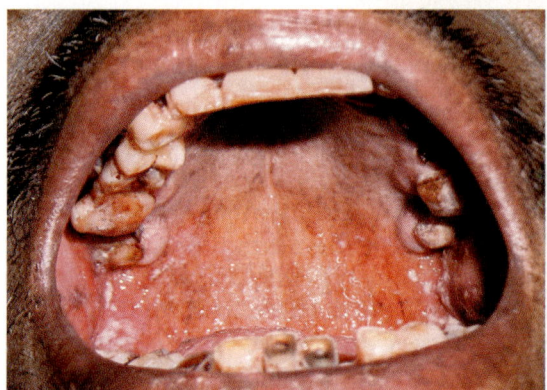

Fig. 6.17: Confluent white scrapable plaques of oral thrush on the retromolar regions, palate and buccal mucosa, that resemble curdled milk

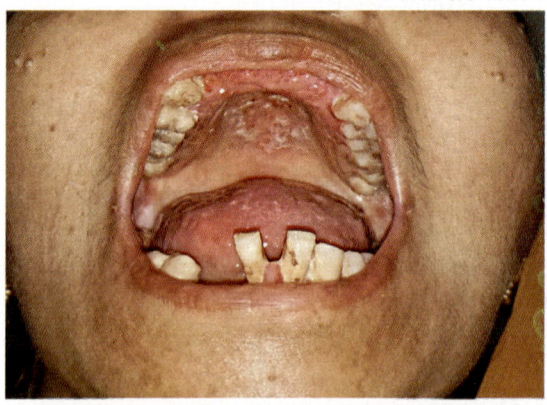

Fig. 6.18: Slightly raised, creamy white patches of acute pseudomembranous candidiasis on the palate in a patient undergoing chemotherapy for carcinoma of gall bladder

Differential diagnosis: A few lesions mimicking pseudomembranous candidiasis could be white coated tongue, thermal and chemical burns, lichenoid reactions, leukoplakia, secondary syphilis and diphtheria.

☛ *Acute Atrophic Candidiasis (Antibiotic sore mouth)*

This typically follows a course of broad-spectrum antibiotic therapy. Clinically, it manifests as a painful localized erythematous area. The lesions are seen on the dorsum of the

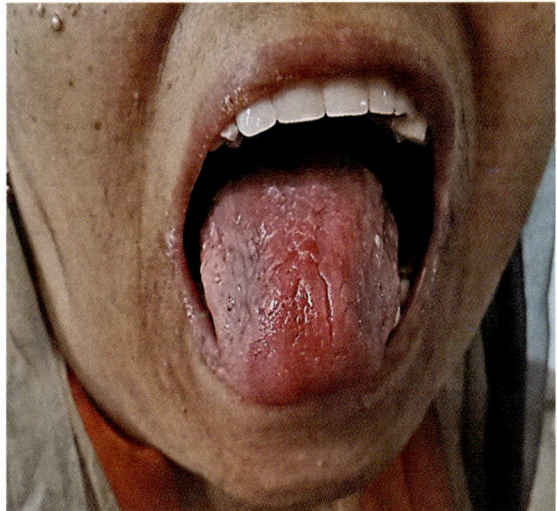

Fig. 6.19: Acute atrophic candidiasis manifesting as redness and depapillation on the tongue

tongue, typically presenting as depapillated areas. The redness is accompanied by pain and burning sensation. Also, patients who suffer from xerostomia for any reason also have an increased prevalence of erythematous candidiasis.

Differential diagnosis: Thermal burns, anemia, erythroplakia, denture stomatitis, erythema migrans.

◈ Chronic Hyperplastic Candidiasis

This condition is also referred to as 'candidal leukoplakia.' Clinically, it may present in two forms.

× Homogenous adherent white plaques
× Erythematous multiple nodular/speckled type

The lesions usually occur bilaterally in the commissural region of buccal mucosa and the tongue. These lesions are non-scrapable associated with smoking and may present with varying degrees of dysplasia. Some cases may be associated with nutritional deficiencies like iron or folate and with defective cell-mediated immunity.

Differential diagnosis: Leukoplakia, lichen planus, angular cheilitis and squamous cell carcinoma.

◈ Candida Associated Lesions

☛ *Denture Stomatitis (Chronic Atrophic Candidiasis)*

This condition is characterized by varying degrees of erythema, sometimes by petechial hemorrhages, localized to denture bearing areas of the maxillary arch. It may also manifest as a granular or papillary type. It is seen in almost 50–65% of denture wearers. It is usually asymptomatic but occasionally patients may complain of burning sensation or soreness. Associated factors include poor oral hygiene, ill-fitting dentures with limited salivary flow.

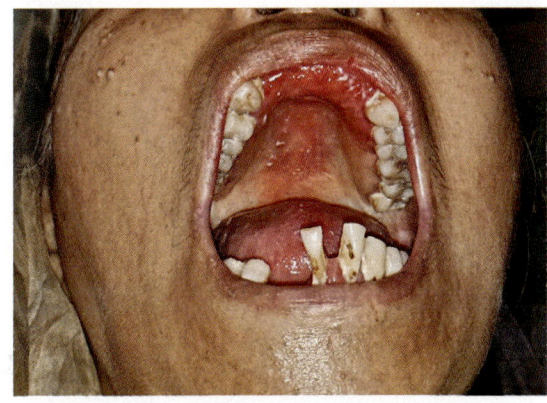

Fig. 6.20: Denture stomatitis manifesting as diffuse erythema of the maxillary alveolus in 11, 21, 22 regions and on the hard palate in a patient wearing removable partial denture

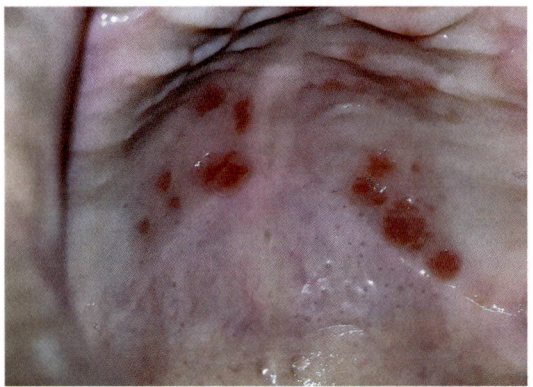

Fig. 6.21: Denture stomatitis of the granular type on the hard palate. Also note the inflamed orifices of the minor salivary glands due to smoker's palate

☛ *Angular Cheilitis (Perleche)*

This condition is characterised by erythema fissuring and scaling seen at commissures of the lip. It is usually seen in older individuals with reduced vertical dimension of occlusion and accentuated folds at the corner of the mouth. It may also be seen in vitamin B_{12} deficiency and in iron deficiency anemia. There is drooling of saliva in these areas, favouring fungal and bacterial growth. Microbiological studies have shown 20% of these cases are caused by Candida alone, by *Staph. aureus* in 20% cases and a combination of the two in the remaining cases.

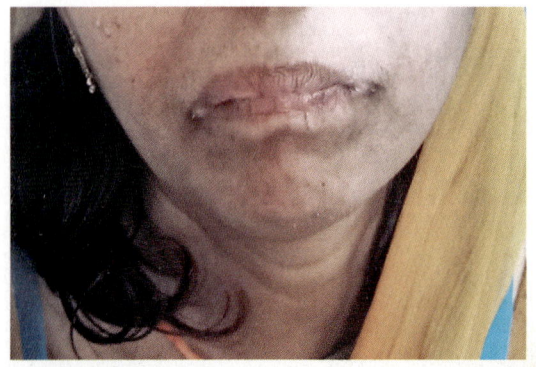

Fig. 6.22: Angular cheilitis appearing as fissuring at the corner of mouth

☛ *Median Rhomboid Glossitis*

The lesions appear as a well-demarcated erythematous, central papillary atrophy of

the tongue and located around the midline of the dorsum of the tongue. The surface may range from smooth to lobulated. The majority of the cases are asymptomatic, some may complain of continuous pain, irritation or pruritis. The lesion is now believed to be a localized chronic infection by *C. albicans*, associated with tobacco smokers and inhalation steroid users.

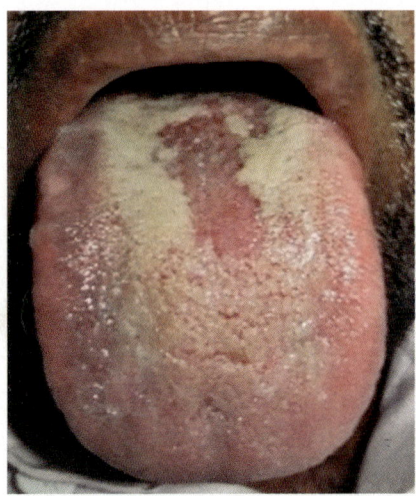

Fig. 6.23: Median rhomboid glossitis

Linear Gingival Erythema

It was referred earlier as HIV gingivitis because of its occurrence with HIV associated periodontal disease. The lesion manifests as a linear gingival erythematous band of 2–3 mm on the marginal gingiva along with petechial or diffuse erythematous lesion on attached gingiva.

C. dubliniensis has been reported to be the emerging pathogen along with *C. albicans*.

Differential diagnosis: Plaque-related gingivitis, herpetic gingivitis, desquamative gingivitis, granulomatous gingivitis, plasma cell gingivitis, leukemia.

SECONDARY CANDIDIASIS

◆ **Mucocutaneous Candidiasis**

This consists of a rare group of immunologic disorders known as mucocutaneous candidiasis. Most cases are sporadic, in some cases autosomal recessive pattern of inheritance has been identified in the families. The immune problem emerges during the first few years of life, with Candida infection of the mouth, nails, skin and other mucosal surfaces. The lesion simulates chronic hyperplastic candidiasis. In some, mutations in the autoimmune regulator (AIRE) gene has been documented with autoantibodies directed against persons own tissues. This immunologic disorder is directed against the endocrine gland, endocrine-candidiasis syndrome, autoimmune polyendocrinopathy-candidiasis syndrome, ectodermal dystrophy syndrome, as well as iron deficiency anemia may develop along with candidiasis. Endocrine disturbances include hypothyroidism, hypoparathyroidism, Addison's disease, diabetes mellitus. Oral cavity involvement is reported in more than 90% cases and the lesions may spread to larynx, pharynx, or oesophagus.

Diagnosis

Fragments of plaque material can be smeared on a microscopic slide, macerated with 20% KOH and examined for typical hyphae. The hyphae can also be appreciated with PAS stain, on exfoliative cytology or biopsy specimen. The PAS method stains carbohydrates contained in abundance on the cell walls. It takes up bright magenta-red color. These hyphae are 2 μm in diameter showing branching along their length. The fungi can be cultured in various media, including blood agar, cornmeal agar and Sabouraud's broth to aid in diagnosis. On histologic sections, Candida hyphae are embedded in the parakeratin layer and rarely penetrate into variable cell layers of epithelium except in extremely immunocompromised patients.

Treatment

General principles
- Early and accurate diagnosis of the infection.
- Correcting the predisposing factors or underlying diseases
- Evaluating the type of Candida infection
- Appropriate use of antifungal drugs, evaluating the efficacy/toxicity ratio in each case which are more effective and have higher salivary concentration and better tolerance for patients with oropharyngeal candidiasis.

Topical antifungals: The topical agents are the treatment of choice for uncomplicated localized lesions in patients with normal immune function. Polyenes are fungicidal drugs that act through binding to ergosterol within fungal cell wall inducing cytoplasmic leakage leading to fungal cell death.
- Nystatin suspension 100,000 units/ml are used for 4–6 ml for 7–14 days.
- Nystatin pastilles 200,000 units each in a dose of 1–4 pastilles a day for 7–14 days.
- Clotrimazole troches 10 mg, 5 times a day for 7–14 days.
- Miconazole can also be used topically and should be used for 1 week also after resolution of symptoms. It also causes altered cell permeability by binding with ergosterol, cytochrome P450 enzyme 14-alpha demethylase. Miconazole in gel form is applied directly to affected area dose 200–500 mg/day 4 times a day. This drug is absorbed by intestine and it inhibits enzyme cytochrome P450, which affects clearance of certain drugs. Mucoadhesive tablets of miconazole are also available, while treating candidiasis four fundamentals should be kept in mind.
- Fluconazole oral suspension in distilled water (10 mg/ml) gives a 95% cure by administering 5 ml daily for 7 to 14 days.

Systemic treatment
- Fluconazole has been used to treat systemic candidiasis because of its efficacy and good tolerability. Dose is 100–200 g daily. This gives good results with immunocompromised patients and cancer patients.
- Itraconazole is used in fluconazole resistant Candida strains.

- The newer antifungal voriconazole (200 mg/day) has been shown to be a potent drug.
- While treating denture stomatitis ketoconazole tablets (200 mg daily with topical 2% ketoconazole have been used but share adverse effects like nausea, vomiting and GIT problems).

Good oral hygiene practices like mechanical cleaning of teeth and dentures with a toothbrush is an effective tool to prevent candidiasis. Oral decontamination using chlorhexidine mouthwashes or cetylpyridinium chloride is equally effective. People using inhalers with corticosteroids should be washing out mouth with water or mouthwash after using inhaler. For susceptible denture wearers, regular cleaning of dentures with removal at night and soaking it in 0.2% chlorhexidine solution helps.

Table 6.6 summarizes the different antifungal medications used systematically.

2. Hairy Leukoplakia

These are white confluent patches of fluffy (hairy) mucosa seen bilaterally, along the lateral borders of the tongue, although other sites may also be involved. It is associated with HIV positive patients and believed to be caused by the Epstein-Barr virus (EBV). It has been less frequently described in immunosuppressed patients following organ transplantation.

Clinical Features

Most often seen in young males. In some instances, the lesion consists of diffuse white plaques with occasional hairy striae. When other sites are involved it may be smooth and homogenous. Most of them are colonised by *C. albicans*. This lesion should be considered as an AIDS prodrome as it is predictive for progression of asymptomatic HIV seropositivity to full-blown syndrome.

Microscopically, the surface parakeratin layer is thickened and colonized with *C. albicans*. The upper spinous layer shows cytopathologically evident altered keratinocytes. The cells show cytoplasmic clearing and nuclear vesiculation with chromatin marginalisation. The spinous layer is of moderate thickness and the submucosa is devoid of inflammation. DNA *in situ* hybridization can be used to detect EBV virions.

Differential diagnosis: Ordinary leukoplakia with Candida infection habit and lichen planus should be considered.

Treatment: As this is a pre-AIDS condition, patients should be referred to ART centres for the treatment and drug therapy.

ALLERGIC REACTIONS

Lichenoid Contact Reactions

There is a subgroup of patients who demonstrate delayed hypersensitivity reaction to

TABLE 6.6: Systemic treatment of oral candidiasis		
	Drug	Dosage
First line	- Fluconazole (per oral or IV)	- 100–200 mg/day for 7–14 days.
Second line	- Itraconazole solution (PO) - Posaconazole (PO) - Voriconazole (PO or IV)	- 200 mg/28 days - 400 mg daily in divided doses - 200 mg twice daily
Agents used in refractory cases	- Caspofungin (IV) - Micafungin (IV) - Anidulafungin (IV) - Amphotericin B oral suspension - Amphotericin B deoxycholate (IV)	- 70 mg loading dose followed by 50 mg daily - 100–150 mg daily - 100 mg loading dose followed by 50 mg daily - 500 mg every 6 hours - 0.3 mg/kg once.

constituents of dental materials; depicting lichenoid lesions adjacent to either dental amalgam filling or dental metals. On patch testing, majority of these patients react to the offending metal and the lesions resolve rapidly after removal of the adjacent dental material. This pathosis is diagnosed as lichenoid contact stomatitis (LCR) and not a true lichen planus.

Etiopathogenesis

It is based on a delayed hypersensitivity reaction. Most commonly, mercury (Hg) is the contact metal which affects the immune system as Hg is not identified initially by T-cell lymphocytes. A delayed reaction which involves APCs, i.e. Langerhans cells and MHC Class II molecule together containing Hg peptide bind on the antigen-specific T-lymphocytes. This is the first signal in the antigen-presenting process. The second signal comprises further cellular interactions which is decisive for clonal expansion of the Hg peptide-specific T-lymphocytes to take place. These cells will migrate into the blood stream to reach the peripheral tissues. At this stage, patient is sensitized to Hg. Once the oral mucosa of the sensitized individual is further exposed to Hg, Langerhans cells are able to present the peptide conjugated Hg to peripheral T-cells with an appropriate T-cell receptor. This interaction will invoke cytokine production and attract inflammatory cells at the site giving rise to clinical reaction pattern of LCR.

Clinical Features

The most commonly affected sites are the posterior buccal mucosa and the ventral surface of the lateral borders of the tongue. Gingival cuffs adjacent to the subgingival metallic restorations and porcelain fused to metal crowns with metal collars may also be affected. The affected mucosa may be white plaque like or erythematous with or without peripheral striae. The difference between OLP and LCR is the extension of the lesion. LCRs are confined to sites that are regularly in contact with dental materials. Most LCRs are asymptomatic, but when erythematous or ulcerative lesions are present, patient may experience discomfort from spicy and warm food.

Diagnosis

The diagnosis is made from adjacent correlation to dental material along with clinical appearance. Patch test is of a little clinical significance. Histopathology, may not be of any assistance in discrimination between OLP and LCR.

Differential diagnosis: The lesions resemble those of oral lichen planus (OLP), and it is therefore necessary to exclude likely lichenoid contact reactions when making a diagnosis of OLP. OLP is a more widespread condition involving many anatomical sites within the oral cavity with or without concurrent skin lesions. Similar oral lesions can occur as a result of drug-related lichenoid reactions or as graft-versus-host disease (GVHD), discoid lupus erythematosus (DLE), and systemic lupus erythematosus (SLE). Diagnosis is facilitated by detailed history, clinical findings, and immunohistological findings. LCRs caused by hypersensitivity to amalgam or its constituents typically have a clear anatomical relationship to the dental amalgam fillings so they are usually unilateral and not symmetrical.

Management

Replacement of dental materials in direct contact with the lichenoid contact reaction will result in cure or marked reduction in 90% of the cases. Most lesions resolve in 1–2 months.

Reactions to Dentifrice and Chlorhexidine

Delayed hypersensitivity reactions to toothpaste and mouthwashes containing flavour additives such as carvone or cinnamon or preservatives are rare. These flavouring agents may be used in chewing gum and produce similar forms of gingivostomatitis. The clinical manifestations include fiery red, edematous gingiva, which may include both white lesions or ulcerations. Labial and buccal mucosa and tongue mucosa may also be involved. The lesions heal after withdrawal of the allergen containing agent.

Differential diagnosis: Desquamative gingivitis due to erosive lichen planus, mucous membrane pemphigoid or pemphigus vulgaris, pubertal or pregnancy-induced gingivitis, and leukaemia associated gingivitis.

TOXIC REACTIONS

Smokeless Tobacco Use (Tobacco Pouch Keratosis)

Tobacco pouch keratosis or smokeless tobacco-induced keratosis in the development of a white mucosal lesion in the area of tobacco contact. The term smokeless tobacco is derived from the fact that tobacco is not burned unlike smoking. Table 6.7 depicts the types of smokeless tobacco.

TABLE 6.7: Forms of smokeless tobacco	
Types of smokeless tobacco	Methods of consumption and description of ingredients
Chewing tobacco/spit tobacco	Chewed in the form of leaves. Placed in between the cheek or lip. Once chewed, the saliva is spit.
Spitless tobacco	Finely milled and dissolves orally. The form of tobacco is chewed and spitting is not required; hence referred to as "spitless tobacco".
Snuff tobacco	Snuffed in the form of fine powdered tobacco. Available in dry and moist.

Clinical Features

The most common location is lower anterior vestibule followed by posterior vestibule. Health and addiction hazards are due to ready absorption of nicotine and other molecules through the oral mucosa. The most common local change is painless loss of gingival tissues in the area of tobacco contact. The gingival recession accompanied by destruction of the facial surface of the alveolar bone. Brownish black extrinsic tobacco stains are seen on the enamel and cemental surface of the teeth adjacent to tobacco. Class five cervical caries in cases of cemental wear and halitosis is present in chronic users. The lesion appears thickened and corrugated and as the condition worsens, it becomes leathery. Smokeless tobacco keratosis usually takes 1–5 years to develop. Once the lesion develops keratosis remains unchanged indefinitely unless the daily tobacco contact with the tissue is altered.

Diagnosis

Histopathology of the lesion shows that the squamous epithelium is hyperkeratinized and acanthotic. Parakeratin 'chevrons' may be seen as pointed projections above or in superficial epithelial layers. Increased subepithelial vascularity and vessel engorgement are seen. Occasionally, significant dysplasia or SCC may be present.

Differential diagnosis: Leukoplakia, frictional keratosis.

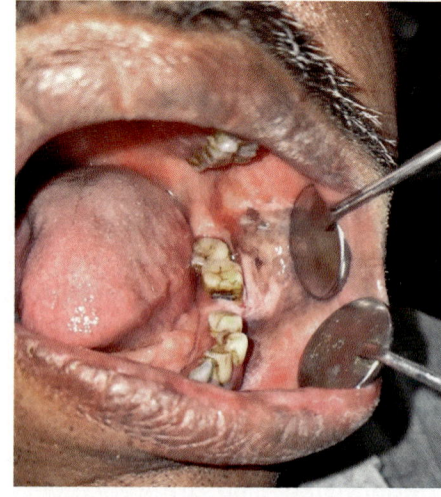

Fig. 6.24: Tobacco pouch keratosis buccal vestibule and buccal mucosa showing a corrugated surface

Management

It includes complete cessation of tobacco chewing habit and follow-up to assess resolution. In maximum number of patients mucosa is resumed to normal in 2–6 weeks after stopping the habit. A biopsy is to be performed if there is any evidence of erythema or ulceration to rule out dysplasia or low-grade oral malignancy and verrucous carcinoma (snuff dippers carcinoma). Nicotine replacement therapy such as nicotine gum and patches can be delivered to patients which acts as a substitute.

Nicotine Stomatitis (Smokers Palate, Nicotina Palatini)

Nicotina palatini is a white keratotic mucosal change of the hard palate associated with tobacco smoking. It does not have a premalignant nature as it develops in response to heat rather than chemicals in tobacco smoke. Pipe smoking generates more heat on the palate, hence often associated with this habit. Similar changes are seen with long-term use of extremely hot beverages.

In some American and southeast Asian cultures, hard rolled cigarettes and cigar are smoked with the lit end held within the mouth producing excessive heat and pronounced palatal keratosis or so-called reverse smokers' palate. This lesion has a significant potential to develop dysplasia or carcinoma.

Clinical Features

This is commonly found in men older than 45 years of age. With long-term exposure to heat, the palatal mucosa becomes diffusely grey or white, with small nodular excrescences having a central red spot corresponding to the inflamed orifices of the minor salivary glands. The palatal surface may become so keratinized and thickened that a fissured or dried mud appearance is impaired. The white appearance involves marginal gingiva and interdental papilla, sometimes leukoplakia may be seen in buccal mucosa. Heavy brown or black tobacco stains may be present on the teeth.

Diagnosis

Microscopic examination reveals that the epithelium is characterized by hyperorthokeratosis and acanthosis along with patchy chronic inflammation of the subepithelial connective tissue and mucous glands squamous metaplasia of the excretory ducts and an inflammatory exudate with the ductal lumina is often noted. In cases of papular elevation, hyperplastic ductal epithelium may be seen near the orifice.

Differential diagnosis: Oral leukoplakia, Darier's disease, discoid lupus erythematosus, oral candidiasis, oral lichen planus, and denture-induced hyperplasia.

Treatment

This condition is completely reversible after stoppage of habit within 1–2 weeks even if it may be present for decades. Although this is not a precancerous lesion, care should be taken to observe any erythematous, ulcerated areas which are to be suspiciously seen and to be biopsied if, persist even after stoppage of the habit.

REACTIONS TO MECHANICAL TRAUMA

Morsacatio buccarum (Chronic Cheek Chewing)

Morsacatio comes from Latin word *morsus* or bite, chronic nibbling produces lesions that are located on buccal mucosa, lip or lateral border of the tongue. The lesions are found in people under stress or exhibiting psychological conditions. It is more prevalent in women and three times more prevalent after 35 years.

Clinical Features

The lesions could be bilateral on anterior buccal mucosa or unilateral combined with lesions on lips and lateral border of tongue.

There are areas of thickened, shredded white areas with intervening zones of erythema, erosion or focal traumatic ulceration.

Diagnosis

Biopsy reveals extensive hyperparakeratosis in an extremely ragged surface with numerous projections of keratin. Surface bacterial colonization is often seen. Sometimes, clusters of vacuolated cells are seen in the superficial portion of prickle cell layer striking similarity to oral hairy leukoplakia. In most cases the clinical presentation is pathognomonic and rarely requires biopsy. However, lesions on the border of the tongue have to be viewed with suspicion to rule out HIV.

Differential diagnosis: White sponge naevus, leukoplakia, lichen planus.

Frictional Keratosis

Frictional keratosis is a common alteration in areas of recurring mild mechanical trauma or irritation from malposed teeth, dental prosthesis, exuberant tooth brushing with an overly firm toothbrush, constant rubbing of the tongue against the teeth (tongue thrust keratosis) or frequent clenching of the facial muscles, thereby pushing cheek and lips firmly against the dentition.

Clinical Features

Frictional keratosis is usually seen in young adults of both genders. There may be presence of a thin, slightly raised, white keratotic line bilaterally along the occlusal plane of the buccal mucosa. This is called *linea alba*, a form of frictional keratosis. At times the surface may be quite rough, and irregular and scalloping may be seen on the buccal mucosa, simulating the contours of adjacent teeth.

A similar linear line of excess keratin may be found along the lateral edges of the tongue, often with crenations from chronically pushing the tongue against the teeth; tongue thrust keratosis. Rounded or irregularly shaped white plaques may be seen in retromolar region from trauma due to maxillary posterior teeth

Alveolar keratosis is another form of frictional keratosis which presents as a thick, white verruciform, keratotic plaque often bilaterally on the edentulous mucosa of the alveolar ridge in the retromolar areas of the mandible. The irregular granular plaque is well demarcated from the surrounding mucosa. Alveolar keratosis has shown to have a low frequency of epithelial dysplasia and much lower risk of malignant transformation than verrucous leukoplakia.

Diagnosis

Microscopically, hyperorthokeratosis and acanthosis are the hallmarks of frictional keratosis.

Differential diagnosis: Alveolar keratosis must be distinguished from oral leukoplakia and tobacco pouch keratosis.

Treatment

No treatment is required for frictional keratosis as there is no malignant potential. The white keratotic plaques will completely disappear within a few days or weeks after elimination of chronic trauma. Any keratosis that persists for more than 4 weeks after stoppage of habit or removal of chronic trauma should be considered as true leukoplakia and biopsy be performed.

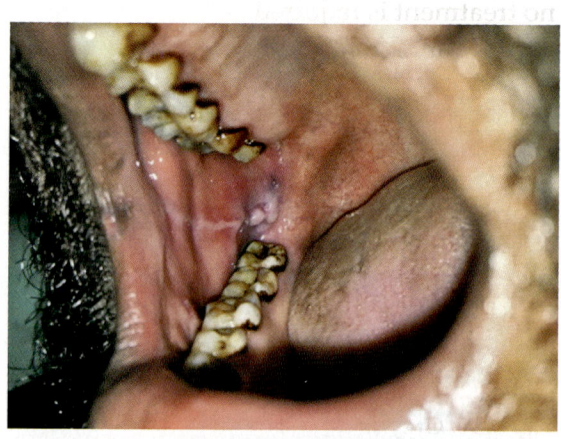

Fig. 6.25: Linea alba on the right buccal mucosa

OTHERS

Leukoedema

Leukoedema is a variant of the normal mucosa that is more prevalent in Caucasians and Black population. The gender distribution is equal. The etiology is not clear.

Clinical Features

It is a bilateral white veil-like alteration of the oral mucosa that is merely considered as a normal variant. These lesions are more prevalent in the Caucasians and Black population. This condition is encountered bilaterally on the buccal mucosa and sometimes the borders of the tongue. The lesions disappear on stretching the mucosa and reappear on stretching the mucosa and reappear on release of the mucosa. This is characteristic feature of leukoedema.

Histopathology shows hyperparakeratosis, acanthosis with intracellular edema in spinous layer of epithelial cells.

Differential diagnosis: Other white lesions of the oral mucosa including leukoplakia, oral candidiasis, oral lichen planus, white sponge nevus, *Morsicatio buccarum* may be confused with leukoedema but can be easily distinguished from these conditions as leukoedema disappears completely on stretching.

Treatment: As the condition is asymptomatic, no treatment is required.

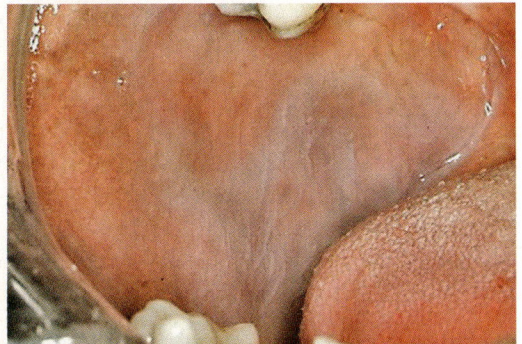

Fig. 6.26: Greyish white veil-like appearance of the right buccal mucosa that characterizes leukoedema

Benign Migratory Glossitis
(Geographic Tongue)

Benign migratory glossitis is a psoriasiform mucositis of the dorsum of the tongue. This is characterized by changing pattern of serpiginous white lines surrounded by smooth, depapillated mucosa. The changing appearance has led to call this as wandering rash or geographic tongue-like continental outlines on a globe. The etiology is unknown but aggravates due to psychological stress and is found with increased frequency in the patients with psoriasis of skin.

Diagnosis

A biopsy taken from prominent serpiginous line at the periphery of a depapillated patch shows thickened layer of keratin infiltrated with neutrophils. These inflammatory cells often produce small microabscess called Munro's abscess in the keratin and spinous layers. Rete ridges are typically thin and elongated with thin layer of epithelium overlying the connective tissue papillae. When rete ridges are not elongated, then

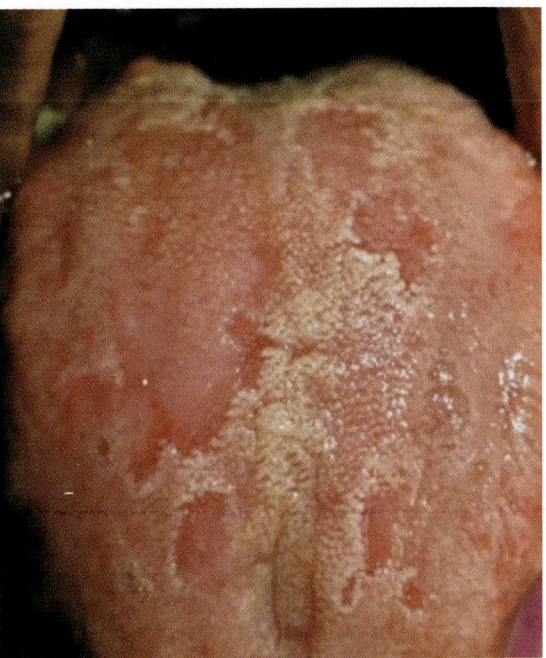

Fig. 6.27: Benign migratory glossitis

Reiter's syndrome could be considered. PAS staining will demonstrate Candida hyphae on the superficial layers of the epithelium. Ulcerations can be seen in Reiter's syndrome.

Differential diagnosis: Red lesions of the mucosa including chemical burns, contact stomatitis, fissured tongue, erosive lichen planus, atrophic candidiasis may be confused with geographic tongue. Proper history taking helps distinguish it from these conditions.

Treatment

No treatment is usually necessary. However, topical prednisolone or topical or systemic antifungal medication can be tried in case of symptomatic lesions and secondary Candida infection.

White Sponge Nevus

This is a rare genodermatosis that is inherited as an autosomal dominant trait with high degree of penetrance and variable expressibility. Mutations in keratin 4 and keratin 13 may be responsible for the clinical manifestations.

Clinical Features

The lesions appear at birth or early childhood, sometimes during adolescence. Symmetrical thickened, white, corrugated or velvety diffuse plaques affect the buccal mucosa bilaterally. Other sites include the ventral surface of the tongue, labial mucosa, soft palate, floor of the mouth. Patients are asymptomatic.

Diagnosis

The microscopic picture is characteristic depicting prominent hyperparakeratosis, acanthosis with the clearing of cytoplasm of the cells in the spinous layer. In some instances, an eosinophilic condensation is noted in the perinuclear region of the cells, in the superficial layers of the epithelium, a feature that is unique to white sponge nevus. No treatment is required for this condition.

Differential diagnosis: Cheek chewing lesion, leukoedema, leukoplakia, pachyonychia congenita, hereditary benign intraepithelial dyskeratosis.

Pachyonychia Congenita

Pachyonychia congenita is a rare genodermatoses inherited as an autosomal dominant trait. Oral lesions are seen only in patients affected by the Jadassohn-Lewandowsky form of the disease (pachyonychia congenita type 1).

Clinical Features

Patients with pachyonychia congenita exhibit characteristic nail changes, either at birth or in the early neonatal period. The free margins of the nails are lifted up because of an accumulation of keratinaceous material in the nail beds. This results in a pinched, tubular configuration of the nails, ultimately leading to nail loss. Other skin changes that may occur include marked hyperkeratosis of the palmar and plantar surfaces, producing thick, callous-like lesions. The oral lesions seen in the Jadassohn-Lewandowsky form consist of thickened white plaques that involve the lateral margins and dorsal surface of the tongue and buccal mucosa.

Diagnosis

Microscopic examination of lesional oral mucosa shows marked hyperparakeratosis and acanthosis with perinuclear clearing of the epithelial cells.

Differential diagnosis: The white keratotic lesions of this condition may be similar to that white sponge nevus and both conditions may be present at birth. However, the presence of the nail anomalies and the skin lesions in pachyonychia congenita distinguishes this entity from white sponge nevus.

Treatment: Because the oral lesions of pachyonychia congenita show no apparent tendency for malignant transformation, no treatment for the oral lesions is required.

Dyskeratosis Congenita

Dyskeratosis congenita is a rare genodermatosis having an X-linked recessive inheritance pattern, and hence a striking male predilection.

Clinical Features

Dyskeratosis congenita usually becomes evident during the first decade of life. A reticular pattern of skin hyperpigmentation develops, affecting the face, neck, and upper chest along with, abnormal, dysplastic changes of the nails. Intraoral, the tongue and buccal mucosa develop bullae, that are followed by erosions and, eventually, leukoplakic lesions. These leukoplakic lesions are potentially malignant. Hematologic complications of thrombocytopenia and aplastic anemia develop in 70 % of the cases.

Diagnosis

Biopsy specimens of the early oral mucosal lesions show hyperorthokeratosis with epithelial atrophy. As the lesions progress, epithelial dysplasia develops.

Differential diagnosis: White sponge nevus, pachyonychia congenita.

Treatment: The discomfort of the oral lesions is managed symptomatically and periodic oral mucosal examinations are recommended to check for evidence of malignant transformation in the leukoplakic lesions. Routine medical assessment is warranted to screen the patient for the development of aplastic anemia.

FREQUENTLY ASKED QUESTIONS

Long Answer Questions

1. Define leukoplakia. Describe the etiology, classification, clinical and dysplastic features of oral leukoplakia. Add a note on its management.
2. Enumerate the potentially malignant disorders of the oral cavity. Describe the etiopathogenesis, clinical features and management of OSMF.
3. Define lichen planus. Describe the etiopathogenesis and the clinical variants of OLP. Add a note on the treatment of oral lichen planus.
4. Classify candidiasis. Describe the etiopathological factors, clinical features and treatment of acute pseudomembranous candidiasis.
5. Classify the red and white lesions of the oral cavity. Describe speckled leukoplakia in detail.

Short Answer Questions

1. Oral thrush
2. Candidal leukoplakia
3. Erosive lichen planus
4. Antibiotic sore mouth
5. Denture stomatitis
6. Proliferative verrucous leukoplakia
7. Speckled leukoplakia
8. Drug-induced lichenoid reactions
9. Smokers palate
10. Hairy tongue
11. Clinical variants of OLP
12. Erythroplakia
13. Systemic lupus erythematosus
14. Angular cheilitis / perlèche

BIBLIOGRAPHY

1. Burket, Greenberg MS, Glick M, Ship J. Burket's oral medicine: diagnosis and treatment. 2008.Hamilton, Ont: BC Decker.
2. Neville BW, Damm DD, Allen CM, Buoquot JE.. Oral and maxillofacial pathology. 2009.St. Louis, Mo: Saunders/Elsevier.
3. Shafer, William G, Maynard K. Hine, Barnet M. Levy. A Textbook of Oral Pathology. 7th edition 2012. Editors Sivapathasundharam S, Rajendran R. Philadelphia: Saunders.
4. Silverman Sol, Eversole L, Truelove E. Essentials of oral medicine. 1st edition, 2005. BC Decker, New York.
5. National Cancer Institute. Cancer Stat Facts: Oral Cavity and Pharynx Cancer. National Cancer Institute, Surveillance, Epidemiology and End Result Program. Available at https:// seer.cancer.gov/statfacts/html/oralcav.html.
6. Priebe S, Aleksejuniene, Dharamsi S, Zed C. Oral cancer and cultural factors in Asia.

Canadian journal of dental hygiene 2008; 42: 291–295.

7. Hashibe M, Jacob BJ, Thomas G, Ramadas K, Mathew B, Sankaranarayanan R, Zhang ZF. Socioeconomic status, lifestyle factors and oral premalignant lesions. Oral Oncology, 2003;39: 664–671.

8. Scully C. Challenges in predicting which oral mucosal potentially malignant disease will progress to neoplasia. Oral Dis. 2014; 20:1–5.

9. Walsh T, Liu JL, Brocklehurst P, Glenny AM, Lingen M, Kerr AR, et al. Clinical assessment to screen for the detection of oral cavity cancer and potentially malignant disorders in apparently healthy adults. Cochrane Database Syst Rev. 2013 Nov 21. 11:CD010173.

10. Sarode SC, Sarode GS, Karmarkar S, Tupkari JV. Oral (mucosal) potentially malignant disorders. Oral Oncol. 2012;48:e35–6.

11. World Health Organization. Geneva: World Health Organization; 1973. Report of a meeting of investigators on the histological definition of precancerous lesions.

12. Sarode SC, Sarode GS, Tupkari JV. Oral potentially malignant disorders: A proposal for terminology and definition with review of literature. J Oral MaxillofacPathol. 2014;18(Suppl 1): S77–80.

13. Barnes L, Eveson JW, Reichart P, Sidransky D. Pathology and Genetics of Head and Neck Tumors. WHO Classification of Tumors 2005, 3rd Edition, Volume 9.

14. Alexander RE, Wright JM, Thiebaud S. Evaluating, documenting and following up oral pathological conditions. A suggested protocol. J Am Dent Assoc 2001;132:329–335.

15. Bagán JV, Jimenez Y, Sanchis JM. Proliferative verrucous leukoplakia: high incidence of gingival squamous cell carcinoma J Oral Pathol Med 2003;32:379–382.

16. Bagán JV, Murillo J, Poveda R, et al. Proliferative verrucous leukoplakia: unusual locations of oral squamous cell carcinomas, and field cancerization as shown by the appearance of multiple OSCCs. Oral Oncol 2004; 40:440–443.

17. Brennan M, Migliorati CA, Lockhart PB et al: Management of oral epithelial dysplasia: a review, Oral Surg Oral Med Oral Pathol Oral Radiol Endod 2007;103:S19.e1-S19.e12.

18. Cabay RJ, Morton TH, Epstein JB: Proliferative verrucous leukoplakia and its progression to oral carcinoma: a review of the literature, J Oral Pathol Med 2007;36:255–261.

19. Eversole LR, Eversole GM, Kopcik J: Sanguinaria-associated oral leukoplakia: comparison with other benign and dysplastic leukoplakic lesions, Oral Surg Oral Med Oral Pathol Oral Radiol, Endod 2000;89:455–464.

20. Fettig A, Pogrel MA, Silverman S Jr, et al: Proliferative verrucous leukoplakia of the gingiva, Oral Surg Oral Med Oral Pathol Oral RadiolEndod 2000;90:723–730.

21. Holmstrup P, Vedtofte P, Reibel J. et al. Oral premalignant lesions: is a biopsy reliable? J Oral Pathol Med 2007; 36:262–266.

22. Lee JJ, Hung CH, Cheng SJ, et al. Carcinoma and dysplasia in oral leukoplakias in Taiwan: prevalence and risk factors, Oral Surg Oral Med Oral Pathol Oral RadiolEndod 2006;110:472–480.

23. Mithani SK, Mydlarz, WK, Grumbine FL et. al. Molecular genetics of premalignant oral lesions 2007; Oral Dis 13:126–133.

24. Lodi G, Sardella A, Bez C, et al. Systematic review of randomized trials for the treatment of oral leukoplakia, J Dent Educ 2002;66:896–902.

25. Garewal HS, Katz RV, Meyskens F, et al. Carotene Produces Sustained Remissions in Patients With Oral Leukoplakia: Results of a Multicenter Prospective Trial. Arch Otolaryngol Head Neck Surg. 1999;125(12): 1305–1310.

26. Ribeiro AS, Salles PR, Da Silva TA, Mesquita RA. A Review of the Nonsurgical Treatment of Oral Leukoplakia. International Journal of Dentistry.https://doi.org/10.1155/2010/186018.

27. Holmstrup P, Vedtofte P, Reibel J, et al: Long-term treatment outcome of oral premalignant lesions, Oral Oncol 2006;42:461–474.

28. Lodi G, Sardella A, Bez C, et al. Interventions for treating oral leukoplakia, Cochrane Database Syst Rev 4:CD001829, 2006.

29. Arruda JAA, Álvares PR, Sobral APV, Mesquita RA. A Review of the Surgical and Nonsurgical Treatment of Oral Leukoplakia. J Dent and Oral Disord. 2016;2: 1009.

30. Mascarenhas AK, Allen CM, Moeschberger ML. The association between Viadent use and oral leukoplakia. Epidemiology 2001;12:741–743.

31. Nielson H, Norrild B, Vedtofte P. et al. Human papillomavirus in oral premalignant lesions. Eur J Cancer B Oral Oncol 1996;32B:264–270.

32. Pandey M, Thomas G, Somanathan T et al. Evaluation of surgical excision of non-homogeneous oral leukoplakia in a screening intervention trial, Kerala, India, Oral Oncol 2001;37:103–109.

33. Petti S. Pooled estimate of world leukoplakia prevalence: a systematic review, Oral Oncol. 2003;39:770–780.

34. Reibel J. Prognosis of oral pre-malignant lesions: significance of clinical, histopathological, and molecular biological characteristics. Crit Rev Oral Biol Med 2003;14:47–62.

35. Sankaranarayanan R, Mathew B, Varghese C, et al. Chemoprevention of oral leukoplakia with vitamin A and beta carotene:an assessment, Oral Oncol 1997;33:231–236.

36. Schoelch ML, Sekandari N, Regezi JA, et al. Laser management of oral leukoplakias: a follow-up study of 70 patients, Laryngoscope 1999;109:949–953.

37. Sciubba JJ. Oral leukoplakia. Crit Rev Oral Biol Med 1995;6:147–160.

38. Shiu MN, Chen TH, Chang SH, et al. Risk factors for leukoplakia and malignant transformation to oral carcinoma: a leukoplakia cohort in Taiwan. Br J Cancer 2000;82:1871–1874.

39. Speight PM, Farthing PM, Bouquot JE. The pathology of oral cancer and precancer. Curr Diag Pathol 1997;3:165–176.

40. Van der Waal I, Axéll T. Oral leukoplakia: a proposal for uniform reporting. Oral Oncol 2002;38:521–526.

41. Van der Waal I, Shepman KP, van der Meij EH, et al. Oral leukoplakia: a clinicopathologic review. Oral Oncol 1998;33:291–301.

42. Zakrzewska JM, Lopes V, Speight P, et al. Proliferative verrucous leukoplakia: a report of ten cases. Oral Surg Oral Med Oral Pathol Oral Radiol Endod 1996;82:396–401.

43. Maria Auxiliadora Vieira do Carmo and Patrícia Carlos Caldeira (January 23rd 2013). Binary System of Grading Epithelial Dysplasia in Oral Leukoplakias, Carcinogenesis, Kathryn Tonissen, IntechOpen, DOI: 10.5772/54466. Available from: https://www.intechopen. com/books/carcinogenesis/binary-system-of-grading-epithelial-dysplasia-in-oral-leukoplakias

44. Swetha P, Supriya NA, Kumar GN. Characterization of different verrucous mucosal lesions. Indian J Dent Res 2013;24:642–4.

45. Diz P, Gorsky M, Johnson NW, Kragelund C, Manfredi M, Odell E, Thongprasom K, Warnakulasuriya S, Bagan J, van der Waal I. Oral leukoplakia and erythroplakia:a protocol for diagnosis and management. EAOM. Diagnostic and therapeutic protocols. Oral leukoplakia and erythroplakia<http://www. kcl. ac.uk/dentistry/about/acad/oral-leukoplakia-anderythroplakia. pdf. 2011

46. Rosebush MS, Anderson MK, Rawal YB. Pre-cancer and Cancer, Diagnosis and Management of Oral Lesions and Conditions: A Resource Handbook for the Clinician, Cesar A. Migliorati and Fotinos S. Panagakos, Intech Open, DOI: 10.5772/57597. Available from:https://www.intechopen.com/books/diagnosis-and-management-of-oral-lesions-and-conditions-a-resource-handbook-for-the-clinician/pre-cancer-and-cancer.

47. See JA, Shumack S, Murrell DF, et al. Consensus recommendations on the use of daylight photodynamic therapy with methylaminolevulinate cream for actinic keratoses in Australia. Australas J Dermatol. 2016;57(3):167–174. doi:10.1111/ajd.12354

48. Vigliante CE, Quinn PD, Alawi F. Proliferative verrucous leukoplakia: Report of a case with characteristic long-term progression. Journal of Oral and Maxillofacial Surgery 2003;61: 626–31.

49. B. Priyadharshni. Classification System for Oral Submucous Grading—A Review. International Journal of Science and Research (IJSR). 2014; 3:740–4.

50. Passi D, Bhanot P, Kacker D, Chahal D, Atri M, Panwar Y. Oral submucous fibrosis: Newer proposed classification with critical updates in pathogenesis and management strategies. Natl J Maxillofac Surg. 2017; 8(2):89–94.

Oral Cancer and Radiologic Considerations of Malignant Lesions

INTRODUCTION

Oral cancer (OC) is the commonest cancer in India, accounting for 50–70% of total cancer mortality.

It also accounts for the highest incidence among Asian countries. OC is the sixth most common cancer worldwide. It can affect anterior tongue, cheek, floor of mouth, gingival or any other part of the oral cavity. The incidence of OC is directly correlated with age of subjects. Rates rise dramatically after the age of 40–49 years, and reach a plateau around the age of 70–79 years. OC is more frequent in men than women, and depending on its location within the oral cavity, males are two to six times more likely to be affected than females, largely owing to their higher intake of alcohol and tobacco. Oral cancer can be divided according to the tissue involvement, such as, epithelial cancer—squamous cell carcinoma, verrucous carcinoma, etc., salivary gland cancer—mucoepidermoid carcinoma, acinic cell carcinoma etc., soft tissue cancer— Kaposi sarcoma, hematolymphoid cancer— Burkitt lymphoma, T cell lymphoma, etc., odontogenic carcinoma—ameloblastic carcinoma, primary intraosseous squamous cell carcinoma developed in cysts, etc. and odontogenic sarcomas—ameloblastic fibrosarcoma.

Epidermal	Carcinoma
Connective tissue	Sarcoma
Fibrous	Fibrosarcoma
Vascular	Angiosarcoma, etc.

ORAL CARCINOMA

Etiopathogenesis/Carcinogenesis

Tobacco: It is used either as smokeless tobacco combined with pan, gutkha, or in cigarettes, cigars, pipe and bidi, i.e. smoking hookah and chillum (a clay pipe used to keep the burning tobacco) are other common forms of smoking in some countries of Asia including India. The most important carcinogens in tobacco smoke are the aromatic hydrocarbon benzpyrene and the tobacco-specific/nitrosamines (TSNs), namely 4-(nitrosomethylamino)-1-(3-pyridyl)-1-butanone (NNK) and N'-nitrosonornicotine (NNN).

Alcohol: Alcohol has additive effect. Alcohol causes dehydration of mucosa. It is shown to increase the permeability of oral mucosa producing an alteration in morphology characterized by epithelial atrophy, which in turn leads to easier penetration of carcinogens into the oral mucosa.

Viruses: Viruses are capable of hijacking host cellular apparatus and modifying DNA and the chromosomal structures and inducing proliferative changes in the cells. **Human papillomavirus** and **herpes simplex** virus (HSV) have been established in recent years as causative agents of OC. The most commonly detected HPV in head and neck squamous cell carcinoma (HNSCC) is HPV-16, which has been demonstrated in 90–95% of all HPV positive HNSCC cases, followed by **HPV-18, HPV-31, and HPV-33**. **Epstein-Barr virus** (EBV), **human herpesvirus-8** (HHV-8) and **cytomegalovirus** have also been reported as risk factors of OSCC in different studies.

Immunosuppression: Immunosuppressed individuals are more prone to develop oral cancers.

Candida

Nodular leukoplakia infected with Candida has a tendency for higher rate of dysplasia and malignant transformation.

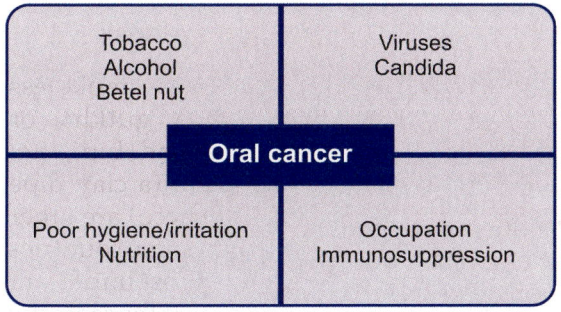

Fig. 7.1: Various predisposing factors for development of oral cancer

Occupational Risks

Occupational risks such as exposure to excessive solar radiation/ultraviolet (UV) light is known to cause lip cancers. UV rays also cause actinic cheilitis which may transform to malignancy. Sulfur dioxide, asbestos, pesticide exposures, and mists from strong inorganic acids and burning of fossil fuels have also been known to cause cancers of posterior mouth, pharynx, and larynx. Certain occupations have been reported to place people at increased risk for the development of salivary gland carcinomas. These include manufacturing of rubber products, plumbing (exposure of metals), and wood working in an automobile industry.

Syphilis

Tertiary syphilis had been known to predispose to the development of oral cancer along with other risk factors such as tobacco and alcohol. However, nowadays, tertiary syphilis is rare in clinical practice as the infection is diagnosed and treated before the onset of tertiary stage.

Dental Hygiene and Related Factors

Poor oral hygiene and prolonged irritation from sharp teeth have been viewed for their possible role in the development of OC. Poor oral hygiene and dental sepsis is thought to promote carcinogenic action of tobacco. This is due to the presence of coexisting risk factors like smoking and alcohol consumption.

Nutritional Factors

Dietary deficiencies are also suggested to play a role in the development of OC. Some researchers have reported lower risk of OC with higher intake of fruits and vegetables.

Pathogenesis: The complete understanding of molecular pathology of OC and its association with causative agent is a complex mechanism. Genetic approach and proteomic approach in recent years have revealed the molecular pathological picture of OC.

The common mechanism for cancer initiation appears to be through damage to DNA resulting in uncontrolled cell proliferation. There are several gene classes involved in carcinogenesis, which are affected by genetic transmission. The major epigenetic modification in tumors is methylation. Changes in the methylation patterns can play an important role in tumor formation.

Genetic susceptibility: Glutathione S-transferase M1 (GSTM1) null genotype appears to be the most consistent polymorphic susceptibility marker for head and neck

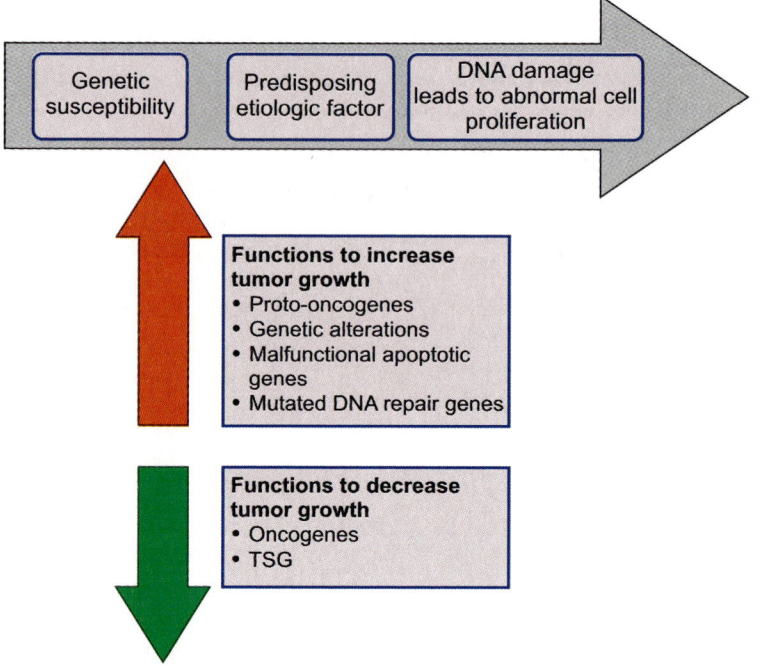

Fig. 7.2: Effects of various genes on oral cancer

cancer including OC. It is found that ALDH1B and ALDH2 (aldehyde dehydrogenase 2) genes were associated with HNSCC and showed significant correlation with alcohol consumption.

Proto-oncogenes increase the cell growth and differentiation and help in carcinogenesis.

Oncogenes act in a positive way in the normal growth regulatory pathway of the cell.

Genetic alterations define molecular basis of carcinogenesis, which includes point mutations, amplifications, rearrangements, and deletions.

Tumor suppressor genes (TSG): Tumor suppressor gene products are involved in the negative control of cell proliferation and differentiation, for example, p53, p16.

Apoptotic genes: The production of tumors includes disturbances of the mechanism that control cell death by apoptosis (cells escape normal aging and death), e.g. myc gene.

DNA repair genes: Mutations in DNA repair genes are known to lead some cancers.

Metastasis genes: Genes involved in metastasis are **nm23-H1 (NME1) and nm23-H2 (NME2).**

Angiogenesis is required for expansion of the primary tumor and new blood vessels penetrating the tumor are frequent sites for entry of tumor cells into the circulatory system. Cells first detach themselves from the primary tumor and circulate in the body.

Clinical Presentations

Sites: High risk oval

A. Buccal mucosa

B. Soft palate

C. Retromolar region

D. Ventral surface of tongue

E. Floor of mouth

F. Lips

G. Tongue lateral borders

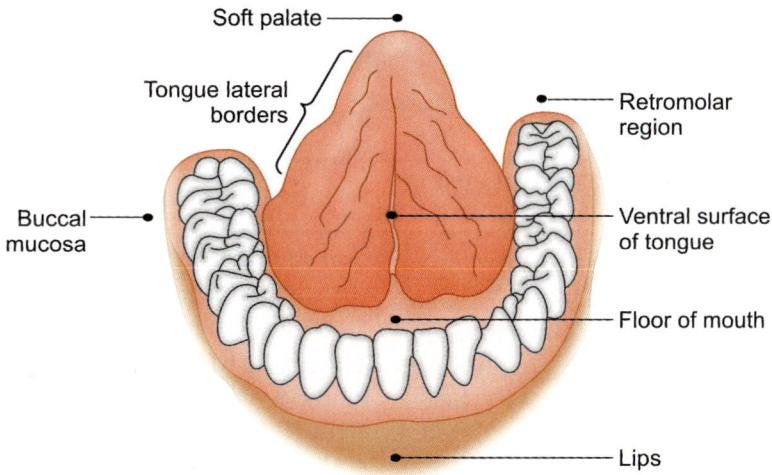

Fig. 7.3: High risk oval

Symptoms
- Lump or swelling/ulcer growth/patch
- Minimally palpable to indurated
- Bleeding
- Loose teeth
- Malfitting denture
- Neck lump or swelling
- Restriction of the tongue movements
- Dysgeusia
- *Change in sensation:* Hyperesthesia, paresthesia, or anesthesia
- Paresis or paralysis
- Chronic cough
- Change in speech
- Change in voice
- Dysphagia
- *Lymphadenopathy:* Submandibular, digastrics and upper cervical nodes

Mode of Spread
- Hematogenous
- Lymphatic

TNM staging: The American Joint Committee on Cancer (AJCC) has developed *tumor nodes metastasis* staging system for cancer. This staging helps clinicians to reflect on prognosis and probable outcome of treatment plan.

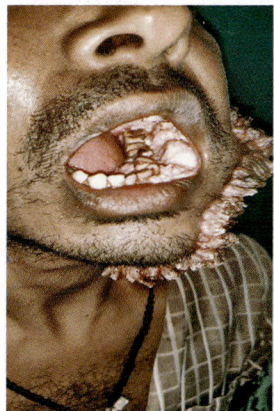
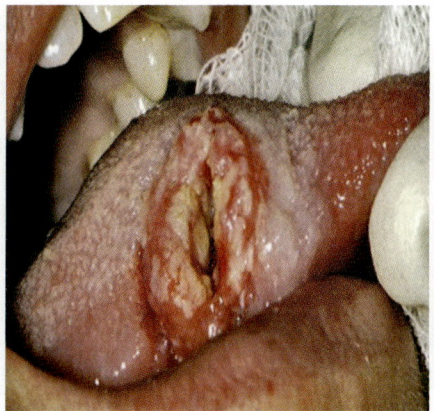
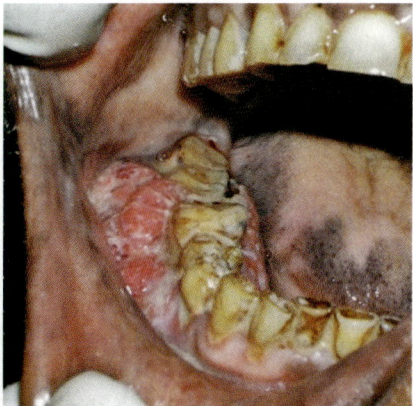

Fig. 7.4: Clinical presentation of oral malignancy

Tumor (T) describes the size of the tumor (area of cancer).

TX: Primary tumor cannot be assessed

T0: No evidence of primary tumor

T1: Tumor 2 cm or less in greatest dimension
T2: Tumor >2 cm, but <4 cm

T3: Tumor >4 cm

T4a: Moderately advanced local disease, means the tumor has grown further than the mouth and oropharynx and into surrounding tissues such as bone, tongue, skin or the facial air cavities (sinuses).

T4b: Very advanced local disease, means the tumor has spread into nearby areas such as the space behind the jaw, the base of the skull, or the area of neck surrounding the arteries (carotid arteries).

Lymph Node (N): Regional Lymph Nodes Affected or Involved

NX: Regional LN cannot be assessed

N0: No regional LN metastasis or there are no cancer cells in the lymph nodes.

N1: Metastasis or cancer cells in 1 lymph node on the same side of the neck (ipsilateral). 3 cm or less in greatest dimension.

N2a: Metastasis or cancer cells in 1 lymph node on the same side of the neck (ipsilateral). >3 cm and <6 cm in dimension.

N2b: Metastasis in more than 1 lymph node on the same side of the neck as the cancer. But none of these nodes are bigger than 6 cm.

N2c: Metastasis in multiple nodes on the opposite side of the neck, or in nodes on both sides. But none of these nodes are bigger than 6 cm.

N3: Metastasis in nodes more than 6 cm.

Metastasis (M): Distant metastasis due to primary tumor.

M describes whether the cancer has spread to a different part of the body.

M0 : Means the cancer has not spread to the other parts of the body.

M1: Means cancer has spread to other parts of the body such as the lungs.

Investigations

There are various diagnostic aids or investigations available for early detection of potentially malignant and malignant lesions of oral cavity. Detail case history with accurate clinical examination is always necessary as an adjunct to investigations.

Toluidine blue: This is a vital tissue staining method. It uses a chromatic dye, which has affinity to bind with DNA. This property is used and the dye is applied directly to suspicious tissue. Positive retention of dye by the lesion helps to identify the site of biopsy.

Fine needle aspiration cytology (FNAC): This diagnostic procedure can be used for neoplastic and non-neoplastic and, for deep seated as well as superficial lesions. It is simple, fairly sensitive and specific procedure, inexpensive and comfortable to the patient. It can be used in conjunction with good clinical and morphological co-relation of the lesion.

Biopsy: Tissue biopsy is gold standard method in detecting malignancy. Incisional or excisional biopsy is performed depending on the criteria of size of the lesion.

Chemiluminescent devices: It involves the use of a hand-held, single-use, disposable chemiluminescent light stick that emits light at 430, 540 and 580 nm wavelengths. The use of the light stick is intended to improve the visual distinction between normal mucosa and oral white lesions. Normal epithelium will absorb light and appear dark, whereas hyperkeratinized or dysplastic lesions appear white. The difference in color could be related to altered epithelial thickness or to the higher density of nuclear content and mitochondrial matrix that preferentially reflect light in the pathological tissues.

Confocal Microscopy

It is an optical imaging technique for increasing optical resolution and contrast of a micrograph by means of using as partial pinhole to block out-of-focus light in image formation. The identification 3000 technology combines anatomical imaging with fluorescence, fiber optics and confocal microscopy to map and delineate the lesion in the area being screened. The advantage of this device is its small size and easy accessibility to all tissues in the oral cavity.

Optical Coherent Tomography (OCT)

It is one of the light-based diagnostic aids which uses back scattered reflections to create images up to a depth of 1.5–2 mm. OCT is a noninvasive real time imaging modality that helps in obtaining images that can be compared to histopathological sections and hence this procedure is also termed optical biopsy.

Oral CDx Brush Biopsy

It uses the concept of exfoliative cytology to provide a cytological evaluation of cellular dysplastic changes. The oral CDx provides a complete transepithelial sample as the brush extends deep in the epithelial layers. The oral cytological epithelial samples are fixed onto a glass slide, stained with a modified Papanicolaou test and analyzed microscopically via a computer-based imaging system.

Molecular Markers

Most tumor markers are proteins and these markers may be detected within exfoliated or distributed cells, or as circulating agents within the peripheral blood or plasma. Other uses of tumor markers are to assess cancer response to:
* Treatment and to check for its recurrence.
* In some types of cancers, tumor marker levels may reflect the presence of the disease but are not predictive of the stage of the disease.

Imaging

Selection of imaging modality depends on the type and location of suspected tumor. It includes:

* Intraoral periapical radiographs, extraoral radiographs like OPG, PA views, etc.
* Ultrasonography, computed tomography, magnetic resonance imaging, positron emission tomography or PET scan.

Other investigations indicated are routine hemogram, ESR, liver function test, kidney function test, X-ray chest

Common radiographic appearances of oral carcinoma involving bone–
* Floating tooth
* Radiolucency with ragged and vague borders
* Band-like widening of PDL
* Mixed radiolucent—radiopaque lesion with vague pattern
* Sunray appearance from the border of the bone, possible combined changes.
* Periosteal reactions
* Onion skin appearance from the border of the bone

Treatment

* Management of oral cancer is a challenge, as it involves multidisciplinary approach to maintain critical functions like mastication, speech, swallowing as well as esthetics of the patient. Treatment of individual case depends on site, location, stage, histology, node status of the lesion and 4Cs, i.e. complication, compliance of patient, cost, convenience (Shah et al 2009).
* There are three basic modalities practiced for the treatment of oral cancer: Surgery, radiotherapy and chemotherapy.

Surgery and radiotherapy: Curative approach: Initial stage (T1 and T2)

Chemotherapy in combination with surgery and radiotherapy—supportive care approach: Surgery/radiotherapy + chemotherapy—advanced stage

Surgery results in a sacrifice of the structure, which can compromise esthetics and function. Surgery involves removal of the primary tumor that may demand for jaw removal with neck dissection. Surgical excision of dysplastic and malignant lesions can also be accomplished with laser

Surgery and radiotherapy—curative approach—initial stage (T1 and T2)

Chemotherapy—in combination with surgery and radiotherapy—supportive care approach

Surgery/radiotherapy+ chemotherapy—advanced stage

Indications for surgery	Indications for radiotherapy	Indications for chemotherapy
✗ For tumors involving bone. ✗ When side effects of surgery are expected to be less significant than those with radiotherapy. ✗ Radio-resistant tumors	✗ Radical treatment (medically inoperable cases) ✗ Post-operative treatment (advanced cases) ✗ As a palliative therapy	✗ Chemoradiation—chemotherapy given with radiotherapy in cases where surgery is not a choice of treatment. ✗ Adjuvant chemotherapy—given after surgery to kill remnant cancer cells. ✗ Induction chemotherapy—given prior to surgery to shrink the tumor. ✗ Sometimes chemotherapy is given to cancers that have metastasized and cannot be treated by surgery.

therapy. Recent advances in surgical field are novel approaches of reconstructions of the jaws such as vascularized flaps and free microvascular reconstruction. These methods help to provide stable implant prosthesis, enhance esthetics and function as a component of rehabilitation.

Radiotherapy is based on principle of interaction of radiation with matter or tissues. It kills cells by reacting with water molecules inside them, causing damage to cells. Cancer cells have less potential to repair after damage compared to normal cells and they are more sensitive to radiations due to higher growth fraction. To achieve better effect of radiation therapy, it is delivered only in fractions for planned days (e.g. 5 days/week with 2 days of gap to repair for 5/6 weeks). Due to this method, central hypoxic cells that are less susceptible to radiations become well oxygenated, as peripheral cells are killed with subsequent fractions of radiation. Exophytic and well-oxygenated tumors are more radiosensitive, whereas large invasive tumors with small growth are less responsive.

Radiotherapy can be administered by methods like external beam radiation therapy (EBRT) and brachytherapy.

External beam radiation therapy (EBRT) directs a beam of radiation externally (outside the body) at tumor inside the body. EBRT delivers high-energy rays to tumors, using a special gamma ray machine called a linear accelerator. Special planning is done to use radiations to reach to the contour of the tumor. The machine moves around the body without touching the patient and aims radiation at the tumor.

Radiation can be delivered to a localized lesion by using implants or needles inside the tumor which is known as brachytherapy.

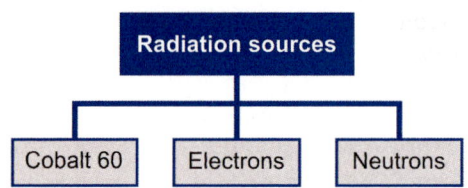

Intensity modulated radiation therapy (IMRT) and image-guided radiotherapy (IGRT) are a few other advance methods of radiotherapy.

Chemotherapy: Chemotherapy refers to the drugs that prevent cancer cells from dividing and growing. It does this by killing the dividing cells. The drug can be administered orally or intravenously depending on the type and stage of malignancy. Commonly used drugs for chemotherapy are 5-Fluorouracil, Cisplatin, Bleomycin, Methotrexate and Taxol.

Complications of Cancer Treatment

Surgery can cause disfigurement of the jaws or face, acute pain, fibrosis due to scarring and neurologic changes. Oral hard and soft tissue structures also respond to radiotherapy and chemotherapy treatment. This occurs due to direct toxicity and secondary bacterial infections occurring in the oral cavity. These oral changes resolve after completion of therapy within a few weeks. Radiation acts by hypovascularity, hypocellularity and hypoxia causing fibrosis and necrosis while chemotherapy suppresses bone marrow activity, which further leads to variable oral manifestations.

TABLE 7.1: Clinical presentation of complication of treatment modalities

Complication	Signs and symptoms	Treatment
Mucositis	⊠ Peripheral erythema ⊠ Dysgeusia	⊠ Maintenance of oral hygiene ⊠ Chlorohexidine gluconate mouthwash.
Hyposalivation/ xerostomia	⊠ Dental caries (often rampant caries) ⊠ Thirst ⊠ Dysphagia ⊠ Dysphonia ⊠ Acid erosion ⊠ Oral candidiasis ⊠ Oral dysesthesia	⊠ Saliva substitute like mucin spray, mucin lozenge, biotene oral balance gel and toothpaste, etc. ⊠ Saliva stimulants such as ascorbic acid, malic acid, parasympathomimetic drugs, etc.
Candidiasis	⊠ Burning sensation in oral cavity ⊠ Pseudomembrane (blisters) formation ⊠ Dysphagia ⊠ Dysphonia	⊠ Antifungal drugs like nystatin, miconazole, gentian violet, amphotericin B, etc.
Caries	⊠ Pain, tooth loss, difficulty in eating. ⊠ Demineralization of calcific structures of teeth.	⊠ Low sugar diet, tooth brushing, fluoride, flossing.
Soft tissue and osteoradio-necrosis	⊠ Pain and swelling. ⊠ A sore or ulcer in the mouth or on the jaw. ⊠ Difficulty opening the jaw or trismus ⊠ An abnormal opening or fistula between the jaw and the surface of the face.	⊠ Antiseptic mouthwashes, antibiotics, ultrasonic therapy, hyperbaric oxygen therapy as a conservative management. ⊠ Removal of small sequestrate, sequestrectomy, alveolectomy with primary closure, closure of orocutaneous fistula and large resections.
Speech and mastication	⊠ Dysphonia ⊠ Dysphagia	⊠ Restoration and rehabilitation.
Taste and smell impairment	⊠ Dysgeusia ⊠ Focal seizure ⊠ Uremia	⊠ Vitamin supplements.
Pain	⊠ Patient's discomfort ⊠ Anxiety	⊠ Administration of analgesics. ⊠ Psychological distress, etc.
Mandibular dysfunction	⊠ Difficulty in mastication ⊠ Dentoalveolar pain ⊠ Malocclusion	⊠ Mouth opening exercises ⊠ Surgical measures to eliminate the cause.
Dentofacial abnormalities	⊠ Malocclusion ⊠ Difficulty in mastication ⊠ Poor esthetics	⊠ Restoring the normal occlusion by orthodontic or by surgical means. ⊠ Rehabilitation

Update

Laser Capture Microdissection (LCM)

This novel technology offers sample purity and complements gene chips by allowing accurate gene profiling studies.

Promising gene therapy strategies have been reported the use of highly efficient adenovirus vectors to deliver therapeutic genes in advanced cases of HNSCC.

"Irressa" is an orally-active selective epidermal growth factor receptor—tyrosine kinase inhibitor, showing anti-tumor activity in HNSCC, in combination with radiation treatment.

Dealing with case history:
✗ Positive history of short duration of lesion with involvement of adjacent vital structures. Absence of pain except in case of secondary infection
✗ History of associated habits
✗ Sudden weight loss, anorexia and malaise

RADIOGRAPHIC STUDY OF MALIGNANT DISEASES OF THE JAWS AND ORAL CAVITY

Malignant tumor is a genetic disorder in the course of its progression in which visible physical changes take place at cellular level and at tissue level.

Radiographic features of malignant tumors of the jaw will be discussed primarily as follows:

- ✗ Primary epithelial tumors, i.e. carcinomas
- ✗ Metastatic [secondary]
- ✗ Sarcoma and
- ✗ Malignancy arising from the hematopoietic system (Table 7.2).

General Radiographic Features of Malignant Tumors of Oral Cavity

Squamous cell carcinomas occur in older age group (>50 years), whereas sarcomas occur in younger age group. They are more common among males. Malignant epithelial tumors of the jaw are commonly present in the following sites, i.e. tongue, floor of the mouth, tonsillar area, lip, soft palate or gingiva. They may spread and invade the adjacent areas involving the upper and lower jaws.

- ✗ Sarcomas are more common in posterior mandible. Some lesions grow in the developing dental follicles and periapical areas of teeth.
- ✗ Metastatic tumors are more seen in posterior mandible and maxilla.

Clinical Features

These tumors are primarily tumors of soft tissue, extending into the bone and thus

TABLE 7.2: Radiographic differences between benign and malignant lesions		
	Benign tumor	*Malignant tumor*
Margins	✗ Well defined	✗ Infiltrative and irregular
Effects on surrounding structures	✗ Displaces the surrounding tissue—no resorption or destruction	✗ Invades and destroys surrounding tissue. Destruction of cortical outlines.
Effects on surrounding structures	✗ There may be periosteal reaction	✗ There is bone destruction and rarely periosteal reaction.
Internal structure	✗ Radiopaque/radiolucent/mixed	✗ Mostly radiolucent except osteosarcoma and some metastatic carcinomas.
Effects on teeth	✗ Displacement and smooth resorption	✗ Resorption is rare. If present, then spiked root resorption. ✗ Floating teeth appearance.

causing radiographic changes. The basic understanding of pattern of growth of malignant tumors reflects in its radiographic presentation. Thus, the clinical features of malignant tumors are discussed pertaining to its radiographic presentation:

- **Ulceroproliferative growth/ulcers/exophytic lesion:** It may sometimes mimic a healing socket after tooth extraction, which however never heals. Presents radiographically as a soft tissue mass with adjacent bone resorption.
- **Uncontrolled uncoordinated growth:** Radiographically ill-defined borders with finger-like extensions
- **Non-encapsulated:** Absence of radiolucent capsule
- **Rapid rate of growth:** Rapid bone destruction and floating teeth appearance
- Persists even after cessation of stimulus
- **Invasion of surrounding structures:** Destruction of cortical outlines
- Displacement and mobility of teeth as compared to contralateral side
- **Regional and distant metastasis:** Metastatic radiolucent lesions
- Exposure of underlying bone presents radiographically as pathological fracture
- Paresthesia may present as invasion of inferior alveolar nerve.

Radiographic Features

These tumors are primarily tumors of soft tissue, extending into the bone and thus causing radiographic changes. There may sometimes be no visible radiographic signs of oral malignant lesions specially when there is only involvement of soft tissues. Radiographic investigations help to determine the extent of the disease and to assess osseous involvement.

Typically, borders are ill-defined with lack of cortication and absence of encapsulation. Evidence of mild ragged border on the alveolar ridge may be seen in initial bony invasion of malignancy arising in soft tissue. The borders may show finger-like projections and uneven extensions of bone destruction, which resembles bays and promontories.

Since epithelial cells are not normal constituents of the bone, thus they do not produce bone, instead cause osteolysis. They are typically radiolucent in most cases. Most malignancies are osteolytic, however, there may be residual islands of bone giving a *salt and pepper appearance* due to rapid destruction of bone. Malignancy causes invasion of surrounding bone.

Metastatic malignant epithelial tumors may sometimes produce bone. Sarcomas which arise from connective tissue elements from which bone forming cells are derived, tend to produce bone. Some metastatic tumors from breast and prostate can induce bone formation, hence appear radiopaque. Osteosarcoma produces bone and may give a patchy radiopaque appearance. Some lesions may stimulate reactive bone formation (osteoblastic).

Malignancy is mostly destructive and rapidly growing. There is destruction of the cortical boundary with adjacent soft tissue mass. It destroys supporting alveolar bone so that teeth may appear to be *floating in space.* Root resorption may be seen. Root resorption is more common in benign tumors, and is smooth. Resorption associated with malignancy is: *Spiked root resorption.*

It penetrates by means of easiest route like periodontal ligament space and causes irregular widening and destruction. It may grow along inferior neurovascular canal and through mental foramen. There is widening of inferior alveolar canal. Inferior border of mandible may be thinned and destroyed resulting in pathologic fracture. Multifocal lesions located at root apices and in the papilla of developing tooth destroying the crypt cortex and displacing the developing tooth in occlusal direction.

Cortical bone destruction of inferior border of mandible, cortical border of inferior alveolar nerve canal, floor of sinus, lamina dura and developing follicles of teeth.

Periosteal reactions in malignant lesions

Onion skin (laminated periosteal reaction)
Formation of *Codman's triangle*

- A spiculated sun-ray/hair on end type of periosteal reaction.

Absence of radiographic features is indicative that the lesion has not invaded the bone or an early lesion involving bone. Careful observation may show superficial mild *surface erosion/cupping* of surface bone described as a *saucer-shaped defect*. Evidence of irregular soft tissue mass adjacent to an area of ill-defined radiolucency is highly suggestive of malignancy.

Squamous cell carcinomas affect the jaws in 2 ways:

1. Primary soft tissue tumor: Arises in soft tissue
2. Central variety: Develops within jaw

RADIOGRAPHIC FEATURES OF SQUAMOUS CELL CARCINOMA/EPIDERMOID CARCINOMA (PRIMARY SOFT TISSUE TUMOR)

Squamous cell carcinomas occur in older age group (>50 years). It occurs most commonly in males. Tongue, floor of the mouth, tonsillar area, lip, soft palate or gingiva are the common sites. Involvement of palate is rare. They may spread and invade the adjacent areas involving the upper and lower jaws. In squamous cell carcinoma of oral mucosa, the malignancy infiltrates the adjacent bone. Thus, the radiographic features are not because of bone tumor, but tumor in bone.

Radiographic Features

Evidence of mild ragged borders on the alveolar ridge may be seen in initial bony invasion of malignancy arising in soft tissue. The borders are ill-defined blending gradually with the normal bone. The borders may show *finger-like projections* and uneven extensions of bone destruction, which resembles *bays and promontories*. There is bone infiltration of tumor in which little bays of bone destruction extend into bone, leaving irregular areas of promontories.

Oral squamous cell carcinoma produces osteolytic lesion which is radiolucent. There may be residual islands of bone giving a *salt and pepper appearance* due to rapid destruction of bone. Initial lesions may show *saucer-shaped* erosions on the alveolar crest. These osteolytic lesions may sometimes resemble alveolar resorption following tooth removal, delaying the diagnosis. There may be presence of pathological fracture in advanced and aggressive lesions.

Malignancy is mostly destructive and rapidly growing causing destruction of the cortical boundary with adjacent soft tissue mass. Evidence of irregular soft tissue mass

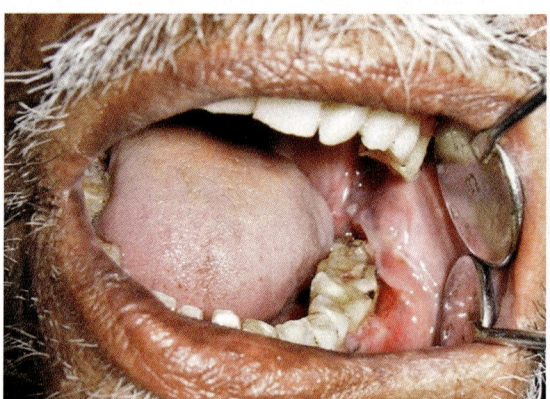

Fig. 7.5: An ulcerative lesion in left cheek region

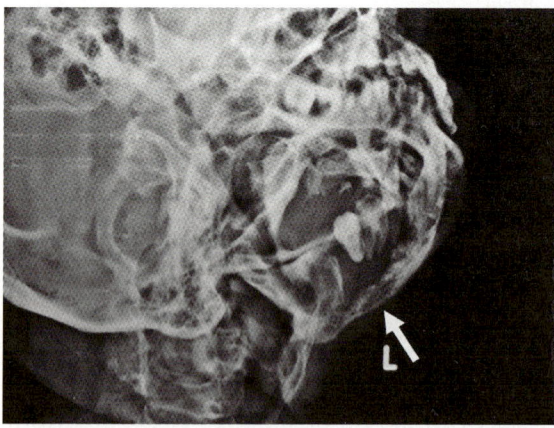

Fig. 7.6: Lateral oblique radiograph of the above case showing floating tooth appearance and ill-defined radiolucent lesion on left side of mandible

adjacent to an area of ill-defined radiolucency is highly suggestive of malignancy. It destroys supporting alveolar bone so that teeth may appear to be *floating* in space. The cortical outlines of maxillary antrum and inferior alveolar canal, etc. are destroyed rather than displaced, as in a benign tumor. There may be evidence of the tumor invasion in the maxillary sinus presenting as a diffuse radiopacity within it with loss of cortical outlines.

Root resorption may be seen rarely and is described as spiked root resorption.

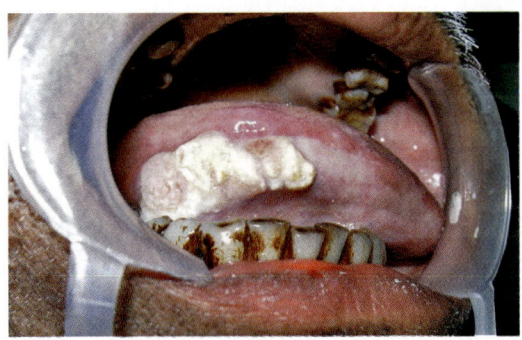

Fig. 7.9: White exophytic lesion on tongue

Differential Diagnosis

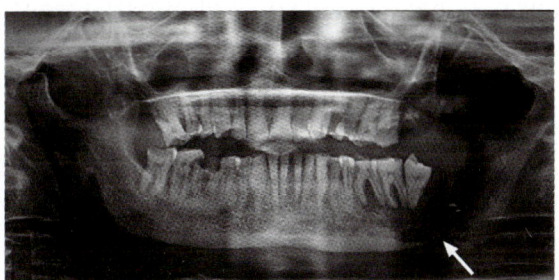

Fig. 7.7: Panoramic radiograph showing severe bone destruction up to the lower border of mandible with ill-defined borders and pathologic fracture

Squamous cell carcinoma	Osteomyelitis
✗ Clinically presence of ulceroproliferative lesion. No evidence of pus discharge.	✗ Clinically presence of non-vital tooth with pus discharge.
✗ No evidence of periosteal reaction	✗ Presence of periosteal reaction
✗ Paresthesia, pathological fracture may be present.	✗ Paresthesia, pathological fracture may be present.
✗ Destruction of cortical structures like inferior alveolar canal.	✗ Cortical structures may be destroyed later.
✗ Floating teeth appearance	✗ Moth-eaten appearance
✗ The borders of the lesion are ill-defined with finger-like extensions.	✗ Borders are ill-defined with radiopaque sequestrum in radiolucent background.

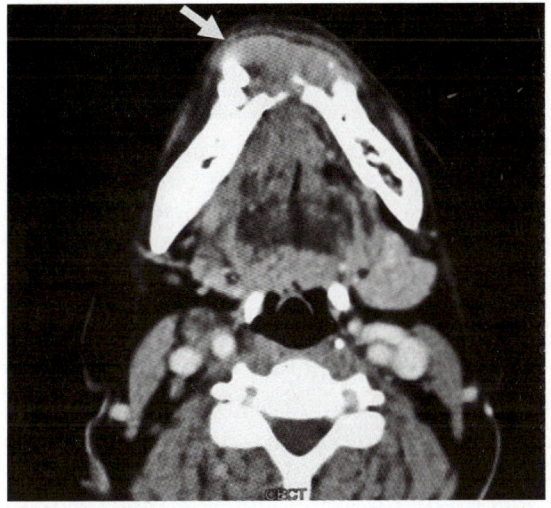

Fig. 7.8: Axial CECT of mandible shows a soft tissue enhancing mass in mandibular anterior region causing erosion of labial and lingual surface of mandible

* In osteoradionecrosis there is previous history of malignancy treated by radiotherapy which resembles osteolytic lesion of squamous cell carcinoma. There may be presence of radiopaque sequestrum.
* Osteosarcoma presents with mixed radiolucent and radiopaque borders. However, there may be some radiographic evidence of sclerotic lesions present. Clinically also, there is no evidence of soft tissue lesion in osteosarcoma.

* **Periodontitis:** The bone destruction in periodontal disease starts at the alveolar crest and extends apically at the root surface. Margins of bone loss in periodontitis are smooth and well-defined as compared to squamous cell carcinoma. Alveolar bone loss in periodontitis is generalized as compared to localized lesion in squamous cell carcinoma. Evidence of mild areas of sclerosis in periodontitis due to chronicity of disease.

* **Langerhans cell histiocytosis:** Epicenter of bone destruction in LCH is in the mid-root region. There is scooped out appearance. It affects patients in younger age group up to 3 decades in contrast to squamous cell carcinoma which affects elderly people.

RADIOGRAPHIC FEATURES OF PRIMARY INTRAOSSEOUS CARCINOMA

Squamous cell carcinoma originating in bone, intra-alveolar epidermoid carcinoma, central squamous cell carcinoma.

The malignant epithelial tumor which arises within the jaw is termed **central or intraosseous carcinoma**. It arises from the intraosseous remnants of odontogenic epithelium like enamel organ or dental lamina, derived from ameloblastoma, odontogenic cysts, etc. It is more common in 4 to 7th decade. It is more common in males.

Mandibular molar region followed by anterior mandible or maxilla is more commonly affected and can occur in the tooth bearing region only.

Radiographic Features

It may be round or irregular in shape with ill-defined periphery and ragged borders.

Internal structure is radiolucent.

Destruction and effacement of adjacent cortical structures and floating tooth appearance.

Differential Diagnosis

Primary intraosseous carcinoma	Metastatic carcinoma
Concentrically destructive	* No uniform pattern of destruction
Usually appears at a single site	* Multifocal
Unilateral	* May be bilateral

Infected periapical cyst or granuloma: The adjacent teeth are non-vital. The borders of infected periapical lesion have lost the cortical outline, however, careful observation may depict the presence of some areas of intact cortical lining of the cyst.

Odontogenic tumors: They are slow growing with well-defined borders causing expansion and thinning of cortex, in contrast to destruction and ill-defined borders.

Carcinoma arising in the cyst: There is presence of a few areas of intact cortical lining of the pre-existing cyst, indicating origin from it.

Multiple myeloma: It is a bilateral lesion with multiple well-defined punched out lesions.

RADIOGRAPHIC FEATURES OF MALIGNANCY ARISING IN A CYST

Epithelial lining of periapical cyst, residual, dentigerous and odontogenic keratocyst may sometimes undergo transformation to form malignant neoplasm. As it is arising from odontogenic epithelium of a cyst, it can appear in tooth bearing region. It is more common in mandible.

The smooth and corticated periphery of the cyst is lost. Initial lesions may show the smooth round oval shape of the cyst, which is lost in advanced lesion. The borders become ragged and ill-defined later.

Internal structure is radiolucent. It causes resorption of corticated lining of maxillary sinus or inferior alveolar nerve canal. Loss of lamina dura of adjacent teeth may occur.

Differential Diagnosis

* **Infected dental cyst:** It may show loss of cortical boundary and ill-defined borders of the cyst, however, some remnants of the intact cortical lining is present. History, previous radiographs and histological examination may confirm the diagnosis.
* Metastatic tumor usually resembles this lesion but are multifocal and history of primary malignancy is present.
* In multiple myeloma multiple punched out well-defined radiolucent lesions are present. Solitary lesion of multiple myeloma may resemble malignancy arising in the cyst.

RADIOGRAPHIC FEATURES OF METASTATIC TUMOR

It affects people of older age with no gender predilection. It is more common in mandibular posterior region of jaw, followed by maxillary sinus, anterior hard palate and mandibular condyle. Paresthesia, without any clinical evidence of a lesion, is the commonest presentation of a metastatic malignancy.

The metastatic lesions may produce either osteolytic or osteoblastic radiographic appearances. The osteolytic lesions may produce

i. Frank bony destruction
ii. Salt and pepper appearance
iii. Multiple areas of bone destruction resembling multiple myeloma.

It has a moderately well-demarcated osteolytic lesion but has no cortication or encapsulation at their tumor margins. It may be polymorphous. Thyroid, prostatic and breast lesions may stimulate sclerotic bone formation and may produce a radio-opaque or mixed radiolucent-radiopaque appearance.

Internal structure is mostly radiolucent if sclerotic metastasis is present and patchy sclerosis is seen.

It stimulates a periosteal reaction in a spiculated pattern resembling *hair on end/* *sunburst appearance*. There is effacement of lamina dura, causing irregular increase in width of periodontal ligament. There may be multiple areas of radiolucencies interspersed with patchy radiopacities giving a *salt and pepper appearance.* Sometimes there may be extensive bone destruction giving a *floating tooth appearance*. In developing teeth there may be effacement of bony crypts. Loss of cortical boundaries of maxillary sinus, nasal fossa, inferior alveolar canal and lower border of mandible.

Differential Diagnosis

Primary squamous cell carcinoma	Metastatic tumor of the jaw
Single lesion is usually present	Multifocal
Clinically presence of exophytic lesion on the alveolar ridge, etc. may be present	Clinically no evidence of pathology in the cavity
Radiographically, presence of soft tissue mass with adjacent ill-defined radiolucent lesion.	Radiographically, multifocal lesions with well-defined borders.
Unilateral	Can be bilateral

Infected odontogenic cyst: It may show loss of cortical boundary and ill-defined borders of the cyst, however, some remnants of the intact cortical lining is present. History, previous radiographs, histological examination may confirm the diagnosis.

Osteomyelitis: Clinical examination, history and presence of infective foci help to rule out. Pus is usually present in osteomyelitis. Moth-eaten appearance, with radiopaque sequestrum, surrounded by involucrum is present.

Squamous cell carcinoma arising in a cyst: There is presence of a few areas of intact cortical lining of the pre-existing cyst, indicating origin from it.

Multiple myeloma: Multiple punched out well-defined lesions.

Periapical lesion: There is periapical periodontal ligament widening in contrast to irregular widening extending up to the side of the root in metastatic carcinoma. The teeth are usually vital in metastatic carcinoma.

Osteopenia and osteoporosis: There is generalized presence of decreased bone radiopacity.

Radiopaque lesions of metastatic malignancy may resemble Paget's disease, however, there is bilateral bony enlargement, which is absent in metastatic malignant lesions.

RADIOGRAPHIC FEATURES OF CENTRAL MUCOEPIDERMOID CARCINOMA

It is a malignancy of the salivary gland, the cells of which are derived from pluripotent cells of odontogenic epithelium or from the lining of a cyst. The tumor behaves like a benign lesion causing displacement of bony walls without destruction. It is more common in mandible, usually in premolar and molar region and occurs above the inferior alveolar canal. It is more common in females.

Radiographically, it appears as a unilocular or *multilocular* expansile mass. Borders are well-defined and well-corticated and often crenated or undulating in nature. Internal structure has a *soap bubble or honeycomb appearance* due to presence of thick or thin cortical septa.

It can cause expansion of adjacent normal bony walls. Teeth are not affected but lamina dura is lost. There is displacement of the mandibular canal inferiorly.

Differential Diagnosis

Radiographically this malignancy resembles multilocular lesions of the jaw-like ameloblastoma, odontogenic myxoma and central giant granuloma which is confirmed histopathologically.

Features of Malignant Ameloblastoma and Ameloblastic Carcinoma

It occurs in middle age up to 6th decade. Males are more commonly affected and more in mandibular posterior region of jaw (premolar and molar).

Well-defined borders with cortication, crenations and scalloping are present. Unilocular or multilocular lesions having *honeycomb or soap bubble appearance* with thick septa are present within the lesion.

Tooth displacement and root resorption by tumor are commonly seen. Cortical boundaries may be effaced or breached. Lesions may erode lamina dura and displace normal anatomic boundaries of floor of mouth and maxillary sinus. Inferior alveolar nerve canal may be displaced or cortical boundaries may show resorption.

Differential Diagnosis

- Multilocular benign lesions like ameloblastoma, central giant cell granuloma, odontogenic myxoma, odontogenic keratocyst
- Malignant lesion of central mucoepidermoid tumor.

The diagnosis of the above lesions is confirmed by histopathology.

RADIOGRAPHIC FEATURES OF OSTEOSARCOMA

It is a malignant tumor of the bone characterized by bone formation. It is known to occur secondary to radiation in Paget's disease and fibrous dysplasia. It occurs commonly in males in 3rd to 4th decade. Lesions are known to occur more commonly in mandibular posterior region and tend to cross the midline.

There are three main radiographic features of osteosarcoma

i. Frankly osteolytic
ii. Lesions producing some bone (mixed radiolucent-radiopaque)
iii. Sclerotic osteosarcomas, almost entirely bone forming.

It is characterized by ill-defined borders with no peripheral sclerosis or encapsulation. When the periosteum is displaced, partially destroyed and disorganized, typical *sun ray spicules or hair on end* trabeculae may be seen. If the periosteum is elevated and maintains its osteogenic potential, but is breached in the center, a *Codman's triangle* is formed.

The internal structure is usually radiolucent, mixed radiolucent-radiopaque or quite radiopaque. Initial radiolucent lesion may give rise to *moth-eaten appearance.* Internal osseous structure may appear as granular or sclerotic and the bone appears as *cotton balls, wisps (sclerotic) or honeycombed* (mixed appearance). Internal structure may show areas of adjacent bone destruction of the pre-existing osseous architecture. The mixed type produces granular or structureless appearing bone. Sclerotic type produces bone of homogenous density and the trabeculae are not clearly seen.

It may be characterized by symmetrical widening of periodontal ligament space of teeth involved in the lesion. This is described as *Garrington's sign.* The antral or nasal wall cortices may be lost/ destroyed in maxillary lesion. Mandibular lesions may destroy the cortex of neurovascular canal and adjacent lamina dura. Subperiosteal reaction may sometimes give rise to *laminated onion peel* appearance. Pathologic fractures may occur in extensive lesion.

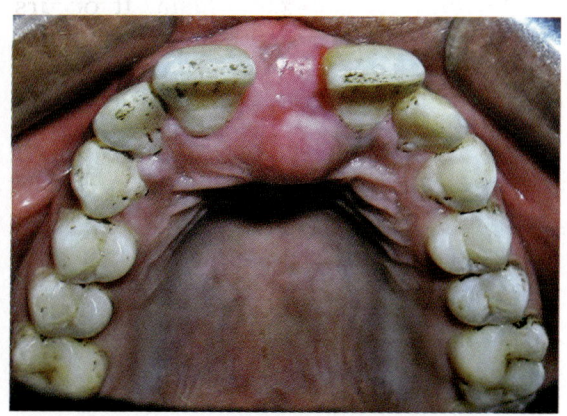

Fig. 7.10: Mild intraoral swelling in maxillary central incisor region showing erythematous area

Differential Diagnosis

Squamous cell carcinoma: Early osteolytic stage of osteosarcoma may resemble squamous cell carcinoma, metastatic carcinoma but can be differentiated by clinical examination and history. There is absence of any soft tissue involvement in osteosarcoma. Sarcoma produces concentric bone destruction as compared to carcinoma.

Chondrosarcoma: It is more common in old age and maxilla.

Osteosarcoma	Chondrosarcoma
Rapid growth rate	Slow growth
Young age	Old age
More malignant potential	Less malignant
High metastasis rate	Slower metastasis
More tendency to recur	Less recurrence
More common	Less common
Mandibular posterior	Anterior maxilla and symphysis and angle of mandible

Ossifying fibroma: It is a benign capsulated lesion with well-defined margins.

Fibrous dysplasia: It occurs in younger age.

Osteomyelitis: Clinical examination, history and presence of infective foci help to rule out. Pus is usually present in osteomyelitis.

Sarcoma is usually rapidly growing.

RADIOGRAPHIC FEATURE OF CHONDROSARCOMA

It is a malignant tumor of cartilaginous tissue. It is of two types: Primary which arises directly from the cartilage and secondary in which malignant transformation occurs in chondroma. Chondrosarcoma is a relatively slow growing malignant lesion.

Primary tumor occurs in younger age, whereas secondary occurs in old age. It affects male and female equally.

It occurs with equal frequency in maxilla and mandible. Maxillary lesions occur in anterior region and mandibular lesions are

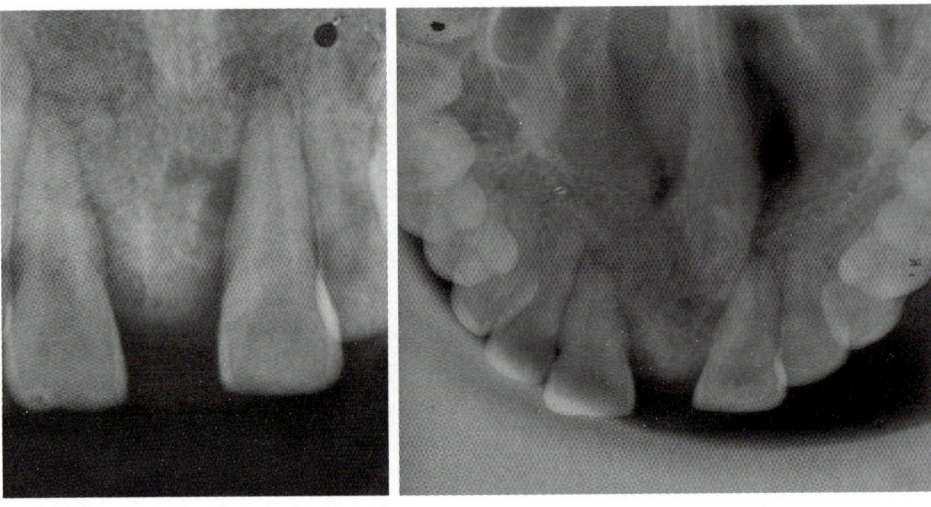

Fig. 7.11: IOPA and occlusal radiograph show irregular radiopacity in upper anterior region

more common in coronoid process, condylar head and neck and symphysis, where cartilaginous tissue is more.

The lesion is slow growing, round, ovoid or lobulated with well-defined corticated borders. Aggressive lesions have infiltrative ill-defined margins. Some form of calcification within the center is seen giving them a mixed radiolucent-radiopaque appearance. Typically described as *moth-eaten appearance*. The central radiopaque structure has been described as *flocculent or snow-like* features.

Since they are slow growing tumors, hence there is expansion of cortical boundaries rather than destruction. Displacement and mobility of teeth is present. In mandible the inferior border is grossly expanded. Maxillary lesions may push the walls of maxillary sinus or nasal fossa and impinge on the infratemporal fossa. Peripheral new bone formation may resemble *sun ray or hair on end* appearance. When condyle is involved, there may be widening of temporomandibular joint space with its remodeling.

Differential Diagnosis

Osteosarcoma: It is relatively more aggressive and has more infiltrative margins.

Fibrous dysplasia: It occurs in younger age with characteristic radiographic appearances.

RADIOGRAPHIC FEATURES OF EWING'S SARCOMA

It mostly affects the long bones and rarely affects the jaw. It is highly invasive tumor with high metastatic potential.

It is more common in mandibular posterior areas and mostly affects in second decade of life. It is common in males.

The borders of the lesion are poorly demarcated and never corticated. Its advancing edge destroys bone in an uneven fashion resulting in ragged borders. The internal structure is entirely radiolucent.

It stimulates the periosteum to produce new bone causing laminar periosteal new bone formation which is described as *onion skin appearance. Codman's triangle or hair on end appearance* may also be seen.

It does not cause root resorption but destroys the supporting bone of adjacent teeth causing mobility. Cortical borders of maxillary sinus, inferior alveolar canal and lower border of mandible may be effaced. There is destruction of dental follicle and lamina dura of adjacent teeth.

Differential Diagnosis

Osteomyelitis: Periosteal reaction is seen in osteomyelitis, however, there is a pus discharge and focus of infection present in it. There is presence of radiopaque sequestrum and moth-eaten appearance.

Eosinophilic granuloma: is characterized by well-defined borders, as compared to ragged borders.

Osteosarcoma: Also shows periosteal reaction. It occurs in one end of the bone, whereas Ewing's sarcoma in center of bone.

Radiographic Feature of Fibrosarcoma

This tumor is more common in mandibular molar and premolar region.

The borders are ill-defined and ragged. They are non-corticated and lack any capsule. They tend to elongate through marrow spaces.

RADIOGRAPHIC FEATURES OF MULTIPLE MYELOMA

It is a malignant neoplasm of plasma cells. The single lesions are called plasmacytoma and multiple lesions are called multiple myeloma.

There is a male predilection and affects commonly at 35–70 years of age.

Posterior mandible is the most common site and lesions are mostly bilateral. It is divided into two varieties:
  i. Solitary (plasmacytoma)
 ii. Multiple

Three main radiographic manifestations are:
  i. Multiple lesions
 ii. Generalized osteoporotic lesions
iii. Solitary lesions

The borders are well-defined and non-corticated. They may sometimes be infiltrative and ill-defined. Multiple radiolucent lesions are present which resemble *punched out radiolucencies*. Solitary lesions may sometimes form sausage-shaped lesions with undulating margins. There may be generalized osteopenia in the bone and the teeth appear conspicuous (to stand out) in the radiolucent jaws.

The surrounding structures may be destroyed. Cortical structures of inferior alveolar canal, lower border of mandible and lamina dura may be obliterated. Root resorption not seen. Teeth are grossly displaced. Widening of periodontal ligament space. There may be a *sun-ray* appearance.

If a large amount of bone is resorbed, the teeth may appear too radiopaque and may stand out conspicuously from their osteopenic background. Lamina dura is lost. Changes are profound if associated with renal disease.

Differential Diagnosis

Benign giant cell tumor: It occurs anterior to the molars and in young people.

Periapical cyst may resemble a plasmacytoma if it is present at the apex of the tooth. The tooth is however vital.

Malignant lesions like histiocytosis X and metastatic carcinoma can be ruled out by histopathology and biochemistry.

Osteomyelitis shows moth-eaten appearance with radiopaque sequestrum.

Hyperparathyroidism also causes multiple radiolucencies of the jaw and occurs in older patients.

MALIGNANT LYMPHOMA

It is a neoplastic process of lymphopoietic cells of reticuloendothelial system involving the lymphocytes and histiocytes. It is of two types: Hodgkin lymphoma and non-Hodgkin's lymphoma.

Radiographic Features of Hodgkin's Lymphoma

It is characterized by painless enlargement of lymphoid tissues of the body.

Cervical lymph nodes are usually involved first followed by other superficial lymph nodes which are painless and rubbery.

It is characterized by severe pruritis and characteristic Pel-Ebstein fever. There is bimodal age incidence and affects young adults and fifth to sixth decade of life. There is no sex predilection. Borders are ill-defined with irregular borders. Internal structure is radiolucent.

Radiographic Features of Non-Hodgkin's Lymphoma

It is a neoplastic proliferation of B lymphocytes and it affects lymph nodes as well as extra nodal sites involving the maxillary sinus, posterior palatal area, posterior mandible and tonsils.

Mostly occur in lymph nodes. Extra nodal sites include maxillary sinus and posterior mandible. It affects all age groups.

There are three radiographic appearances associated with Hodgkin's disease
1. Bone destruction
2. Bone destruction with bone formation
3. Bone formation alone

The most common lesion is the osteolytic one, producing ill-defined radiolucent areas. Initially it takes shape and form of host bone. It has the capability of destroying overlying cortex. The borders are ill-defined and invasive. There may be multiple areas of destruction. In the sclerotic lesions, radiopaque masses may be seen in the maxillary sinus with ill-defined borders. There may be distinct areas of frank sclerosis filling in the narrow spaces.

It is almost always entirely radiolucent. In maxillary sinus lesions the antral walls may be effaced. Lesions involving mandible destroy the cortex of neurovascular canal. There may be *floating teeth appearance* due to destruction of underlying bone. Crypt of dental follicles and lamina dura may be lost. The tumor occurring in younger age group has tendency to shift or displace developing teeth occlusally which may cause their premature eruption and sometimes their exfoliation. There may be a laminated periosteal reaction present.

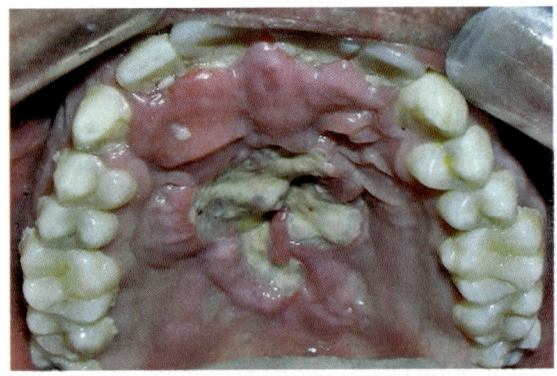

Fig. 7.12: Clinical presentation of NHL as chronic ulcer in the palate

Differential Diagnosis

Ewing sarcoma has similar osteolytic lesions, however, there may be presence of periosteal reaction in it.

Multiple myeloma: Histopathology and presence of Bence-Jones proteins.

Leukemia and Langerhans cell histiocytosis which occur in younger age group, may displace the teeth occlusally.

Osteomyelitis: It is characterized by pus formation and normal appearing bone adjacent to radiolucent lesion in contrast to absence of acute inflammation in Hodgkin's lymphoma.

Sclerotic areas may resemble metastatic breast or prostate carcinoma.

Radiographic Features of Burkitt's Lymphoma

Burkitt's lymphoma is also known as African jaw lymphoma. It is a B cell lymphoma and is the fastest growing tumor with a tumor doubling time less than 24 hours. The endemic form is known as African type and the non-endemic form is the American type.

African cases may involve one jaw or both and affect its posterior parts. It mostly affects young children. There is no sex predilection. Lesions begin as multiple ill-defined large, non-corticated radiolucencies that coalesce later into larger ill-defined radiolucencies with expansile periphery. This expansion breaches its outer cortical limits, causing gross **balloon-like expansion** with thinning of adjacent structures.

Osteolytic radiolucent lesions are present in almost all cases. It grows rapidly to involve adjacent structures like maxilla, ethmoidal and sphenoidal sinuses, nasal and orbital cavity when involving the upper jaw. The teeth in tumor area are grossly displaced. After tumor involvement of the developing dental structures occurs, root development ceases. Lamina dura of teeth is destroyed and cortical boundaries of maxillary sinus, nasal floor are thinned out. There may be an adjacent soft tissue mass.

Differential Diagnosis

Non-Hodgkin's lymphoma radiographically appears similar and it is more common in older age group.

Cherubism: It is common in children and shows floating tooth appearance and is bilateral.

Ewing's sarcoma: Periosteal reaction may be present.

Osteosarcoma: The osteolytic type resembles lesion of Burkitt's lymphoma.

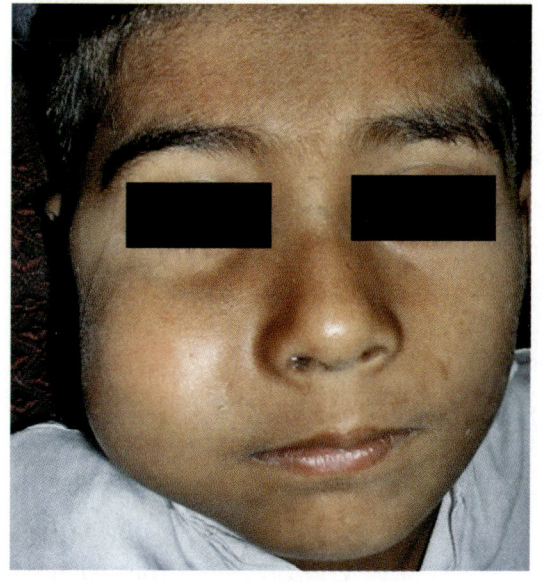

Fig. 7.13: Extraoral swelling associated with Burkitt's lymphoma

RADIOGRAPHIC FEATURES OF LEUKEMIA

Leukemia is a malignancy of immature neutrophils which increase at the expense of other cells in the bone marrow resembling preapical pathology.

Its manifestations are seen in jaws in areas of tooth development, mostly in the periapical area. Leukemic infiltrates called chloromas (greenish in color) may be present in the skull and facial bones. Leukemic infiltration in bone marrow causes ill-defined radiolucent areas in the jaws which are usually bilateral. The radiolucent areas produce osteopenia in which the teeth appear to stand out conspicuously from their surrounding bone. Patchy radiolucent areas are also seen in the jaws.

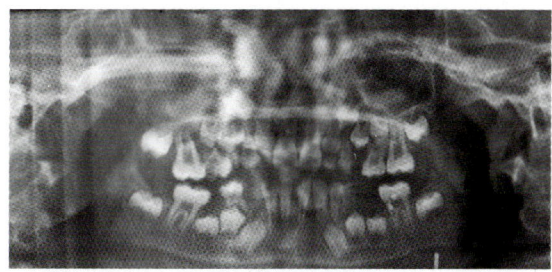

Fig. 7.14: Radiogaraphic presentation of Burkitt's lymphoma

Developing teeth and bony crypts may be displaced occlusally. Premature loss of teeth is seen. Lamina dura and bony outline of dental crypts may be lost. There may be periosteal reaction causing new bone formation without bony expansion.

Differential Diagnosis

Hyperparathyroidism may cause generalized bony radiolucency. Blood investigation may reveal endocrinal imbalance.

Malignant disorders like multiple myeloma and leukemia may cause similar picture on the radiograph.

Radiolucent areas at the apex of tooth may resemble periapical pathology.

Common appearances of malignant lesions involving jaws:

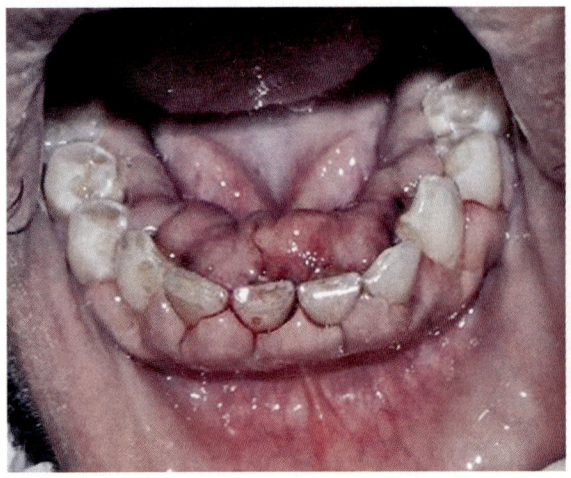
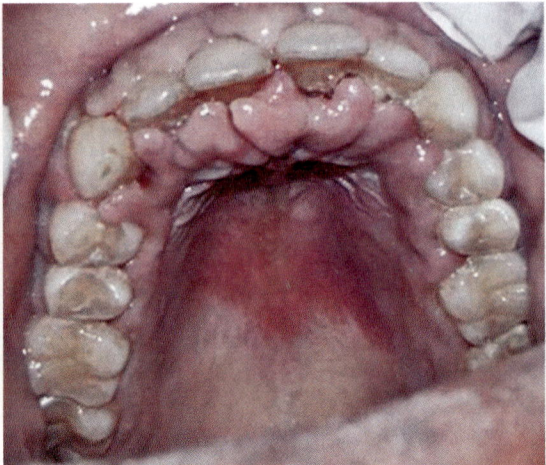

Fig. 7.15: Leukemic gingival enlargement

Sunray/Sunburst appearance
1. Osteosarcoma
2. Hemangioma
3. Thalassemia
4. Sickle cell anemia

Onion peel appearance
1. Ewing sarcoma
2. Osteosarcoma
3. Garre's osteomyelitis
4. Syphilis
5. Infantile cortical hyperostosis

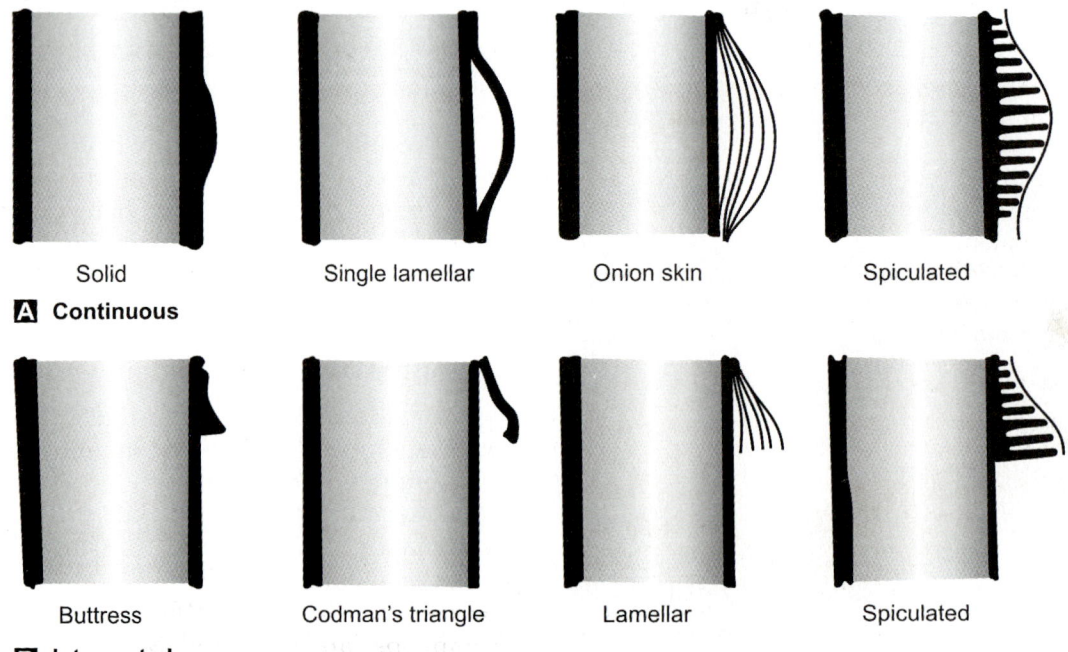

Solid   Single lamellar   Onion skin   Spiculated

A Continuous

Buttress   Codman's triangle   Lamellar   Spiculated

B Interrupted

Fig. 7.16: Various types of periosteal reactions

FREQUENTLY ASKED QUESTIONS

1. Write clinical features, radiographic features, investigations and treatment protocols for malignancy/squamous cell carcinoma.
2. Write a note on radiographic features of malignant lesions in maxillofacial region.
   × Notes: TNM classifications
3. Adverse effects of radiotherapy/chemotherapy.
4. Stages of malignancy.

BIBLIOGRAPHY

1. Malay Kumar, Ronak Nanavati, Tapan G Modi, Chintan Dobariya. Oral cancer: Etiology and risk factors: A review. Jr ICRT 2016, vol 12, Iss.2, 458–463.
2. Hari Ram, Jayanta Sarkar, Hemant Kumar, Rituraj Konwar M.L.B. Bhatt, Oral Cancer: Risk Factors and Molecular Pathogenesis. Jr Maxillofac Oral Surg. 2011 Jun; 10(2): 132–137.
3. Mei Syafriadi. Pathogenesis of oral cancer. Indonesian Journal of Dentistry. 2008; 15(2):104–110.
4. Diana V. Messadi Diagnostic aids for detection of oral precancerous conditions Int J Oral Sci. 2013 Jun; 5(2): 59–65.
5. S Chliephake H. Prognostic relevance of molecular markers of oral cancer--a review. Int J Oral Maxillofacial Surg. 2003 Jun; 32(3): 233–45.
6. Reddy RS, Sai Praveen KN. Optical coherence tomography in oral cancer: A transpiring domain. J Cancer Res Ther.2017 Oct–Dec; 13(6):883–888.doi:10.4103/0973–1482.180684
7. Muralee Mohan Choontharu, Arpit Binda, Smitha Bhat, Sampathila Mahalinga Sharma. Role of tumor markers in oral squamous cell carcinoma: Review of literature and future consideration. Jr SRM Research in Dental Sciences 2012, Volume 3. Iss 4 pg:251–256.
8. Glick M. Burket's Oral Medicine. 12th edition Shelton, USA: Peoples Medical Publishing House; 2015.
9. Woud N., Goaz P. Differential Diagnosis of Oral & Maxillofacial lesions. 5th edition, Elsevier; 2007.
10. Greenberg M. Glick M. Burket's Oral Medicine Diagnosis & Treatment. 10th edition: BC Decker Inc; Elsevier; 2003.
11. Karjodkar F. Essentials of Oral & Maxillofacial Radiology. 1st edition New Delhi: Jaypee Brothers Medical Publishers; 2014.
12. Glick M. Burket's Oral Medicine. 11th edition Shelton, USA: Peoples Medical Publishing House; 2015.
13. Karjodkar F. Textbook of Dental & Maxillofacial Radiology, 2nd edition: Jaypee Brothers Medical Publishers; 2009.
14. Whaites E. Essentials of Dental Radiography & Radiology, 4th edition, Spain: Churchill Livingstone, Elsevier; 2007.
15. White S. Pharoah Medicine Oral Radiology. Principles & Interpretation. 6th edition: Elsevier Inc; 2011.
16. White S. Pharoah Medicine Oral Radiology. Principles & Interpretation. 5th edition: Mushy; 2004.
17. Venkataraman BK. Diagnostic Oral Medicine 1st edition: Wolters Kluwer; 2013.
18. Goaz Paul W. Oral Radiology Principles & Interpretation. 2nd edition: BI Publishers; 1998.
19. Whaites E. Essentials of Dental Radiography & Radiology, 2nd edition, Churchill Livingstone; 1997.

Benign Tumors of the Jaw

According to Rupert Willis, neoplasm is

"An abnormal mass of tissue, the growth of which exceeds and is uncoordinated with that of the normal tissues and persists in the same excessive manner after cessation of the stimuli that evoked the change."

Neoplasms can be classified as benign and malignant.

General characteristics of benign tumors are:
1. They are insidious in onset, are slow growing and spread by direct extension and not by metastases.
2. They have an unlimited growth potential
3. They are well-defined masses of regular, smooth outline with a fibrous capsule.
4. They usually resemble the tissue of origin histologically.
5. Clinically they show enlargement of the jaws or are found during a radiographic examination.

General Symptoms

1. Benign tumors are painless unless they are secondarily infected and do not metastasize.
2. They produce symptoms due to swelling and pressure effect on the surrounding structures.
3. A slow growing benign lesion towards the lower border of the mandible causes the cortex to expand.

4. Some tumors of the bone invade the adjacent normal bone like ameloblastoma.
5. Roots usually may be resorbed.
6. They sometimes recur as their complete removal is difficult.

General Radiographic Features

1. The tumors have a specific anatomic predilection
   × Odontogenic tumors occur in the alveolar process above the inferior alveolar nerve canal.
   × Vascular and neural lesions may originate inside the mandibular canal.
   × Cartilaginous tumors occur in jaw locations where residual cartilaginous cells lie such as in the condyle.
2. They are usually well defined, corticated or hyperostotic. Some tumors are demarcated by a radiolucent band of soft tissue or capsule at the periphery which separates more mature internal radiopaque portion from the surrounding normal bone.
3. The internal structure may be completely radiolucent, radiopaque or mixture of radiopaque-radiolucent structures.

There radiolucent tumors show various appearances. Some are radiolucent unilocular, multilocular, cystic, honeycomb or soap bubble (ameloblastoma, myxoma, hemangioma, central giant cell granuloma).

Mixed Radiopaque-Radiolucent Lesions

- Curved septae that are characteristics in ameloblastoma represent residual bone trapped into the tumor that has remodeled into curved septa.
- Reactive bone lesions seen in central giant cell granuloma.
- Numerous scattered radiopaque foci of varying size giving a snow-driven appearance seen in CEOT, milky-way lumen appearance seen in AOT.
- Complete radiopaque structures usually represent either residual bone or a calcified material that is being produced by the tumor-like osteoblastoma has an internal granular radiopaque pattern which produced by abnormal bone due to tumor.
- Benign tumors can be odontogenic and non-odontogenic tumors.

TABLE 8.1: Classification according to WHO
A. Benign odontogenic tumors
I. Odontogenic epithelial tumors without ecto-mesenchymal origin: a. Ameloblastoma b. Squamous odontogenic tumor c. Calcifying epithelial odontogenic tumor (CEOT)/Pindborg tumor. d. Adenomatoid odontogenic tumor (AOT) e. Keratocystic odontogenic tumor
II. Odontogenic epithelial tumors with ectomesenchymal origin with or without hard tissue formation. a. Ameloblastic fibroma b. Ameoblastic fibro-dentinoma c. Ameloblastic fibro-odontoma d. Compound and complex odontoma e. Odontoblastoma f. Calcifying cystic odontogenic tumor g. Dentinogenic ghost cell tumor
III. Odontogenic ectomesenchymal tumors with or without odontogenic epithelium a. Odontogenic fibroma b. Odontogenic myxoma

c. Cementoblastoma: It is a solitary, slow growing hamartomatous tumor comprising of disorganized cementum at the apical end of the root. It is more common in males and younger adults, with no racial predilection. The involved tooth is vital and painful without any mobility. The adjacent teeth may get displaced. Cementum-like material or abnormal bone with invasion of root canal is seen in the histopathological sections.

Source: Pathology and Genetics of Head and Neck tumors, edited by Leon Barnes, Published by WHO in 2005.

B. Nonodontogenic tumors
I. Benign epithelial tissue origin a. Papilloma b. Keratoacanthoma
II. Connective tissue origin a. Fibroma b. Epulis c. Pregnancy tumor
III. Adipose tissue origin: a. Lipoma
IV. Cartilage tissue origin: a. Chondroma b. Chondroblastoma
V. Bone tissue origin: a. Osteoma b. Torus
VI. Lymphatic and vascular tissue origin: a. Hemangioma b. Sturge-Weber syndrome
VII. Neural tissue origin: a. Neuroma b. Neurofibroma c. Neuroblastoma
VIII. Muscle tissue origin: a. Leiomyoma b. Rhabdomyoma

Source: Collected and modified from Textbook of Oral Pathology. Shafer, Hine, Levy. Edited by B Sivapathasundaram, 8th edition. 2016. Elsevier Inc.

TABLE 8.2: Differences between benign and malignant tumors

	Benign tumors	Malignant tumors
1.	Usually single mass	Multiple masses may be seen
2.	Usually round	Irregular masses
3.	Slow growth	Rapid growth
4.	No necrosis	Necrosis may be seen, so fetid odour
5.	Lymph nodes may not be enlarged	Lymph nodes may be enlarged, fixed
6.	No metastasis	Distant metastasis
7.	Recurrence uncommon	Recurrence common
8.	Good prognosis	Poor prognosis
9.	Tumor cells similar to parent cells	Tumor cells are undifferentiated
10.	Well-defined fibrous capsule present	Fibrous capsule absent
11.	No invasion in connective tissue	Connective tissue invasion seen
12.	Normal nuclei	Abnormal nuclei
13.	No dysplastic changes	Dysplastic changes like abnormal mitosis, increased nuclear–cytoplasm ratio seen
14.	Well capsulated and defined margins	No capsule with ill-defined margins
15.	Root resorption may be seen	Root resorption may not be seen
16.	Displacement of adjacent structures like floor of maxillary sinus, inferior alveolar canal	Invasion of adjacent structures
17.	No floating tooth appearance	Floating tooth appearance due to severe bone destruction
18.	No pathologic fractures	May lead to pathologic fractures

I. EPITHELIAL TISSUE ORIGIN

A. Benign Odontogenic Tumors

I. Odontogenic epithelium tumors without ectomesenchymal origin:

◈ Ameloblastoma

According to Robinson, ameloblastoma is defined as "a tumor of the odontogenic epithelium, which is unicentric, non-functional, intermittent in growth anatomically benign and clinically persistent lesion which does not undergo differentiation to the extent of hard tissue formation."

It arises from remnants of dental lamina and dental organ (odontogenic epithelium).

Clinical features: Ameloblastoma is more commonly seen beyond the age of 40 years, in the molar ramus region. Males are more commonly affected than females. It gives rise to expansion of buccal and lingual cortical plates. Displacement of teeth in the involved region may be seen. Occasionally, pain or paresthesia is noticed. The surrounding bone is thinned out, so on palpation 'egg shell crackling' is felt.

Radiographic features: It is mostly seen in mandibular posterior region in molar-ramus area. The radiolucency is usually well-defined and delineated by a cortical border. In the maxilla it is usually more ill-defined.

Roots of the involved teeth may show resorption.

According to HM Worth, 4 types of appearance are seen.
1. **Unicystic type:** It appears as a unilocular radiolucency resembling the cyst.
2. **Spider variety:** From the center of the lumen, coarse strands of trabeculae radiate peripherally giving size to a *gross caricature of a spider.*
3. **Multilocular radiolucency:** Ameloblastomas which are seen as multilocular radiolucencies have a *soap-bubble appearance.*

4. **Solid ameloblastoma:** Multiple small radiolucencies are seen surrounded by polygonal or hexagonal thick-walled bony cortices giving rise to a *honeycomb* appearance.
   - Tooth displacement is common. An occlusal radiograph may demonstrate cyst-like expansion and thinning of a cortical plates leaving a thin "egg shell" of bone.

Variations

Malignant ameloblastoma is defined as that particular ameloblastoma which has given evidence of truly malignant behavior judged chiefly by the occurrence of metastasis, but in which the metastatic lesions have no significant differences from the primary tumor.

Ameloblastic carcinoma: It is defined as that type of ameloblastoma in which there has been obvious histologically malignant transformation of the epithelial component and in which the tumor has behaved in a malignant fashion, so that the metastatic lesions do not resemble the primary odontogenic tumor.

Mural ameloblastoma: It is unicystic variant arising from the lining of dentigerous cyst.

Recurrent ameloblastoma: Recurrent tumor has typical characteristic appearance of multiple small cyst-like structures with very coarse sclerotic cortical margins.

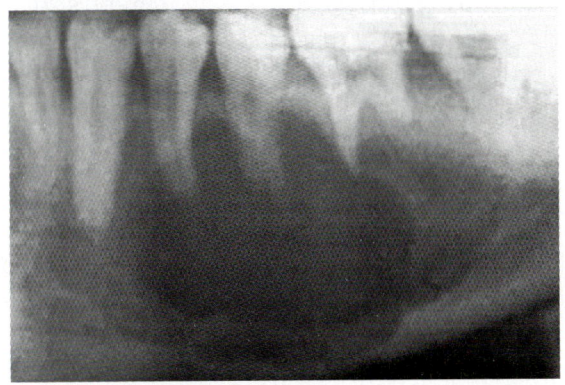

Fig. 8.1: Radiograph showing ameloblastoma

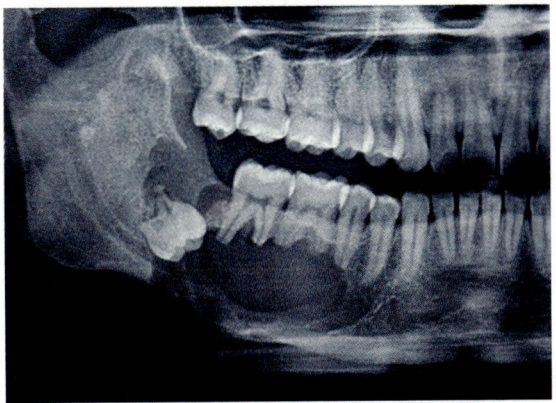

Fig. 8.2: OPG showing ameloblastoma

Management: Complete resection.

Differential diagnosis:

Residual cyst	History of tooth extraction
Central giant cell granuloma	More common in anterior to premolar region
Dentigerous cyst	Radiolucency surrounds CEJ
KOT	Has curved septae, minimal expansion
Giant cell granuloma	Anterior to molars, younger age
Odontogenic myxoma	Sharp, thin septae

◈ Calcifying Epithelial Odontogenic Tumor (CEOT): Pindborg's Tumor

It is an epithelial odontogenic tumor originating from the reduced enamel epithelium.

Clinical features: The frequent age group affected is adults over 40 years of age. Males are common affected than females. Mandible is twice more affected than maxilla with a predilection for premolar–molar region, the swelling is hard, painless and shows slow expansion of buccal and lingual cortical plates. Sometimes may be associated with impacted tooth.

Radiographic features: The lesion is unilocular or multilocular with a well-defined cortex. Initially the lesion is radiolucent. In the mixed stage, numerous scattered radiopaque foci are seen giving a *driven snow appearance.* The trabeculae are irregularly arranged in all directions. It may displace erupting tooth or cause impaction.

On CT examination, expansion of the jaw bone with thinning of buccal and lingual cortex may be seen because of the well-defined mass.

Histologically they are not capsulated. Round eosinophilic masses which undergo calcification, in the form of Liesegang's rings are seen within the tumor.

Management: Enucleation and curettage

Differential diagnosis

Dentigerous cyst	Impacted tooth
Ameloblastoma	Middle age, molar-ramus region

◆ Adenomatoid Odontogenic Tumor (AOT)

It is also called adenoameloblastoma. The tumor is a noninvasive hamartoma arising from enamel organ epithelium and is sometimes as a mixed tumor as it contains connective tissue stroma and sometimes calcifications that have been interpreted as enamel like or dentinoid material. It is commonly associated with an unerupted maxillary cuspid.

- **Follicular type:** Associated with impacted tooth
- **Extrafollicular type:** Not associated with impacted tooth

Clinical features: The average age range is 5 to 50 years with an average age of below 20 years with a female predilection. It is slow growing, gradually expanding, and asymptomatic swelling, associated with unerupted or impacted tooth. It is observed in the anterior region of the jaw mostly.

It is most commonly seen in the cuspid region in the maxilla. The cortex may be expanded. This tumor has follicular relationship with an impacted tooth, it often does not attach at the cemento-enamel junction but surrounds a greater part of the tooth. Often a tooth may be missing in the region affected by the tumor.

Peripheral lesions have been observed on the gingiva as painless masses.

Radiographic features: It is associated with impacted tooth, usually canine. The lesion shows a unilocular radiolucency with well-defined corticated borders. The small radiopaque flecks give rise to *milky way lumen* appearance to the lesion. Most commonly AOT shows a pericoronal radiolucency with well-defined margins. Rarely root resorption is seen. The adjacent teeth may be displaced.

Management: Resection

Differential diagnosis:

Follicular cyst	Radiolucency from CEJ
CEOT	Posterior mandible and older age group
Ameloblastic fibro-odontoma	Multilocular, radio-opacities of enamel and dentine seen in radiolucent area.

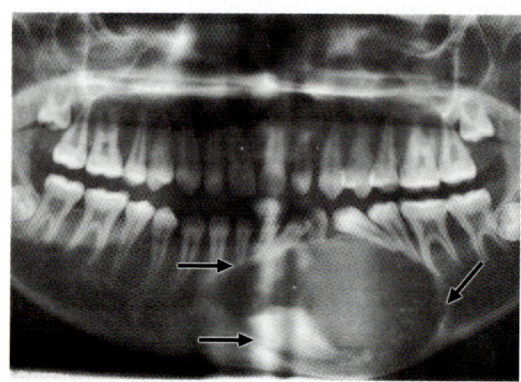

Fig. 8.3: OPG showing AOT associated with impacted canine

◆ Odontogenic Keratocyst (Keratocystic Odontogenic Tumor—KOT)

WHO, in 2005, reclassified KOT as odontogenic tumors from its earlier nomenclature as odontogenic keratocyst which was first explained by Philipsen in 1945. It is also grouped as primordial cyst. It is derived from the remnants of dental lamina. KOTs can be associated with nevoid basal cell carcinoma.

The tumor arises from the dental lamina.

Clinical features: The tumor is more common in 2nd to 3rd decade, with a more male predilection and with a mandibular molar ramus predilection. It is usually asymptomatic. There is minimal swelling and expansion of bone and expands along the bone.

The lumen filled with thin straw colored fluid.

The condition shows high recurrence rate because of:
- Thin epithelium
- Presence of daughter cysts
- No rete pegs in epithelium which is difficult to scrape

Radiographic features: The common site is the posterior mandible, superior to the inferior alveolar canal. The lesion has corticated margins with a scalloped outline. It is smooth, round or oval in shape. It shows radiolucent internal structure with curved septae giving it a multilocular appearance. There is minimal expansion as the tumor grows along the internal aspect of the bone. The roots may get displaced. The inferior alveolar canal may be displaced inferiorly. Radiologically these variations can be noted
- *Envelopmental type:* Envelops an unerupted tooth
- *Replacement type:* Replaces normal teeth
- *Collateral type:* Adjacent to roots of teeth

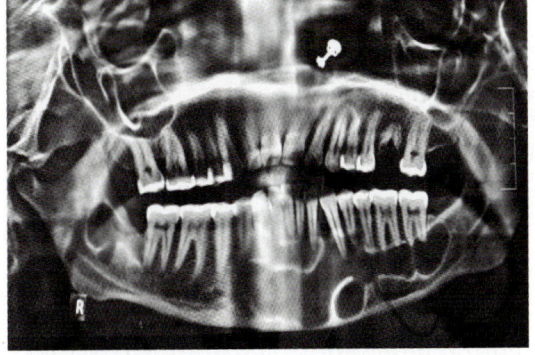

Fig. 8.4: OPG showing OKC

Management: Marsupialization or enuclea-tion. Carnoy's solution is used to irrigate larger lesions and thus has been observed to reduce the size of the lesion.

Differential diagnosis

Dentigerous cyst	Radiolucency involving the CEJ of unerupted teeth
Ameloblastoma	Expansion of cortex, middle age, no straw colored fluid on aspiration
Primordial cyst	Missing tooth seen
Traumatic bone cyst	Usually unilocular with scalloped margins, mostly positive history of trauma

II. Epithelial tumors with ectomesenchymal origin

◈ Ameloblastic Fibroma

It is a tumor of the odontogenic epithelium of the enamel organ and odontogenic mesenchyme of the primitive dental pulp. It is non-invasive as it is well encapsulated. Histopathologically the epithelium is odontogenic in nature and shows focal areas of calcifications. The connective tissue contains randomly oriented fibroblasts.

Clinical features: It is an asymptomatic, slow growing tumor commonly seen in younger age group with an average of 14 years with no sex predilection. The frequent site is mandibular molar region, often associated with an unerupted tooth.

Radiographic features: They are seen as unilocular or multilocular well corticated radiolucencies with indistinct curved septa. Expansion may be noted with an intact cortex.

Management: Surgical excision.

Differential diagnosis:
- Ameloblastoma—middle age, coarse septa
- Giant cell granuloma—anterior to first molars, granular, ill-defined septa.

◈ Ameloblastic fibro-odontoma

It is an expansile tumor with soft tissue component as fibroma and hard tissue component as odontoma. It has a higher growth potential with local destruction. Histopathologically, a well-encapsulated lesion, with the epithelium resembling dental lamina with the connective tissue showing fibroblasts is observed. In the adjacent areas, complex odontomas are seen.

Clinical features: It is seen in the first and second decade of life. It is an asymptomatic, slow growing tumor with swelling, commonly seen in the posterior mandible.

Radiographic features: A well-defined, corticated, large unilocular or multilocular, mixed radiopaque-radiolucent lesion is seen. It may be associated with an impacted tooth.

Management: Surgical enucleation.

Differential diagnosis:
* Ameloblastic fibroma—no calcification
* Odontoma—has no radiolucent component

◈ Odontoma

Odontomes are believed to be hamartomas of dental origin which are derived from the primordial odontogenic cysts during the period of tooth development and they do not grow beyond a particular point.

Mixed variety of odontoma can be classified into:
* Compound composite odontoma
* Complex composite odontoma
* Germinated odontoma
* Dilated odontoma: Further classified as (HM Worth)
  ▪ dens in dente
  ▪ root dilation
  ▪ inverted open umbrella
  ▪ fleur-de-lis which resembles the French emblem

Clinical features: Compound odontoma is made up of two or more tooth-like bodies with enamel capped crowns known *as denticles,* whereas the complex odontoma appears as a single mass with haphazard distribution of enamel, dentine and cementum. Most of compound type occur in the anterior maxilla mainly in association with the

crown of an unerupted canine. In contrast, 70% of complex odontome are found in the mandibular first and second molars.

Dilated odontoma is seen as a single calcified structure with a more radiolucent central portion that has an overall form similar to a doughnut.

Radiographic features:
* *Compound odontome:* It is more common in anterior maxilla, around crowns of unerupted teeth. It appears as multiple radiopaque bodies surrounded by a radiolucent fibrous capsule which is in turn surrounded by a corticated border.
* *Complex odontome:* It is more common in mandibular molar region. It appears as a dense, irregular radiopaque mass, the density of which is equal to that of the dental tissues. It is surrounded by a radiolucent halo which in turn is surrounded by a corticated well-defined border.

Radiographically dilated odontome shows tooth within a tooth appearance because of enamel lined tract within the tooth.

Management: Simple excision

Differential diagnosis:

Complex odontome:

Cemento-ossifying fibroma	More radiopaque, younger patients
Periapical cemental dysplasia	Multiple, common in lower anterior periapical region, wider uneven sclerotic border
Calcifying epithelial odontogenic tumor	Fleks of calcification seen, less opaque.
Enostosis	Do not have soft tissue capsule

◈ Dentinogenic Ghost Cell Tumor

Dentinogenic ghost cell tumor (DGCT) is a rare odontogenic tumor with a locally invasive behavior. It is proposed that DGCT is a neoplastic variant of calcifying epithelial odontogenic cyst. It was renamed by Práetorius et al. and more recently categorized as a separate entity in the updated classification of the World Health Organization (WHO).

Clinical features: It usually affects elderly people and 75% occur in males. Two variants have been recognized: Intraosseous (central) and extraosseous (peripheral). Intraosseous lesions show locally invasive behavior and mostly affect the canine to first molar region. Peripheral DGCT usually shows predilection for the anterior portion of the jaw.

DGCT is characterized by a peculiar histology composed of ameloblastoma like islands of epithelial cells in a fibrous connective tissue stroma with variable amounts of keratin production or dentinoid material. Connection between tumor cells and the overlying oral mucosa has been described in the peripheral lesions.

The condition shows a high recurrence rate.

Radiographic features: DGCTs usually appear as unilocular, mixed radiolucent and radiopaque lesions. Usually the lesions show well-defined borders, but poorly defined borders have been observed in cases.

Management: Radical treatment of peripheral or segmental resection

III. Odontogenic ectomesenchymal tumors with/without odontogenic epithelium

◈ Ossifying Fibroma

It is classified as a fibro-osseous lesion. The term cemento-ossifying fibroma was discarded as it was not easy to differentiate between cementum and bone histologically and radiographically.

Peripheral and central variety can be observed.

Peripheral ossifying fibroma: Calcifications or ossifications seen in the hypercellular fibroblastic stroma.

Clinical features: It is more common in young adults, females than males. It is well-demarcated focal mass exclusively on the gingiva, in the interdental papillae region, sessile or pedunculated. It is pale pink or cherry red. The surface may be intact or ulcerated.

Radiologic features: No underlying bone involvement seen. It rarely shows mild erosion.

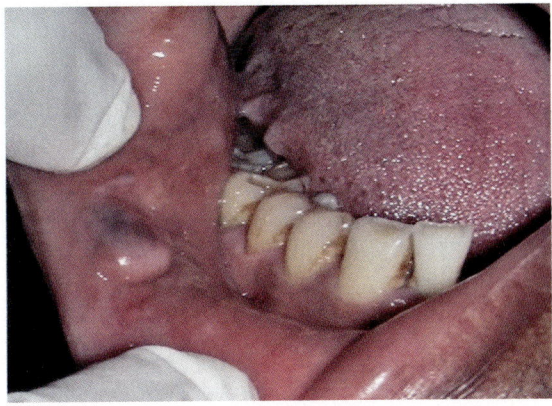

Fig. 8.5: Odontogenic ectomes enchymal tumors

◈ Central Ossifying Fibroma

Clinical features: It is more common in young adults with equal occurrence males and females and more common in the mandibular premolar molar region. It is asymptomatic. Facial asymmetry may be noted because of the swelling. Displacement of teeth is common.

Radiographic features: It is an expansile lesion with a clearly defined cortical margin which enlarges concentrically. Radio-opaque foci appear in later stages which tend to coalesce. The teeth in the region may get displaced and may get resorbed. It grows into cavities like nasal, antral and destroys surrounding bone. It can be subclassified as:
- Ossifying form
- Cementifying or psammomatoid form
- Aggressive or juvenile form: More aggressive form
- Familial gigantiform fibroma

Management: Surgical enucleation

Differential diagnosis:

Ameloblastoma	Age, location
Central giant cell granuloma	Anterior to molars, granular, ill-defined septae
Odontogenic myxoma	Straight sharp septae

◈ Odontogenic Myxoma

Myxomas are rare benign tumors of mesenchymal in origin occurring only in facial bones. These are not encapsulated and tend to infiltrate into the surrounding tissues.

Clinical features: Myxomas are more common in females, usually occur at younger age between 10 and 30 years. It is a slow growing painless swelling, mainly affects mandible in the premolar–molar region. Teeth involved are loosened.

Radiographic features: A well-defined multilocular lesion associated with impacted tooth. The internal structure is made up of thin, straight bony trabeculae arranged at right angles to the periphery giving rise to a *tennis racket or step ladder like pattern*. The lesion also frequently scallops between the roots of adjacent teeth similar to a simple bone cyst.

Histologically, myxomas show loosely arranged spindle cells with long fibrillary processes, which mix with the odontogenic epithelium.

Management: Resection with wider margins

Differential diagnosis:

Ameloblastoma	Septae are not thin and straight, older age, molar ramus region
Central giant cell granuloma	Common in anterior mandibular region
Central hemangioma	Calcifications in larger lesions, no missing teeth
Odontogenic sarcoma	Cortex not intact

Cementoblastoma

It is a solitary, slow growing hamartomatous tumor comprising of disorganized cementum at the apical end of the root. It is more common in males and younger adults, with no racial predilection. The involved tooth is vital and painful without any mobility. The adjacent teeth may get displaced. Cementum like material or abnormal bone with invasion of root canal is seen in the histopathological sections.

Radiologic features: They are commonly seen in the mandibular premolars or first molars. A well-defined radiopacity with corticated margins surrounded by a well-defined radiolucent rim because of the soft tissue capsule is seen at the apical end of the root obliterating the root outline. The internal structure is amorphous and gives a wheel spoke appearance. The roots may show resorption. Larger lesions cause the cortex to expand. Jaw expansion is seen only in larger lesions.

Management: Extraction of involved tooth

Differential diagnosis
* Focal cemental dysplasia—irregular shaped, not attached to root
* Periapical sclerosing osteitis—no radiolucent rim
* Hypercementosis—surrounding periodontal ligament space is thinner, no root resorption.

B. Non-odontogenic Tumors

I. Epithelial tissue origin

◈ Papilloma

It is a rare neoplasm of respiratory epithelium. The most common site is nasal cavity and para-nasal sinuses. Chronic trauma is a major etiology. Oral papillomas are caused by HPV virus.

Clinical features: It is more common in men, third and fourth decade of life. It is an exophytic, cauliflower-like growth. The maxillary and ethmoidal sinus are more commonly affected. It can cause unilateral nasal obstruction, nasal discharge, pain and epistaxis. There is usually a history of recurrent sinusitis. The other sites could be tongue, cheek, lip or oesophagus. It rarely grows more than 1 cm. Oral papillomas do not undergo malignant changes.

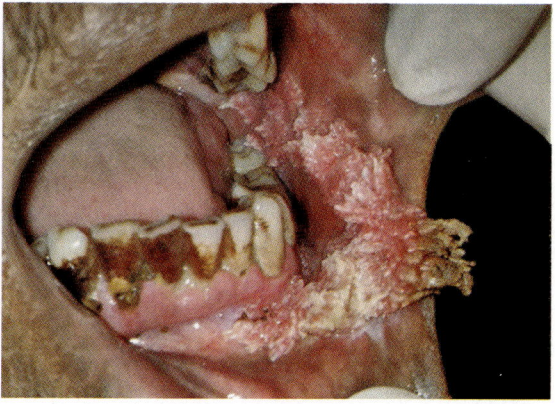

Fig. 8.6: Papilloma

Radiographic features: It is a small homogeneous mass of soft tissue density. The pressure effect may lead to erosion of bone.

Management: Surgical excision, laser.

Differential diagnosis:

Squamous cell carcinoma	More exophytic appearance.
Verrucous carcinoma	Seen in elderly patients with a history of tobacco smoking habit, flat, wide-based lesion.

◈ Keratoacanthoma

It is a localized lesion, usually found in the sun-exposed region, tar, HPV virus, immunocompromised status. It has a rapid growth. It is fixed to surrounding tissue with a pseudoepitheliomatous periphery and a thick keratin cap. 40% of the lesions regress spontaneously.

Clinical features: It occurs at any age group. Men more commonly affected. The common sites are face, neck and dorsum of upper extremities. The lesions are usually solitary, round or dome-shaped. The surface is shiny with a central keratin plug.

Management: Surgical excision, lasers.

Differential diagnosis:

Oral squamous cell carcinoma	Larger lesions, more exophytic.

◈ Fibroma

It is not a true neoplasm with a limited growth potential. Histologically, it appears as a hypocelluar mass with hyperkeratinized epithelium.

Clinical features: It presents as a rounded, painless, firm non-blanching mass on the intact mucosa. it could be seen on the cheek, lips, lateral border of the tongue. It is referred to as traumatic fibroma if it is secondary to trauma.

Management: Surgical excision

Differential diagnosis: Lipoma—soft in consistency

◈ Lipoma

It is a rare intraoral benign tumor of adipocytes. The etiology could be trauma, chronic irritation, infection and hormonal imbalance.

Clinical features: It is more common in age above 30 with no gender predilection. It has been observed on the tongue, buccal mucosa and floor of the mouth. Two variants are: Superficial and diffuse form.

Superficial form is single, sessile or pedunculated mass and diffuse is a deeper version usually. Lipomas are soft in consistency with a yellowish appearance.

Multiple lipomas in head and neck region are common in neurofibromatosis and Gardner's syndrome.

Histologically, collection of multiple adipocytes, well-demarcated from the surrounding connective tissue is seen. Depending upon the involvement of tissues, the lipoma is defined, e.g. small vasculature-angiolipoma.

Management: Lipomas are excised with no recurrence.

◈ Chondroma

These are extremely rare benign tumors of mature cartilage. Histopathologically, lobulated hyaline cartilage is seen which contains small, regular chondrocytes.

Clinical features: They are seen in the anterior maxilla, nasal septum or the body of mandible. They don't have any sex predilection and are painless.

Radiographic features: They appear as well demarcated radiolucent expansions of the bone. At times, calcification of cartilages is seen as radiopacities.

Management: Surgical excision, if required.

◈ Osteoma

Most common mesenchymal neoplasm of bone and commonly seen in the para-nasal sinuses.

Clinical features: It is more common in males, 2nd–4th decade. It is a slow growing, asymptomatic, bony hard swelling. The mucosa is normal over the swelling. It is more common in frontal and ethmoidal air sinuses. The symptoms depend on extent of the growth. Osteoma of maxillary sinus may cause nasal obstruction, swelling on the face or orbital proptosis.

In the jaws, mandibular posterior region is common and could be exophytic.

Soft tissue osteomas are rare and known as osteoma mucosae.

Radiographic features: It is usually round or lobulated homogeneous radiopacity with sharp-defined margins. Larger lesions can displace adjacent structures.

Histologically, osteomas are composed of dense compact bone or coarse cancellous bone.

Management: Surgical resection

Differential diagnosis:

× Fibrous dysplasia—diffuse borders, homogeneousness of bone differs
× Torus—usually bilateral, diffuse

◈ Torus

A bony overgrowth in the body of the bone is a torus. It is the most common exostosis of bone. It develops due to genetic or environmental factors. It may sometimes obstruct in the making of a denture.

Clinical features: It is more common in females, around 30 years of age. It is asymptomatic and may appear single or multiple, unilateral or bilateral, flat, lobulated, or nodular. The overlying mucosa is normal or may get ulcerated due to trauma. The most common sites in maxilla is hard palate and in mandible is lingual surface of the alveolar ridge.

Radiographic features

Torus palatinus: It is well-defined, homogeneous dense radiopacity attached to the palate. The borders are usually well defined.

Torus mandibularis: It could be unilateral or bilateral, homogeneous radiopacity. It is well-demarcated anteriorly and poorly demarcated in the posterior region.

Management
× No treatment if asymptomatic
× Surgical excision if obstructs in denture making or routine activities

Differential diagnosis

Exostosis	Diffuse margins, density of bone

◈ Peripheral Giant Cell Granuloma

It is a reactive lesion of the oral cavity. The etiology could be local irritation, dental plaque, calculus, faulty restoration, ill-fitting dental appliances. Histologically, it is non-capsulated lesion with giant cells resembling osteoclasts in the connective tissue. Numerous capillaries around the periphery of the lesion.

Clinical features: It occurs at around the 4th to 6th decade. Females are more affected than males. It is usually asymptomatic, has a rapid growth rate. It occurs on gingiva or alveolus anterior to the molars. It is pedunculated or sessile, 0.5 to 1.5 cm, red, vascular and granular in appearance. It may get ulcerated due to trauma.

Radiographic features: It may not show any bony involvement. It shows mild superficial erosion or peripheral cuffing of the bone is seen sometime.

Management: Conservative excision.

Differential Diagnosis:
- Other inflammatory lesions—history, biopsy
- Hemangioma—by birth
- Metastatic carcinoma—has a primary lesion elsewhere

◈ Lymphangioma

It is a benign developmental hamartomatous hyperplasia of lymphatic vessels. It is a developmental malformation of vessels. It can be classified as:
 a. Simple lymphangioma
 b. Cavernous lymphangioma
 c. Cellular or hypertrophic lymphangioma
 d. Diffuse systemic lymphangioma
 e. Cystic hygroma lymphangioma

Clinical features: Usually present at birth or before the age of 10. Head and neck lymphangiomas are on the lateral side of the neck and termed cystic hygromas which appear as large, diffuse swellings. Intraorally the common sites are tongue, buccal mucosa and lips. Superficial lesions appear papillary with slightly reddish hue, deeper lesions are diffuse nodules without any significant superficial changes. Tongue involvement may show macroglossia.

Histologically, multiple coalesced lymph vessels in a fibrovascular stroma are seen.

Surgical debulking is the typical line of management.

◈ Central Hemangioma

It is a hamartoma. Proliferation of blood vessels is seen. It is rare in the jaws. It could be developmental or traumatic.

Clinical features: The male: female ratio is 1:2. It is more common in the first decade. The mandible is twice more affected than the maxilla. The ramus and body of mandible is the most common location. It is slow growing, painless bony hard expansion. The adjacent teeth may be displaced or loosened. The tumors are sometimes compressible and show bruit on auscultation. Aspiration shows arterial blood.

Types
- *Capillary:* Aggregation of smaller capillaries.
- *Cavernous:* Dilated blood vessels mainly arteries.

Radiographic features: Larger lesions show expansion of cortex. Well-defined corticated margins are seen. A sun-ray appearance is seen because spicules of bone seen coming out of the bony surface. The marrow spaces are enlarged. Coarse, dense, well-defined trabeculae are seen giving a honeycomb appearance. Phleboliths are seen when the soft tissues are involved. Roots are resorbed sometimes. The inferior alveolar canal follows a tortuous course.

Management: *En bloc* resection, use of sclerosing agents to reduce the size of the lesion.

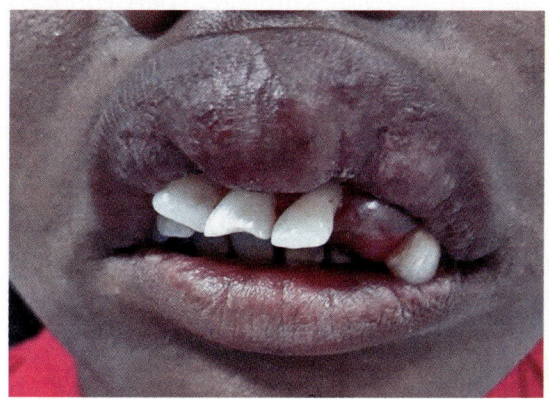

Fig. 8.7: Hemangioma involving upper lip

Differential diagnosis:

Ameloblastoma	Age, location, no calcifications

II. Neural tissue origin

◈ Neuroma

It is not a true neoplasm. There is abnormal proliferation of the peripheral nerve due to mechanical or chemical irritation in an attempt to regenerate.

Clinical features: There is no sex predilection. It is more common in 2nd and 3rd decade. The most common site is inferior alveolar canal. It is a slow growing tumor with swelling, severe pain, paresthesia or neuralgia.

Radiographic features: The mental foramen is the most common location. It is a radiolucent lesion with well-defined corticated margins. There is expansion of the inferior alveolar canal.

Management: Surgical excision along with the proximal portion of the nerve.

◈ Neurofibromatosis: (von Recklinghausen disease)

It is a genetic disorder of the skin. It has two subtypes: Neurofibromatosis 1 (NF-1) and neurofibromatosis 2 (NF-2).

NF-1 is an autosomal dominant condition and appears early in life as 1.5 cm or larger café-au-lait macules in the axilla (axillary freckle sign or Crowe sign) and freckles. These grow in size with age. There could be associated skeletal abnormalities like bone erosion, pigmented hamartomas of the iris or Lisch nodules are observed.

Well-circumscribed, firm growths are seen originating from Schwann cells. In the jaw they may occur in the mandibular canal.

Intraorally, discrete, non-ulcerated nodules are seen on the buccal mucosa, palate, alveolar ridge floor of the mouth and gingiva occurs when tongue is involved.

Diagnostic criteria:
1. Six or more café-au-lait macules
2. Two or more neurofibromas of any type
3. Freckling of axial or inguinal region
4. Optic glioma
5. Two or more Lisch nodules
6. Distinctive osseous lesion
7. Seen in first degree relations.

Shows no or a few peripheral signs. Intracranial or intraspinal neural tumors in the form of schwannomas or meningiomas are seen.

Diagnostic criteria:
- Bilateral VIII nerve tumors OR
- First degree relative OR
- Two of the following criteria:
  - Dermal or subcutaneous neurofibromas
  - Plexiform neurofibromas
  - Schwannoma, glioma
  - Meningioma

Radiographic findings: Unilocular radiolucencies with sharp borders around the nerve region are seen. The nerve canal may show fusiform enlargement.

Differential diagnosis:

Vascular lesions	The whole canal may be enlarged.

Management: Solitary lesions can be surgically excised. Recurrence is observed with malignant transformation in a few cases.

III. Muscle tissue origin

◈ Leiomyoma

It is a benign tumor of the smooth muscles and are uncommon in the oral cavity, except in the blood vessels or excretory ducts of salivary glands.

Clinical features: They are seen in adults over the age of 30 years. It is a slow growing, painless, occasionally pedunculated lesion. It resembles normal mucosal surface.

Management: Surgical excision

◈ Rhabdomyoma

It is a hamartoma rather than a true neoplasm.

Clinical features:
- **Adult type:** It is found in females and older age group. Symptoms are seen depending upon their location. If it occurs on the tongue, it may cause protrusion and if it is seen in the pharyngeal muscles, it may lead to obstruction. The other sites where it could be seen are floor of the mouth or soft palate
- **Fetal type:** It is rare and presents as a painless mass within the muscles usually beneath the intact skin or mucosa
- **Genital type:** It is the rarest and seen as a polypoid mass on the genitalia.

Management: Excision

Differential diagnosis: Lipoma—soft consistency

TABLE 8.3: Differences between cysts and benign tumors

	Cysts	Benign tumors
1.	Usually radiolucent	Mixed radiolucency seen usually
2.	Smooth, round, continuous, corticated	Scalloped borders
3.	Trabeculae absent	Trabeculae may be present
4.	Septae may be present	Septae are absent
5.	Buccal expansion may be seen, rarely lingual expansion	Buccal and lingual expansion may be seen
6.	Root resorption uncommon	Root resorption may be seen
7.	Rarely splaying of roots	Splaying of roots common

FREQUENTLY ASKED QUESTIONS

1. Classify benign tumors. Write about clinical features, radiographic features and differential diagnosis of ameloblastoma / AOT / PGCG / ossifying fibroma.
2. Write a short note on fibroma, osteoma, torus.

BIBLIOGRAPHY

1. Essentials of Oral and Maxillofacial Radiology. Freny R. Karjodkar. Jaypee Brothers Medical Publishers (P) Ltd. 2nd ed. 2014.
2. Differential diagnosis of oral and maxillofacial lesions. Reed Elsevier India Pvt Ltd. .Norman K. Wood, Paul W Goaz. 5th edition. (1997 reprinted 2013).
3. Oral and Maxillofacial Pathology. Quintessence Publishing Co. Inc. Robert E. Marx, Diane Stern. 2003.
4. Buchner A, Akrish SJ, Vered MJ. Central Dentinogenic Ghost Cell Tumor: An Update on a Rare Aggressive Odontogenic Tumor. Oral Maxillofac Surg. 2016 Feb;74(2):307–14. doi: 10.1016/j.joms.2015.08.001. Epub 2015 Aug 7.
5. Candido, Germano Angarani et al. Peripheral dentinogenic ghost cell tumor: a case report and review of the literature. Oral Surgery, Oral Medicine, Oral Pathology, Oral Radiology and Endodontics, Volume 108, Issue 3, e86–e90
6. Woud N., Goaz P. Differential diagnosis of Oral and maxillofacial lesions. 5th edition, Elsevier; 2007.
7. Greenberg M., Glick M. Burket's Oral medicine diagnosis and treatment. 10th edition: BC Decker Inc; Elsevier; 2003.
8. Greenberg M., Brightman V. Burket's Oral medicine diagnosis and treatment. 9th edition: Lippincott

Pigmentation

The oral mucosa and peri-oral tissues can assume a variety of appearances, showing color variations in health and disease. The normal color of gingival tissues has traditionally been described as coral pink, whereas the color of the buccal mucosae and oral vestibules has been described as moist pink. The causes of oral mucosal pigmentations are varied. Broadly stating the oral pigmentations can arise as a result of endogenous or exogenous causes. Endogenous pigmentation arises as a result of intrinsic colored complexes present in the body. Exogenous pigmentation results from extrinsically administered drugs, chemicals, etc. or chromogenic bacteria. Figure 9.1 presents a simple classification of oral pigmentation.

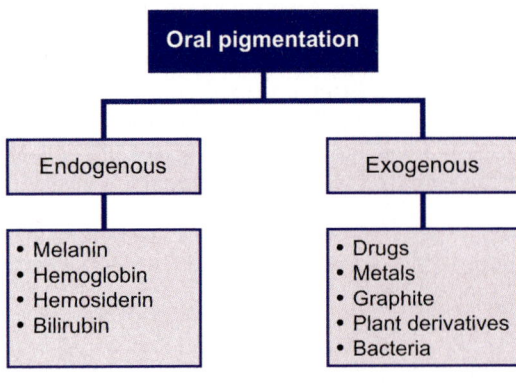

Fig. 9.1: Classification of oral pigmentation

ENDOGENOUS ORAL PIGMENTATION

Colored molecular complexes synthesized within the human body are the causes of endogenous oral pigmentation. Melanin, is a brown-black pigment synthesized by melanocyte, residing near the basal layer of the epithelium. As a general rule, the amount of melanin pigment normally present imparts the skin tone or color. It follows that, any disturbance in the melanin metabolism leads to blackish or brownish appearance of the oral mucosa.

Hemoglobin is a red compound present in the red blood cells. Any factors causing extravasation of blood and lysis of RBCs and vascular overgrowth may hence manifest as reddish/reddish blue appearing lesion on the oral mucosa. Hemosiderin is a hemoglobin-derived granular pigment that is golden yellow to brown and accumulates in tissues when there is a local or systemic excess of iron.

Bilirubin, a yellow orange pigment, is basically a catabolic product synthesized due to the breakdown of hemoglobin. Hyperbilirubinemia causes jaundice, i.e yellowish appearance of skin and mucous membranes.

Table 9.1 enlists in detail the various causes of endogenous oral pigmentation.

TABLE 9.1: Causes of endogenous oral pigmentation (adapted from Burket's Oral Medicine, 11th edition)

Pigment	Etiology	Associated lesion/condition
Melanin	Physiologic, developmental, idiopathic, neoplastic, reactive, drugs, hormones, genetic, autoimmune, infectious	× Ephelis × Melanotic macule × Actinic lentigo × Melanocytic nevus × Malignant melanoma × Physiologic pigmentation × Chloroquine-induced pigment × Lichen planus pigmentosus × Laugier-Hunziker pigmentation × Smoker's melanosis × Peutz-Jeghers disease × Adrenal insufficiency × Cushing's syndrome × Oral submucous fibrosis × HIV/AIDS
Hemoglobin and hemosiderin	Developmental, hamartomatous, neoplastic, genetic, autoimmune, trauma, idiopathic, inflammatory	× Varix × Hemangioma × Lymphangioma × Angiosarcoma × Kaposi's sarcoma, × Hereditary hemorrhagic telangiectasia × CREST syndrome × Hematoma, ecchymosis, purpura, petechiae × Vasculitis × Hemochromatosis
Bilirubin	Trauma, alcohol, infection, neoplasia, genetic, autoimmune	× Jaundice

MELANIN ASSOCIATED ENDOGENOUS ORAL PIGMENTATION

Melanin is the pigment derivative of the amino acid tyrosine. It is synthesized by the melanocytes, which reside near the basal cell layer of the oral epithelium. Melanin is synthesized within specialized structures known as melanosomes. Melanin is composed of eumelanin, which is a brown-black pigment, and pheomelanin, which has a red-yellow color. The melanocytes present in the skin serve as protection against actinic radiation and act as scavangers against cytotoxic metabolites, however, their role in the oral mucosa is obscure. Light, hormones, and genetic constitution influence the amount of pigment produced. Melanin pigmentation may be physiologic or pathologic. It may be focal, multifocal, or diffuse in its presentation. Figure 9.2 highlights the various causes of oral melanotic hyperpigmentation. Biopsy is definitively mandated whenever a clear-cut cause of oral hyperpigmentation cannot be ascertained.

Focal Melanocytic Pigmentation

Freckle (Ephelis)

The cutaneous freckle, or ephelis is a common, asymptomatic, small (1–3 mm), well-circumscribed, tan- or brown-colored macule that is often seen on the sun-exposed regions of the facial and perioral skin.

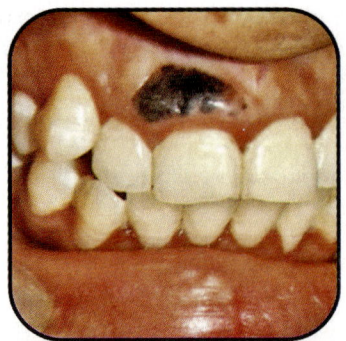

Focal
- Freckle/ephelis
- Oral/labial melanotic macule
- Oral melanoacanthoma
- Melanocytic nevus
- Malignant melanoma

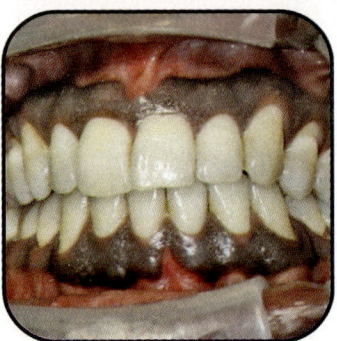

Multifocal/diffuse
- Physiologic
- Smokers melanosis
- Drug-induced melanosis
- Postinflammatory hypermelanosis
- Melasma

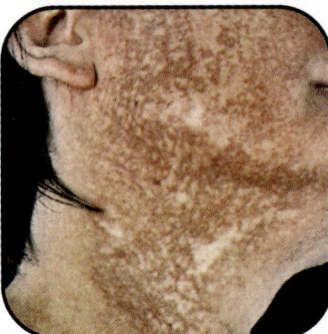

Associated with systemic disease
- Hypoadrenocorticism
- Cushing's syndrome/Cushing's disease
- Hyperthyroidism
- Primary biliary cirrhosis
- Vitamin B$_{12}$ deficiency
- Peutz-Jegher's syndrome
- Café au lait pigmentation
- HIV associated melanosis

Fig. 9.2: Causes of melanotic oral hyperpigmentation

Etiopathogenesis: Freckles are developmental in origin and a genetic basis for their formation has been identified that includes polymorphisms in the ***Melanocortin 1 receptor gene (MC1R)*** and an another freckles-predisposition gene which has been mapped to chromosome ***4q32–q34***.

Clinical features: These innocuous macules are most commonly observed in light-skinned individuals and in red- or light blond-haired individuals. Although the pigmentation itself is focal, most patients have multiple freckles. These are usually more in number and darker in intensity during childhood and adolescence. Freckles tend to become darker during periods of prolonged sun exposure (spring, summer) and less intense during the autumn and winter months. They arise as a result of temporary overproduction of melanin by a normal quota of melanocytes due to stimulation by UV radiation. With increasing age, the number of freckles and their color intensity tends to reduce.

Treatment: No therapeutic intervention is needed as the lesions tend to spontaneously resolve over a period of time.

Oral Melanotic Macule

The oral melanotic macule is defined as a benign, pigmented lesion exclusive to the oral mucosa, with no known dermal counterpart. It is the most common oral lesions of melanocytic origin, that is relatively innocuous in nature.

Etiopathogenesis: The etiology of the melanotic macule remains largely obscure. Trauma has been postulated to be an elucidating factor. In a rare instance, the lesion has also been reported after external beam radiotherapy. However, exposure to sunlight has no role whatsoever in the development of these lesions.

Clinical features: Melanotic macules develop more common in females with a predisposition for the lower lip and gingiva though any intra-oral mucosal site may be involved. It is usually a solitary lesion that occurs mostly in light-skinned individuals. Although the lesion may develop at any age, it generally tends to present in adulthood, mean patient ages being between 31.5 and 44 years. Congenital melanotic macules have also been reported.

The lesions usually present as small (<1 cm), well-circumscribed, oval macules that are uniformly pigmented, brown to black in color (Fig. 9.3). Most of the lesions remain constant in size and do not tend to become malignant. Their size is unaffected by sun exposure. They do not recur after surgical removal. Microscopically, increased melanin is seen in the basal cell layer with many lesions also showing melanin in the lamina propria, some of which is contained in melanophages.

Differential diagnosis: The differential diagnosis includes melanocytic nevus, malignant melanoma, amalgam tattoo, and focal ecchymosis. If such pigmented lesions are present after a 2-week period, ecchymosis can usually be ruled out, and a biopsy specimen should be obtained to secure a definitive diagnosis. Since oral mucosal malignant melanomas have no defining clinical characteristics, a biopsy of any persistent solitary pigmented lesion is always warranted.

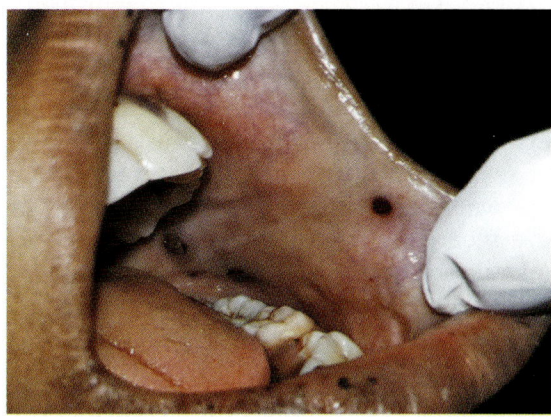

Fig. 9.3: Melanotic macule present on the left buccal mucosa

Treatment: The incisional biopsy is diagnostic as well as curative for the lesion.

Oral Melanoacanthoma

Oral melanoacanthoma is a benign, relatively uncommon pigmented lesion of the unique to the oral mucosa. The lesion is innocuous in nature, with many cases showing spontaneous regression. Oral melanoacanthoma is an entity clearly distinct from the melanoacanthoma of skin. The cutaneous melanoacanthoma represents a pigmented variant of seborrheic keratosis and typically occurs in older Caucasian patients.

Etiology and pathogenesis: The oral melanoacanthoma is essentially a reactive lesion. Patients often report a history of acute trauma or a chronic irritation usually prior to the development of the lesion.

Clinical features: Oral melanoacanthoma is seen almost exclusively in the individuals of the negroid race, has a definite a female predilection, and is most common during the third and fourth decades of life. The buccal mucosa is the most common site of occurrence. The lips, palate, gingiva, and alveolar mucosa also may be involved. Most patients exhibit solitary lesions, although bilateral or multifocal involvement is possible as well. Oral melanoacanthomas typically are asymptomatic; however, pain, discomfort, burning, and pruritus have been reported in a few cases. The lesion may be smooth, flat or slightly raised, and dark-brown to black in color. Lesions often demonstrate an increase in size rapidly, reaching a diameter of several centimeters within a period of a few weeks. The borders are typically irregular in appearance, and the pigmentation may or may not be uniform.

Differential diagnosis: The clinical presentation and a rapid increase in the size of the lesion often gives rise to the suspicion of malignant melanoma. Since, clinically it is not distinguishable from other melanocytic lesions, a nevus and melanotic macule could also be considered in the differential diagnosis.

Treatment: Because of the alarming growth rate of oral melanoacanthoma, incisional biopsy is usually indicated. Microscopically, the oral melanoacanthomas are characterized by a proliferation of benign, dendritic melanocytes throughout the full thickness of an acanthotic and spongiotic epithelial layer. A mild lymphocytic infiltrate with exocytosis is also characteristic. Once the diagnosis has been established, no further treatment is necessary. The biopsy procedure itself may lead to spontaneous regression of the lesion. Recurrence or development of additional lesions has been reported only rarely. There is no potential for malignant transformation. In cases where a source of irritation is present, it must be removed to prevent any future recurrence.

Melanocytic Nevus (Mole)

The term 'nevus' encompasses a varied group of pigmented lesions occurring on the skin or oral mucosa. Nevi could be congenital or developmental in origin. As opposed to ephelides and melanotic macules, which result from an increase in melanin pigment synthesis, nevi arise due to proliferation of melanocytes.

In general, both genetic and environmental factors are thought to play a role in the formation of nevi. Sun exposure is a well-recognized factor for the development of nevi on the skin. The role of genetics in nevogenesis, has been evidenced by the occurrence nevi in a number of inherited diseases, e,g. Turner's syndrome and Noonan syndrome, etc.

Acquired Melanocytic Nevus

The most commonly recognized nevus is the **acquired melanocytic nevus,** or common **mole**—so much so that the simple term *nevus* is often used synonymously for these pigmented lesions. The acquired melanocytic nevus represents a brownish black pigmented lesion of the skin and mucous membrane that arises due to a benign, localized proliferation of the *nevus cells* (Fig. 9.4). The nevus cells are the derivatives of neural crest cells.

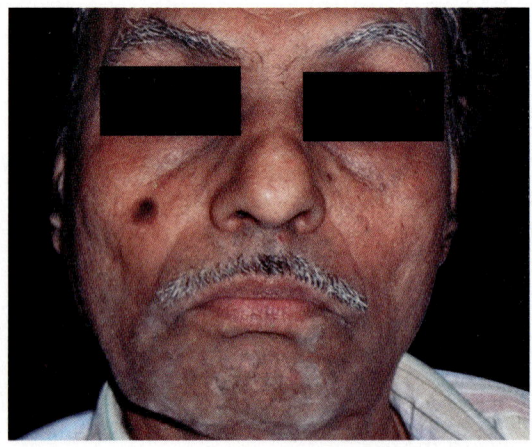

Fig. 9.4: A melanocytic nevus on the face in a middle aged Indian man

Clinical features: The development of the acquired melanocytic nevi on the skin usually begins in childhood, and most lesions are present before 35 years of age. There is a slight female predilection for their development. It has also been found that there is an increased occurrence of these lesions in Caucasians. The head and neck region is relatively a common site, with most lesions.

Acquired melanocytic nevi advance through several clinical stages, which tend to correlate with specific histopathologic features. The foremost clinical presentation is that of a sharply demarcated, brown or black macule, typically less than 6 mm in diameter, **the junctional nevus**. As the lesion progresses over time, the nevus cells proliferate to produce a slightly elevated, soft papule with a relatively smooth surface, **the compound nevus.** Further, the amount of visible pigmentation becomes less and the lesion appears brown or tan. As time passes, the nevus gradually loses its pigmentation, the surface may become somewhat papillomatous, and hairs may be seen growing from the center, **the intradermal nevus.** Figure 9.5 shows the prototypical clinical appearance of these three types. However, the nevus usually remains less than 6 mm in diameter. Ulceration does not occur usually, unless the nevus is located where it is constantly subjected to irritation by clothing like belts, etc. Many of the acquired melanocytic nevi undergo spontaneous involution and disappear with ageing.

Intraoral melanocytic nevi are relatively uncommon. Common intra-oral locations are the hard palate, buccal mucosa, and gingiva, though any oral mucosal site may be affected. Roughly two-thirds of intraoral examples are found in females and the average age at diagnosis is 35 years. Intraoral lesions progress through same stages as the skin lesions and have a similar appearance, but papillary surface change does not occur even in mature lesions. Some intra-oral nevi may lack clinical pigmentation.

Microscopically, the acquired melanocytic nevus is characterized by a benign, unencapsulated proliferation of small, ovoid cells called the nevus cells. These cells demonstrate a variable capacity to produce melanin, with the pigment primarily evident in the superficial aspects of the lesion. Nevus cells typically lack the dendritic processes that melanocytes possess.

Halo nevus (as the name suggests surrounded by a halo) and spitz nevus (solitary, dome-shaped pink/red nevus typically seen in children) are cutaneous nevi with distinct clinical characteristics.

Treatment and prognosis: No treatment is indicated for a cutaneous melanocytic nevus unless it is needed for esthetic considerations, is chronically irritated by clothing, or shows clinical evidence of a change in size or color. By midlife, cutaneous melanocytic nevi tend to regress. If removal is indicated, then conservative surgical excision is the treatment of choice and any recurrence is unlikely. There have been incidences of skin **melanomas** arising from long standing or irritated nevi of the skin. Overall, the risk of transformation of a particular acquired melanocytic nevus to melanoma is approximately 1 in 1 million.However, because any oral melanocytic nevi clinically can mimic an early malignant melanoma, it is generally advised that biopsy be performed for all unexplained pigmented oral lesions, especially because of the extremely poor prognosis for oral melanoma discovered in its later stages.

Congenital Melanocytic Nevus

Congenital melanocytic nevus as the name suggests affects the newborns. Depending on its size, it is divided into two types: (1) Small (<20 cm in diameter) and (2) large (>20 cm in diameter). Approximately 15% of congenital nevi are found in the head and neck area, although intraoral involvement is quite rare.

Clinical features: The small congenital melanocytic nevus may be similar in appearance to an acquired melanocytic nevus, but it is frequently larger in diameter. The large congenital lesion classically appears as a brown to black plaque, usually with a rough surface or multiple nodular areas. Early lesions are flat and light tan, becoming elevated, rougher, and darker with age. A common feature is the presence of **hypertrichosis** (excess hair) within the lesion, which may become more prominent

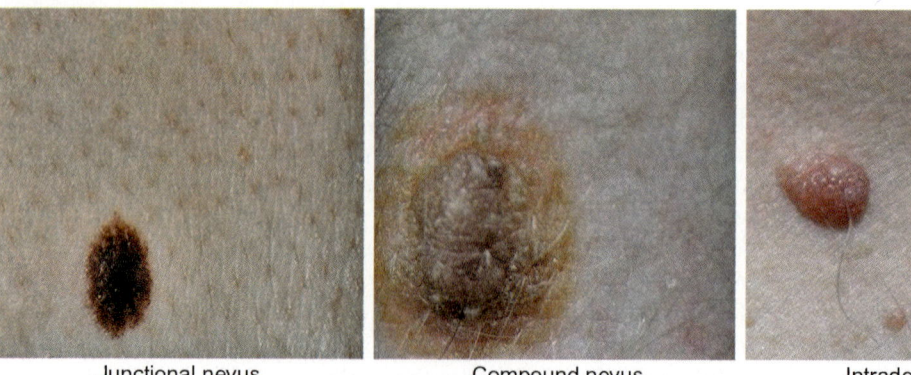

Junctional nevus   Compound nevus   Intradermal nevus

Fig. 9.5: Typical clinical appearance of the three types of cutaneous nevi

with age **(giant hairy nevus).** A very large congenital nevus sometimes may be referred to as **bathing trunk nevus** or **garment nevus,** because it gives the appearance of the patient wearing an article of clothing.

The histopathologic appearance of the congenital melanocytic nevus is similar to that of the acquired melanocytic nevus, and some small congenital nevi cannot be distinguished microscopically from the acquired nevus. In addition, congenital nevus cells often are seen intermingled with neuro-vascular bundles in the reticular dermis and surrounding normal adnexal skin structures (e.g. hair follicles, sebaceous glands).

Treatment and prognosis: Many congenital melanocytic nevi are excised for aesthetic purposes. In addition, 3% to 15% of large congenital nevi may undergo malignant transformation into melanoma. Therefore, whenever feasible, these lesions should be removed completely by conservative surgical excision. Close follow-up is required for lesions not removed. Patients with multiple large congenital nevi also are at risk for developing neurocutaneous melanosis, a rare congenital syndrome in which patients may develop melanotic neoplasms of the central nervous system (CNS), including meningeal melanosis or melanoma. Unfortunately, no effective therapy is currently available for patients with symptomatic neurocutaneous melanosis.

Blue Nevus (Dermal Melanocytoma; Jadassohn-Tièche Nevus)

Blue nevus is an uncommon, benign proliferation of dermal melanocytes, usually deep within subepithelial connective tissue. Two major types of blue nevus are recognized: (1) The **common** blue nevus and the **cellular** blue nevus. The common blue nevus is the second most frequent melanocytic nevus encountered intraorally. The blue color of this lesion can be explained by the **Tyndall effect,** which relates to the interaction of light with particles in a colloidal suspension. In the case of a blue nevus, the melanin particles are deep to the surface, so that the light reflected back has to pass through the overlying tissue. Colors with long wavelengths (reds and yellows) tend to be more readily absorbed by the tissues; the shorter-wavelength blue light is more likely to be reflected back to the observer's eyes. Most common intraoral location is the hard palate.

Malignant Melanoma

Malignant melanoma is a malignancy of melanocytic origin that arises from a benign melanocytic lesion or *de novo* from melanocytes within otherwise normal skin or mucosa. It is the deadliest of all primary cancers of skin.

Etiopathogenesis: The etiopathogenesis of malignant melanoma, like any malignancy is an interplay of both environmental and intrinsic factors. Damage from ultraviolet radiation and acute sun damage, in the form of history of multiple sunburns especially at a young age are considered a major causative factor. Oral lesions, however, are not related to sun exposure. A positive family of melanoma is also a strong risk factor. Additional predisposing factors include a fair complexion and light hair and a history of dysplastic or congenital nevus.

In recent years, there have been many discoveries regarding recurrent genetic alterations in melanomas, including those involving the *Ras-Raf-ERK*, mitogen activating protein (MAP) kinase, and phosphatidylinositol 3-kinase *(Pl3K)* pathways. Melanoma-prone families have a high incidence of germline mutations in the tumor suppressor genes, CDKNA2 and CDK4 and BRAF, HRAS, and NRAS proto-oncogenes.

Clinical Features

Cutaneous malignant melanoma: Malignant melanomas of the skin occur usually in white individuals living in the sunbelt regions. The age range is 30–80 years with the average age at diagnosis being 55 years. 91% of all melanoma lesions arise on the skin and of all cutaneous lesions, about 25% arise in the head and neck regions. Overall, there is a male predilection, but melanoma is one of the most commonly occurring cancers in women of child bearing age. On the facial skin, the malar region is a common site for melanoma since this area is subject to significant solar exposure. Melanomas may develop either *de novo* or arise from a pre-existing nevus. As many clinical similarities exist between melanoma and its benign counterpart, the melanocytic nevus, an "ABCDE" system of evaluation has been developed. The ABCDE criteria include: A symmetry, irregular borders, color variegation, diameter greater than 6 mm, and evolution or surface elevation.

Four main clinico-pathologic subtypes of melanoma have been described.
1. Superficial spreading melanoma
2. Nodular melanoma
3. Lentigo maligna melanoma
4. Acral lentiginous melanoma

In the first three varieties, the initial growth is characterized by radial extension of the tumor cells **(radial growth phase).** In these lesions, the malignant melanocytes have a tendency to spread horizontally through the basal layer of the epidermis. These lesions have a good prognosis if they are detected early and treated. Eventually, however, the malignant cells begin to invade the underlying connective tissue, thus initiating **the vertical growth phase**. The development of nodularity in a previously macular lesion is often an ominous sign. In the nodular melanoma, the vertical growth phase predominates.

Superficial Spreading Melanoma

Superficial spreading melanoma is the most common variety found on the skin, representing about 70% lesions. The site predilections are, the interscapular area in males and the back of the legs of females. The lesion essentially appears as a macule which may be tan, brown, gray, black, blue, white or pink in color. Usually, the lesion is smaller than 3 cm in greatest diameter at diagnosis, but it may be larger. The lesional surface may show slight elevated. Clinically, invasion is indicated by the appearance of surface nodules or induration. Satellite macules or nodules may develop around the primary lesion.

Lentigo Maligna Melanoma

Lentigo maligna melanoma develops from a precursor lesion called **lentigo maligna (Hutchinson's freckle).** It accounts for 5% to 10% of cutaneous melanomas, lentigo maligna occurs almost exclusively on the sun-exposed skin of fair-complexioned older adults, particularly in the midfacial region. The lesion appears as a large, slowly expanding macule with irregular borders and a variety of colors, ranging from tan, brown, black, and even white.

Acral Lentiginous Melanoma (Mucosal Lentiginous Melanoma)

Acral lentiginous melanoma is the most common form of oral melanoma. It is commonly seen in blacks. The usual sites involved are palms, soles, subungual area, and mucous membranes. It begins as a darkly pigmented, irregularly marginated macule, which later develops a nodular growth phase that is invasive.

Nodular Melanoma

Nodular melanoma represents 15% of cutaneous melanomas, and one-third of such lesions develop in the head and neck area. Nodular melanoma is thought to begin almost immediately in the vertical growth phase; therefore, it typically appears as a nodular elevation that rapidly invades into the connective tissue. Nodular melanoma is usually a deeply pigmented exophytic lesion, although sometimes the melanoma cells are so poorly differentiated that they no longer can produce melanin, resulting in a non-pigmented **amelanotic melanoma.**

ORAL MALIGNANT MELANOMA

Primary mucosal melanomas comprise less than 1% of all melanomas. The majority develop in the head and neck, mostly in the sinonasal tract and oral cavity. The prevalence of oral melanoma is higher among black-skinned individuals and Japanese people. The etiology of the oral malignant melanoma is obscure and mutations in BRAF gene are less common as compared to the skin lesions. A definite male predilection has been reported, with two-thirds of the affected individuals being males. Most patients are older than 50 years of age at the time of diagnosis. The hard palate and the maxillary gingiva are the sites most commonly involved. An oral lesion typically begins as a brown to black macule with irregular borders (Fig. 9.6) though most melanomas are often nodular at the time of diagnosis. The macule

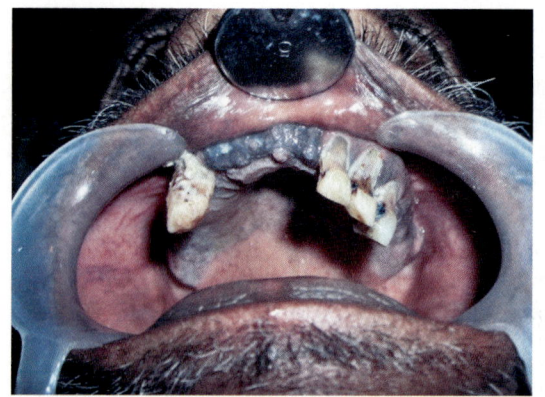

Fig. 9.6: Malignant melanoma of the maxillary anterior region presenting as pigmented patch

extends laterally, and a lobulated, exophytic mass develops once the vertical growth is initiated. Up to one-third of oral melanomas may exhibit a little or no clinical evidence of pigmentation a phenomenon termed amelanosis. Most lesions remain relatively soft to palpation. Other signs and symptoms that may be associated with oral melanoma are nonspecific including ulceration, pain, tooth mobility or spontaneous exfoliation, root resorption, boneloss, and paresthesia/ anesthesia may be evident. Underlying or adjacent bone may show radiographic evidence of irregular or "moth-eaten" destruction. The mucosal melanomas are usually diagnosed at a more advanced stage and are much more aggressive than their cutaneous counterpart. Regional lymphatic metastases are frequently identified. Melanoma occasionally affects the parotid gland, usually as a metastatic deposit from a scalp, conjunctival, or paranasal tumor.

In a few cases, oral melanomas may appear as diffuse multifocal areas of pigmentation. This particular appearance can be attributed to the presence of both melanotic and amelanotic areas within a lesion. Lesions of the oral cavity that do not involve the hard palate or gingiva and exhibit amelanosis are more likely to be metastatic lesions from another primary site.

Thus, the clinical differential diagnosis may be quite exhaustive and could include melanocytic nevus, oral melanotic macule, and amalgam tattoo, as well as various vascular lesions and other soft tissue neoplasms. Hence a biopsy of any persistent solitary pigmented lesion is always warranted. Oral mucosal malignant melanoma usually has a grave prognosis with 5-year survival rates between 15 and 40%.

Histopathologically, oral mucosal melanomas may show a radial or a vertical growth pattern. The radial pattern is often seen in macular lesions wherein clusters of pleomorphic melanocyte exhibiting nuclear atypia and hyperchromatism proliferate within the basal cell region of the epithelium. As the vertical growth into the connective tissue starts, the lesions appear clinically as nodular mass.

Treatment

1. *Surgery:* For primary oral melanomas, ablative surgery with wide margins is the first line of treatment. Adjuvant radiation therapy may also be required.
2. *Chemotherapy and immunotherapy:* Chemo- and immunotherapeutic strategies are often used if metastases are identified and as a palliative measure. Adjuvant interferon-alpha-2B therapy has been approved for the treatment of primary cutaneous melanomas greater than 4 mm in thickness. The role of an anti-tumor vaccine against malignant melanoma is also under exploration owing to its immunogenic nature.

MULTIFOCAL/DIFFUSE PIGMENTATION

Physiologic Pigmentation

Physiologic pigmentation remains the most common source of multifocal oral mucosal pigmentation. It is frequently observed in dark-skinned individuals. Clinically it appears as patchy to generalized hyperpigmentation of the oral mucosal tissues usually involving the gingiva and buccal mucosa (Fig. 9.7). The pigmentation begins in childhood itself. The pigmentation is considered a variation of normal and has no particular clinical relevance. Surgical intervention may be indicated if the pigmentation is compromising the esthetics. Gingivectomy and laser therapy have been used to remove pigmented oral mucosa. However, repigmentation may occur.

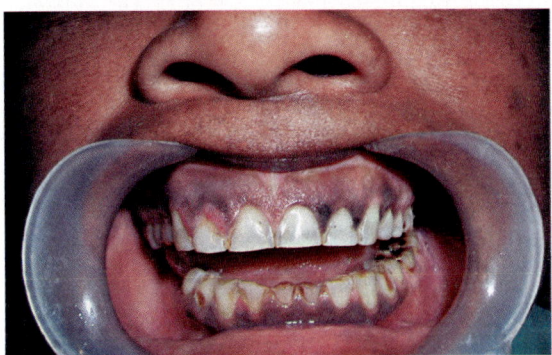

Fig. 9.7: Physiologic gingival pigmentation in an Indian female of wheatish complexion

Differential diagnosis: Idiopathic, drug-induced, or smoking-induced pigmentation. Hyperpigmentation associated with endocrinopathic and other systemic disease

Drug-induced Melanosis

Etiology and pathogenesis: Medications may induce oral melanosis or cause oral pigmentation due to the soft tissue deposition of drug metabolites. The later kind of pigmentation is discussed with exogenous pigmentation further in the chapter. Table 9.2 shows the list of drugs commonly implicated in inducing oral mucosal melanosis. Of these, the most common offenders are the antimalarials including chloroquine, hydroxychloroquine, quinacrine. Although the mechanisms by which melanin synthesis is increased remains unknown, one theory is that some drugs may stimulate melanogenesis and others may physically bind to melanin which results in retention of the drug within melanocytes and may contribute to the oral pigmentation.

TABLE 9.2: Drugs that may induce diffuse oral melanosis

✗ Amiodarone	✗ Imipramine
✗ Amodioquine	✗ Ketoconazole
✗ Aziodothymidine	✗ Mepacrine
✗ Bleomycin	✗ Methacycline
✗ Busulfan	✗ Methyldopa
✗ Chloroquine	✗ Minocycline
✗ Chlorpromazine	✗ Oral contraceptives
✗ Clofazamine	✗ Premarin
✗ Cyclophosphamide	✗ Quinacrine
✗ Gold	✗ Quinidine
✗ Hydroxychloroquine	✗ Tacrolimus
✗ Hydroxyurea	

Clinical features: Clinically, the pigmentation can be localized to one mucosal surface, often the hard palate and gingiva (Fig. 9.8), or it can be multifocal and involve multiple surfaces. The diffuse lesions are flat and without any evidence of nodularity (Fig. 9.9). The lesions present on the skin may be exacerbated by sun exposure. Microscopically, there is evidence of basilar hyperpigmentation and melanin incontinence without a concomitant increase in the number of melanocytes.

Diagnosis: In most cases, the pigmentation resolves and subsides within a few months after the offending drug is identified and discontinued. Nonetheless, pigmentation caused by hormone therapy may persist longer.

Differential diagnoses include other causes of diffuse mucosal pigmentation.

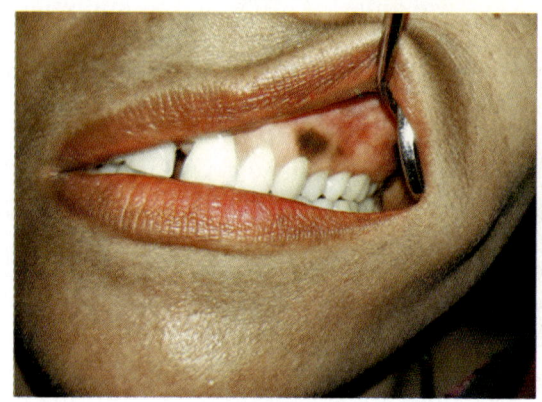

Fig. 9.8: Localized gingival pigmentation; patient gave a history of homeopathic medicine used for arthritis

Smoker's Melanosis

Multifocal oral pigmentation involving the anterior maxillary and mandibular gingiva, buccal mucosa, lateral borders of the tongue, hard palate, and floor of the mouth is reported among cigarette smokers (Fig. 9.10). Melanin synthesis is thought to be stimulated by tobacco smoke products. It is also postulated that one or more of the chemical compounds incorporated within cigarettes, along with

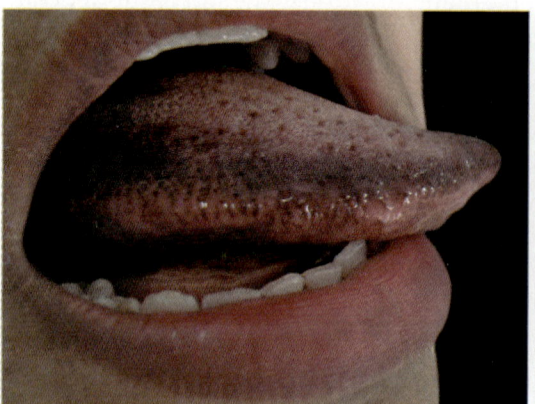
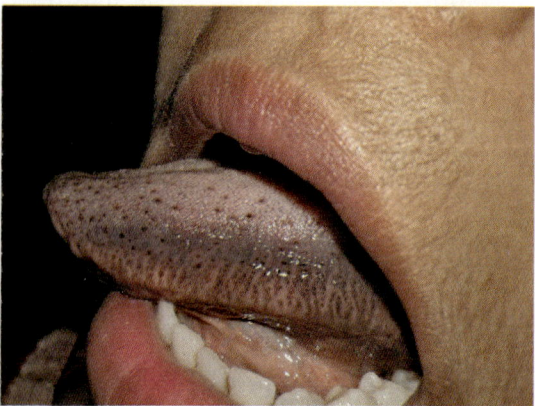

Fig. 9.9: Pigmentation seen on the lateral borders of the tongue post-chemotherapy for a case of misdiagnosed breast cancer

the heat generated, rather than the actual tobacco, may be causative.

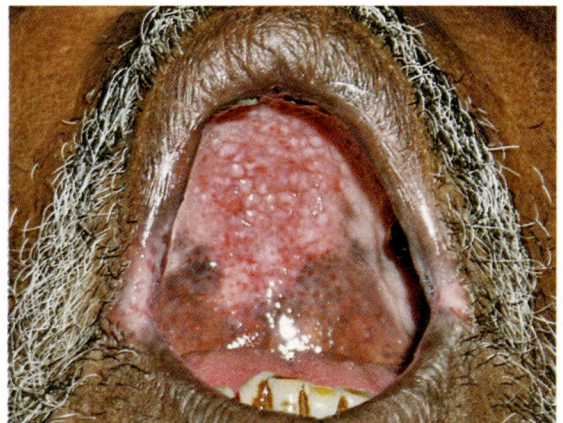

Fig. 9.10: Grayish black pigmentation of the soft palate in a smoker

Clinical features: The pigmented areas are brown, flat, and irregular or map-like in configuration, prominently during the first year of smoking. Spontaneous resolution is reported with the cessation of the smoking habit. Smoker's melanosis is not a potentially malignant condition. In addition to smoking, alcohol abuse has also been associated with diffuse oral mucosal pigmentation particularly in the posterior regions of the mouth and soft palate. Diffuse patchy pigmentation may also be seen in oral submucous fibrosis caused by areca nut chewing habit.

Histologically, basilar melanosis with melaninin continence is observed.

Postinflammatory Hyperpigmentation

Postinflammatory hyperpigmentation is the presence of focal or diffuse pigmentation in sites that have been subjected to previous injury or inflammation. It is more commonly observed in dark individuals. The areas of healed acne on the face are a relatively common site for this phenomenon.

Postinflammatory pigmentation in the oral cavity has been observed in the following instances:

× **Oral lichen planus (lichen planus pigmentosus):** Pigmentation has been observed along with lesions of oral lichen planus (Fig. 9.11). Upon resolution of these lesions, the pigmentation may or may not disappear. Histologically, along with the typical histopathological changes of lichen planus basilar hyperpigmentation and melanin incontinence are seen.

× The overlying mucosa in a nonmelanocytic malignancy may become pigmented.

Melasma (Chloasma, Pregnancy Mask)

The term 'melasma' is used to describe the hyperpigmentation changes seen on the

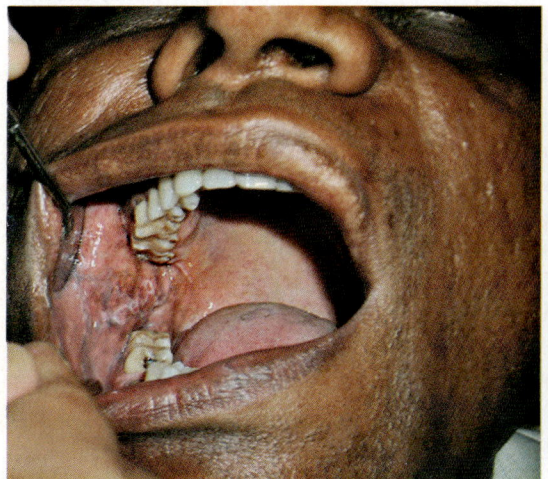
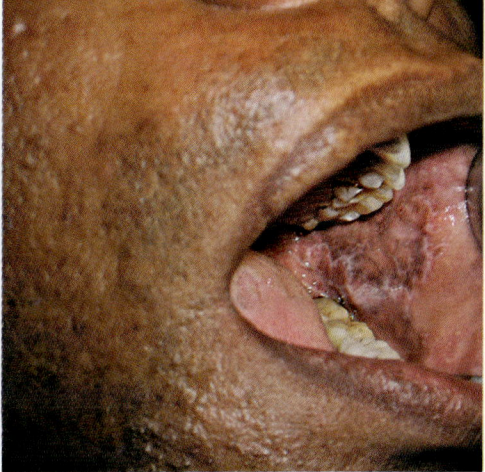

Fig. 9.11: Pigmentation associated with reticular lichen planus on buccal mucosae

face that are associated with pregnancy or ingestion of contraceptive hormones in females. It develops as acquired, symmetric areas of diffuse hyperpigmentation on sun-exposed areas of the skin and the face. The forehead, cheeks, upper lips, and chin are the most commonly affected. Melasma tends to evolve rapidly over a period of a few weeks. Sun exposure excerabates the condition further. Rare cases of idiopathic melasma have also been described in females. It is believed that the combination of estrogen and progesterone hormones induces the melanosis. The condition may spontaneously resolve after parturition, or cessation of the exogenous hormones. Biopsy reveals basilar melanosis with no increase in the number of melanocytes.

MELANOSIS ASSOCIATED WITH SYSTEMIC OR GENETIC DISEASE

Hypoadrenocorticism (Addison's Disease)

Hypoadrenocorticism is an endocrinal disorder characterised by a decrease in endogenous corticosteroid levels, which can have grave consequences. The causes of hypoadrenocorticism include autoimmune disease, infection, malignancy, trauma, medications, genetic disease and iatrogenic causes. As a result of low steroid levels, there is a compensatory activation of adreno-corticotropin hormone (ACTH) secretion from the pituitary gland. With persistently low steroid levels, there is a loss of feedback mechanism, resulting incontinuous secretion of ACTH. Along with the ACTH the serum levels of alpha-melanocyte-stimulating hormone also increase. This phenomenon is due to the fact that ACTH and alpha-MSH share the common precursor gene called pro-opiomelanocortin. Both these hormones are also thought to have stimulatory effects on melanocytes.

Clinical features: The first sign of disease may be mucocutaneous hyperpigmentation. Generalized bronzing of the skin and diffuse but patchy melanosis of the oral mucosa are the prototypical features of hypoadrenocorticism. Other important symptoms include weakness, fatigue, and depression. Diffuse hyperpigmentation is more commonly associated with chronic form hypoadrenocorticism. Evaluation of serum cortisol and electrolyte levels is necessary to make a diagnosis of addisonian hyperpigmentation. Treatment consists of exogenous steroid replacement therapy. With appropriate therapy, the pigmentation eventually resolve.

The differential diagnosis includes other causes of diffuse oral pigmentation as discussed earlier.

Cushing's Syndrome/Cushing's Disease

Cushing's syndrome results from high levels of circulating endogenous or exogenous corticosteroids. Causes include injudicious and poorly monitored steroid therapy, pituitary tumor (Cushing's disease), adrenal pathology (hyperadrenocorticism), as well as ectopic secretion of corticosteroids in certain malignancies like small cell lung carcinoma.

Clinical features: Cushing's syndrome is more common in female patients. Signs and symptoms include truncal obesity, weight gain "moonfacies," and diffuse mucocutaneous pigmentation in some cases. Hyperpigmentation is common in patients where the etiology is a primary pituitary neoplasm, that leads to increased ACTH secretion. Oral pigmentation appears similar to as seen in hypoadrenocorticism. Serum steroid and ACTH levels help in the diagnosis, and the pigmentation tends to resolve after appropriate treatment of the underlying cause.

Hyperthyroidism

It has been reported that more than one-third of the patients diagnosed with hyper-thyroidism and thyrotoxicosis present with diffuse mucocutaneous hyperpigmentation. This phenomenon is relatively common amongst dark skinned individuals. The trigger mechanism in this situation remains largely unexplained, but the pigmentation spontaneously resolves following correction of the thyroid disorder.

Primary Biliary Cirrhosis

Primary biliary cirrhosis is an autoimmune disorders that result from damage to small intrahepatic bile ducts. This condition may cause generalized melanotic as well as non-melanotic hyperpigmentation (yellowish discoloration, due to jaundice). The exact mechanism by which melanosis develops in this condition is unknown.

Vitamin B₁₂ (Cobalamin) Deficiency

Vitamin B_{12} deficiency essentially causes megalobastic anemia and various other neurologic deficits. Diffuse mucocutaneous hyperpigmentation is an uncommon manifestation of vitamin B_{12} deficiency. The pigmentation regresses the following correction of deficiency.

HIV infection Associated Melanosis

Hyperpigmentation has been frequently observed as an oral manifestation of HIV infection. This may be due to anti-retroviral/anti-fungal drugs or as a result of adrenocortical destruction by the virus. It has also been reported that the immune dysregulation in HIV infection leads to increased secretion of alpha-MSH from the anterior pituitary gland, which may also stimulate increased melanin synthesis.The buccal mucosa is the most frequently affected site, but the gingiva, palate, and tongue may also be involved.

Peutz-Jeghers Syndrome

The Peutz-Jeghers syndrome is an autosomal dominant disorder. Mutations in the *STK11/LKB1* tumor suppressor gene have been postulated as the cause. Clinical features of this syndrome include multiple intestinal polyposis that have a malignant potential, and multiple, pigmented macules of the lips, perioral skin, and extremities. The macules are usually small measuring <0.5 cm in diameter. The oral and peri-oral pigmentations are quite characteristic. Histologically, these lesions show increased basilar melanin without an increase in the number of melanocytes. The color intensity and number of macules is unaffected by sun exposure. Other syndromes with similar clinical manifestations include Cowden syndrome and Cronkhite-Canada syndrome.

Café-au-lait Pigmentation

Cafe-au-lait ("coffee with milk") macules are discrete melanin-pigmented patches of skin that have irregular margins and a brown coloration. The lesions are noted at birth or soon thereafter and may also be seen in normal children. No treatment is required, but they may be indicative of a syndrome of greater significance. It is obscure how the gene mutations that give rise to the various genetic diseases stimulate melanin production.

Genetic disorders where café-au-lait spots are seen include the following syndromes:

Neurofibromatosis Type I

Individuals with six or more large (>1.5 cm in diameter) café-au-lait macules should be suspected of possibly having neurofibromatosis (NF). Neurofibromatosis type I is an autosomal dominant disease that is associated with the development of multiple neurofibromas of the skin, oral mucosa, nerves, central nervous system, and occasionally the jaw. The genetic abnormality is in the neurofibromin gene located on chromosome 17q 11.2. In addition, the size, number, and age at onset of the cutaneous café-au-lait spots are of diagnostic importance for this disease. Axillary and/or inguinal freckling (Crowe's sign) and pigmented lesions of the iris (Lisch nodules) are also highly characteristic of neurofibromatosis type I.

McCune-Albright Syndrome

This syndrome is characterized by multiple café-au-lait spots, polyostotic fibrous dysplasia and endocrinal disturbances. This sporadic disorder is considered to be strongly associated with mutation of the Gs, alphagene. The café-au-lait spots in McCune-Albright syndrome appear distinct from those associated with neurofibromatosis. The café-au-lait macules of Albright's syndrome tend to be large and unilateral and have irregular borders, whereas in neurofibromatosis, the borders are typically smooth and soft tissue myxomas.

Mazabraud Disease

This entity is genetically and phenotypically similar to McCune-Albright syndrome. It is characterised by polyostotic fibrous dysplasia, café-au-lait pigmentation and soft tissue myxomas.

Microscopically, café-au-lait macules are not particularly remarkable. They generally show excess amounts of melanin in basal keratinocytes and subjacent macrophages. Melanocytes are normal in appearance and may be slightly increased in number.

Noonan's syndrome and the allelic **Leopard syndrome** (multiple lentigines, electrocardiographic-conduction abnormalities, ocular hypertelorism, pulmonary stenosis, abnormal genitalia, retardation of growth, and sensineural deafness) are autosomal dominant disorders that are also associated with pigmented mucocutaneous macules.

IDIOPATHIC ORAL PIGMENTATION

Laugier-Hunziker Pigmentation

The Laugier-Hunziker pigmentation decribed as an acquired, idiopathic, macular hyperpigmentation of the oral mucosal tissues specifically involving the lips and buccal mucosae (Fig. 9.12). In majority of the cases pigmentation of the nail in the form linear melanotic streak is seen (Fig. 9.13).

This condition is essentially a diagnosis of exclusion when all other systemic and genetic causes of oral pigmentation have been ruled out after a thorough diagnostic work up. Oral involvement presents as multiple, discrete, brown black macules of varying sizes.

HEMOGLOBIN AND IRON-ASSOCIATED PIGMENTATION

Ecchymosis

Ecchymosis occurs due to extravasation of blood in the submucosal tissues.

Causes of Ecchymosis

Trauma: This is the single most common cause. Traumatic ecchymosis usually occurs on the lips and face. Intraoral ecchymosis due to trauma can be seen in cases of blunt trauma and oral intubation. The lesion appears bright red in cases of fresh trauma and gradually changes to brown in 2–3 days.

Hemorrhagic diasthesis and coagulation disorders: Presence of multiple ecchymotic patches in the absence of trauma should raise a strong suspicion of an underlying hematological disorder.

Anticoagulant therapy, leukaemia, end stage renal disease and cirrhosis of the liver may also be associated with oral ecchymosis.

Purpura/Petechiae

These lesions arise as a result of focal capillary hemorrhages. The difference between the two lies essentially in their size. Petechiae are typically described as pinpoint hemorrhages, whereas purpura as multiple, small 2 to 4 mm collections of extravasated blood. Causes include platelet deficiency and aggregation disorders, viral infections and trauma.

Hemochromatosis

Hemochromatosis is a chronic, progressive disease that is characterized by excessive iron deposition, in the form of hemosiderin in the liver and other organs.

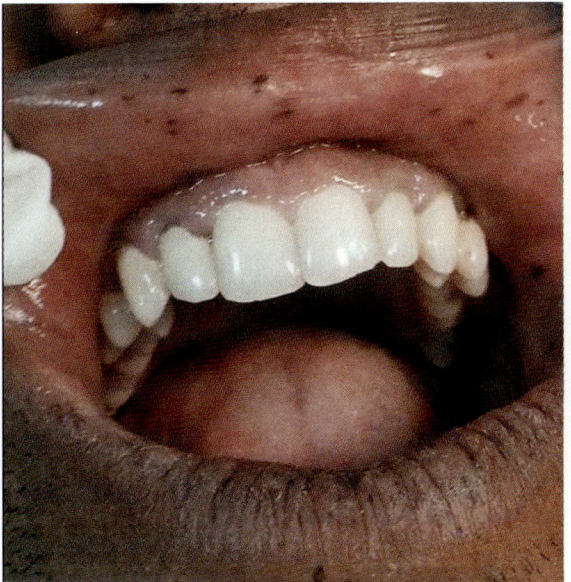 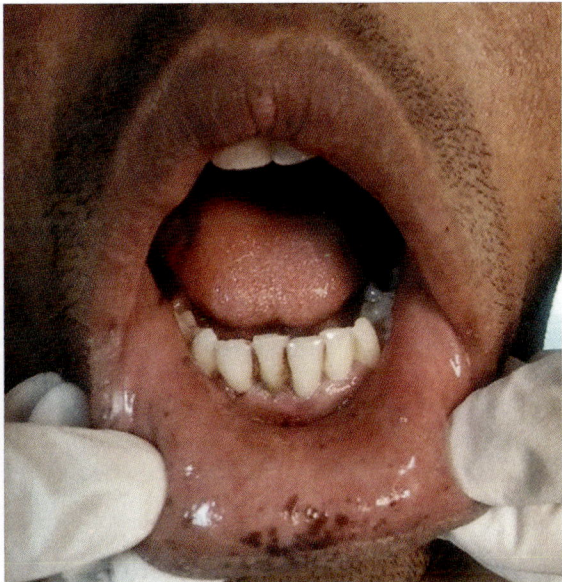

Fig. 9.12: A case of Laugier-Hunziker pigmentation showing multiple macules on upper and lower labial mucosa and vermilion border

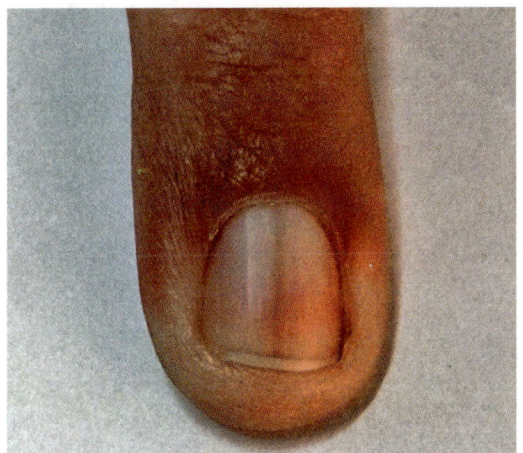

Fig. 9.13: Longitudinal melanotic streak on the nail in LH pigmentation

Causes

× Idiopathic
× Neonatal hemochromatosis
× Blood transfusion
× Hereditary

The cutaneous pigmentation is a hallmark of the disease. The oral mucosal though less common, appears as diffuse and brown to gray pigmentation involving the palate and gingiva. Iron deposition within the adrenal cortex may lead to hypoadrenocorticism with its impending complications.

Other sequelae of hemochromatosis may include liver cirrhosis, diabetes, anemia, heart failure, hypertension, and bronzing of the skin. Lower labial gland biopsy has been shown to be an effective method for the diagnosis of hemochromatosis, where golden or brown-colored hemosiderin can be seen diffusely scattered throughout the submucosal and salivary gland tissues, which can be further confirmed by Prussian blue stain for iron.

EXOGENOUS PIGMENTATION

Amalgam Tattoo

Etiology and pathogenesis: Amalgam tattoo is the single most common source of solitary or focal pigmentation in the oral mucosa. It occurs as a result of the inadvertent deposition of amalgam restorative material into the submucosal tissue.

This can occur in several ways.

- Mucosal abrasions can be contaminated by amalgam dust within the oral fluids.
- Broken amalgam fragments can fall off into extraction sites.
- If dental floss becomes contaminated with amalgam particles of a recently placed restoration, then linear areas of pigmentation can be created in the gingival tissues as a result of hygiene procedures.
- Amalgam from endodontic retrofill procedures, accidentally left within the soft tissue at the surgical site.
- Fine metallic particles can be driven through the oral mucosa from the pressure of high speed air turbine drills.

Clinical features: Amalgam tattoos appear small macules that are black, blue or gray in color with borders that may be well-defined or diffuse. The lesions are usually asymptomatic. They may be found on any mucosal surface. However, the gingiva and buccal mucosa are the most common sites. In some cases, the lesions may be slightly raised. Lateral spread may occur for several months after the implantation. In most cases, solitary site is involved, although multiple tattoos in a single patient may be present. The lesions are often found in the vicinity of teeth with large amalgam restorations or crowned teeth that probably had amalgams, around the apical region of endodontically treated teeth with retrograde restorations or obturated with silver points, and in areas in and around healed extract ion sites.

Theoretically, the use of the rubber dam should decrease the risk of amalgam tattoos, however, immediately after removal of the dam, the occlusion often is adjusted with the potential for amalgam contamination of any areas of mucosal damage.

Pathology: Microscopically, pigmented fragments of the metal are seen within the connective tissue. Often a fine brown granular stippling of reticulum fibers is seen with a particular affinity for vessel walls and nerve. The tissue response appears related to particle size and the elemental composition of the amalgam. Large fragments often become surrounded by dense fibrous connective tissue with mild inflammation. Smaller particles typically are associated with a more significant inflammatory response that may be granulomatous or a mixture of lymphocytes and plasma cells.

Differential diagnosis: Intra-oral radiograph may reveal well-defined radiopacity in the involved region, suggestive of the embedded metallic fragments in the soft tissue. For this purpose the radiographic film should be such that it provides high detail, since some fragments are extremely minute. If there is no radiographic evidence of amalgam and the lesion is not in proximity to any restored tooth, a biopsy is necessary. A typical differential diagnosis often includes melanotic macule, nevus, and melanoma. Pigmentation associated with other dental restorative materials like cast alloy, has also been described. Titanium has been associated with pigmentation of the skin, specifically in areas around orthopaedic implants.Thus, it is justifiable that dental implants may also be a potential source of exogenous oral pigmentation.

Management: Amalgam tattoos are innocuous, their removal is not always mandated. Occassionally, the amalgam implantation may occur in a cosmetically objectionable location such as the anterior maxillary facial gingiva. In such cases, conservative surgical excision can be performed; alternatively amalgam tattoos have been removed successfully with Q switched ruby or alexandrite lasers.

Graphite Tattoo

Graphite tattoos mainly result from accidental injury involving pencils, in which graphite from the tip of the pencil is inserted into the oral mucosa. The lesions are most common on the palate. Clinically they appear similar to amalgam tattoos, presenting as a solitary gray or black macule. Since the traumatic event often occurs in childhood, many patients may not report a history of injury. Thus, a biopsy may be necessary to confirm the diagnosis. Microscopically, graphite particles resemble those of amalgam. Treatment is recommended only in cases with esthetic considerations.

Ornamental Tattoos

Amateur tattooing on the mucosa in the form of designs has gained a considerable amount of popularity. Such tattoo inks are basically composed of simple, carbon particles derived from burnt wood, paper, etc and from a variety of inks, such as India ink, pen ink, and plant-derived matter. Such tattoos are permanent, unless a therapeutic intervention in the form of lasers is sought for to attempt their removal.

In certain tribal cultures, ornamental mucocutaneous tattooing with plant derived pigments is considered an aesthetics enhancing, custom particularly among female members.

A rare South African female tribal custom includes brushing the teeth and gums with a chewed root of the tree *Euclea natalensis*, for its purported antibacterial effects. This plant contains pigmented naphthoquinones that impart a bright orange to the teeth and mucosa. Contrary to the ornamental tattoos, this form of pigmentation is transient and reversible.

Medicinal Metal-induced Pigmentation

Metals and metallic salts are constituents of a number of therapeutic and medicinal agents used for treating a variety of conditions. Oral mucosal pigmentations can result from such treatments in different forms.

Gold: Gold therapy (used for the treatment of rheumatoid arthritis) has been shown to cause diffuse cutaneous pigmentation. Gold-induced pigmentation called chyriasis may appear blue-gray or purple. Chyriasis is uncommon in the oral cavity, nonetheless, oral lichenoid eruptions have been reported with systemic gold therapy. The pigmentation resulting in such instances may be persistent, even after discontinuation of the therapy.

Silver: Oral pigmentation more often results due to ingestion of silver. Colloidal silver is used as a nutritional supplement and has been shown to cause diffuse cutaneous pigmentation. Silver nitrate cautery has been used to treat recurrent aphthous stomatitis. Silver may cause a generalized blue-gray discoloration (argyria).

Salts of metals are also found in topical medications, examples include silver nitrate and zinc oxide, and zinc oxide is a common component of suntan lotions. They have also been associated with focal mucocutaneous pigmentation that often appears grayish black. Bismuth subsalicylate tablets, a commonly used antacid, has also been associated with a diffuse blackish pigmentation of the tongue. Maintenance of tongue hygiene and discontinuation of the bismuth-based antacid are remedial.

Heavy metal pigmentation: Lead, mercury, bismuth, and arsenic have all been shown to be deposited in oral tissue if ingested in sufficient quantities or over an extended period of time. Such a chronic exposure to these heavy metals usually occurs as a result of an occupational and health hazard for individuals who work in certain industrial plants and for those who live in the environment in and around these types of facilities. These ingested metal salts tend to extravasate from vessels in areas of chronic inflammation. Thus, in the oral cavity, the pigmentation is usually found along the free marginal gingiva. This metallic line is a gray to black in color.

Drug-induced pigmentation: Minocycline and methacycline, both tetracycline derivatives, have been implicated in causing oral pigmentation, due to the deposition of the drug complexes within the developing bones, imparting the bone a grayish or brownish color, which is reflected through the overlying mucosa. Minocycline may also cause actual soft tissue pigmentation which appears clinically as patchy or diffuse grayish black hyperpigmentation.

Hairy tongue: Hairy tongue is a fairly common condition of the tongue with no known etiology. A change in the oral microflora due to prolonged antibiotic therapy has been suggested as a possible cause. The discoloration typically involves the dorsum of the tongue. The filiform papillae are severely enlarged and elongated. These hyperplastic papillae then become pigmented by the colonization of chromogenic bacteria, which can impart a variety of colors, including green, brown, or black. Food items and beverages can also contribute to the diffuse discoloration. Smoking of tobacco, cocaine and use of psychotropic medications has also been linked to black hairy tongue. Treatment consists of maintaining the tongue hygiene and limiting the ingestion of color-forming foods and drinks.

Conclusion

Thus oral pigmentation can arise due to multifactorial causes. A thorough clinical examination with proper diagnostic work up and investigations is often necessary to ascertain the right cause behind the pigmented lesion. Treatment is often warranted for cosmetic purposes and in rare cases of malignancy as a life-saving measure.

EXPECTED QUESTIONS

Short Answer Questions

1. Define macule. Add a note on oral melanotic macule.
2. Amalgam tattoo
3. Peutz-Jeghers syndrome
4. Café-au-lait pigmentation
5. Blue nevus
6. Drug-induced pigmentation
7. Amelanotic melanoma
8. Hairy tongue
9. Enumerate two syndromes associated with café-au-lait pigmentation. Describe any one.

Long Answer Question

1. Classify oral pigmentation, enumerate the various causes of endogenous oral pigmentation and describe malignant melanoma in detail.

BIBLIOGRAPHY

1. Burket, Greenberg MS, Glick M, Ship J. Burket's Oral Medicine: Diagnosis and Treatment. 2008.Hamilton, Ont: BC Decker.
2. Neville BW, Damm DD, Allen CM, Buoquot JE.. Oral and maxillofacial pathology. 2009.St. Louis, Mo: Saunders/Elsevier.
3. Regezi JA, Sciubba JJ, Jordan, RCK. Oral pathology: Clinical pathologic correlations 2003. St. Louis, Mo: Saunders.
4. Valášková, P, Muchová L. Metabolism of bilirubin and its biological properties Klin. Biochem. Metab., 2016;24:198–202.
5. Burns, Tony, Stephen Breathnach, Neil Cox and Christopher Griffiths (eds). Rook's Textbook of Dermatology 2010. Blackwell Publishing.
6. Cichorek M, Wachulska M, Stasiewicz A, Tymińska A. Skin melanocytes: biology and development. Advances in Dermatology and Allergology/Postępy Dermatologii I Alergologii. 2013;30:30–41.
7. Kauzman A, Pavone M, Blanas N, Bradley G. Pigmented lesions of the oral cavity: review, differential diagnosis, and case presentations. J Can Dent Assoc. 2004; 70:682–683.
8. Müller S. Melanin-associated pigmented lesions of the oral mucosa: presentation, differential diagnosis, and treatment. Dermatol Ther. 2010;23:220–9.
9. Barrett AW, Porter SR, Scully C, et al: Oral melanotic macules that develop after radiation therapy. Oral Surg. 1994;77: 431–434.
10. Kaugers GE, Heise AP, Riley WT, et al: Oral melanotic macules: a review of 353 cases, Oral Surg 1993;76:59–61.
11. Gaeta, GM, Satriano, RA, Baroni, A. "Oral pigmented lesions". Clin Dermatol. vol. 20. 2002; 20;286–288.
12. Hicks MJ, Flaitz CM. Oral mucosal melanoma: epidemiology and pathobiology. Oral Oncol. 2000 Mar. 36(2):152–69.
13. Torres Fernández G. Pigmented lesion of the oral cavity with eight years follow-up. PR Health Sci J. 2000;19(2):165–168.

14. Andrews BT, Trask DK: Oral melano-acanthoma: a case report, a review of the literature, and a new treatment option, Ann Otol Rhinol Laryngol 2005;114:677–680.
15. Chandler K, Chaudhry Z, Kumar N et al: Melanoacanthoma: a rare cause of oral hyperpigmentation, Oral Surg Oral Med OralPathol Oral Radiol Endod 1997;84:492–494.
16. Contreras E, Carlos R: Oral melanoacanthosis (melanoacanthoma): report of a case and review of the literature, Med Oral Patol Oral Cir Bucal 2005;10:9–12.
17. Gupta AA, Nainani P, Upadhyay B, Kavle P. Oral melanoacanthoma: A rare case of diffuse oral pigmentation. J Oral Maxillofac Pathol 2012;16:441–3
18. Amérigo-Góngora M, Machuca-Portillo G, Torres-Lagares D, Lesclous P, Amérigo-Navarro J, González-Cámpora R. Clinicopathological and immunohistochemical analysis of oral melanocytic nevi and review of the literature. J Stomatol Oral Maxillofac Surg2017;118 (3):151–155.
19. Allen CM, Pellegrini A: Probable congenital melanocytic nevus of the oral mucosa: case report, Pediatr Dermatol 1995;12:145–148.
20. Barnhill RL: The Spitzoid lesion: the importance of atypical variants and risk assessment. Am J Dermatopathol 2006;28:75–83.
21. Bett BJ: Large or multiple congenital melanocytic nevi: occurrence of cutaneous melanoma in 1008 persons. J Am Acad Dermatol 2005; 52:793–797.
22. Casso EM, Grin-Jorgensen CM, Grant-Kels JM: Spitz nevi, J Am Acad Dermatol 1992;27:901–913.
23. Oral compound nevus. Cardoso BL, Consolaro Alberto, Santos P, Sampieri M, Araújo J. Dermatology Online Journal.2014; 20: 9.
24. Chuang WY, Hao SP, Yeh CJ et al: Blue nevi of the sinonasal mucosa: a report of two cases and review of the literature, Laryngoscope; 117:371–372.
25. Dorji T, Cavazza A, Nappi O et al: Spitz nevus of the tongue with pseudoepitheliomatous hyperplasia: report of three cases of a pseudomalignant condition, Am J Surg Pathol 2002;26:774–777.
26. Fistarol SK, Itin PH: Plaque-type blue nevus of the oral cavity, Dermatology 2005.211:224–233.
27. Marques YM, de Lima Mde D, Raitz R, Pinto Ddos S Jr, de Sousa SO. Blue nevus: report of a case. Gen Dent. 2009;57(1):1–3.
28. Flaitz CM, McCandless G: Palatal blue nevus in a child. Pediatr Dent 2001;23:354–355.
29. Hale EK, Stein J, Ben-Porat L et al: Association of melanoma and neurocutaneous melanocytosis with large congenital melanocytic naevi—results from the NYU-LCMN registry.Br J Dermatol2005;152:512–517.
30. Buchner A, Merrell PW, Carpenter WM. Relative frequency of solitary melanocytic lesions of the oral mucosa. J Oral Pathol Med 2004; 33(9):550–7.
31. Cardoso LB, Consalaro A, da Silva Santos PS, da Silva Sampieri MB, Tinoco-Araújo JE. Oral compound nevus. Dermatol Online J. 2014;20:2.
32. Le Boit P: Spitz nevus: a look back and a look ahead. Adv Dermatol 2000;16:81–109.
33. Seehra J, Sen P, Lloyd R, Sloan P. Intraoral Spitz naevus: a case report. Int J Oral Maxillofac Surg 2007;36:661–662.
34. Piperi EP, Tosios KI, Sklavounou A, Stich E, Koutlas IG. Junctional spitz tumor (nevus) of the upper lip. Head Neck Pathol. 2014 Sep. 8(3):354–8.
35. Marghoob, AA, Agero ALC, Benvenuto-Andrade C et al: Large congenital melanocytic nevi, risk of cutaneous melanoma, and prophylactic surgery.J Am Acad Dermatol 2006;54:868–870.
36. Meleti M, Mooi WJ, Casparie MK et al: Melanocytic nevi of the oral mucosa—no evidence of an increased risk for oral malignant melanoma: an analysis of 119 cases. Oral Oncol 2007;43:976–981.
37. Ojha J, Akers JL, Akers JO, Hassanein AM, Islam NM, Cohen DM, et al. Intraoral cellular blue nevus: report of a unique histopathologic entity and review of the literature. Cutis. 2007;80(3):189–192.
38. Mones JM, Ackerman AB: "Atypical" Spitz's nevus, "malignant" Spitz's nevus, and "metastasizing" Spitz's nevus: a critique in historical perspective of three concepts and flawed fatally. Am J Dermatopathol 2004;26:310–333.
39. Pinto A, Raghavendra S, Lee R et al: Epithelioid blue nevus of the oral mucosa: a rare histologic variant.Oral Surg Oral MedOral Pathol 2003;96:429–436.

40. Takata M, Saida T: Genetic alterations in melanocytic tumors.J Dermatol Sci 2006; 43:1–10.

41. Weyers W, Euler M, Diaz-Cascajo C, Schill WB, Bonczkowitz M. Classification of malignant melanoma. Cancer. 1999; 86: 288–299.

42. Abassi NR, Shaw HM, Rigel DS et al: Early diagnosis of cutaneous melanoma. Revisiting the ABCD criteria. Journal of American Medical Association 2004;292:2771–2776.

43. Balch CM, Buzaid AC, Soong SJ et al: Final version of the American Joint Committee on Cancer staging system for cutaneous melanoma. J Clin Oncol 2001;19:3635–3648.

44. Chidzonga MM, Mahomva L, Marimo C et al: Primary malignant melanoma of the oral mucosa.J Oral Maxillofac Surg 2007;65:1117–1120.

45. Curtin JA, Fridlyand J, Kageshita T et al: Distinct sets of genetic alterations in melanoma, N Engl J Med 2005;353:2135–2147.

46. Garbe C, Eigentler TK: Diagnosis and treatment of cutaneous melanoma: state of the art Melanoma Res 2006; 17:117–127.

47. Garzino-Demo P, Fasolis M, Maggiore GM et al: Oral mucosal melanoma: a series of case reports.J Craniomaxillofac Surg2004;32:251–257.

48. Gorsky M, Epstein JB: Melanoma arising from the mucosal surfaces of the head and neck, Oral Surg Oral Med Oral Pathol OralRadiol Endod 1998;86:715–719.

49. Gray-Schopfer V, Wellbrock C, Marais R: Melanoma biology and new targeted therapy, Nature 2007;445:851–857.

50. Hicks MJ, Flaitz CM: Oral mucosal melanoma: epidemiology and pathobiology. Oral Oncol 2000;36:152–169,.

51. Kahn M, Weathers DR, Hoffman JG: Transformation of a benign oral pigmentation to primary oral mucosal melanoma, Oral Surg Oral Med Oral Pathol Oral Radiol Endod ;100:454–459.

52. Zembowicz A, Mihm MC: Dermal dendritic melanocytic proliferations: an update, Histopathology.2004;45:433–451.

53. Haresaku S, Hanioka T, Tsutsui A, Watanabe T. Association of lip pigmentation with smoking and gingival melanin pigmentation. Oral Dis. 2007;13 (1):71–6.

54. Teja R, Devy AS, Nirmal MR, Sunil PM, Deepasree M. Cytomorphometric analysis of exfoliated cells in oral lichen planus CytoJournal 2014; q2:3–7.

55. Takeda Y. Congenital nevocellular nevus of the oral mucosa. Ann Dent. 1988 Winter. 47(2):40–2.

56. Gilbert ML, Hanna W, Ghazarian D, Dover D, Klieb HB. Congenital melanocytic nevus of the oral mucosa: report of a rare pigmented lesion and review of the literature. Clin Pract2011; 29:17.

57. Hanna A, Rawal SY, Anderson KM, Rawal YB. The epithelioid blue nevus: A rare intraoral nevomelanocytic tumor. J Oral Maxillofac Pathol. 2011;15(1):88–90.

58. Ajagbe O. Halo nevus: an unusual upper lip presentation in a black patient and a review of the subject. NDA J. 1994 Jan-Feb. 45(1):19–23.

59. Cerrato F, Wallins JS, Webb ML, McCarty ER, Schmidt BA, Labow BI. Outcomes in pediatric atypical spitz tumors treated without sentinel lymph node biopsy. Pediatr Dermatol. 2012;29 (4):448–53.

60. Lambertini M, Patrizi A, Fanti PA, Melotti B, Caliceti U, Magnoni C, et al. Oral melanoma and other pigmentations: when to biopsy?. J Eur Acad Dermatol Venereol. 2017; 1:10–16.

61. Lanza A, Heulfe I, Perillo L, Dell'Ermo A, Nicola. Oral Pigmentation as a Sign of Addison's Disease: A Brief Reappraisal. The Open Dermatology Journal. 2009; 3: 3–6.

62. R. Chandran, L. Feller, J. Lemmer, and R.A. G. Khammissa. HIV-Associated Oral Mucosal Melanin Hyperpigmentation: A Clinical Study in a South African Population Sample. AIDS Research and Treatment 2016. https://doi.org/10.1155/2016/8389214

63. Moraes, R.M, Gouvêa Lima, G.D, Guilhermino, M., Vieira, M. S, Carvalho, Y. R, and Anbinder, A. L. Graphite oral tattoo: case report. Dermatology Online Journal 2010;21;10

64. Molini PRB, Velloso TRG, Silva DN, Bertollo RM, Azevedo SLV, Pereira TCR. Pigmented lesion in hard palate: a graphite tattoo. J. Oral Diag. 2016;1;1–5

Salivary Gland Disorders— Clinical and Radiologic Considerations

INTRODUCTION

Salivary gland is a secretary gland that secretes tasteless, clear fluid called saliva. Salivary glands can be classified into major and minor. There are three pairs of major salivary glands, namely parotid glands, submandibular salivary gland and sublingual gland in addition to minor salivary glands which are dispersed throughout the oral mucosa. Saliva plays an important role in lubrication of food, integrity of mucosa, prevention of tooth decay, antimicrobial effect and in digestion. The main constituent of saliva is water with organic and inorganic components.

DEVELOPMENT OF SALIVARY GLANDS

The development of salivary gland starts between 4th–6th week of intrauterine life with parotid being first gland to initiate followed by submandibular gland at 6th week and sublingual gland including minor salivary gland at 8th–12th week. Parotid gland is the largest salivary gland which is ectodermal in origin. Submandibular gland and sublingual gland are endodermal in origin.

ANATOMY OF SALIVARY GLANDS

Parotid Gland

It is the largest salivary gland. The parotid lobe lies on the lateral aspect of the ramus of the preauricular region. The parotid gland wedges in between sternocleidomastoid muscle and masseter muscle. The gland is enclosed in deep fascia of neck.

Relations of Gland

a. **Superiorly:** External auditory meatus
b. **Inferiorly:** Lies over the posterior belly of the digastric muscle
c. **Anteriorly:** Ramus of the mandible and masseter muscle
d. **Posteriorly:** Sternocleidomastoid muscle
e. **Medially:** Facial nerve. Retromandibular vein and external carotid artery lies medial to the parotid lobe

The duct of parotid gland, called Stenson's duct, opens into buccal vestibule opposite to upper second molar. The secretion of parotid gland is generally serous (primarily watery) in nature.

Submandibular Gland

Submandibular gland lies medially to the body of mandible with large superficial lobe and small deep lobe. Both the lobes are connected around the posterior aspect of mylohyoid muscle. Superficial lobe is wedged between mandible and mylohyoid muscle and lies within deep fascia of neck. Submandibular gland is separated by parotid gland by stylomandibular ligament.

Relations of the Gland

a. **Superficially:** Platysma and cervical branch of facial nerve.
b. **Deep:** Mylohyoid muscle, lingual nerve and hypoglossal nerve.
c. **Medially:** Deep part or small lobe of gland projects along hyoglossus.

Submandibular gland's duct, called Wharton's duct, opens in floor of the mouth in the midline along the frenulum of the tongue on the summit of sublingual papilla. The secretion of submandibular gland is mixed (serous and mucous) in nature.

Sublingual Gland

Sublingual gland is the smallest salivary gland and is almond-shaped gland which lies deep to the submandibular gland.

Relations

a. **Medially:** Separated from base of the tongue by submandibular duct and lingual nerve.
b. **Laterally:** Sublingual groove on the medial aspect of the mandible.

Its secretions are mainly drained through numerous small ducts called Rivinus duct that opens along the sublingual fold in floor of mouth. Sometimes few anterior ducts may join to form a common duct called Bartholin's duct. Sublingual and minor salivary glands secretion is predominantly mucous in nature.

Saliva

Saliva is produced and secreted by salivary glands out of which submandibular gland secretes approximately 60% of total salivary volume. Total volume of saliva secreted in a day by an adult is 600–1000 ml. In the resting (unstimulated) state, approximately two-thirds of the total volume of the whole saliva is produced by submandibular glands. Upon stimulation, the parotid glands are responsible for at least 50% of the total volume of saliva from the mouth. The average rate of unstimulated whole saliva is 0.3–0.4 ml/min.

TABLE 10.1: Major constituents of saliva

Electrolytes	Sodium, potassium, chloride, bicarbonate, calcium, magnesium, phosphate, thiocynate, and fluoride
Secretory proteins/ peptides	Amylase, proline rich proteins, mucins, histatin, cystatin, peroxidase, lysozyme, lactoferrin, glycoproteins, lysozyme, defensins
Secretory immuno-globulins	IgA, IgG, IgM
Organic constituents	Glucose, amino acids, urea, uric acid, and lipid molecules
Biological active peptides	Leptin, ghrelin and endothelin
Other constituents	Epidermal growth factors, epithelial cells, insulin, cyclic adenosine monophosphate, binding proteins and serum albumin

SIALOGRAPHY

Sialography is a technique where retrograde injection of dye is instilled into the duct of major salivary gland. Following injection a series of radiographs are taken in order to evaluate the salivary glands. Prior to the advent of CT and MRI, sialography is the only technique to assess the ductal and parenchymal tissue of salivary glands. Today MRI has largely replaced sialography in evaluation of salivary glands.

The first sialogram was performed by Carpy in 1902 on isolated parotid gland using mercury as contrast agent. Subsequently,

Arcelin reported the first ever *in vivo* human sialogram using bismuth as contrast agent.

Contrast Agents

The contrast agents used in sialography are either fat soluble or water soluble, containing approximately around 37% of iodine.

Fat soluble media: Fat soluble dyes were used due to its virtue of higher viscosity and excellent contrasting agent, however, higher viscosity requires extra pressure to push the dye into the ductal system. Also, fat soluble dye may remain inside the gland and can initiate inflammatory process leading to change in texture of gland. Some of the fat soluble dyes are lipoidal, ethiodol and pantopaque.

Ethiodol is one of the popularly used fat soluble dyes due to lower viscosity and excellent contrast properties. Ethiodol is insoluble in saliva and not absorbed in the glandular mucosa. That is why it was frequently used as contrast agent. Sooner, fat soluble dye was replaced by water soluble dyes.

Water soluble dyes: The most common water soluble dyes are angiographic dyes. Water soluble dyes are less viscous and can be easily injected into the gland. The major drawback of these dyes is saliva soluble and can be absorbed by the gland. This often results in poor radiographic contrast and suboptimal demonstration of ducts. However, the good quality is liquid-based dyes do not provoke any inflammatory process inside the gland.

Most commonly used liquid-based sialographic dye is **Sinograffin** composed of **Diatrizoate meglumine** and **Iodipamide meglumine**. It is highly viscous dye with sufficient contrast property as it has 38% of iodine content.

Armamentarium for Sialography

Sialography is comparatively easier procedure. It requires following things:
1. Sialographic catheters
2. Lacrimal probes
3. Iodinated contrast agent
4. Dental cotton rolls

Sialographic Procedure

Sialography should ideally be performed under direct fluoroscopy, however, most of the times it is performed without fluoroscopic observation. Thorough examination of salivary gland should be performed before carrying out the procedure. All procedural steps should be explained to the patient and written consent form should be signed by the patient before the start of the procedure.

First step in sialography is dilation of ductal opening using lacrimal probes. The injection containing dye should be given with steady, constant pressure. The injection should be ceased once patient shows discomfort. Normally, parotid can accommodate around 0.5–0.75 ml of contrast and submandibular accommodates 0.3 ml of contrast agent.

Phases of Salivary Gland

Sialography can be divided into three phases
1. Ductal
2. Acinar
3. Evacuation

Ductal phase: The ductal phase starts with injection and terminates on acinar opacification. Ductal opacification is intended to demonstrate abnormalities in ductal system.

Acinar opacification: It starts after ductal opacification and ends at increased density of gland. This phase demonstrates intraglandular and extraglandular masses in parenchyma.

Evacuation and postevacuation phase: This phase shows secretory function of the gland and ductal pathology, if any, present in the gland. Normally all contrast agent leaves the gland during this phase. Any residual dye inside the gland may indicate any pathology in the ductal system.

Indications of Sialography

1. Acute obstructive and/or chronic recurrent sialadenitis

2. Autoimmune sialadenitis
3. Sialosis
4. Post-trauma evaluation
5. Mandibular lesions like Stafne's cyst.

Contraindications of Sialography

1. Acute infection of the gland
2. Hypersensitivity to the iodine dye

Diseases of Salivary Gland

Salivary glands are involved in number of conditions. The diseases of salivary glands can occur from within the gland or can be manifestation of any systemic diseases. Various conditions of salivary gland can be classified as given in Table 10.2.

Developmental Disorders

Aplasia/Agenesis and Related Aberrancy of Salivary Glands

Aplasias/agenesis of major salivary gland is rare finding. It can occur unilaterally or bilaterally, involving either single salivary gland or multiple salivary glands. It can be syndromic or non-syndromic.

Aplasia/Agenesis: Agenesis/aplasia refers to congenital absence of salivary gland(s). The first case of agenesis/aplasia was reported by Gruber in 1885. It is a rare condition of unknown etiology. Usually, it is present bilaterally, however, some cases of unilateral agenesis were also reported in literature. Agenesis/aplasia of parotid gland can occur independently or in association with agenesis of submandibular gland, lacrimal gland, first branchial arch developmental disturbances or any other developmental disturbance. The true incidence of agenesis/aplasia cannot be determined as majority of cases goes unnoticed. Syndromes associated with aplasia/agenesis are **Treacher Collins syndrome, hemifacial microsomia, lacrimo-auriculo-dento-digital syndrome (LADD).**

Atresia: It is a congenital absence/occlusion of salivary gland duct which can lead to mucocele or mucus retention phenomenon.

Aberrancy: It is an anatomic variation where the gland is found at unusual position. Example is Stafne's bone cyst. Stafne's bone cyst is the accumulation of abnormal salivary gland tissue at medial surface of body of mandible causing indentation in the medial aspect of body of mandible.

Clinical features: Often, cases of aplasia/agenesis are asymptomatic due to partial manifestation of the disease. The clinician should look out for ductal openings of major salivary glands in case of suspicion of salivary gland aplasia/agenesis. Thorough history from siblings is mandatory to rule out any familial tendency.

The clinical features of aplasia/agenesis include hyposalivation, frequent dental caries, enamel hypoplasia, occlusal wearing of teeth or congenital absence of teeth, difficulty in swallowing, poor oral hygiene. Besides oral features, ophthalmologic dryness and association of aplasia/agenesis with other syndromes should be considered.

Radiologic features: Radiological examination includes ultrasonography (USG), computed tomography (CT) of parotid and submandibular areas and pertechnetate scintingraphy. USG and CT will reveal partial to complete absence of one or more gland. Scintingraphy will show reduced or no uptake of radioisotope in the major salivary gland areas.

Management: Management of such cases will include periodical dental examinations, salivary substitutes, meticulous home care and frequent fluoride application to prevent dental caries.

Hyperplasia of Salivary Glands

Hyperplasia of salivary glands is a pseudo tumor, generally manifested in minor salivary glands located in hard and soft palate in oral cavity. It is a rare lesion with unknown etiology. Although, some authors think local trauma could be the cause.

Clinical features: It is characterized by localized, indolent swelling in hard and soft

TABLE 10.2: Classification of salivary gland disorders

Developmental	Functional disorders	Inflammatory disorders	Autoimmune disorders	Non-inflammatory disorders	Tumors benign	Tumors malignant
✗ Aplasia/ agenesis and related aberrancy of salivary glands ✗ Hyperplasias	✗ Xerostomia ✗ Sialorrhea	✗ Mucocele ✗ Ranula ✗ Salivary duct cyst ✗ Sialolithiasis, sialadenitis *Viral infections* ✗ Mumps ✗ HIV ✗ Subacute necrotizing sialadenitis ✗ Cheilitis glandularis ✗ Necrotizing sialometaplasia	✗ Sjögren's syndrome ✗ Mikulicz's disease	✗ Sialoadenosis ✗ Orofacial granulomatosis	✗ Pleomorphic tumor ✗ Warthin's tumor ✗ Oncocytoma ✗ Canalicular adenoma ✗ Basal cell adenoma	✗ Mucoepidermoid carcinoma ✗ Acinic cell adenocarcinoma ✗ Malignant mixed tumor ✗ Metastasizing mixed tumor ✗ Adenoid cystic carcinoma

palate. The most common presentation of adenomatoid hyperplasia is painless swelling which may be soft to firm on palpation. It generally occurs in 4th to 6th decades of life. The overlying mucosa may be normal in color. The diagnosis can be confirmed by biopsy.

Management: After confirmation of diagnosis by biopsy, patient should be kept under observation for 6 months. Any change in size or change in color should be investigated further.

Functional Disorders of Salivary Gland

Xerostomia

Xerostomia refers to "dry mouth" which may be associated with decrease in quality or quantity of saliva. Hypofunction means decreased function of saliva. However, both these terms have been used interchangeably. The prevalence of the hypofunction/ xerostomia varies in different population as xerostomia is subjective sensation of oral dryness. Hyposalivation refers to decreased flow rate of saliva from salivary glands.

The flow rate of saliva varies with daytime so defining the normal rate is difficult. However, salivary rate less than 0.15 ml/ min is considered as reference for decreased flow rate. Sometimes patients with decreased salivation have no complaints. Conversely, patients with dry mouth complaints have normal salivary production.

Xerostomia has great impact on one's quality of life. Patients with complains of Xerostomia have difficulty in chewing, speaking, swallowing and wearing dentures. Patients complaining of dry mouth comes with chief complains of need to sip frequently, difficulty in swallowing without water or burning sensation in oral cavity.

Various causes of dry mouth are listed in Table 10.3.

Mouth breathing, tobacco smoking, alcohol use and beverages containing caffeine also cause decrease in salivary production. In the past, aging was considered as reason for decreased salivary secretion, however, recent studies revealed that there is no significant decrease in salivary production as age advances. It might be due to medications taken during old age.

TABLE 10.3: Various causes of dry mouth

Developmental	Salivary gland aplasia
Medications	Tricyclic antidepressants, antipsychotic drugs, diuretics, antihistamines, proton pump inhibitors, opioids, benzodiazepines, selective serotonin reuptake inhibitors, anticholinergics
Radiotherapy/ chemotherapy	Radiotherapy to salivary glands and related structures
Autoimmune diseases	Sjögren's syndrome, systemic lupus erythematosus
Infections	Viral infections like HIV, hepatitis C induced salivary diseases
Other systemic diseases	Diabetes mellitus, sarcoidosis, Parkinson's disease, cystic fibrosis, vitamin A deficiency

Clinical Features

Examination of patients with dry mouth demonstrates a reduction in salivary secretion and saliva appears to be 'thick and ropy". The dorsal aspect of tongue is fissured with atrophic filliform papillae. Patients complain of food sticking in oral membranes while eating. The amount of saliva secretion can be determined by assessing stimulated and unstimulated salivary flow.

In xerostomic patients there is increase incidence of caries and oral candidiasis because of reduction in quantity and quality of saliva. The xerostomia related caries commonly occur in cervical and root area.

Various chair side procedures could be done in order to diagnose dry mouth condition. These are:

1. **Lack of pooling** of saliva in floor of the mouth is the basic sign of dry mouth.
2. **Cracker sign:** If patient tells that he was unable to chew cracker without sipping water, then it is indication of decreased salivary secretion.
3. **Lipstick sign:** If lipstick remains adhered to upper incisors in females, indicates dry mouth.
4. **Mouth mirror test:** The clinician places the mouth mirror on buccal mucosa or on dorsal tongue and check for mouth mirror sticking to surface. If it sticks, then clinician can deduce diagnosis of dry mouth.

Radiological features: All patients with dry mouth do not require radiological investigations. Depending upon the cause of dry mouth, radiological investigations should be prescribed. If decreased secretion is due to medication, radiotherapy/ chemotherapy, then apparently there is no need for radiographic investigation. For other conditions, special radiological procedures should be advised. Radionuclide salivary imaging will show reduced uptake of pertechnetate in Sjögren's syndrome. Sialosis usually demonstrates enhanced pertechnetate uptake and in cases of post-radiotherapy patients, there is reduced uptake of radionuclide dye.

Treatment: The treatment of dry mouth is very difficult and unsatisfactory. Artificial saliva and frequent water sipping may help patients with decreased saliva secretion. In addition, sugarless candy or vitamin C candy (limcee, celin lozenges) can be used in order to stimulate saliva. Use of oral hygiene products containing lactoperoxidase, lysozyme and lactoferrin (biotene toothpaste, oral balance gel) should be prescribed to patients.

Systemic pilocarpine 5 to 10 mg three to four times a day may also be given to the patients. Pilocarpine is parasympathomimetic agonist that can be used as sialogogue. Another cholinergic agonist with affinity for M3 receptor is cevimeline hydrochloride which can be prescribed to increase the secretion from salivary glands. Both these drugs are contraindicated in patients with narrow angle glaucoma.

If dryness is secondary to patient's medications, then patient should be asked to consult his/her physician for either modulation of dose or substitution of drug. As patients with dry mouth have increased risk for caries, frequent fluoride applications are recommended with chlorhexidine mouth-wash to minimize plaque accumulation.

SIALORRHEA (PTYALISM)

Sialorrhea or ptyalism is a condition with excessive salivation. Sialorrhea is not only a medical issue but also a social stigma. It generally occurs secondary to any underlying condition. Various causes include neurological disorders, infections, heavy metal poisoning, Wilson's disease, drug-induced, rabies, familial dysautonomia. In most of the patients with neurological disorders, drooling of saliva is not related to increased production of saliva but due to decreased neurosensory control of orofacial muscles to retain saliva.

Minor sialorrhea results from local irritation from new or ill-fitting dentures, aphthous ulcer. Episodic excess salivation or "water brash" occurs as a result from gastrointestinal reflux (GERD). Drugs involved with increased salivation are antipsychotic drugs such as clozapine, cholinergic agonist used in treatment of Alzheimer's disease and myasthenia gravis. Another hypersecretion of saliva of unknown etiology is idiopathic paroxysmal sialorrhea. Individuals with this condition exhibit increased salivation for small burst of time lasting from 2 to 5 minutes. These episodes are usually associated with nausea or vomiting.

Clinical features: Patients with excessive secretion of saliva complain of soiling of clothes and bed linens. In children with decreased intellectual disability or cerebral palsy, uncontrolled salivary drooling may result in maceration sores around mouth, chin or neck that may become secondarily infected.

Treatment: The treatment of sialorrhea depends upon its cause. Transitory or mild sialorrhea does not require any intervention. Patients with increased salivation due to GERD may be referred to physician to manage underlying cause. For persistent severe drooling, therapeutic intervention may be indicated. Anticholinergic medication can decrease salivary production, however, side effects are unacceptable. Intra-glandular injection of botulinium toxin has been shown to be successful in decreasing saliva secretion.

Besides, medicinal treatment, surgical interventions like relocation of parotid and submandibular duct, ligation of ducts and bilateral tympanic neuroectomy with sectioning of chorda tympani may help in managing these patients.

INFLAMMATORY DISORDERS OF SALIVARY GLAND

Inflammatory disorders are most common lesions affecting salivary glands. The etiology of these inflammatory conditions can be obstruction, infection, granulomatous disease or unknown. Below is the description of common inflammatory pathology of major and minor salivary glands.

Mucocele (Mucus Extravasation Cyst)

Mucus extravasation cyst is a pesudocyst which results from rupture of salivary gland duct and secretion of gland spills into the surrounding connective tissue. That is why it is called mucus extravasation cyst. The most common cause for development of mucocele is local trauma. However, in some cases trauma could not be found to be the cause.

Clinical features: Mucocele generally occurs in minor salivary glands present on the lower lip (Fig. 10.1). The chance of trauma is more in younger age group and on lower lip that is why it is more common in lower lip with younger age group. However, case reports with involvement of all age groups have been documented in literature. Other sites for mucocele are buccal mucosa, floor of the mouth, ventral tongue, palate and retromolar.

Mucocele typically presents as lesion with 1–2 mm to several centimeters in diameter, dome-shaped with smooth surfaced (non-ulcerated) and fluctuant swelling. The color of swelling is bluish if it is presented superficially. Deep swelling may have normal mucosal color. The duration of lesion can vary from a few days to several years. Sometimes, patients present with history of recurrent swelling that periodically ruptures and spill its fluid contents.

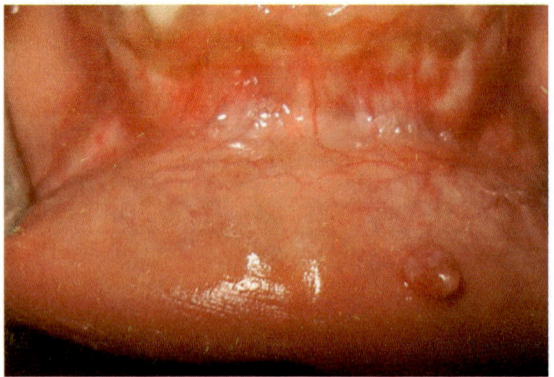

Fig. 10.1: Mucocele of lower lip

Differential diagnosis: Differential diagnosis will include lipoma, mucus producing salivary gland tumor, lymphangioma, hemangioma, vesicobullous lesion like cicatricial pemphigoid. Lipoma would be normal in color and its margins will slip during palpation. Lymphangioma and hemangioma would be present in younger age group and cicatricial pemphigoid would leave scar once it has healed. Also in pemphigoid other systemic features will also be present.

Treatment: Mucocele are chronic in nature, therefore, require surgical intervention. Careful surgical excision with removal of feeding gland should be done as this will decrease the chances of recurrence. Some mucoceles are short spanned that ruptures and heal by its own. The excised tissue should be sent to histopathological examination to rule out the possibility of any tumor.

Ranula

The term **Ranula** is derived from Latin word Rana means "frog". As the swelling resembles the translucent underbelly of frog, the term ranula has been coined. Ranula is the swelling of floor of the mouth, commonly arising from the sublingual gland. Ranula is primarily a mucocele; however, it has been discussed separately due to its bigger size and different characteristics. The etiology of ranula is local trauma or any obstruction or aneurysm of the duct.

Clinical features: The ranula usually presents as dome-shaped, fluctuant swelling with bluish tinge on the floor of the mouth (Fig. 10.2). The size of ranula is much larger than commonly occurring mucocele and it can raise the tongue causing considerable discomfort to the patients. Ranula appears in children and in young adults. The ranula is generally located lateral to the midline, thus can be distinguished from midline dermoid cyst.

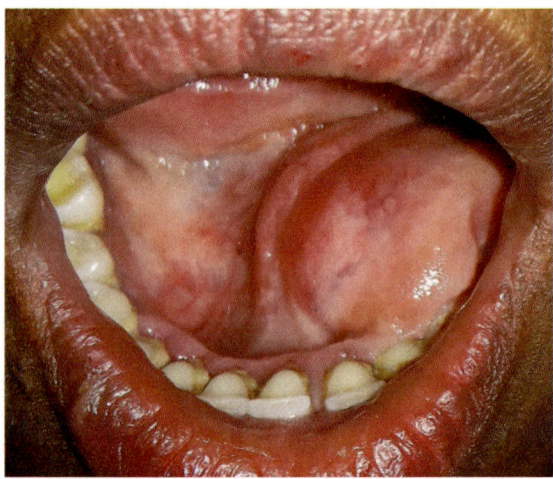

Fig. 10.2: Ranula of floor of mouth

A variant of ranula is "**Plunging ranula**" which occurs when leaked mucin divides mylohyoid muscle and produces swelling in the neck which can be seen extra-orally.

Radiological features: Imaging can help in supporting the clinical diagnosis and in determining the origin and extent of the lesion. Computed tomography (CT) and magnetic resonance imaging (MRI) can be taken before surgery. The "tail sign" is characteristically seen in plunging ranula cases. It is the slight extension of lesion in to the sublingual space.

Treatment: The treatment of ranula/plunging ranula is surgical. Removal of feeding sublingual gland and/or marsupialization can be done for small and superficial ranulas. For larger lesions, the removal of involved gland is important in order to prevent recurrence of the lesion.

Salivary Duct Cyst (Sialocyst)

Salivary duct cyst is true cyst arising from the salivary gland tissue. Unlike mucocele, sialocyst is lined by epithelium and separated from salivary ducts. The cause of occurrence of such cyst is unknown. Some researchers refer such lesions as mucus retention cyst however, it is different from retention cyst.

Clinical features: Salivary duct cyst can occur in major salivary glands and in minor salivary glands as well. Among major salivary glands, parotid gland is commonly involved. Cyst is presented as slowly growing, painless swelling. In minor glands, the swelling can occur in floor of the mouth buccal mucosa and in lips. The consistency of these cysts are same as that for mucocele, however, some cysts are firm in consistency. In some patients multiple sialocysts can also develop which often is presented as painful nodules with dilated ductal orifices on mucosal surface.

Radiological features: Smaller lesions do not require any imaging procedures. Larger lesions in major salivary gland would require CT/MRI to confirm the diagnosis and to see the extent of lesion. Ultrasonography can also be used to see the nature of the lesion.

Treatment: Isolated salivary gland cyst should be treated by conservative surgery. For cysts in major glands partial or total gland removal may be necessary. The chances of recurrence are very minimal. For multiple lesions, only symptomatic lesions should be removed surgically as and when required.

Sialolithiasis (Salivary Calculi: Salivary Stones)

Sialolithiasis is a condition where calcified structures are developed in the salivary ductal system. The cause for formation of sialoliths is still unclear but their formation can be supported by the chronic sialadenitis or partial obstruction. The composition of sialolith may consist of calcium and phosphorus salts which get deposited around the nidus of debris in the ductal system. The debris may include mucin, bacteria, ductal epithelial cells or any foreign body. The development of the sialolithiasis does not have any systemic implication and typically not related with calcium or phosphorous level imbalance.

Clinical features: Sialolithiasis can occur in major and minor salivary glands of which about 80% of sialoliths develop in submandibular gland ductal system. The reason for frequent formation of sialoliths in submandibular salivary gland is its long, tortuous duct with path which is against the gravity, causing stasis of saliva. Also, the secretion of submandibular gland is more mucous and thick.

Sialolithiasis can occur in any age group, however, young and middle-aged affect more often. There is no sex predilection for sialolith formation. Sialolithiasis in major salivary gland is frequently associated with episodic pain and swelling which increases during meal (Fig. 10.3). The severity of the symptoms depends upon the extent of obstruction and amount of resultant back pressure produced on the structures. If the obstruction is partial, then saliva may pass through the obstruction and relieves the symptoms associated.

The stone can be easily palpated in the floor of the mouth if it is present in terminal portion of the submandibular duct. Sometimes, in long standing cases, the ductal opening is also inflamed in sialolithiasis. Chronic obstruction of the saliva may lead to infection, fibrosis or glandular atrophy.

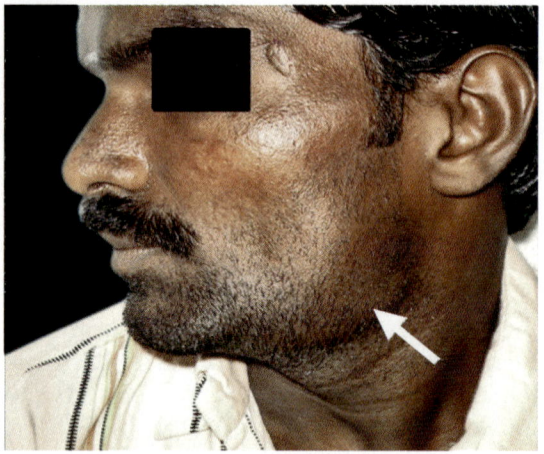

Fig. 10.3: Submandibular gland sialolithiasis

Radiological features: Plain radiography is still a convenient and inexpensive way of confirming diagnosis of sialolithiasis. The stones present in the terminal portion of the duct can be visualized as radio-opaque mass in occlusal radiograph. The submandibular stones which are formed away from the ductal opening can be visualized in panoramic radiographs. They may be superimposed on the mandibular body and should not be confused with any bony pathology.

Multiple parotid gland stones can be seen in PA view, lateral view (Fig. 10.4). These multiple stones should not be confused with calcified lymph nodes which are present in cases of tuberculosis. Sometimes, the obstruction in ductal system may occur due to mucus plug which cannot be seen on

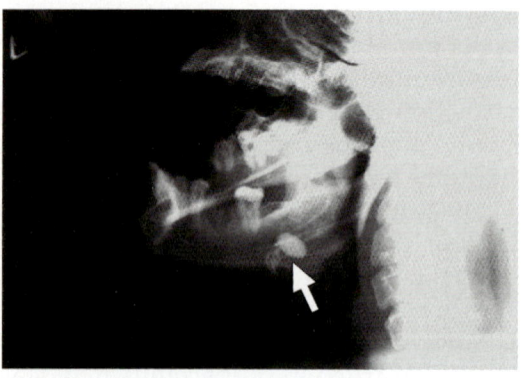

Fig. 10.4: Stone in submandibular gland

radiographs. Radiolucent sialoliths can be diagnosed using sialography. Radiolucent stone appears as filling defect in contrast filled ducts. Sialography can also easily differentiate between radiolucent sialolith and stricture formation.

Besides sialography, ultrasonography is an effective tool in detecting stones in the ductal system. USG of parotid or submandibular gland can be done as it is non-invasive and non-ionizing. Contrast enhanced CT and MRI can also be advised, however, they should be kept reserved for the cases which could not be diagnosed through plain radiography or USG.

Diagnostic sialoendoscopy is newer tool used in evaluation and diagnosis of ductal obstructions. In this technique, a miniaturized endoscope is introduced into the duct through ductal orifice, allowing direct visualization of ductal system for any stones, strictures or adhesions.

Treatment: The stones present near the ductal opening should be treated conservatively by massage of the gland. Sialogogues (drugs that increase salivary flow) and increased fluid intake may also promote passage of stone. Larger sialoliths should be removed surgically. Extracorporeal shock wave lithotripsy (ESWL) and interventional sialoendoscopy are newer, non-invasive way of removal of stones from the ducts.

Sialadenitis

Sialadenitis is an inflammation of salivary glands, whereas sialodochitis is an inflammation of salivary ductal system. There are various causes of sialadenitis which include bacterial, viral, radiation therapy, Sjögren's syndrome, medications, ductal obstruction, sarcoidosis and congenital anomalies. Viral etiology of sialadenitis is the most common.

Other causes may include recent surgery (especially abdominal surgery) after which acute parotids may develop. Sialadenitis may be acute or chronic depending upon duration.

Bacterial Sialadenitis

Bacterial sialadenitis is common during pre-antibiotic era. However, with the advent of newer and potent antibiotics the incidence of bacterial sialadenitis has decreased. Most bacterial infections result due to ductal obstruction or decreased salivary flow. Sialolithiasis, congenital strictures, compression by adjacent tumor or any surgery can lead to ductal blockade. Decreased salivary flow may result from medications, dehydration, or conditions like diabetes mellitus.

Common bacteria involved in bacterial sialadenitis are *Staphylococcus aureus*, *Streptococcus viridians*, *Strep. pneumonia*, *Escherichia coli*, and *Haemophilus influenzae*.

Clinical features: Acute bacterial sialadenitis most commonly affects parotid gland unilaterally or bilaterally. The affected gland is painful, swollen with raised temperature. Patient may experience mild or low grade fever associated with chills and sweating. A purulent discharge may be seen from the ductal opening when gland is milked (Fig. 10.5). Patient may also complain of limited mouth opening and change in taste sensation.

Chronic or recurrent sialadenitis may result from ductal obstruction or stricture.

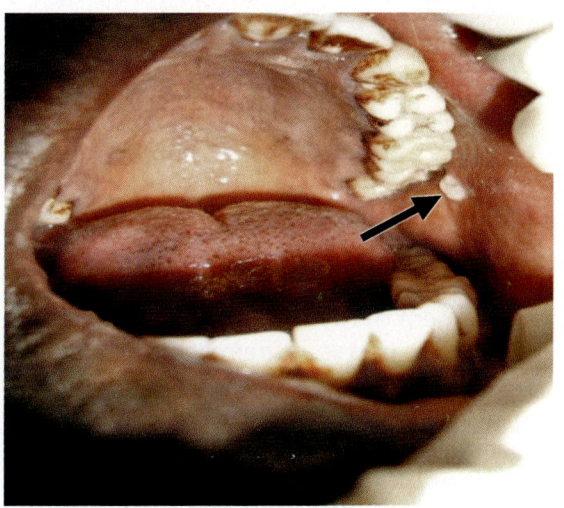

Fig. 10.5: Suppurative parotitis

Periodic swelling and pain may occur in the affected gland which usually increases during meal time. Pain may not be as severe as in acute sialadenitis patients. Generally, chronic adenitis occurs in older age group. Constitutional signs of fever, chills and sweating may be absent. Purulent discharge may or may not be present.

Juvenile recurrent parotitis is the most common condition affecting children in United States and second common worldwide after mumps. It usually affects children with age between 3 and 6 years. The etiology of this condition is unknown; however, congenital malformations, genetic factor or immunological factors are described in literature. Clinically, it manifests as recurring episodes of unilateral or bilateral, non-purulent parotid gland swelling. The condition may resolve around the puberty by its own.

Radiographic features: Patients with sialadenitis should have panoramic radiograph screening to rule out sialolith. Additional imaging studies include sialography, CT and MRI. Sialography is an important tool in diagnosis of sialadenitis and can differentiate chronic obstructive sialadenitis with autoimmune sialadenitis. However, with the introduction of advanced imaging techniques, Sialography is not such popular nowadays.

Acute sialadenitis shows minimal changes on sialography. However, evidence of obstruction might be seen in sialography. The sialographic findings of chronic sialadenitis patients vary with number and severity of previous infections. The sialographic pattern ranges from minimal changed to extensively altered ductal system. The pattern shows multiple areas of focal stricture and dilatation involving main duct (Fig. 10.6). Involvement of secondary duct may occur in advanced cases. Areas of fusiform dilatation and stricturing of main duct shows "sausage" or "string of sausages" like pattern.

On CT sialography studies, sections through the primary duct will demonstrate marked dilatation of primary duct.

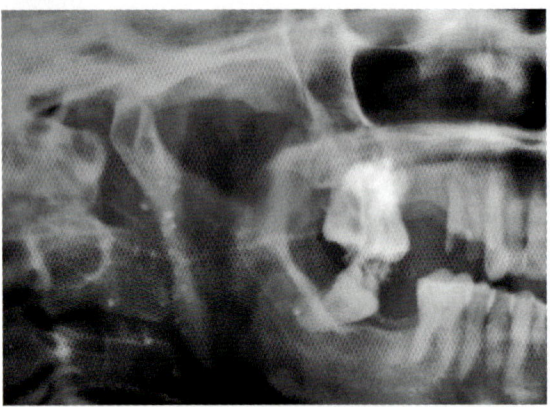

Fig. 10.6: Sialography showing chronic recurrent parotitis

Treatment: The treatment includes antibiotic therapy and rehydration. Surgical drainage may be done if required. Treatment of chronic sialadenitis includes various factors like number and times of previous episodes. The treatment ranges from conservative management to surgical intervention. Conservative management includes antibiotics, analgesics, sialogogues, and sometimes, corticosteroids. The cases which develop secondary to ductal blockage should be treated with removal of sialolith.

If strictures are present, then patient might be prone for recurrent inflammation of the gland. Sialoendoscopy and ductal irrigation are employed in such patients in order to eliminate any stasis, sialolith or mucus plug in the duct. If conservative method cannot alleviate the symptom, then gland removal may be done.

Viral Infections

The most common viral infection involving salivary glands is mumps. It is caused by paramyxovirus. Other viruses involved in salivary gland pathology are coxsackie A virus, cytomegalovirus, human immunodeficiency virus (HIV) and parainfluenza virus.

◆ Mumps (Epidemic Parotitis)

Mumps is an infection of exocrine glands like salivary gland, pancreas, choroid plexus and mature ovaries and testes. Among all exocrine glands major salivary glands are affected usually. Mumps is a contagious, self-limiting disease which spreads through respiratory droplets, saliva and urine. The incubation period of this virus is 16–18 days with range of about 2–4 weeks.

Mumps can occur in epidemic form, however, its incidence has been brought down after introduction of two-dose regimen of MMR vaccination.

Clinical features: Mumps is a self-limiting disease with approximately 30% of subclinical cases. It affects adolescence population but recent trend shows more young adults involvement. The disease usually starts with pro-dromal symptoms such as low grade fever, malaise, anorexia and myalgia. Parotid gland is most commonly affected major salivary gland followed by submandibular and sublingual gland. It is presented as unilateral/bilateral parotid painful swelling. The glandular enlargement typically peaks in 2–3 days. Patient complains of difficulty in mouth opening and in chewing food.

Epididymo-orchitis is other common finding in young adult patients. It affects about 25% of males. The testicles are swollen and tender. Unilateral involvement of testes is more common as compared to bilateral involvement. On resolution, testes might show atrophy leading to sub-fertility. The condition may involve other organs also leading to pancreatitis, arthritis, carditis meningoencephalitis and decreased renal function.

The common oral manifestation of mumps is inflammation of Stenson's and Wharton's ductal openings. Apart from this, sublingual gland swelling may lead to bilateral enlargement of floor of the mouth.

The diagnosis of epidemic parotitis can be easily done clinically, however, isolated cases require laboratory confirmation. Mumps specific IgG and IgM titers may be elevated up to four times. The swab from secretion of salivary glands can be used for viral culture or real time PCR.

Treatment: The treatment of mumps is symptomatic. Analgesics and lots of fluid intake is recommended to the affected patients. The children should be immunized using two-dose MMR vaccination.

◆ HIV Infections and Salivary Glands

Another virus which affects salivary gland is HIV. It is evident in 5–10% of HIV affected individuals. The affected individuals have xerostomia which in turn leads to unilateral or bilateral salivary gland enlargement. The underlying pathogenesis may be autoimmune dysregulation and viral opportunistic infection. The incidence of salivary gland disease in HIV individuals is more in homosexuals and in intravenous drug abusers.

Clinical features: Salivary gland swelling is less commonly associated with HIV infection. Bilateral salivary gland swelling with lymphadenopathy is seen in majority of affected individuals. Patient may also complain of dry mouth. Dry mouth may occur either due to disease progression or due to antiretroviral therapy.

Radiographic features: CT and MRI of individuals may show multiple cystic masses in major salivary glands.

Treatment: The treatment of HIV associated salivary gland disease is symptomatic. Patient should be asked to sip water frequently with periodic dental examination. Fluoride application may be undertaken in order to prevent dental caries. Some investigators have reported that use of prednisone and antiretroviral therapy may regress the swelling. Other treatment options are removal of gland or radiotherapy.

◆ Subacute Necrotizing Sialadenitis

Subacute necrotizing sialadenitis is a self-limiting lesion which involves minor salivary glands of hard palate. The cause of subacute necrotizing sialadenitis is unknown, however, some investigators believe it to be allergic or infectious in origin.

Clinical features: Subacute necrotizing sialadenitis typically affects patient in their teens. It is represented as localized palatal swelling covered by erythematous, smooth, intact mucosa. Abrupt pain may be associated with this condition. It can be differentiated from necrotizing sialometaplasia on the basis of smooth surface, whereas latter has ulcerated surface.

Treatment: Though it is a self-limiting disease but the patient should be kept under observation for 2–3 weeks. If it does not heal, biopsy should be taken to confirm the diagnosis.

◆ Cheilitis Glandularis

In 1870 Volkmann first used the term "cheilitis glandularis" to describe a disorder which is suppurative inflammation of lower lip. It is an uncommon inflammatory lesion of minor salivary glands. Although cause for this condition is unknown, but investigators have pointed actinic damage, tobacco, poor hygiene and hereditary as etiologic factors.

Clinical features: Cheilitis glandularis occurs in middle aged and older with male sex predilection. It characteristically involves vermillion border of lower lip. Affected individuals have swollen lower lip with eversion due to hypertrophy and inflammation of minor salivary glands. Secondary infection of inflamed minor salivary glands in lower lip may lead to suppuration and mucopurulent discharge from the ductal openings. Based on its severity, it is classified into three progressive types:
 a. Simple
 b. Superficial suppurative (Baelz disease)
 c. Deep suppurative lesion (cheilitis glandularis apostematosa)

  Biopsy may be done in order to confirm the diagnosis of cheilitis glandularis.

Treatment: Depending upon the severity of lesion, the lesion may be treated with topical steroids, intralesional steroids or systemic steroids and antihistaminics. If conservative treatment fails, then surgical treatment with resection or vermillonectomy should be considered.

Deep suppurative type of cheilitis glandularis has potential to convert into squamous cell carcinoma. This might be due to actinic damage due to solar radiation.

◆ Necrotizing Sialometaplasia

Necrotizing sialometaplasia is a self-healing, local infiltrative, rare inflammatory disorder of the salivary gland. It mainly affects minor salivary glands. The exact cause for lesion is unknown but local ischemia of salivary gland may play role in the etiopathogenesis. Some of the authors have enlisted a few predisposing factors which might play role in its etiopathogenesis. These are traumatic injuries, ill-fitting dentures, dental infections, upper respiratory tract infections, adjacent trauma and previous history of surgery, etc. Necrotizing sialometaplasia mimics squamous cell carcinoma clinically and histopathologically due to its infiltrative nature.

Clinical features: Necrotizing sialometaplasia is a condition which frequently develops in 4th decade of life and older individuals. Males are affected nearly twice as females. The usual site of involvement is palate with hard palate more commonly involved than soft palate. It mainly presents in midline, however, it can also occur unilaterally. Submandibular gland and sublingual glands are rarely affected.

The lesions appear as non-ulcerated swelling in midline palate associated with pain or paraesthesia. In due course, the surface of lesion undergoes necrosis and ulcer-like defect is created which mimic malignant process. The pain may reduce after ulcer formation. Underlying palatal bone might get involved in latter stages.

Radiological features: Computed tomography can be done in order to see any bony resorption and also to differentiate from squamous cell carcinoma. In malignancy, bony destruction with lymph nodes involvement may be seen on CT sections.

Treatment: Since this condition mimics malignancy, biopsy should be done in order to rule out the possibility. Once the diagnosis has been established, patient should be given symptomatic treatment and should be kept under observation as this disease is self-limiting. The lesion may heal on its own in 5–6 weeks.

AUTOIMMUNE DISEASES

Sjögren's Syndrome

Sjögren's syndrome is chronic autoimmune disease affecting salivary gland and lacrimal gland. The population prevalence of primary Sjögren's syndrome is 0.5% with women affecting more as compared to men in ratio of 9:1. About 15% of rheumatoid patients suffer from secondary Sjögren's syndrome. It is the second common autoimmune disease worldwide with prevalence of 1–3%.

The cause of Sjögren's syndrome is unknown. It has been postulated that human histocompatibility antigens (HLA-DRw52, HLA-DR3) might play role in etiopathogenesis of this condition. Additionally some researchers have described the role of viruses like Epstein-Barr virus and human T cell lymphotropic virus, in the pathogenesis of Sjögren's syndrome but substantially it has not been confirmed. The condition is not hereditary disease *per se*. Traditionally, the disease is divided into two forms:

1. **Primary Sjögren's syndrome:** It is also known as sicca syndrome with clinical feature of xerostomia and xerophthalmia meaning dry mouth and dry eyes. Dry eyes are also called keratoconjunctivitis sicca. No other autoimmune disorder is present.
2. **Secondary Sjögren's syndrome (sicca syndrome + autoimmune disorders):** The patients manifest other autoimmune disorders like rheumatoid arthritis, systemic lupus erythromatosus or scleroderma, in addition to sicca syndrome.

Clinical Features

Sjögren's syndrome is a rare condition which occurs in middle-aged individuals. There is preponderance for females. The classification criterion was proposed by American-European consensus group which is being discussed below.

The main symptom which patient presents is oral dryness due to decreased salivary secretion. The salivary acini are destroyed by the lymphocytic infiltration. The patients often find difficulty in chewing, swallowing, speaking, wearing dentures and have altered taste sensation. The tongue may become fissured and exhibits atrophy of papillae. The oral mucosa may become red due to candidal infection. There are increased chances of caries in such patients.

Some patients may exhibit diffuse enlargement of salivary glands unilaterally or bilaterally. The swelling is painless and persistent in nature. More is the severity of disease and more are the chances of appearance of salivary gland swelling. These patients may have possibility of retrograde bacterial sialadenitis due to decreased salivary secretion.

Above described features along with dry eyes are seen in patients with primary Sjögren's syndrome. Keratoconjunctivitis sicca develops as a result of less secretion from lacrimal glands. The lacrimal inflammation causes decrease in water content of tears and makes tears more mucinous. Patient may complain of dry, gritty sensation or perceived presence of foreign body in eyes. The eye problem worsens as day progresses.

Apart from xerostomia and xerophthalmia patient with secondary Sjögren's syndrome may have other connective tissue disorders. The skin is often dry as are the nasal and vaginal mucosae. Lymphadenopathy, primary billiary cirrhosis, Raynaud's phenomenon, interstitial nephritis, intestinal lung fibrosis, vasculitis and peripheral neuropathy may be noticed in patients with secondary Sjögren's syndrome.

TABLE 10.4: European–American consensus group criteria for Sjögren's syndrome

1.	Ocular symptoms (at least 1 of 3) a. Daily dry eyes >3 months b. Recurrent sand or gravel sensation in eyes c. Use of tear substitute for more than 3 times a day
2.	Oral symptoms (at least 1 of 3) a. Feeling of dry mouth >3 months b. Recurrent or persistent swelling of major salivary glands c. Need frequent sipping of fluid during swallowing of food
3.	Ocular signs (1 of 2) a. Schirmer's test performed without anesthesia ($\leq$ 5 mm in 5 mins) b. Rose Bengal score or other ocular dye score ($\leq$ 4 according to van Bijsterveld's scoring system)
4.	Histopathology In labial gland biopsy: Focus score $\geq$ 1 focus/4 mm^2 of glandular tissue
5.	Salivary gland involvement (at least 1 of the following) a. Unstimulated salivary flow ($\leq$ 1.5 ml in 15 mins) b. Parotid sialography shows presence of disuse sialectasia without evidence of ductal obstruction c. Salivary scintigraphy shows delayed uptake, reduced concentration and/or delayed excretion of tracer
6.	Autoantibodies: presence of anti-Ro and anti-LA antibodies
7.	Diagnosis of primary Sjögren's syndrome a. Presence of any 4 items out of 6 as long as item 4 and item 6 are positive b. Presence of any 3 out of four items (items 3, 4, 5, 6)
8.	Diagnosis of secondary Sjögren's syndrome a. Presence of item 1 or item 2 with any two items from items 3, 4, 5 is considered positive for secondary Sjögren's syndrome.

Exclusion Criteria	
× Past head and neck radiation treatment × Hepatitis C infection × AIDS × Sarcoidosis	× Pre-existing lymphoma × Graft-versus-host disease × Use of anticholinergic drugs

Laboratory Tests

In Sjögren's syndrome patients have increased ESR and have high levels of circulating IgG immunoglobulins. Reduction in salivary gland flow using Lashley cups, less than 1.5 ml in 15 mins is considered positive for decreased secretion. Sialochemistry can also be done as there is decreased phosphate concentration and increased sodium concentration in saliva.

Various antibodies are positive in blood, however, none of the test is specific for diagnosis of the disease. The antibodies which are positive in Sjögren syndrome is anti-Ro (SS-A) and anti-La (SS-B), antinuclear antibodies (ANAs) and rheumatoid factor (RF). Occasionally antibodies against salivary gland duct can also be demonstrated.

For keratoconjunctivitis sicca Schirmer's test and Rose Bengal dye test can be performed. In Schirmer's test, a standardized strip of sterile filter paper is placed such that the margin of strip lies over the lower eyelid. Subsequently, the length of wetting is measured after 5 minutes. Values less than 5 mm are indicative of positive Schirmer test.

In Rose Bengal dye test, the cornea of eye is stained with Rose Bengal dye and examined using slit lamp for any ulceration. Histopathologically, labial gland biopsy shows lymphocytic infiltration of minor salivary glands with focus: 1 focus/4 mm^2.

American College of Rheumatology proposed classification criteria for Sjögren's syndrome.

TABLE 10.5: European–American consensus: Patients must have at least two of the following three objectives:

1.	Positive autoantibodies to Ro (SS-A) and/or La (SS-B) antigens, or positive rheumatoid factor and antinuclear antibodies titer $\geq$ 1:320
2.	Labial salivary gland biopsy exhibiting focal lymphocytic sialadenitis with focus score $\geq$ 1 focus/4 mm^2
3.	Keratoconjunctivitis sicca with ocular staining score $\geq$ 3

Radiographic features: Sialographic examination reveals punctuate, cavitatory or destructive pattern and lack of normal architecture of ductal tissue, demonstrating "fruit laden branchless tree" pattern.

Scintigraphy with radioactive technetium-99m pertechnetate characteristically shows decreased uptake, retention and/or excretion of isotope.

Treatment: The treatment of Sjögren syndrome is primarily supportive. Salivary substitute or sialogogues should be used along with sugarless candies and daily fluoride application to prevent dental caries. Topical antifungal agent such as clotrimazole or miconazole may be used in order to prevent any fungal candidiasis. Pilocarpine or cevimeline may be used to enhance the saliva secretion from unaffected salivary gland.

Artificial tears may be used topically to prevent eyes from drying. Sealing of lacrimal punctum may prevent normal drainage of lacrimal secretion into nose and in turn, helps in keeping eyes moist.

Patients with Sjögren's syndrome have risk of 5 to 15% for developing lymphoma. Recent literature reveals that all salivary gland infiltrates are not benign lymphoepithelial lesions but some of them are low grade non-Hodgkin B cell lymphomas of mucosa associated lymphoid tissue. The detection of immunoglobulin gene rearrangements in labial salivary gland biopsy may serve as useful marker for predicting development of lymphoma.

Mikulicz's Disease (IgG4 Related Disease)

Mikulicz's disease was first described by Johann von Mikulicz-Radecki in late 1800s. Mikulicz's disease is characterized by chronic inflammatory infiltrate in the salivary glands. Histopathologically, some of the lesion's presentation is confusing and same as benign lymphoepithelial lesions associated with Sjögren syndrome. Therefore, these types of lesions are classified as IgG4 related lesions which are a fibroinflammatory disorder.

IgG4 related diseases are the group of sclerosing inflammatory disorders in which IgG4 levels are elevated in serum along with presence of IgG4 positive plasma cells. Serum levels of IgG4 can shoot up to 25 times greater than normal levels.

Clinical features: IgG4 related diseases may present as unilateral/bilateral salivary gland painless swelling. It affects in middle aged and older individuals in 6th decade of life. After pancreas, head and neck region is second most common region to be affected by this condition. There is slight predilection for men than women. IgG4 related disease affects submandibular gland more frequently. The severity of disease depends upon the site of involvement.

Treatment: IgG4 related diseases should be treated aggressively. Systemic corticosteroid is the mainstay of treatment to avoid further damage of organ. Most of the patients show rapid response to immunosuppressive therapy. Other steroid sparing immuno-suppressive drugs are azathioprine, mycophenolate mofetil and methotrexate.

NON-INFLAMMATORY DISORDERS OF SALIVARY GLANDS

Sialadenosis (Sialosis)

Sialadenosis is non-inflammatory, non-neoplastic disorder involving major salivary glands. The condition arises majorly due to any systemic cause like endocrinal, nutritional or neurogenic. Most common systemic conditions which cause sialadenosis are diabetes mellitus, malnutrition, alcoholism and bulimia.

The cause for sialadenosis is believed to be dysregulation of autonomic nervous system supplying salivary glands. The condition leads to excessive accumulation of secretory granules with marked enlargement of acinar cells. In addition, there is atrophy of supporting myofilaments around acinar cells

due to reduced innervations of myoepithelial cells.

TABLE 10.6: Conditions associated with sialadenosis

1.	Endocrine disorders
	a. Diabetes mellitus
	b. Diabetes insipidus
	c. Acromegaly
	d. Hypothyroidism
	e. Pregnancy
2.	Nutritional
	a. General malnutrition
	b. Alcoholism
	c. Cirrhosis
	d. Anorexia nervosa
	e. Bulimia
3.	Neurogenic medications
	a. Antihypertensive drugs
	b. Psychotropic drugs
	c. Sympathomimetic drugs used for treating asthma

Clinical features: Sialadenosis represents as bilateral or unilateral, painless, slow growing swelling. The saliva secretion is decreased. Sometimes, it may present as painful swelling. The most common major gland which is involved is submandibular salivary gland. Minor salivary glands are rarely affected. It may be differentiated from Sjögren syndrome on the basis of systemic history and laboratory tests.

Radiographic features: Sialadenosis generally spares the ductal system and involves acinar tissue of major salivary glands. Therefore, sialography examination reveals "leafless pattern" with splaying of ductal system. CT scan studies demonstrate generalized increase in size and density of parenchyma caused by infiltration of fatty and fibrous tissue.

Treatment: Treatment will include patient reassurance and education. Many times treatment is often unsatisfactory. Underlying cause should be corrected first. Mild swelling of parotid gland does not cause many problems. Bigger swelling is a concern from cosmetic point of view. Therefore, surgically, partial/complete removal of involved gland can be undertaken. Pilocarpine might be used to increase the secretion in case of salivary output.

Orofacial Granulomatosis

Wiesenfeld introduced the term orofacial granulomatosis in the year 1985 which comprises variety of clinical presentations. Histopathologically, all orofacial granulomatoses share some pictures of non-caseating giant cell granulomas. Various orofacil granulomatosis pathologies are Melkersson-Rosenthal syndrome, cheilitis granulomatosa, Crohn's disease, sarcoidosis and tuberculosis.

Sarcoidosis is a multisystem immune-related disorder primarily affecting lymph nodes. Heart, liver, spleen, bones, kin eyes, parotid gland may also get involved in some patients.

Clinical Features

Painless, asymptomatic or mildly sympto-matic enlargement of major salivary gland may be the first sign of sarcoidosis. Facial nerve involvement may present and can be wrongly diagnosed as malignancy. Salivary gland milking may yield delayed response, however, sialometry is normal in this condition. It may also affect other parts of orofacial region such as gingiva, buccal mucosa, floor of the mouth and tongue. Biopsy of lesion should be carried out in order to diagnose sarcoidosis.

Serum angiotensin converting enzyme (sACE) is considered as diagnostic for sarcoidosis. Elevated level of sACE is found in 80–90% of the cases as sACE is secreted by granulomas.

Treatment: Spontaneous regression is seen in most of the patients. Some patients may require systemic corticosteroids. Refractory cases may be treated with azathioprine, mycophenolate mofetil and cyclosphosphamide or methotrexate.

Consultation with dentist should be done in order to prevent dental caries and dry mouth.

TUMORS OF SALIVARY GLANDS

General Considerations

1. The annual incidence of salivary gland tumor worldwide is 1.0–6.5/100,000. That means salivary gland tumor is not a rare entity.
2. **Parotid glands:** Around 60–80% of salivary gland tumors occur in parotid gland and relatively low percentage of tumors are malignant in nature. Around 2/3rd to 3/5th parotid tumors are benign in nature. Pleomorphic adenoma is most common tumor occurring in parotid gland followed by Warthin's tumor.
3. **Submandibular gland:** Approximately 8–11% of salivary glands tumors occur in submandibular gland. The incidence of malignant tumor involving submandibular gland is more as compared to parotid gland. Pleomorphic tumor followed by adenoid cystic carcinoma is most common tumors of salivary gland.
4. **Sublingual gland:** The occurrence of tumor in sublingual salivary gland is rare. However, the chances of malignant tumors are more in sublingual gland as compared to other two major salivary glands.
5. **Minor salivary glands:** Minor salivary gland tumor is the second most common site for salivary neoplasia. The frequency of malignant tumors in minor salivary gland is far more common as compared to major salivary gland tumors.
6. Mucoepidermoid carcinoma is the most common malignant tumor of minor salivary gland.
7. Palate is the most common site for salivary gland tumors accounting for about 50% of tumor occurring at this site. The density of minor salivary gland is more in posterolateral hard or soft palate that is why more tumors occur at postero-lateral aspect of palate.

8. Although CT and MRI have replaced the sialography in evaluation of salivary masses, the reader should be aware of some sialographic patterns obtained in cases of neoplasia. In tumors, sialography will show the following patterns:
   a. Ductal splaying or "ball in hand" appearance
   b. Ductal displacement, buckling or cut off
   c. Abrupt ductal irregularities or displacement and contrast spilling within gland
   d. Filling defects on parenchymal opacification.

The above sialographic signs are non-specific and could not be able to differentiate between low grade malignancies and benign tumors. Sialographic pattern suggestive of malignancy is abrupt ductal irregularity and displacement and contrast spilling in tissue parenchyma.

Classification

Benign

- Pleomorphic adenoma (mixed tumor)
- Myoepithelioma
- Basal cell adenoma
- Canalicular adenoma
- Warthin tumor (papillary cyst adenoma lymphomatosum)
- Oncocytoma
- Sebaceous adenoma
- Sebaceous lymphadenoma
- Ductal papillomas
- Sialadenoma papilliferum
- Intraductal papilloma
- Inverted ductal papilloma
- Papillary cyst adenoma

Malignant

- Malignant mixed tumors
- Carcinoma ex pleomorphic adenoma
- Carcinosarcoma
- Metastasizing mixed tumor
- Mucoepidermoid carcinoma
- Acinic cell adenocarcinoma
- Adenoid cystic carcinoma
- Polymorphous low-grade adenocarcinoma
- Basal cell adenocarcinoma
- Epithelial-myoepithelial carcinoma
- Mammary analogue secretory carcinoma
- Salivary duct carcinoma
- Myoepithelial carcinoma
- Cyst adenocarcinoma
- Sebaceous adenocarcinoma
- Sebaceous lymph adenocarcinoma
- Clear cell adenocarcinoma
- Oncocytic carcinoma
- Squamous cell carcinoma
- Malignant lymphoepithelial lesion (lymphoepithelial carcinoma)
- Small cell carcinoma
- Sialoblastoma
- Adenocarcinoma, not otherwise specified (NOS)

BENIGN TUMORS OF SALIVARY GLANDS

Pleomorphic Adenoma

Pleomorphic adenoma is most common tumor of salivary gland. It is also called mixed tumor of salivary gland because it is derived from ductal and myoepithelial elements and microscopically it presents wide variation from one tumor to another. However, it does not originate from more than one germ layer. Cytogenetic analysis revealed that 70% of adenoma primarily involves translocation of pleomorphic adenoma gene 1 (PLAG1) located on chromosome 8q12.

Clinical Features

Pleomorphic adenoma can occur in major and minor salivary glands. It is painless, slow growing, firm mass with well distinct borders. Most common age is between 30–60 years. However, it can develop in any age group. There is slight female predilection.

Parotid gland pleomorphic adenoma presents as swelling on the ramus of mandible. Initially the swelling becomes less movable. In most cases superficial lobe of parotid gland is involved and in about 10% of cases deep lobe of parotid gland is involved. The lesion does not show fixation either to the deeper tissues or to the overlying skin. Associated features of facial nerve palsy and pain are less evident in literature.

Pleomorphic adenoma of minor salivary gland generally occurs in palate (Fig. 10.7) followed by upper lip and buccal mucosa. It presents as smooth surfaced firm swelling in posterolateral portion of palate. The swelling might get ulcerated if it is traumatized.

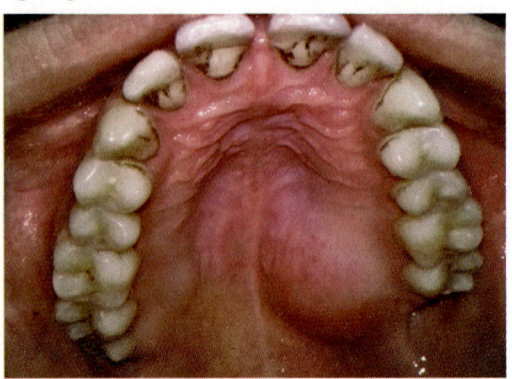

Fig. 10.7: Pleomorphic adenoma of minor salivary gland

Radiographic features: Computed tomography will show pleomorphic adenoma as enhancing, well-circumscribed lesions with fibrous capsule around it. The tumors are well-demarcated from sound parenchymal tissue. Lesions smaller than 1 cm usually rounded and lesions above 1 cm are lobulated. To rule out any malignant changes, evaluation of facial nerve involvement is essential. On ultrasonography, lesion are well circumscribed, hypoechoic and non-enhancing masses.

Treatment: Pleomorphic adenomas are best treated by surgical removal. Parotidectomy with identification and preservation of facial nerve is recommended. The prognosis of pleomorphic adenoma is excellent and chances of recurrence are less.

Warthin's Tumor

Warthin's tumor or papillary cystadenoma lymphomatosum, is the second most common tumor of parotid gland. It accounts for about 5–22% of parotid gland tumors. The pathogenesis of the lesion is controversial. One theory believes that it arises from salivary gland tissue found in the parotid lymph node. However, other researchers believe that the tumor may develop from salivary gland duct cells. The incidence of Warthin's tumor is found to be more in smokers than non-smokers.

Clinical Features

Warthin's tumor occurs in older age group between 6th and 7th decades of life. Male preponderance was seen in previous literature (10:1), however, recent studies show frequency of occurrence is similar in female and males. Smoking is considered as one of the important etiological agents and nowadays frequency of smoking is more or less equal in male and female probably, that is why the male and female predilection is similar in recent studies.

Warthin's tumor presents as slow growing, painless swelling in the tail end of parotid gland. Rarely, it can involve sub-mandibular and sublingual gland also. The consistency on palpation is fluctuant or firm. Warthin's tumor can occur bilaterally with one swelling appearing after another.

Radiographic Features

Sialographic studies in Warthin's tumor show indistinguishable features from other benign tumors of salivary gland such as pleomorphic adenoma. It can also occur in inferior aspect of superficial lobe of parotid gland.

Computed tomography examination show tumor as enhancing, rounded and well-demarcated lesion in posteroinferior segment of parotid gland. Radionuclide scan shows increased uptake of radionuclide dye and presents as "hot spot" on the scans. This might be due to the fact that Warthin's tumor is composed of secretory cells not excretory cells so the dye gets accumulated in the gland. Ultrasound studies show hypoechoic areas with echogenic line and may also demonstrate lobulated outline.

Treatment: Surgical excision is the choice of treatment in cases of Warthin's tumor. Some surgeons excise with minimal surrounding tissue and others prefer parotidectomy. The chances of recurrence are minimal.

Oncocytoma (Oxyphillic Adenoma)

Oncocytoma is a rare, benign tumor of salivary gland mainly composed of oncocytes. The word onco (derived from Greek word onkoustai) means to swell. In this tumor, swollen granular cytoplasm with accumulation of mitochondria is seen in salivary gland cells. Sometimes, metaplasia of ductal and acinar cells is also noted. Besides salivary gland, oncocytes are also seen in other organs like thyroid, parathyroid, and kidney.

Clinical features: Oncocytoma occurs in older age group, around 6th–7th decade of life. It commonly involves parotid gland although, cases involving submandibular gland and minor salivary glands are also reported in literature. The tumor appears as firm, slow growing and painless swelling in parotid gland. It majorly affects superficial lobe of parotid gland and clinicians find it difficult to distinguish it from other benign tumors of parotid gland.

Radiographic features: CT images of oncocytoma usually reports well-circum-scribed enhancing lesion in the parotid gland. It can be multifocal or bilateral. MRI usually demonstrates well-circumscribed, low signal intensity on T1 and T2 weighted images. Homogenous enhancement of lesion is seen after intravenous injection of contrast.

Treatment: The oncocytoma is benign in nature, therefore, surgical excision with partial parotidectomy can be done. Facial nerve should be preserved while operating. Oncocytoma affecting submandibular gland should be excised completely with gland removal. The chance of recurrence is rare. Some cases of oncocytoma are locally aggressive and should be considered for low grade malignancy.

Canalicular Adenoma

Canalicular adenoma is an uncommon tumor of minor salivary gland. Histopathologically, it shows uniform pattern, therefore, it is also called monomorphic adenoma.

Clinical Features

Canalicular adenoma occurs in older age group peaking in 7th decade of life with slight female preponderance. Canalicular adenoma is one of the rare tumors that occur on upper lip. The buccal mucosa is the second common affecting site. It usually affects major salivary glands and also predilection for minor salivary gland.

It presents as slow growing, fluctuant, painless swelling with bluish surface. This tumor is often mistaken as mucocele. The mucocele of upper lip is very uncommon, therefore, swelling on the upper lip should be considered for canalicular adenoma.

Radiographic features: CT findings will show well-defined, enhancing, homogenous lesion in the major salivary gland. MRI can also be done revealing same finding as that of CT scan.

Treatment: Local surgical excision is the choice of treatment for canalicular adenoma. Recurrence of the lesion is rare.

Basal Cell Adenoma

Basal cell adenoma is an uncommon tumor accounting for about 1–4% of all salivary gland tumors. As canalicular adenoma, it is also categorized under monomorphic adenoma of salivary gland, however, some histopathological study reveals presence of more than one cell type. Previously canalicular and basal cell adenoma were used synonymously but recent literature termed them different entity.

Clinical Features

Basal cell adenoma is a tumor of major salivary gland with basaloid appearance microscopically. It may occur in minor salivary glands also. The tumor can occur at any stage of life with peak prevalence of 7th decade of life. Females are more affected than male counterparts (2:1).

Clinically, basal cell adenoma shows features like pleomorphic adenoma. The swelling usually slow growing and painless in nature. Superficial lobe of parotid gland is involved commonly. One subtype, termed membranous basal cell adenoma, is hereditary and often occur with dermal tumors like cylindromas and trichoepitheliomas. Membranous basal cell adenoma bears resemblance to the dermal counterparts microscopically, therefore, termed dermal analogue tumors.

Radiographic features: CT scan shows well-defined, enhancing, homogenous lesion. It may be round to oval in shape. Sometimes, CT findings reveal inhomogenous mass due to presence of cystic spaces within the lesion.

Treatment: Like pleomorphic adenoma, basal cell adenoma is also treated surgically and prognosis is very good with less chance of recurrence.

MALIGNANT TUMORS OF SALIVARY GLAND

Mucoepidermoid Carcinoma

Mucoepidermoid carcinoma is the most common malignancy arising from salivary glands. Mucoepidermoid carcinoma may be graded according to aggressiveness of the tumor into low grade, intermediate grade and high grade tumor. The etiopathogenesis of the tumor is not clear, however, some researchers reported radiation exposure as one of the causes. Reciprocal translocation (11:19) is also been reported by some authors in low grade and intermediate type of mucoepidermoid carcinomas.

Clinical Features

Mucoepidermoid carcinomas commonly occurs in parotid gland followed by minor salivary glands on palate (Fig. 10.8), lower lip and floor of the mouth. The tumor may occur during wide age range but it is very rare in first decade. Mucoepidermoid carcinoma generally starts as painless swelling which may involve facial nerve in later stages. The swelling is usually smooth surfaced but may get ulcerated due to secondary trauma.

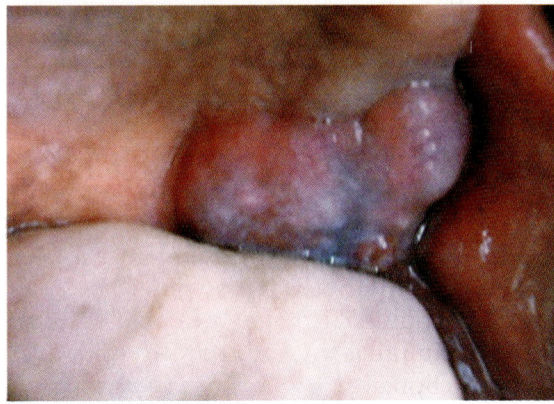

Fig. 10.8: Mucoepidermoid carcinoma of palate

Clinically, low grade carcinomas are associated with a slower growth rate, longer duration and good prognosis as compared to high grade carcinomas. About two-thirds of mucoepidermoid carcinomas are low grade. Low grade carcinomas generally present as cystic swelling, whereas high grade are more solid in consistency. High grade malignancy may infiltrate surrounding structures and may metastasize to the regional lymph node.

Radiographic features: Clinically suspected case of mucoepidermoid carcinoma should be investigated using contrast enhanced CT. In low grade malignancy CT images will show well-circumscribed mass with cystic degeneration in some areas. More or less, these tumors have appearance like benign mixed tumors. High grade malignancy will show poorly demarcated, solid lesion which is infiltrating locally.

Ultrasonography and MRI studies can also be done. MRI studies may be done in order to rule out perineural spread of tumor into base of skull.

Treatment: Patients with low grade malignancy should be treated surgically with wide excision. Facial nerve may be conserved while operating. Patients with high grade tumor should be treated aggressively. Parotidectomy with wide excision along with facial nerve dissection and neck dissection may be required. Radiotherapy and/or chemotherapy may be done after surgical treatment.

Prognosis for low grade is generally good with survival chance of 90–98%, however, survival rate is reduced in cases with high grade malignancy.

Intraosseous Mucoepidermoid Carcinoma

Intraosseous salivary gland tumors may develop in the jaws and anterior tumor can arise in bone, however, mucoepidermoid carcinoma is most common tumor to arise inside bone. Many theories had been proposed for the intrabony presence of salivary tumor but none has been found to be good enough to explain the reason. Some intraosseous mucoepidermoid carcinoma develops in association with impacted teeth or odontogenic cysts.

Clinical features: Intraosseous mucoepidermoid carcinoma occurs in middle age group with mandible more commonly involved than maxilla. There is slight predilection for females as compared to males. The tumor presents as swelling with cortical expansion, like in benign tumors. The swelling may be associated with pain, trismus and paraesthesia.

Radiographic features: Radiographically, it represents as unilocular or multilocular radiolucency with well-defined borders. However, in some cases ill-defined borders are also noted with osteolytic lesion depending upon tumor's aggressiveness. Contrast enhanced CT scan shows in homogenous enhancement with well-defined borders.

Treatment: Intraosseous carcinomas are treated by surgery first followed by radiotherapy or chemotherapy or both. The recurrence chance is high if surgery with conservative approach is done. Metastasis has also been reported in some cases.

Acinic Cell Carcinoma

Acinic cell carcinoma is low grade malignancy where salivary gland cells undergo serous acinar differentiation. Previously, this entity was considered as tumor and was termed acinic cell tumor. But these tumors can metastasize, recur and can cause mortality. Therefore, now researchers have kept this tumor into low grade malignancy.

Clinical features: Predominately, acinic cell carcinoma occurs in parotid gland. Superficial lobe affects more than deep lobe of parotid gland. Other sites of involvement are submandibular gland, minor salivary gland in buccal mucosa, lip and palate. Majority of cases occur in parotid gland as this is the largest salivary gland and is serous in nature. The tumor occurs in wide age range from 4th–7th decade of life. The tumor usually appears as slow growing mass and can attain large size. Most of the time it is asymptomatic and facial nerve involvement is rare.

Radiographic features: Radiographic features of acinic cell carcinoma are overlapping with benign tumor. CT scan findings show enhancing, irregular lesion which may be associated with necrotic areas.

Treatment: Acinic cell carcinoma is treated by lobectomy if the lesion is confined to superficial lobe and parotidectomy if deep lobe is involved. Submandibular gland tumor may be treated by total gland removal. The prognosis of the patients with acinic cell carcinoma is generally good with some chances of recurrence.

Malignant Mixed Tumors

Malignant mixed tumors present malignant counterpart of pleomorphic adenoma. It is comparatively rare carcinoma comprises 2–4% of all salivary gland tumors. Malignant

mixed tumors are categorized into three categories:
1. Carcinoma ex pleomorphic adenoma
2. Carcinosarcoma
3. Metastasizing mixed tumor

Carcinoma ex pleomorphic adenoma is the most common variant among three. Histopathologically, it shows dysplastic features in the epithelial component of pleomorphic adenoma. Carcinosarcoma is rarest of the three and shows both epithelial and connective tissue component undergoing dysplasia, whereas metastasizing mixed tumor does not show any dysplasia in the epithelial or connective tissue part but metastasize to other parts of body. The microscopic features of metastasize lesion shows benign appearance.

Clinical Features

◈ Carcinoma ex pleomorphic adenoma

This variant develops in long standing cases of pleomorphic adenoma. It commonly occurs in parotid gland and suddenly benign tumor starts to grow at rapid pace. Rapid growth may be associated with surface ulceration. It may be painful or painless. Facial nerve involvement can be seen in this variant. It may also occur in minor salivary glands and palate is the most common site for its occurrence. It generally occurs in middle age group in 6–7th decade of life.

◈ Carcinosarcoma

Carcinosarcoma is one of the rare malignant tumors of salivary gland. It either occurs in long standing pleomorphic adenoma or *de novo*. It most commonly involves parotid gland although cases of submandibular gland are also reported. The clinical signs and symptoms are more or less similar to carcinoma ex pleomorphic adenoma.

◈ Metastasizing mixed tumor

Metastasizing mixed tumor is also rare tumor, commonly occurring in parotid gland. It shows benign nature and frequently metastasizes to bones, lungs, regional lymph nodes, liver and skin. It may develop in previously treated mixed tumor also.

Radiographic features: Both CT and MRI can be done to investigate the malignant mixed tumors. Radiographic findings of malignant mixed tumors are similar to the other malignant tumors. Carcinoma ex pleomorphic adenoma and carcinosarcoma shows large, ill-defined, heterogeneous lesion with infiltrative margins. The tumor may infiltrate into surrounding tissues. Regional lymph node metastasis can also be noted. Metastasizing mixed tumor shows well-defined borders, homogeneous and enhancing lesion. However, other parts like bones, liver, skin, lungs may show similar kind of lesion therefore, whole body CT scan or PET scan should be done in order to see distant lesions.

Treatment: Treatment of carcinoma ex pleomorphic adenoma and carcinosarcoma comprises surgery with radiotherapy and chemotherapy. The excision of the lesion should be done with wide margins with regional lymph node removal. The chances of survival after treatment are not so good in both the tumors. Metastasizing mixed tumor should be treated by surgical excision of primary and secondary tumors.

Adenoid Cystic Carcinoma

Adenoid cystic carcinoma is also called cylindroma. It is the relatively common malignancy of salivary gland. Adenoid cystic carcinoma shows myoepithelial and ductal cells in varied arrangement.

Clinical features: Adenoid cystic carcinoma commonly occurs in minor salivary gland with palate being common site (Fig. 10.9). Male to female ratio is 1:1.4. The age group for this malignancy is 4–5th decade and comparatively rare in age below 20. It presents as slow growing lesion associated with pain and facial nerve involvement. Patients often complain of constant, low grade, dull ache which increase in intensity as time progress.

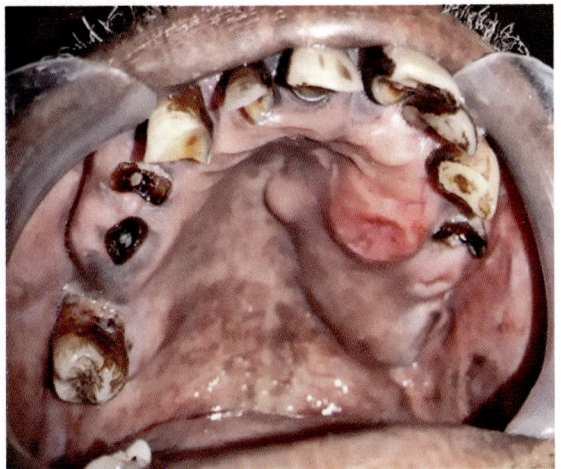

Fig. 10.9: Adenoid cystic carcinoma

Radiographic features: CT scan shows enhancing, heterogeneous mass, locally destructured lesion with involvement of palate and maxillary. The borders are ill defined. Regional metastasis to lymph nodes is comparatively uncommon.

Treatment: Surgical resection with wide borders is the treatment of choice for these tumors. As regional metastasis is uncommon, so the need for neck dissection is not indicated. Adenoid cystic carcinoma is prone to local recurrence and distant metastasis. Both these features increase the mortality index in this carcinoma.

FREQUENTLY ASKED QUESTIONS

Long Answer Questions

a. Classify salivary gland tumors. Write in detail about clinical features, radiographic features and treatment of pleomorphic adenoma.

b. Describe in detail about etiopathogenesis, clinical features, laboratory findings and treatment of Sjögren's syndrome.

c. Describe in detail about indications, contraindications, contrast agents and procedure of sialography.

d. Write in detail about causes, clinical features, chair side tests and treatment of xerostomia.

Short Answer Questions

a. Contrast agents in sialography
b. Sialorrhea
c. Causes of xerostomia
d. Bacterial sialadenitis
e. Mumps
f. Sialolithiasis
g. Mucoepidermoid carcinoma
h. Sialosis
i. Necrotizing sialometaplasia
j. Classify salivary gland disorders.

BIBLIOGRAPHY

1. G.S. Kumar. Orban's Oral Histology and embroyology. 14th edition: Elsevier 2018.
2. Sivapathasundharam B, Rajendran A. Shafer's textbook of Oral Pathology. 7th edition: Elsevier 2012.
3. Michael Glickman. Burket's Oral Medicine: 12th edition, People's Medical Publishing House, 2015.
4. Neville BW, Damm DD, Allen CM, Bouquot J. Neville's Oral and Maxillofacial Pathology: 3rd edition. WB Saunders 2008.
5. Wood NK, Goaz PW. Differential Diagnosis of Oral and Maxillofacial Lesions. 5th edition. Mosby Publications, 1997.
6. Mallya S, Lam E. Oral Radiology: Principles and Interpretations: A Southeast Asia Edition. 1st edition: Elsevier India, 2014.
7. Delbalso AM. Maxillofacial Imaging. 1st edition. WB Saunders 1990.

Temporomandibular Joint Diseases and Radiologic Considerations

INTRODUCTION

The term *temporomandibular disorders* (TMDs) is a collective term embracing a number of clinical problems that involve the masticatory muscles, the temporomandibular joints (TMJs) and the associated structures or both. These disorders are characterized by facial pain in the region of the TMJs or muscles of mastication, limitation or deviation in mandibular movements, and TMJ sounds during jaw movement and function. This chapter presents a general approach to the diagnostic assessment and nonsurgical management of the most common TMDs.

Functional Anatomy

Temporomandibular joint, the TMJ articulation is a joint that is capable of hinge type and gliding movements.

The bony components are enclosed and connected by a fibrous capsule. The mandibular condyle forms the lower part of the bony joint and is generally elliptical, although variations in shape are common. The articulation is formed by the mandibular condyle occupying a hollow in the temporal bone (mandibular or glenoid fossa).

The S-shaped form of the fossa and eminence develops at about 6 years of age and continues into the second decade. During wide mouth opening, the condyle rotates around a hinge axis and glides, causing it to move beyond the anterior border of the fossa, which is identified as the articular eminence.

TABLE 11.1: Anatomy of TMJ	
Bony component of TMJ Fibrous capsule	⚹ The capsule is lined with synovium, joint cavity is filled with synovial fluid. The synovium is a vascular connective tissue lining the fibrous joint capsule extending to the boundaries of the articulating surfaces covering upper and lower joint cavities.
	⚹ The synovial membrane consists of macrophage-like type A cells and fibroblast-like type B cells.
	⚹ Synovial fluid is a filtrate of plasma with added mucins and proteins. Its main constituent is hyaluronic acid. Fluid forms on the articulating surfaces decrease friction during joint compression and motion.
	⚹ Joint lubrication is achieved by weeping lubrication and boundary lubrication. Weeping lubrication occurs as fluid is forced laterally during compression and expressed through the unloaded fibrocartilage. Boundary lubrication is function of water that is physically bound to the cartilaginous surface by a glycoprotein.

Contd.

TABLE 11.1: Anatomy of TMJ *(Contd.)*

Articular disc	⚹ A fibrocartilage is made up of dense collagen and referred to as a disc which occupies the space between the fibrocartilage coverings of each of condyle and mandibular fossa. ⚹ The disc consists of collagen fibers, cartilage like proteoglycans, and elastic fibers and number of cells that resemble fibrocytes and fibrochondrocytes. ⚹ The disc is primarily avascular and has sensory nerve penetration. It is attached by ligaments to the lateral and medial poles of the condyle. The ligaments consist of both collagen and elastic fibers. These ligaments permit rotational movement of the disc on the condyle during mouth opening and closing. ⚹ The disc and its attachments divide the joint into upper and lower compartments which do not communicate. The passive volume of the upper compartment is estimated to be 1.2 ml and that of the lower compartment is estimated to be 0.9 ml. The roof of the superior compartment is the mandibular fossa, and floor is the superior surface of the disc. The roof of the inferior compartment is the inferior surface of the disc and the floor is the articulating surface of the mandibular condyle. At its margins, the disc blends with the fibrous capsule. ⚹ Fibers of the posterior one-third of the temporalis muscle and the deep masseter muscle attach on the anterolateral aspect, and fibers of the superior head of the lateral pterygoid insert into the anteromedial two-thirds of the disc. 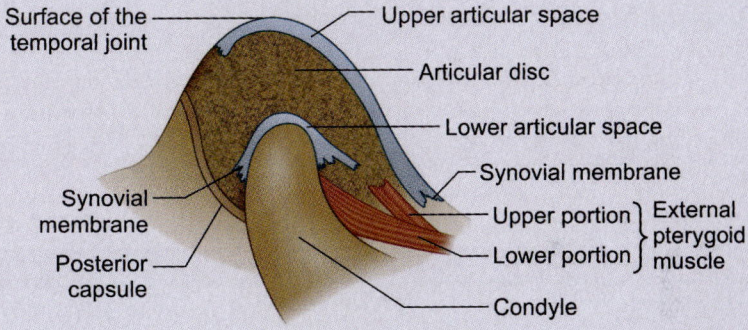 **Fig. 11.1**
Retrodiscal tissue	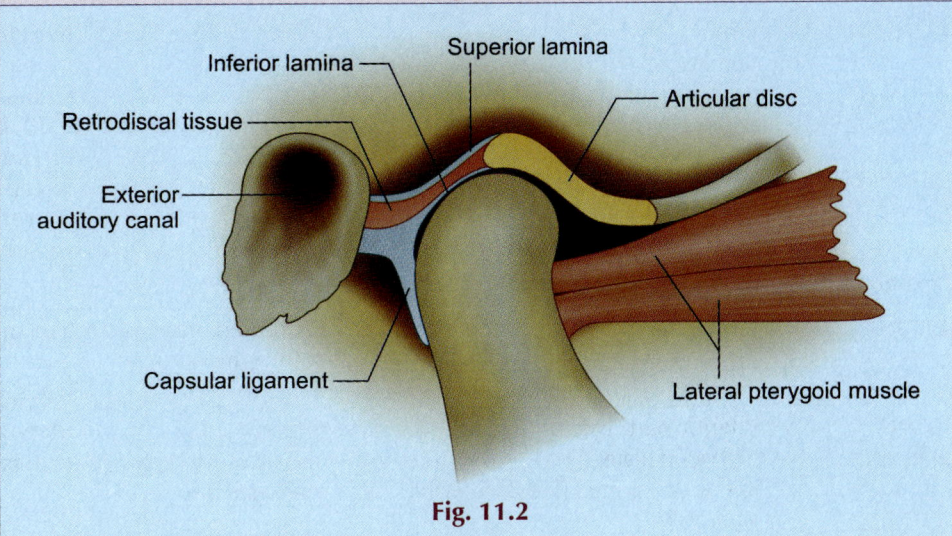 **Fig. 11.2**

Contd.

TABLE 11.1: Anatomy of TMJ *(Contd.)*

	⤬ A mass of soft tissue occupies the space behind the disc and condyle. It is referred to as the posterior attachment; a loosely organized system of collagen fibers, branching elastic fibers, fat, blood and lymph vessels, and nerves. Synovium covers the superior and inferior surfaces with a loose areolar, highly vascular, and well-innervated tissue. ⤬ The superior lamina arises from the posterior band of the disc and attaches to the squamo-tympanic fissure and tympanic part of the temporal bone consists of elastin. The inferior lamina arises from the posterior band of the disc and inserts into the inferior margin of the posterior articular slope of the condyle composed of collagen fibers.
Temporomandibular ligaments	
Capsular ligament	The capsular ligament is a thin inelastic fibrous connective tissue envelope that attaches to the margins of the articular surfaces and neck of the condyle.
Lateral temporo-mandibular ligament	The lateral temporomandibular ligament is the main ligament of the joint. Its fibers pass obliquely from bone lateral to the articular tubercle in a posterior and inferior direction and insert in a narrower area below and behind the lateral pole of the condyle.
Spheno-mandibular ligament	The sphenomandibular ligament arises from the sphenoid bone and inserts on the medial aspect of the mandible at the lingula.
Stylo-mandibular ligament	The stylomandibular ligament extends from the styloid process to the deep fascia of the medial pterygoid muscle. It is thought to become tense during protrusive movement of the mandible and limits protrusive movement.

TABLE 11.2: Muscles of mastication

Muscle of mastication	Origin	Insertion	Function
Masseter	⤬ From maxillary process of zygomatic bone. ⤬ Superficial part of maxillary process of zygomatic bone and the anterior two-thirds of the inferior part.	⤬ Lateral aspect of ramus	⤬ Masseter and medial pterygoid join together to form a sling that cradles the ramus of the mandible and produces the powerful forces required for chewing.
Medial pterygoid	⤬ Medial surface of lateral pterygoid plate	⤬ Medial aspect of ramus.	⤬ Closing of mandible.
Temporalis	⤬ Temporal fascia	⤬ Coronoid process and mandibular ramus.	⤬ Fan-shaped opening and retrusion of mandible.
Lateral pterygoid	⤬ Inferior part: Lateral surface of lateral pterygoid plate. ⤬ Superior part: Greater wing of sphenoid.	⤬ Anteromedial aspect of condylar neck and disc.	⤬ Main protrusive and opening muscle.

Contd.

TABLE 11.2: Muscles of mastication *(Contd.)*

Muscle of mastication	Origin	Insertion	Function
Digastric (accessory muscle)	✗ Anterior belly from digastric fossa of mandible. ✗ Posterior belly from mastoid notch of temporalis.	✗ Together they insert on the hyoid bone.	✗ Depression and retrusion of mandible.
Buccinator (accessory muscle)	✗ From the alveolar processes of maxilla and mandible, and pterygo-mandibular raphae.	✗ Orbicularis oris	✗ Compresses cheek into the teeth for chewing.

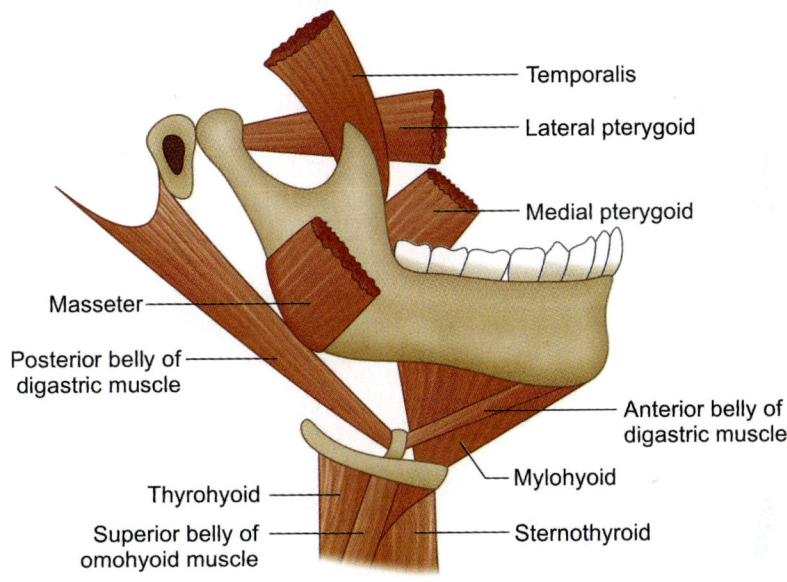

- Temporalis
- Lateral pterygoid
- Medial pterygoid
- Masseter
- Posterior belly of digastric muscle
- Anterior belly of digastric muscle
- Mylohyoid
- Thyrohyoid
- Sternothyroid
- Superior belly of omohyoid muscle

Fig. 11.3

Flowchart 11.1

Diagnostic classification of temporomandibular disorders

Cranial bones
Congenital and developmental disorders:
- Aplasia
- Hypoplasia
- Hyperplasia
- Dysplasia (e.g. first and second branchial arch anomalies, hemifacial microsomia, Pierre Robin syndrome, Treacher Collins syndrome, condylar hyperplasia, prognathism)

Acquired disorders:
- Neoplasia
- Fracture

Temporomandibular joint
- Deviation in form
- Disc displacement (with reduction, without reduction)
- Dislocation
- Inflammatory conditions (synovitis, capsulitis)
- Arthritides (osteoarthritis, osteoarthrosis, polyarthritides)
- Ankylosis (fibrous, bony)
- Neoplasia

Masticatory muscle
- Myofacial pain
- Myositis spasm
- Protective splinting
- Contracture

(Adapted from McNeill C.127) *(Courtesy:* Classification from Burett, 12th ed)

CLASSIFICATION

TABLE 11.3: Taxonomic classification for temporomandibular disorders

Temporomandibular joint disorders

1. **Joint pain**
   A. Arthralgia
   B. Arthritis

2. **Joint disorders**
   A. Disc disorders
      1. Disc displacement with reduction
      2. Disc displacement with reduction with intermittent locking
      3. Disc displacement without reduction with limited opening
      4. Disc displacement without reduction without limited opening
   B. Other hypomobility disorders
      1. Adhesions/adherence
      2. Ankylosis
         a. Fibrous
         b. Osseous
   C. Hypermobility disorders
      1. Dislocations
         a. Subluxation
         b. Luxation

3. **Joint diseases**
   A. Degenerative joint disease
      1. Osteoarthrosis
      2. Osteoarthritis
   B. Systemic arthritides
   C. Condylysis/idiopathic condylar resorption
   D. Osteochondritis dissecans
   E. Ostronecrosis
   F. Neoplasm

Vascular supply of masticatory system structures : The external carotid artery is the main blood supply for the masticatory system structures. The artery sends two important branches, the lingual and facial arteries to the region. At the level of the condylar neck, the external carotid bifurcates into the superficial temporal artery and the internal maxillary artery. These two arteries supply the muscles of mastication and the TMJ.

Nerve supply of masticatory system structures: The masticatory structures are innervated primarily by the trigeminal nerve, but cranial nerves VII, IX, X, and XI and cervical nerves 2 and 3 also contribute. The mandibular division of the trigeminal nerve supplies motor innervation to the muscles of mastication and the anterior belly of the digastric muscle. Branches of the auriculotemporal nerve supply the sensory innervation of the TMJ; this nerve arises from the mandibular division in the infratemporal fossa and sends branches to the capsule of the joint.

The deep temporal and masseteric nerves supply the anterior portion of the joint. The auriculotemporal nerve, a branch of the mandibular portion (V3) of the trigeminal nerve, provides innervation of the TMJ.

ANATOMIC CORRELATION WITH FUNCTIONAL MOVEMENTS

Jaw jerk reflex : The jaw jerk reflex, analogous to the knee jerk reflex, is a stretch reflex that occurs by applying a downward tap on the chin. The tap produces a monosynaptic reflex contraction of the jaw closing muscles. This reflex is thought to relate to the fine control of jaw movements required to masticate different consistencies of food.

Jaw-opening reflex: Stimulating mechanoreceptors or nociceptors in the mouth triggers the jaw-opening reflex. The pathway is polysynaptic; the first synapse is in either the trigeminal sensory nuclei or the adjacent reticular formation and the final synapse is in the trigeminal motor nucleus. The reflex results in an inhibition of the activity of the jaw-closing muscles. This reflex is thought to help in preventing injury while biting or chewing objects.

Rest position: When the mandible is not functionally active, it adopts rest position in which the condyle occupies a relatively neutral position in the glenoid fossa with the teeth separated. The rest position is

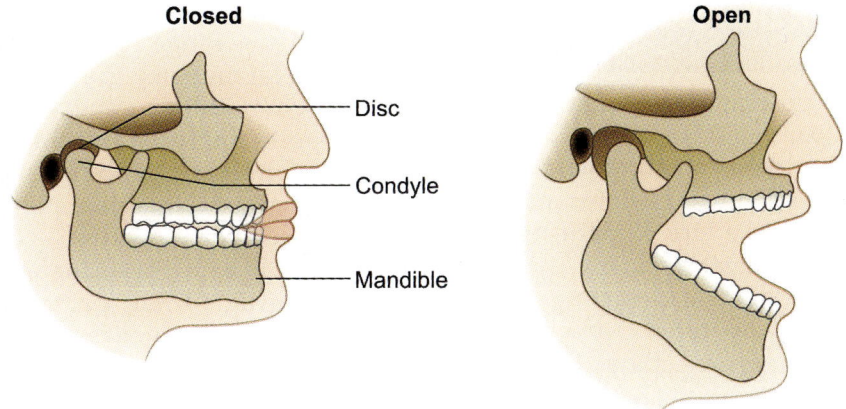

Fig. 11.4: Disc in close and open mouth position

considered to be associated with minimum muscular activity and with the articulating surfaces of the mandibular teeth a few millimeters from the occlusal contact position with the opposing teeth.

Mandibular range of motion: Mandibular motion during normal function is composed of rotation and translation of the condyles. During translation, the disc and condyle move downward and forward along the posterior slope of the articular eminence. The articular disc translates with the condyle, and simultaneously it rotates posteriorly as the condyle moves anteriorly; consequently, the movement of the disc across the fossa is limited to a range of 5–9 mm. The temporomandibular, sphenomandibular, and stylomandibular ligaments, together with the articular eminence, have been suggested as the main constraints of jaw opening.

CASE HISTORY TAKING FOR TMDs

Pain is subjective measure provided by the patient. It is measured in several ways like VAS using 10 cm line scale (left side of scale: No pain, right side: Worst pain). Other means of assessment of pain can be through pain diaries or pain diagram which can be drawn to locate and define the extent of pain.

Symptoms to be asked while examining the Patient

1. Do you feel dizziness or nausea?
2. Do you experience ringing in ears?
3. Any earache, headache, cheek pain?
4. Restricted mouth opening or deviation or does your jaw get lock or stuck often?
5. Do you experience any tingling or burning sensation, etc?
6. Do you experience any jaw misalignment or altered occlusion while opening or closing?
7. Check for mandibular movements: Lateral/protrusive.
8. Do you have any pain in the joint while clenching?

Physical Examination

1. Any facial asymmetry, swelling, mouth deviation while closing and opening mouth.
2. Range of mandibular movements: Any discomfort while opening or lateral and protrusive movements.
3. Palpate masticatory, TMJ, lymph nodes, neck muscles to rule out other causes.
4. Pain in the joint or muscle while clenching the teeth or chewing wax and sugarless gum.
5. Any parafunctional habits, tooth mobility, all the hard and soft tissues to be examined in particular.

EXAMINATION OF MUSCLES OF MASTICATION

The primary finding of masticatory muscle palpation is pain.

The TMD guidelines recommend to apply 1 lb pressure for joint and 2 lb for muscles.

Other things like site of pain, whether referred pain to distant site, etc. should be ruled out while taking case history.

A. **Temporalis:** Palpated in 3 areas:
   1. *Anterior region:* Palpated above zygomatic arch and anterior to TMJ
   2. *Middle region:* Palpated above the TMJ and superior to zygomatic arch
   3. *Posterior region:* Above and behind the ear
B. **Masseter:** Palpated bilaterally
   1. *Superior attachment:* The fingers are placed on each zygomatic arch and dropped down to the portion of the masseter attached to zygomatic arch.
   2. *Deep attachment:* Fingers dropped down from zygomatic arch .

Palpation of TMJ:
 a. Any pain or irregularities during condylar movements like crepitus or clicking?
 b. Any joint noises or pain?

Diagnostic imaging: TMJ imaging should be done when clinical presentations suggest pathological condition of TMJ. Any recent injury, sensory or motor abnormality, altered occlusion; degenerative changes are to be examined.

Usually examination of TMJ is carried by plain film radiography, tomography, arthrography, CT, MRI, single photon emission computed tomography and radioisotope scanning.

Other factors of TMD should also be considered like psychological factors, musculoskeletal problems, incidence of trauma, etc:

Dawson's criteria: Six ways to verify that the TMJs are healthy:
 1. Screening history
 2. Load test

3. **Range and path of movements:** Normal protrusive range 10–14 mm.
   × Lateral movement: 10 mm
   × Max. mouth opening: 40–60 mm
4. **Doppler analysis:** Intact healthy joint is quiet on rotation and translation
5. **Radiography/imaging:** Not necessary, if other tests are negative.
6. **Anterior bite plane for muscle deprogramming:** If flat, permissive anterior bite plane does not relieve pain, suspect intracapsular disorder.

MYOFACIAL PAIN DYSFUNCTION SYNDROME

The temporomandibular joints (TMJ) are complex joints that need to work in concert, essential for mastication, and probably the most used joints in the body.

The temporomandibular joint pain dysfunction syndrome (TMPD; myofascial pain dysfunction (MFD), facial arthromyalgia (FAM), mandibular dysfunction, or mandibular stress syndrome) refers to the common joint symptoms which together comprise the Laskin's criteria:
 1. Facial pain in the region of TMJ.
 2. Limitation or deviation in mandibular movements.
 3. Hyperalgesia of musculoskeletal structures.
 4. TMJ sounds during jaw function and movement.

Incidence: The prevalence is at least 12% of the general population, but these symptoms have been reported at some time by up to 88%—with as many as 25% reporting severe symptoms.

Age: This disorder afflicts young adults mainly, typically teenagers and up to 20–30 years of age.

Gender: Most of the patients are females compared to males.

Etiology: The etiology of the most common TMDs is unknown. The literature has been dominated by several hypothesized causes like occlusal disharmony, muscle hyperactivity, central pain mechanisms, psychological distress and trauma. Premature contacts such as faulty restorative dentistry are traditionally believed to initiate sleep bruxism.

Given the available evidence, the factors that have supporting evidence and at least some biological plausibility, from local to systemic causes are as follows:

The occlusal condition: It is an etiology of temporomandibular disorder, a contributing factor to TMD that has been strongly debated for many years is the occlusal condition. If occlusal factors are related to TMD, the dentist is responsible for providing proper therapy, since dentists are the only health care professionals trained to change the occlusion. On the other hand, if occlusal factors are not related to TMD, the dentist should refrain from treating TMD with occlusal changes.

Trauma: Road accidents, sports injuries, fights and dental treatment or extractions is common and can occasionally be followed by TMJ dysfunction. Trauma can result in muscle spasm or hyperactivity.

Muscle hyperactivity: Psychological stress can also cause muscle hyperactivity. 50–70% of patients (twice as common as controls) have experienced stressful life events in the 6 months before onset. These problems concerning work, money, health loss and interpersonal relationships probably have a causative role by inducing anxiety, which then produces increased jaw muscle activity.

Other risk factors for TMPDs are:
1. TMJ hypermobility
2. Parafunctional behaviors (e.g. sleep bruxism, tooth clenching, jaw guarding, lip or cheek biting)
3. Sleep disturbance
4. Comorbidity in the form of other rheumatic, musculoskeletal, or pain disorders
5. Emotional distress
6. Poor general health and an unhealthy lifestyle

Depression and shortage of sleep are also considered as important risk indicators.

Clinical Features

Symptoms are highly variable, but dysfunction is usually unilateral and characterized by one or more of the following features:
1. **Recurrent clicking in the TMJ:** Clicking occurs either on attempted mouth opening or closing. Often the click allows the completion of that phase of mandibular movement. Clicks are not diagnostic, since they are common in normal TM joints. A grating noise (crepitus) may signify intra-articular arthritic change, there may be crepitus at any point of jaw movement, especially with lateral movements.
2. **Jaw locking or limitation of movement:** Limitation of opening may be intermittent, with jaw 'locking'. There may be deviation of the jaw to the affected side on attempted opening with variable jaw deviation or locking. If there is reduced mouth opening, this often suggests bilateral disease. Limitation may be more obvious on awakening, especially after nocturnal grinding. In some the limitation increases throughout the day.
3. **Pain in the joint and/or surrounding muscles and elsewhere ipsilaterally:** The main site is usually preauricular, but can radiate to back of the mouth, down the neck, up to the temple or behind the ear.

Pain may occur at an early stage or sometimes after the onset of clicking or stiffness of the jaw. It may range from a vague dull ache to an acute pain. The symptoms of individuals who clench or grind during working hours tend to worsen towards evening, and sometimes have a psychogenic basis.

The pain may be aggravated by chewing or other jaw movements. Muscles like masseter, temporalis and pterygoid muscles may be tender to palpation. Sometimes pain is more clearly sited in a single jaw muscle, and sometimes trigger points can be located. Some patients may also complain of headaches, neck aches, and lower back pain

Flowchart 11.2

Treatment of myofacial pain

⬇

Patient education explanation and reassurance about diagnosis

⬇

Self care—eliminating oral habits like clenching, jaw exercises

⬇

Physical therapy—education regarding biomechanics of jaw, neck and head posture

⬇

Passive modalities like heat and cold therapy, ultrasound, laser and TENS

⬇

Intraoral appliances—such that it covers all the teeth on the arch the appliance is seated on

⬇

Pharmacotherapy—NSAIDs, muscle relaxants and tricyclic anti-depressants

⬇

Behavioral/relaxation techniques—relaxation, hypnosis, biofeedback cognitive-behavioural therapy

Flowchart 11.3

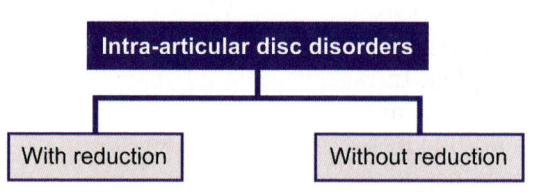

Etiological factors of disc displacements

1. Chronic low grade microtrauma from long-term bruxism or clenching of teeth
2. Generalized laxity of joints
3. Craniofacial morphological alterations
4. Indirect trauma from cervical flexion extension injuries
5. Chronic loading of joint increases suscepti-bility of certain individuals to restraining of ligaments and displacement of disc
6. Pain is severe when it is accompanied by capsulitis and synovitis

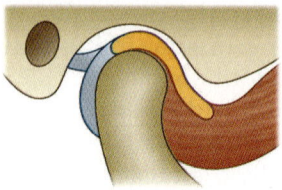
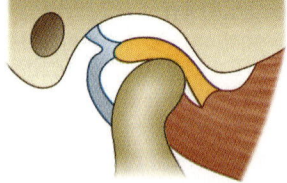
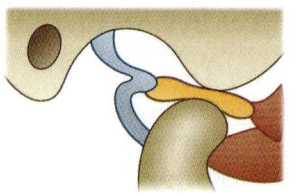

A   **Normal relationship between condyle and disc: They move together**

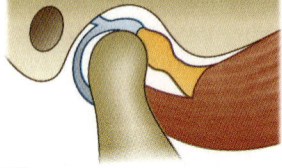
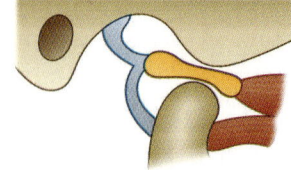
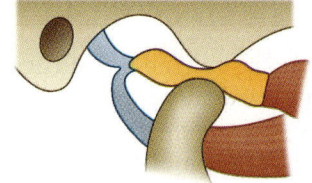

B   **Disc displacement with reduction**

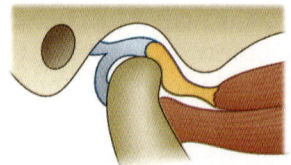
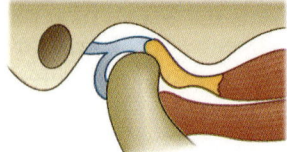
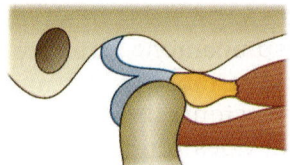

C   **Anterior disc displacement without reduction: No translatory movement**

Fig. 11.5: Disc displacement with and without reduction

1. Disc Displacement with Reduction

Clinical features: An intracapsular biomechanical disorder involving the condyle—disc complex. In the closed mouth position, the disc is in anterior position relative to the condylar head, and the disc reduces upon opening of the mouth. Medial and lateral displacement of the disc may also be present. Clicking, popping or snapping noises may occur with disc reduction. A history of prior locking in the closed position coupled with interference in mastication precludes this diagnosis.

2. Disc Displacement With Reduction With Intermittent Locking

Clinical features: An intracapsular biomechanical disorder involving the condyle—disc complex. In the closed mouth position, the disc is in an anterior position relative to the condylar head, and the disc intermittently reduces with opening of the mouth. When the disc does not reduce with opening of the mouth, intermittent limited mandibular opening occurs. When limited opening occurs, a maneuver may be needed to unlock the TMJ. Medial and lateral displacement of the disc may also be present.

Clicking, popping, or snapping noises may occur with disc reduction.

3. Disc Displacement Without Reduction With Limited Opening

An intracapsular biomechanical disorder involving the condyle-disc complex. In the closed mouth position, the disc is in an anterior position relative to the condylar head, and the disc does not reduce with opening of the mouth. Medial and lateral displacement of the disc may also be present. This disorder is associated with persistent limited mandibular opening that does not resolve with the clinician or patient performing a specific manipulative maneuver. This is also referred to as **"closed lock."**

Clinical Features

1. Jaw lock or catch so that the mouth would not open all the way; and
2. Limitation in jaw opening which is severe enough to limit jaw opening and it also interferes with ability of eating.

Maximum assisted opening (passive stretch) <40 mm including vertical incisal overlap.

4. Disc Displacement without Reduction without Limited Opening

An intracapsular biomechanical disorder involving the condyle–disc complex. In the closed mouth position, the disc is in an anterior position relative to the condylar head and the disc does not reduce with opening of the mouth. Medial and lateral displacement of the disc may also be present. This disorder is not associated with limited mandibular opening.

Clinical features: Same as specified for disc displacement without reduction with limited opening.

Maximum assisted opening (passive stretch) >40 mm including vertical incisal overlap.

5. Subluxation

It is a hypermobility disorder involving the disc-condyle complex and the articular eminence.

In the open mouth position, the disc–condyle complex is positioned anterior to the articular eminence and is unable to return to a normal closed mouth position without a specific manipulative maneuver. The duration of dislocation may be momentary or prolonged. When prolonged, the patient may need the assistance of the clinician to reduce the dislocation and normalize jaw movement; this is referred to as "Open lock".

Clinical Features

1. In the last 30 days, a jaw locking or catching in a wide open mouth position,

	Closed mouth position	Open mouth position
Normal		
Disc displacement with reduction		
Disc displacement without reduction		

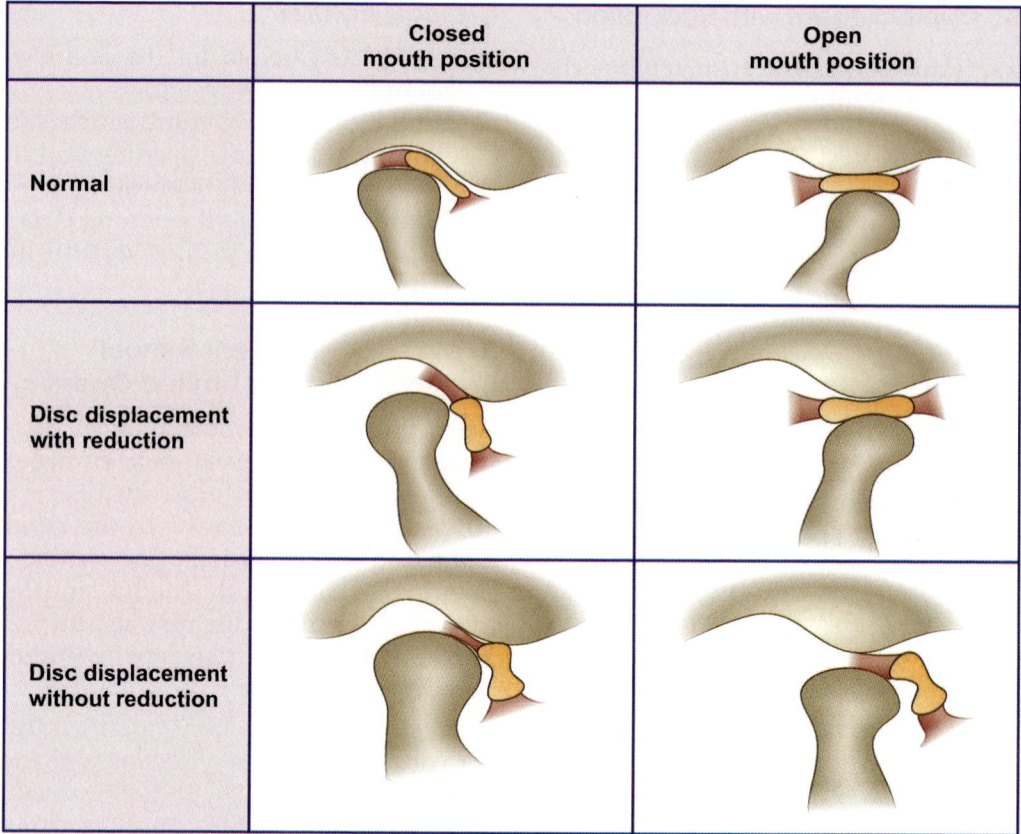

Fig. 11.6: Disc derangements in closed and open mouth position

even for a moment, so that the mouth cannot be closed from the wide open position.

2. Inability to close the mouth without a specific manipulative maneuver.

Although no findings are required, when this disorder is present clinically, examination is positive for inability to return to a normal closed mouth position without the patient performing a specific manipulative maneuver.

6. Dislocation

In dislocation of the mandible, the condyle is positioned anterior to the articular eminence and cannot return to its normal position without assistance. This disorder contrasts with subluxation, in which the condyle moves anterior to the eminence during wide opening but it is able to return to the resting position without manipulation. It has been demonstrated that subluxation is a variation of normal function and that the normal ROM of the condyle is not limited to the fossa.

1. Dislocations of the mandible usually result from muscular incoordination in wide opening during eating or yawning and less commonly from trauma;
2. They may be unilateral or bilateral.
3. The typical complaints of the patient with dislocation are an inability to close the jaws and pain related to muscle spasm.
4. On clinical examination, a deep depression may be observed in the preauricular region corresponding to the condyle being positioned anterior to the eminence.
5. The condyle can usually be repositioned without the use of muscle relaxants or general anesthetics. If muscle spasms are

severe and reduction is difficult, the use of intravenous diazepam (approximately 10 mg) can be beneficial.

Treatment: The practitioner who is repositioning the mandible should stand in front of the seated patient and place his or her thumbs lateral to the mandibular molars on the buccal shelf of bone; the remaining fingers of each hand should be placed under the chin.

The condyle is repositioned by a downward and backward movement. This is achieved by simultaneously pressing down on the posterior part of the mandible while raising the chin. As the condyle reaches the height of the eminence, it can usually be guided posteriorly to its normal position.

POSTREDUCTION RECOMMENDATIONS

1. Consist of limiting mandibular movement and the use of NSAIDs to lessen inflammation.
2. The patient should be cautioned not to open wide when eating or yawning because recurrence is common, especially during the period initially after repositioning.
3. Chronic recurring dislocations have been treated with surgical and nonsurgical approaches.
4. Injections of sclerosing solutions have been used but they are not used as often now because of difficulty in controlling the extent of fibrosis and condylar limitation.
5. Various surgical procedures have been advocated for treating recurrent dislocations of the mandible; these include bone grafting to the eminence, lateral pterygoid myotomy, eminence reduction, eminence augmentation with implants, shortening the temporalis tendon by intraoral scarification, plication of the joint capsule, and repositioning of the zygomatic arch.

Treatment of Disc Displacements and Disorders

1. Anterior positioning appliances
2. NSAIDs
3. Application of moist heat or ice depending on symptoms

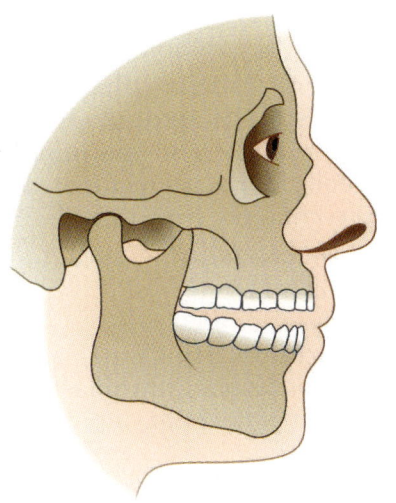 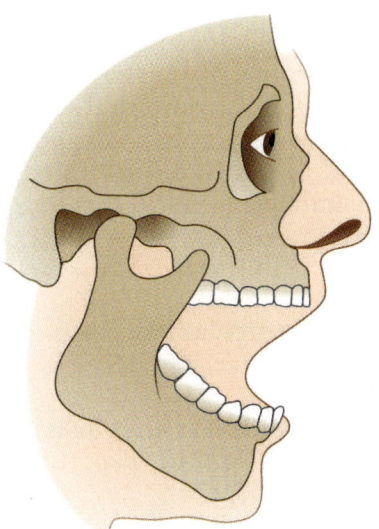

Fig. 11.7: TMJ dislocation

4. Physiotherapy
5. Surgical procedures
6. Prosthesis
7. Orthodontics for facial deformity
8. Soft diet during acute exacerbation

Fractures

Fractures of the condylar head and neck often result from a blow to the chin. The patient with a condylar fracture usually presents with pain and edema over the joint area and limitation and deviation of the mandible to the injured side on opening.

Bilateral condylar fractures may result in an anterior open bite. The diagnosis of a condylar fracture is confirmed by diagnostic imaging. Intracapsular nondisplaced fractures of the condylar head are usually not treated surgically. Early mobilization of the mandible is emphasized to prevent bony or fibrous ankylosis.

Ankylosis

Ankylosis can be defined as *a pathological fusion between two articulating surfaces.* TMJ ankylosis involves fusion between condylar head and temporal bone. Trauma to the chin is the most common cause of TMJ ankylosis, although infections also may be involved. Children are more prone to ankylosis because of greater osteogenic potential and an incompletely formed disc. Ankylosis frequently results from prolonged immobilization following condylar fracture.

Classification

A. **True or intra-articular ankylosis**
   × Fibrous
   × Bony
B. **False or extra-articular ankylosis**
   × Fusion of coronoid process with zygomatic arch
   × OSMF
   × Muscle fibrosis
   × Myositis ossificans

Clinical Features

Mouth opening is gradually decreased, limited mandibular movement, deviation of the chin to the affected side, fullness of the face on the affected side are some of the common clinical features seen in TMJ ankylosis. The inability to open the mouth may also lead to poor oral hygiene. Characteristic *bird face deformity* is seen in cases of bilateral ankylosis.

Radiographic Features

× **Fibrous ankylosis**
   ▪ The articulating surfaces are usually irregular due to erosions.
   ▪ The joint space is usually very narrow and the two irregular surfaces may appear to fit into one another like jigsaw puzzle.
× **Bony ankylosis**
   ▪ The joint space may be completely or partially obliterated by the osseous bridge.
   ▪ Secondary degenerative changes of the joint components are common.
   ▪ Compensatory elongation of the coronoid processes is seen.
   ▪ Deepening of the antegonial notch in the mandibular ramus of the affected side as a result of muscle function during attempted mandibular opening.

Treatment: Ankylosis has been treated by several surgical procedures. Gap arthroplasty using interpositional materials between the cut segments is the technique most commonly performed.

Treatment modalities
× Brisement force
× Condylectomy
× Gap arthroplasty
× Interpositional arthroplasty with reconstruction of the joint

Sleep Bruxism

Sleep bruxism is thought to aggravate or contribute to the persistence of pain symptoms associated with TMD.

1. The etiology is not understood, but the evidence suggests that occlusal abnormalities are not the cause. Occlusal appliances may protect the teeth from the effects of bruxism but cannot be expected to prevent or decrease the bruxism activity.
2. When bruxism is considered to be the cause or a factor of TMD symptoms, oral appliance therapy is effective.
3. Symptoms of bruxing is resolved when the dosage is decreased or when buspirone is added. Buspirone has a postsynaptic dopaminergic effect and may act to partially restore suppressed dopamine levels associated with the use of SSRIs.
4. Severe bruxers in the masseter muscles with botulinum toxin in an open-label prospective trial have reported significant improvement in symptoms and minimal adverse effects. Botulinum toxin exerts a paralytic effect on the muscle by inhibiting the release of acetylcholine at the neuromuscular junction.

TEMPOROMANDIBULAR JOINT ARTHRITIS OSTEOARTHRITIS (DEGENERATIVE JOINT DISEASE)

Degenerative Joint Disease (DJD) also referred to as osteoarthrosis, osteoarthritis, and degenerative arthritis. It is primarily a disorder of articular cartilage and subchondral bone, with secondary inflammation of the synovial membrane.

1. It is a localized joint disease without systemic manifestations. The process begins in loaded articular cartilage that thins, clefts (fibrillation), and then fragments leading to sclerosis of underlying bone, subchondral cysts, and osteophyte formation.
2. The articular changes are essentially a response of the joint to chronic microtrauma or pressure. Microtrauma may be in the form of continuous abrasion of the articular surfaces as in natural wear associated with age or due to increased loading possibly related to chronic parafunctional activity.

Etiology: DJD may be categorized as primary or secondary.

Etiology of degenerative joint diseases
- Primary DJD is of unknown origin, but genetic factors play an important role.
- Secondary DJD results from a known underlying cause, such as trauma, congenital dysplasia or metabolic disease.
- The possibility that a diet of excessively hard or chewy foods might cause increased loads on the joints and lead to degenerative changes.
- Psychological stress leading to parafunctional activities such as tooth clenching or bruxing has been proposed as one of the factors.
- Biologic, biochemical, and hormonal changes that might contribute to changes in the joints, leading to osteoarthritis.

Pathogenesis: The present model suggests that excessive mechanical loading on the joints produces a cascade of events leading to the failure of the lubrication system and destruction of the articular surfaces. These events include the generation of free radicals, the release of proinflammatory neuropeptides, signaling by cytokines, and the activation of enzymes capable of matrix degradation.

Clinical manifestations: DJD of the TMJ begins early and has been observed in over 20% of joints in individuals older than 20 years.

1. The incidence of degenerative changes increases with age.
2. Many patients with mild to moderate DJD of the TMJ have no symptoms, although arthritic changes are observed on radiographs.
3. Degenerative changes of the TMJ detected on radiographic examination may be incidental and may not be responsible for facial pain symptoms or TMJ dysfunction; however, some degenerative changes may be underdiagnosed by conventional

radiography because the defects are confined to the articular soft tissue. These soft tissue changes are better visualized with MR.

4. Patients with symptomatic DJD of the TMJ experience pain directly over the affected condyle, limitation of mandibular opening, crepitus, and a feeling of stiffness after a period of inactivity. Examination reveals tenderness and crepitus on intra-auricular and pre-auricular palpation. Deviation of the mandible to the painful side may be present.

5. Radiographic signs of DJD include signs of previous remodeling, such as flattening and subchondral sclerosis or degenerative changes can be observed.

   × DJD may have a spectrum of appearance ranging from substantial subchondral sclerosis and osteophyte formation (proliferative component) to extensive erosions (degenerative component).
   × The osteophytes may break and lie free within the joint space (joint mice).
   × In maximal intercuspation position, the joint space may appear narrow or absent, which correlates with internal derangement. Perforation of the disk or posterior attachment, resulting in bone to bone contact of the joint components is common.
   × The enlargement of the fossa and reduced size of the condylar head allows the latter to move forward and superiorly into an abnormal anterior position that may result in an anterior open bite.
   × Sometimes small, round radiolucent areas with irregular margins surrounded by a varying increased density are visible deep to the articulating surfaces, these are called Ely's cysts.

Rheumatoid Arthritis (RA)

RA is an inflammatory disease primarily affecting periarticular tissue and secondarily bone. The percentage of RA patients with TMJ involvement ranges from 40% to 80%, depending on the group studied and the imaging technique used.

The disease process starts as a vasculitis of the synovial membrane. It progresses to chronic inflammation marked by an intense round cell infiltrate and subsequent formation of granulation tissue. The cellular infiltrate spreads from the articular surfaces eventually to cause an erosion of the underlying bone.

Clinical manifestations: The TMJs in RA are usually involved bilaterally.

Pain is usually associated with the early acute phase of the disease. Other symptoms often noted include morning stiffness, joint sounds, tenderness and swelling over the joint area.

The symptoms are usually transient in nature, the most consistent clinical findings include pain on joint palpation, limited mouth opening, and crepitus, micrognathia.

Radiographic changes
× The initial changes are seen as generalized osteopenia (decreased density) of the condyle and the temporal component.
× Diminished joint space due to destruction of the disk by the pannus.
× The pannus also causes bone erosions of the articular eminence and the anterior aspect of the condylar head, which permits antero-superior positioning of the condyle when the teeth are in maximal intercuspation, this results in an anterior open bite.

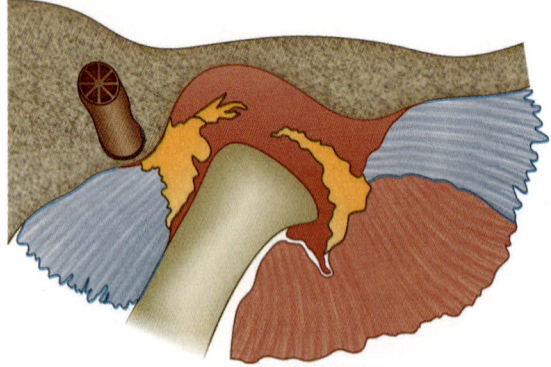

Fig. 11.8: Degenerative lesions in TMJ with disc perforation

* There is a little evidence of marginal proliferation in RA in contrast to the radiographic changes often observed in DJD.
* High resolution CT of the TMJs in RA patients shows erosions of the condyle and glenoid fossa that are not detected on conventional radiography.
* There may be sharpened pencil appearance of the condylar head due to erosion of the anterior and posterior condylar surfaces at the attachment of the synovial lining.

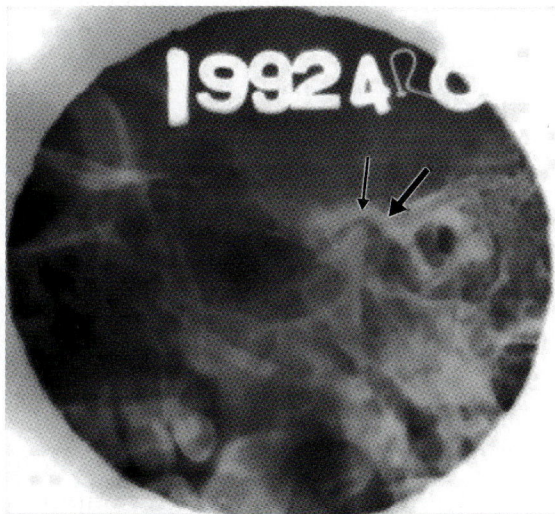

Fig. 11.9: Erosion of condylar surfaces

Connective Tissue Disease

Connective tissue diseases that affect the TMJ include systemic lupus, systemic sclerosis (scleroderma), undifferentiated connective tissue disease and mixed connective tissue disease. When the TMJ is involved, the clinical presentation is similar to other disorders causing inflammation and subsequent degenerative changes.

Clinical Features

A clinical examination supplemented with diagnostic imaging is usually adequate to confirm involvement of the TMJ.
1. Diseases associated with crystal deposits in joints; Gout is a disease that includes hyperuricemia, recurrent arthritides, renal disease and urolithiaisis, effecting men.
2. Acute pain in a single joint is the characteristic clinical presentation. The TMJ is not commonly involved. Calcium pyrophosphate deposition is also known as pseudogout. Deposits of microcrystals in affected joints are responsible for the clinical manifestations.
3. Examination of aspirated synovial fluid from the involved joint by polarized light and detection of monosodium urate crystals confirm the diagnosis.

Treatment: It includes colchicine, NSAIDs, and intra-articular steroid injection. Pseudogout affecting the TMJ has been treated with colchicine and arthrocentesis. Treatment is directed toward the systemic disease with supportive local therapy consisting of jaw self-care, physiotherapy, oral appliance therapy, topical NSAID, and intra-articular corticosteroid injection.

Nonsurgical management may consist of jaw self-management, including behavior modification, heat application, soft diet, physical therapy including jaw exercises, NSAID, and oral appliance therapy.

Arthroscopy, arthroplasty, and arthrotomy are surgical procedures that may be indicated depending on the response to more conservative treatment and the severity of pain and disability. Surgical treatment of the joints, including placement of prosthetic joints is indicated in patients who have severe functional impairment or intractable pain not successfully managed by other means. Orthognathic surgery and orthodontics are required for correction of facial deformity resulting from arthritis during growth.

ARTHROSCOPY

Seronegative Spondyloarthropathies

Several arthropathies that are distinct from RA are not associated with positive serology (rheumatoid factor).

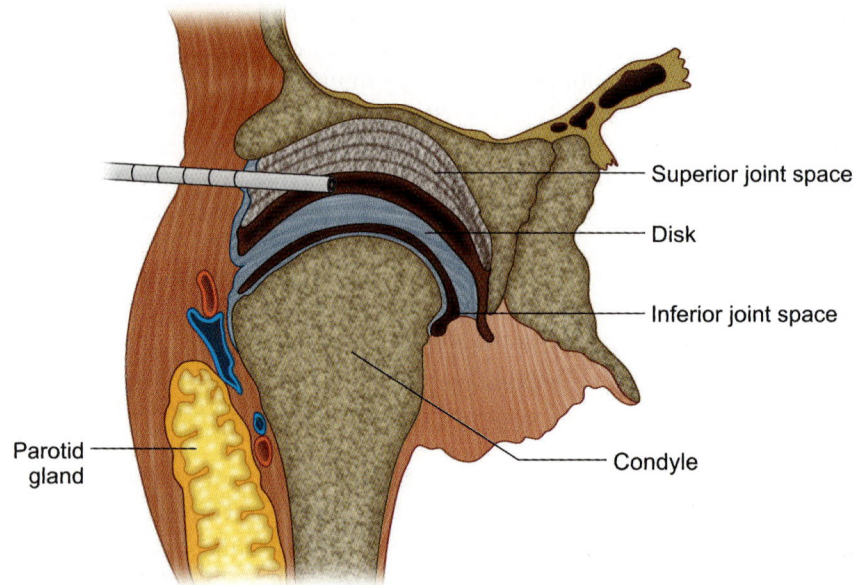

Fig. 11.10: Seronegative spondyloarthropathies

These disorders, characterized by arthritis, are known as the seronegatives spondyloarthropathies and include ankylosing spondylitis (AS), psoriatic arthritis (PA), and Reiter's syndrome. The TMJs can be involved in these arthropathies.

Clinical Features

The clinical manifestations are joint pain with function, limited mouth opening, and erosion of the superior surface of the condyle on radiography. There are no specific findings that are pathognomonic of involvement of the TMJs. It causes inflammation that can lead to new bone formation, causing the spine to fuse, reducing mobility, and producing a forward, stooped posture. The disease usually involves the sacroiliac joints where the spine joins the pelvis.

1. PA is a chronic disease characterized by psoriasis and inflammation of the joints. Approximately 10% of patients who have psoriasis develop joint inflammation. The skin lesions may precede the joint involvement by several years. PA commonly involves the fingers and spine, pitting of the nails is common. The cause is unknown, and the disease presents in a variety of forms.

2. Reiter's syndrome includes polyarthritis, urethritis, and conjunctivitis. It is thought to be triggered by infection, but the arthritis is not septic. It occurs more frequently in males in the third decade. The syndrome usually follows venereal infection most often involving Chlamydia, Mycoplasma, or Yersinia. Approximately 25% of male patients with Reiter's syndrome reported recurrent pain, swelling, and/or stiffness of the TMJ.

Synovial Chondromatosis (SC)

It is an uncommon benign disorder characterized by the presence of multiple cartilaginous nodules of the synovial membrane that break off resulting in clusters of free floating loose calcified bodies in the joint.

It is theorized that SC originates from embryonic mesenchymal remnants of the subintimal layer of the synovium that becomes metaplastic, calcify, and break off into the joint space; most commonly involves one joint, but cases of multiarticular SC have been reported.

Clinical Features

It includes slow progressive swelling in the preauricular region, pain and limitations of mandibular movement which are the most common presenting features. TMJ clicking, locking, crepitus and occlusal changes may also be present.

Radiographic features: Conventional radiography may not lead to the diagnosis due to superimposition of cranial bones that may obscure the calcified loose bodies.

Diagnosis: In a CT scan the lesion may appear as a single mass or as many small loose bodies. Arthroscopy may be necessary for accurate diagnosis, particularly when the loose bodies are not calcified and cannot be visualized by conventional radiology or CT.

Treatment: It should be conservative and consists of removal of the mass of loose bodies. This may be done arthroscopically when only a small lesion is present, but arthrotomy is required for larger lesions.

Septic Arthritis

Septic arthritis of the TMJ most commonly occurs in patients with previously existing joint disease such as RA or underlying medical disorders (particularly diabetes). Patients receiving immunosuppressive drugs or long-term corticosteroids also have increased incidence of septic arthritis. The infection of the TMJ may result from blood-borne bacterial infection or by extension of infection from adjacent sites such as the middle ear, maxillary molars and parotid gland. *Gonococci* are the primary blood-borne agents causing septic arthritis in a previously normal TMJ, whereas *Staphylococcus aureus* is the most common organism involved in previously diagnosed arthritic joints.

Clinical Features

Symptoms of septic arthritis of the TMJ include trismus, deviation of the mandible to the affected side, severe pain on movement, and inability to occlude the teeth, owing to the presence of inflammation in the joint space. Signs and symptoms of gonorrhea such as purulent urethral discharge or dysuria. The affected TMJ should be aspirated and the fluid obtained must be tested by Gram's stain and cultured for *Neisseria gonorrhoeae*.

Treatment of septic arthritis of the TMJ consists of surgical drainage, joint irrigation, and four to six weeks of antibiotics.

Oral Dyskinesia and Dystonia

Oral dyskinesias are abnormal, involuntary movements of the tongue, lips, and jaw.

Etiology: Oral dyskinesias may be a factor contributing to muscle stiffness, TMJ degenerative changes, mucosal lesions, damage to teeth and dental prostheses. Complete loss of teeth is considered to be one cause of oral dyskinesia. Ill-fitting dentures or the lack of replacements may initiate dyskinesia.

Clinical Features

Dyskinesias are characterized clinically by the observation of involuntary mouth movements and the effects of these movements on the jaw muscles, TMJs, oral mucosa, and teeth.

Emphasis on management is prevention because none of the treatment is predictably effective and safe.

A dentist observing dyskinesia in a patient taking conventional antipsychotics should inform the physician managing the medication. Palliative treatment using tetrabenazine, a central monoamine depleter, clonazepam, and baclofen has been tried.

Oromandibular dystonia produces involuntary and excessive contractions of tongue, lip, and jaw muscles. The etiology and pathophysiology are unknown.

The proposed mechanism is related to defective inhibitory control of the basal ganglia of the forebrain, thalamus and brainstem. Injection of botulinum toxin has been used in cases of oromandibular dystonia.

Radiographic Features of TMJ Disorders

1. Condylar Hyperplasia

* The condyle may appear relatively normal but symmetrically enlarged.
* Sometimes an altered shape: Conical, spherical, elongated, lobulated or irregular in outline.
* There may be an elongation of the condylar head and neck with a compensating forward bend, forming an inverted L.
* The cortical thickness and trabecular pattern of the enlarged condyle is normal.

* The affected ramus may have an increased vertical height and may be thicker in the anteroposterior dimension. This prevents the occlusion of the posterior teeth.

2. Condylar Hypoplasia

The condyle appears normal, slightly diminished in size and the mandibular fossa is also proportionately smaller.

The condylar neck and coronoid process are very slender and in some cases shortened or elongated.

* The posterior portion of the ramus and condylar neck may have a dorsal (posterior) inclination.
* The ramus and the mandibular body on the affected side may also be small,

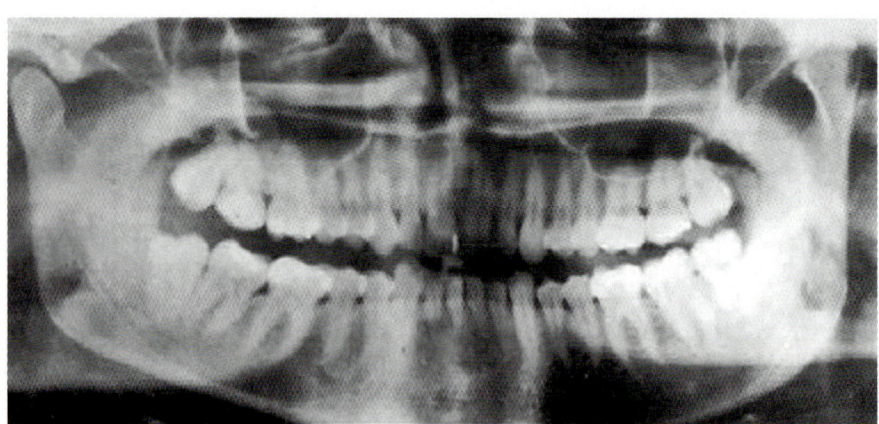

Fig. 11.11: Condylar hyperplasia

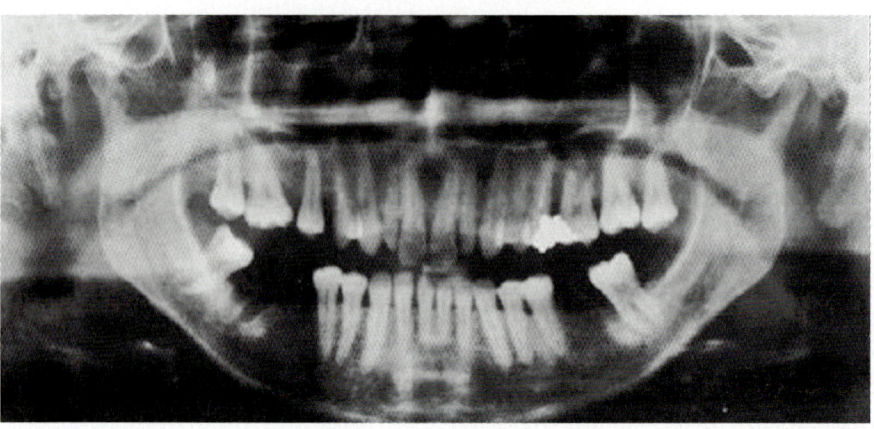

Fig. 11.12: Condylar hypoplasia

resulting in a mandibular asymmetry and dental crowding.The antegonial notch is deepened.

3. Agenesis of the Condyle

Absence of the condyle: The condyle is not seen.

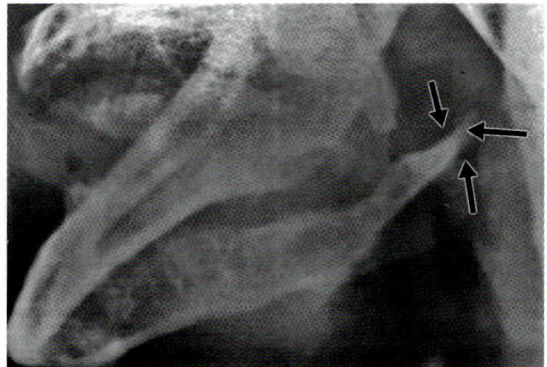

Fig. 11.13: Condylar hypoplasia

4. Juvenile Arthrosis

The condylar head has a typical toad stool appearance, with marked flattening and apparent elongation of the articulating condylar surface and dorsal (posterior) inclination of the condyle and neck.

5. Coronoid Hyperplasia

This is best seen on the panoramic, Water's and lateral tomographic views and CT scan.The coronoid appears elongated and may have a large but normal shape or may curve anteriorly and may appear very radio-opaque.

6. Remodeling and Arthritic Conditions

The radiographic appearance may include one or a combination of the following:
× Flattening
× Cortical thickening of articulating surfaces
× Subchondral sclerosis

TMJ Radiography

The diagnosis and management of temporo-mandibular disorders (TMD) require both clinical and imaging examinations of the temporomandibular joint (TMJ). A variety of modalities can be used to image the TMJ.

Because of the anatomic complexity of the TMJ imaging can be difficult. Choosing the proper imaging technique is essential. Conventional radiography nowadays is of limited interest. The use of flat plane films for TMJ pathology is not sufficient, because this joint requires three-dimensional imaging views.

Temporomandibular joint is bounded laterally by zygomatic arch and medially by petrous ridge of temporal bone. In TMJ radiography, we should be able to identify:
× The external auditory meatus of the ear.
× Articular eminence.
× Articular fossa.
× The neck of condyle.
× Mandibular condyle.

The articular disk (soft tissue) appears radiolucent so it needs specialized imaging techniques.

Radiography for TMJ can be classified into:
A. **Non-invasive radiography**
   1. Conventional radiography
     a. Orthopantomogram and sectional view
     b. Transcranial radiography
     c. Transpharyngeal radiography
     d. Transorbital radiography
   2. Specialized radiography
     a. Computed tomography
     b. Magnetic resonance imaging
     c. Cone beam computed tomography
     d. Ultrasonography
B. **Invasive radiography**
   1. Arthrography

Conventional Radiography

Conventional radiographs have a limited role in evaluation of the TMJ. The shortcomings are:
a. They can be used to evaluate only the bony elements of the TMJ.
b. They also do not give useful information concerning joint effusions, which are

commonly associated with pain and disc displacements.

c. Another disadvantage concerning conventional radiographs is the problem of superimposition of adjacent structures.

❖ Orthopantomogram

It permits visualization of both the joints in one film and can be used to assess only lateral part of condyle.

Sectional view of TMJ helps to visualize condyles laterally. This view is best utilized in cases of hypermobility as it shows position of condyles in relation to fossae in open and closed mouth position. In case of hypermobility, condyle moves beyond articular eminence in open mouth position.

❖ Trans Pharyngeal View
(Infracranial/McQueen Dell)

Indications
× Osteoarthritis and rheumatoid arthritis, cysts and tumors
× Cyst and tumor
× Fracture of neck and condyle

Area of joint seen

Lateral view: Condylar head and neck articular surface

Film placement: Patient holds the cassette flat against patient's ear centered over TM joint of interest against facial skin parallel to sagittal plane / 2 inch anterior to EAM.

Position of patient: Occlusal plane parallel to transverse axis of film—soft parts are in a line with nasopharynx and joint.
× Patient instructed to inhale slowly through nose
× Open mouth—condyles move away from base of skull and mandibular notch is enlarged on opposite side.
× Central ray—directed from opposite side cranially at angle (–5 to –10 degrees)
× Beneath the zygomatic arch, through sigmoid notch posteriorly across pharynx at the condyle.

❖ Transorbital View (Zimmer)

Indication
× Trauma
× Fracture cases

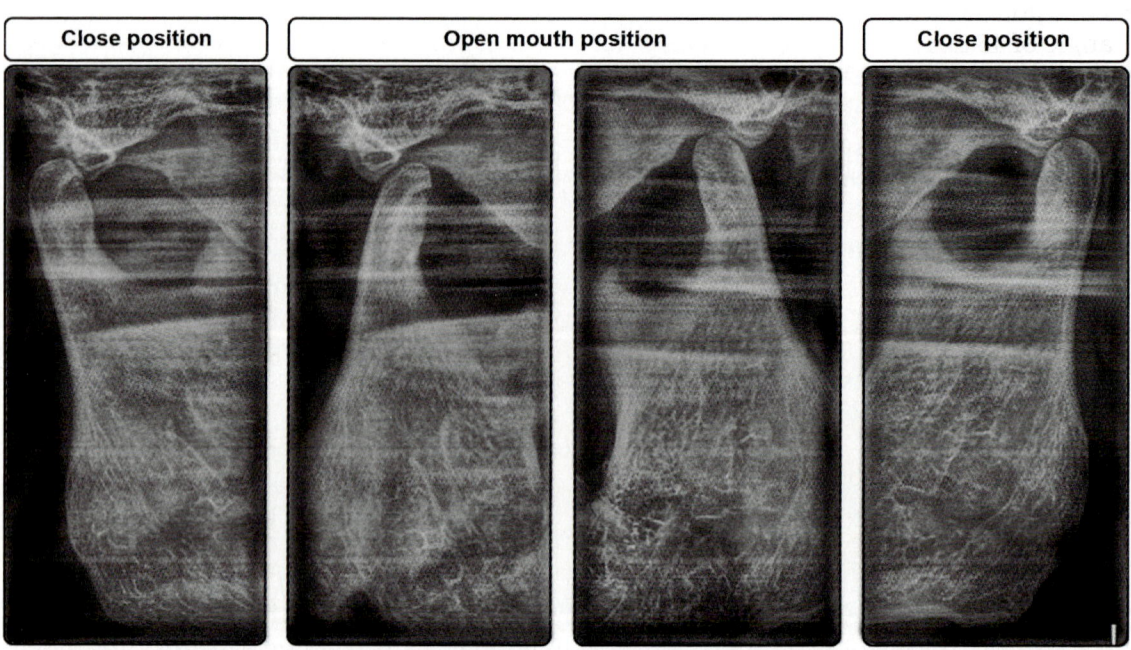

| Close position | Open mouth position | Close position |

Fig. 11.14: Sectional view showing open and closed joint positions in a single tomogram

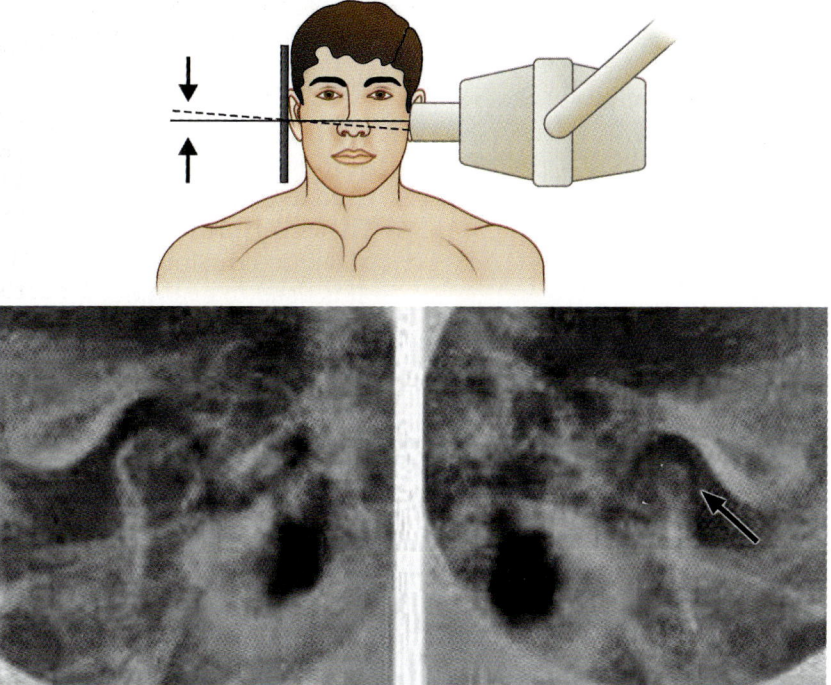

Fig. 11.15: Transpharyngeal view showing medial pole of condyle

Area of joint seen

× Anterior view of TMJ

× Mediolateral displacement of condyle

× **Film position:** Behind patients head at an angle of 45 degree to sagittal plane

× **Position of patient:** Sagittal plane vertical canthomeatal line should be 10 degree to the horizontal with head tipped downwards

× **Central ray—tube head—front of patient's** face directed to joint of interest at an angle of +20 degrees to strike cassette at right angles

Point of entry may be taken as pupil of the indicated side eye by asking patient to look straight ahead.

Disadvantage: If the patient cannot open wide, areas of the joint articulating surfaces will be obscured because of mutual superimposition (Fig. 11.16).

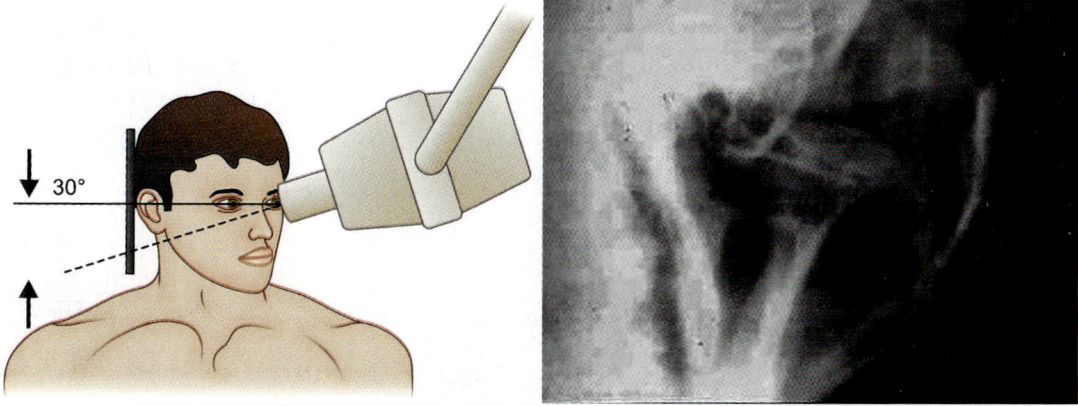

Fig. 11.16: Transorbital view showing mediolateral positioning of condyle

◈ Transcranial View

Indication
1. TMJ dysfunction syndrome
2. Internal derangement

Area of joint seen
1. Lateral aspect of glenoid fossa
2. Articular eminence
3. Joint space
4. Condylar head

Film position: Flat against patient's ear; against facial skin parallel to sagittal plane.

Patient position: Head is adjusted such that sagittal plane is vertical to the floor and ala-tragus line is parallel to the floor.

Central ray 0.5 inch behind and 2 inch above auditory meatus. It should be directed posteriorly so that it passes along the long axis of condyle. This is postauricular/Lindblom technique.

Grewcock approach: Central ray passes through a point 2 inches above external auditory meatus.

Gill's approach: 0.5 inch anterior and 2 inches above external auditory meatus.

Central ray aimed downwards at 25° to the horizontal, across the cranium, centering through the area of interest.

Disadvantages
1. Superimposition of ipsilateral petrous ridge over the condylar neck.

SPECIALIZED RADIOGRAPHY

Ultrasound
- Ultrasound is a less expensive and easily performed imaging modality that can be used to evaluate the TMJ.
- This is simple way to look for the presence of a joint effusion.
  It is used to evaluate:
  1. Cartilage and disk.
  2. It is used for image-guided injections for both diagnostic and therapeutic purposes.

Computed Tomography and Cone Beam Computed Tomography (CBCT)

It is considered to be the best method for assessing osseous pathologic conditions of TMJ. It allows a multi-planar reconstruction (sagittal, axial, coronal) of TMJ structures, obtaining 3D images in closed and opened-mouth positions.

Magnetic Resonance Imaging

MRI is currently considered the reference method for imaging the soft tissue structures of the TMJ (articular disc, synovial membrane, muscles). It has been pointed out as the best imaging modality in diagnosing disc displacements.

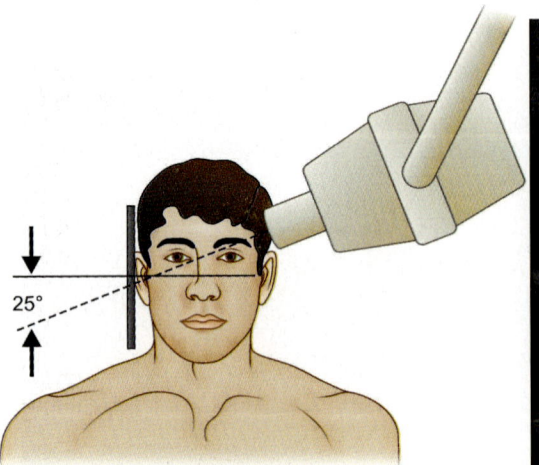

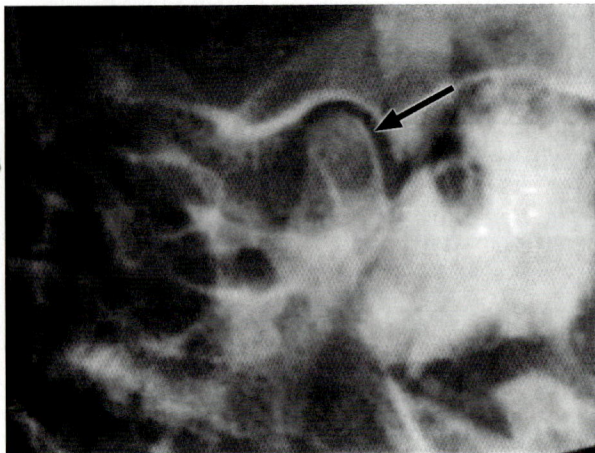

Fig. 11.17: Transcranial view showing lateral pole of condyle

MRI can detect the early signs of TMJ dysfunction, like thickening of anterior or posterior band, rupture of retrodiscal tissue, changes in shape of the disc and joint effusion.

Invasive Radiography

Arthrography is an invasive imaging technique to evaluate the TMJ. This imaging modality requires injection of radiopaque contrast into the TMJ under fluoroscopic guidance. Once the contrast is injected, the joint can be evaluated for adhesions, disk dysfunction, as well as disk perforation based on how contrast flows in the joint. This modality is rarely used today because MRI can be used to evaluate the TMJ without being invasive, exposing the patient to a possibility of allergic reaction from the contrast, possibility of infection.

Treatment Modalities for TMJ Disorders

Instructions to Patients for Self-Care as Part of Initial Therapy

1. Be aware and control oral parafunctional behaviors.
2. Teeth should only contact during chewing and swallowing.
3. Monitor jaw at regular intervals through the day for any clenching, grinding, touching, or tapping of teeth or any tensing or rigid holding of the jaw muscles.
4. Monitor jaw for parafunctional behaviors during specific situations such as while driving, studying, using computer, reading, engaging in athletic activities, when at work, or in social situations, and when experiencing overwork, fatigue, or stress.
5. Practice neutral jaw posture: Place the tip of the tongue behind the top teeth or in the floor of the mouth, separate the teeth slightly, and allow the jaw to "hang" in this position; maintain this position when the jaw is not being used for functions such as speaking and chewing.
6. Modify the food texture in your diet.
7. Choose softer foods and only those foods that can be chewed without pain.
8. Cut foods into smaller pieces; avoid foods that require wide mouth opening and biting off with the front teeth or foods that are chewy and sticky and that require excessive mouth movements.
9. Do not chew gum. Avoid certain postures or movements.
10. Do not lean on or cup the chin when performing desk work or at the dining table.
11. Do not test the jaw by opening wide or moving the jaw around excessively to assess pain or motion.
12. Avoid habitually maneuvering the jaw into positions to assess its comfort or range.
13. Avoid habitually clicking the jaw if a click is present.
14. Do not sleep on the stomach or in postures that place stress on the jaw.
15. Avoid elective dental treatment while symptoms of pain and limited opening are present.
16. During yawning, support the jaw by providing mild counter-pressure underneath the chin with the thumb and index finger or with the back of the hand.
17. Use thermal agents to control pain.
18. Apply moist hot compresses to the sides of the face and to the temple areas for 10–20 min twice daily.
19. Apply ice packs to targeted areas for 10 min; can alternate with heat.

Managing TMD Patients with Necessary Dental Procedures:

Prior to the procedure:

1. Use hot compresses to masseter and temporalis areas 10–20 min two to three times daily for 2 days.
2. Use a minor tranquilizer or skeletal muscle relaxant (e.g. lorazepam, 1 mg;

cyclobenzaprine, 10 mg) on the night and day of the procedure.

3. Start a nonsteroidal anti-inflammatory analgesic the day of the procedure.

During the procedure:

1. Use a child-sized surgical rubber mouth prop to support the patient's comfortable opening; remove periodically to reduce joint stiffness. Alternatively, an extra oral device that supports the jaw can be used.
2. Consider intravenous sedation and/or inhalation analgesia.
3. Provide frequent rest periods to avoid prolonged opening.
4. Apply moist heat to masticatory muscles during rest breaks.
5. Gently massage masticatory muscles during rest breaks.
6. Perform the procedure in the morning, when reserve is likely to be greatest.

After the procedure

1. Extend the use of muscle relaxant and NSAID medication as necessary.
2. Apply cold compresses to the TMJ and muscle areas during 24 hrs after the procedure.

FREQUENTLY ASKED QUESTIONS

1. Classify TMJ disorders. Write in detail about MPDS.
2. Osteoarthritis
3. Ankylosis
4. Disc derangement

BIBLIOGRAPHY

1. Burket's, Michael, Glick. Textbook of Oral Medicine, 12th ed.
2. Freny Karjodkar. Textbook of Oral Radiology 2nd edition.
3. Jeffrey P. Okeson. Management of TMJ Disorders and Occlusion, 6th ed.
4. Peck CC, Goulet JP, Lobbezoo F, et al. Expanding the Taxonomy of the Diagnostic Criteria for Temporomandibular Disorders (DC/TMD). J Oral Rehabil. 2014;41:2–23.
5. Stuart C.White, Michael J. Pharoah Oral Radiology Principles and Interpretation South Asia 1st ed.
6. Wright EF, North SL. Management and Treatment of Temporomandibular Disorders: A Clinical Perspective J Man ManipTher. 2009; 17(4): 247–254.
7. Gauer Rl, Semidey MJ. Diagnosis and Treatment of Temporomandibular Disorders. Am Fam Physician. 2015 Mar 15; 91(6):378–386.

Orofacial Pain

Pain can be defined as 'an **unpleasant emotional experience** usually initiated by noxious stimulus and transmitted over a specialized neural network to the CNS where it is interpreted as such'.

Tissue damage and the activation of nociceptors

↓

Transmission of a noxious stimulus to the brain.

However, due to the rich innervation of the head, face and oral structures, orofacial pain entities are often very complex and can be difficult to diagnose.

Orofacial pain interferes with daily life activities, impacting negatively on quality of life.

The most important aspect in orofacial pain is in understanding the problem and arriving at a proper diagnosis. It is only by proper diagnosis that an appropriate treatment can be selected.

The objective of diagnosis is to accurately identify the what, where, how and why of the patients complaints.

There can be different reasons of having orofacial pain which can be classified as follows:

NEURALGIAS

1. Primary trigeminal neuralgia (tic douloureux)
2. Secondary trigeminal neuralgia (CNS lesion or facial trauma)
3. Herpes zoster
4. Post-herpetic neuralgia
5. Geniculate neuralgia (cranial nerve VII)
6. Glossopharyngeal neuralgia (cranial nerve IX)
7. Superior laryngeal neuralgia (cranial nerve X)
8. Occipital neuralgia

Pain of Musculoskeletal Origin

1. Cervical osteoarthritis
2. Temporomandibular joint disorders
3. TMJ rheumatoid arthritis
4. TMJ osteoarthritis
5. Myofascial pain dysfunction
6. Fibromyalgia
7. Cervical sprain or hyperextension
8. Stylohyoid (Eagle's) syndrome

Primary Vascular Disorders

1. Migraine with aura
2. Migraine without aura
3. Cluster headache
4. Tension-type headache
5. Hypertensive vascular changes (aneurysm, emboli)
6. Cranial arteritis
7. Carotidynia
8. Thrombophlebitis

Psychogenic Pains

1. Delusional/hallucinatory
2. Hysterical/hypochondriac

Generalized Pain Syndromes

1. Post-traumatic pains
2. Sympathetically maintained pain (causalgia)
3. Phantom pain
4. Central pain

Lesions of the Ear, Nose, and Oral Cavity

1. Maxillary sinusitis
2. Otitis media
3. Dentin defects
4. Pulpitis
5. Periapical pathology/abscess
6. Cracked tooth/restoration
7. Atypical odontalgia
8. Periodontal pathology
9. Occlusal trauma
10. Dental impaction
11. Cysts and tumors
12. Osteitis
13. Mucocutaneous diseases
14. Salivary gland diseases
15. Atypical facial pain
16. Glossodynia
17. Malignancy associated pain

Steps in diagnosing a pain complaint, consists of:

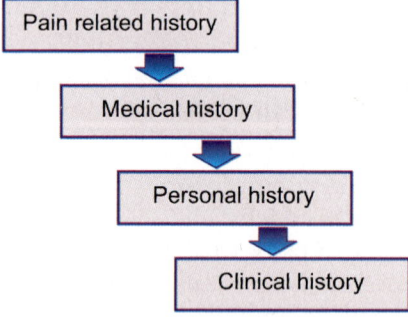

A. **Thorough history of pain:** Questions to facilitate the history taking for pain:
   i. Onset
   ii. Frequency
   iii. Duration
   iv. Provoking factors
   v. Site of initiation of pain
   vi. Radiation and referral of pain
   vii. Is the pain deep or superficial
   viii. Aggravating or exacerbating factors
   ix. Relieving factors
   x. Characteristics of the pain
   xi. Severity
   xii. Other associated features, for example, lacrimation or other autonomic signs and symptoms
   xiii. Previous management strategies attempted
   xiv. Patient's perceived cause(s) of pain

B. **Medical history**
   i. History of systemic disease
   ii. History of medications
   iii. History of major surgery
   iv. History of trauma

C. **Personal history**
   i. History of any deleterious habits
   ii. History of mood imbalances
   iii. History of any psychological illness

D. **Clinical examination**
   i. Accurately identifying the location from which the pain originates
   ii. Imaging can be used to confirm a suspected abnormality. It is the best method to evaluate a suspected tumor, infection, or inflammation.
   iii. *Diagnostic anesthetic blocking:* Skilful anesthetic blocking of muscles of masticatory system, maxillofacial region and TMJ are especially useful in the diagnosis of masticatory pain and non-masticatory myofascial pain disorders. Nerve block injections are especially helpful in identifying whether the painful structure is a site or source of pain.
   iv. *Utilization of diagnostic drugs/Trial therapy:* A short period of trial therapy is a good means of confirming a diagnosis. Oxcarbazepine can be used to confirm a doubtful diagnosis of paroxysmal neurologic conditions.

For proper identification of the pain disorders on occasion, pain problems require medical, otolaryngologic, orthopedic, neurologist, rheumatologic, or psychological consultation.

In the assessment of pain intensity, rating scales often used are:
Different scales can be used depending on cause and site of pain
- Numerical rating scale
- Visual analogue scale (VAS)
- McGill pain questionnaire
- Behavioral rating scale

Amongst these scales the VAS has been shown to be more sensitive to change and is therefore more widely used. It consists of a 10 cm line with anchor points at each end.

The pain management generally covers following factors:
- Elimination of causative noxious stimuli
- Interception of nociceptive circuits
- Enhancement of neural mechanism of pain inhibition.

Physical therapy modalities which are generally included in pain management are sensory stimulations, massage, vapocoolant therapy, mechanical vibration, hydrotherapy, transcutaneous stimulation (TENS), electroaccupuncture, cryotherapy, ultrasound, diathermy, electrogalvanic stimulation, deep heat and other methods.

Management of Specific Orofacial Pain Disorders

Trigeminal Neuralgia (TN)

The term 'neuralgia' means pain in the nerve. Trigeminal neuralgia also known as *"ticdoulourex"*.

Trigeminal neuralgia is a sudden, unilateral, brief, stabbing, recurrent pain in the distribution of one or more branches of the fifth cranial nerve. It is localized most often to the second and third distributions of the trigeminal nerve (V2 and V3) intraorally and extraorally.

The diagnosis is made using the history alone, based on characteristic features of the pain.
- Pain occurs in paroxysms, which can last from a few seconds to several minutes. The frequency of the paroxysms ranges from a few to hundreds of attacks per day.
- Periods of remission can last for months to years, but tend to get shorter over time.
- The condition can impair activities of daily living and lead to depression. Symptoms may worsen also over time and become less responsive to medication, despite dose increases and adding further agents.

Pain usually elicited by momentary stimulation of "Trigger Zones".

Etiology
- Peripheral causes
  - Nerve compression
  - Nerve trauma
  - Nerve back talk
  - Aneurysm around the nerve
  - Demyelination of the nerve
  - Herpes zoster infection
- Central causes
  - Microaneurysm around the nerve root
  - Cerebro-pontine angle tumors
  - Multiple sclerosis
  - Demyelination of the nerve
  - Pulsation of basilar artery
  - High petrous ridge

The etiology of TN is often related to vascular compression that may result in focal demyelination. The superior cerebellar artery compression on the trigeminal root has been shown to be responsible for attacks of TN pain; however, nonvascular compression by a cerebellopontine angle neoplasm, such as acoustic neuromas, meningiomas, cholesteatomas, and neurofibromas, have also been shown to result in TN attacks. A cranial nerve exam can demonstrate other neural deficits that may be present due to a mass pressing on the trigeminal root. Therefore, magnetic resonance imaging (MRI) and computed tomography (CT) imaging of the brain should be requested in order to rule out any intracranial pathology. Furthermore, myelin loss due to multiple sclerosis has been shown to be a causative disorder related to the paroxysmal pain firing of TN attacks.

Clinical Features

There is gender variability in the incidence of TN with a female to male ratio of 1.74:1 with majority cases occurring after 50 years of age. Clinical history, examination, investigations, and imaging are necessary to make a correct diagnosis.

TN is characterized by an abrupt onset and short-lived unilateral shock-like pain, in the distribution of the trigeminal nerve. Usual triggers for classical TN (CTN) include mastication, touch, tooth brushing, eating, talking, and cold wind on the face. Trigger zones are present in more than 90% of the patients, with touch and vibrations being the most common stimuli in provoking pain. Pain is usually distributed along the V2 and V3 branches. Right side of the face is often associated with pain and rarely it is bilateral.

Diagnostic criteria for TN from The International Classification of Headache Disorders (ICHD-3) are summarized below.

TN is orofacial pain restricted to one or more divisions of the trigeminal nerve. It is abrupt in onset and typically lasts only a few seconds (2 min at maximum). Patients may report their pain as arising spontaneously, but these pain paroxysms can always be triggered by innocuous mechanical stimuli or movements. Patients usually do not experience pain between paroxysms. If they do report additional continuous pain, in the same distribution and in the same periods as the paroxysmal pain, they are considered to have TN with continuous pain.

Management

* Medical
* Surgical
  - Peripheral: Injections, neurectomies, cryosurgery
  - Central

* **Classical TN:** Caused by vascular compression of the trigeminal nerve root resulting in morphological changes of the root.
* **Secondary TN:** Caused by major neurological disease, e.g. a tumor of the cerebello-pontine angle or MS idiopathic
* **TN:** No apparent cause
A. At least three attacks of unilateral facial pain fulfilling criteria B and C
B. Occurring in one or more divisions of the trigeminal nerve, with no radiation beyond the trigeminal distribution
C. Pain has at least three of the following four characteristics:
   1. Recurring in paroxysmal attacks lasting from a fraction of a second to 2 min
   2. Severe intensity
   3. Electric shock-like, shooting, stabbing or sharp in quality
   4. Precipitated by innocuous stimuli to the affected side of the face
D. No clinically evident neurological deficit.
E. Not better accounted for by another ICHD-3 diagnosis
13.1.1.1 Classical TN (classical TN, purely paroxysmal; classical TN with concomitant continuous pain)
13.1.1.2 Secondary TN (TN attributed to MS; TN attributed to space-occupying lesion; TN attributed to other cause
13.1.1.3 Idiopathic TN (idiopathic TN, purely paroxysmal; idiopathic TN with concomitant continuous pain).
(IASP—International Association for the Study of Pain; ICHD—International Classification of Headache Disorders; MS—Multiple Sclerosis, TN—Trigeminal Neuralgia)

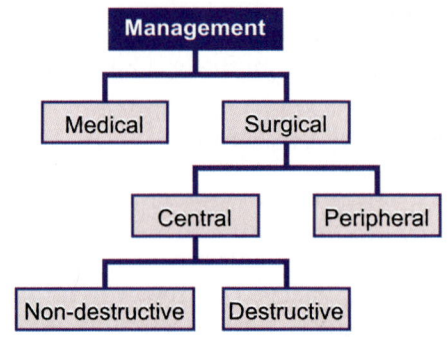

A. **Non-destructive**
- Microvascular decompression (MVD)

B. **Destructive**
- Percutaneous balloon compression
- Glycerol rhizotomy
- Radiofrequency thermocoagulation
- Gamma knife radiosurgery

Medical Management

Antiepileptic medications are the drugs of choice for the management of trigeminal neuralgia.

First line drugs
- Carbamazepine: 100 to 1200 mg, two weeks followed by review
- Oxycarbazepine: 600–1800 mg, two weeks followed by review
- Gabapentine: 900–1200 mg, two weeks followed by review

Carbamazepine, the first-line agent provides pain relief in 72% of patients. Suggested dose is 100 mg twice daily; increase if necessary by 50–100 mg every 3–4 days; target range 400–1200 mg/day.

If these medications are not effective or if the therapeutic range cannot be achieved due to side effects, then doses should be lowered and second-line drugs, such as baclofen and lamotrigine, may be added to reduce the pain attacks.

Second-line drugs
- Lamotrigine: 50–100 mg
- Baclofen: 8 mg
- Pregabalin: 50–100 mg

Side Effects of Medicinal Drugs
- Dizziness
- Confusion
- Drowsiness
- Vision problems
- Nausea
- Gingival hypertrophy
- Neutropenia

If medications are no longer effective or if unmanageable side effects develop, then neurosurgical options, such as microvascular decompression or gamma knife radio surgery may be considered.

Peripheral Management

Alcoholic injections: 95% Absolute alcohol in small quantities 0.5 to 2 ml is given in peripheral branches of trigeminal nerve.

Neurolytic agents
- Long acting local anesthesia
- Ropivacaine with gabapentin
- Absolute alcohol 0.5–2 ml
- Botox type A (25–75 U)

Side effects
Repeated injections may cause:
- Local tissue toxicity
- Inflammation
- Fibrosis
- Burning alcohol neuritis

Peripheral Neurectomies
(Nerve Avulsion)

Indicated in patients in whom craniotomy is contraindicated due to age, debility, limited life expectancy and no respond to medication.

It can be done under local anesthesia in which partial avulsion of offending nerve is done. After avulsion of nerve from bone and soft tissue nerve end is cauterized or suture into viable muscle, periosteum or bone and later foramen is plugged with non-absorbable material.

Cryotherapy for Peripheral Nerve

In this method direct application of cryotherapy probe, i.e. nitrous oxide probe is done. Temperature colder than –60°C, for 2–3 minutes and procedure is repeated for three times. It produces Wallerian degeneration without destroying the nerve sheath.

GLOSSOPHARYNGEAL NEURALGIA

Definition: Glossopharyngeal neuralgia is a rare condition associated with pain in the area supplied by the glossopharyngeal nerve.

Painful sites may include the nasopharynx, posterior part of the tongue, throat, tonsil, larynx, and ear.

Signs: This disorder presents shooting paroxysms of pain that can occur multiple times a day with stimulation of the oropharyngeal region. Common triggers may include mechanical stimulation of the trigger zone as well as activities including chewing, swallowing, coughing, talking, and head movement. The painful episodes may continue for months and then spontaneously go into remission.

Associated pain: Due to the proximity of the vagal sensory nerves, glossopharyngeal neuralgia may coincide with a cardiac dysrhythmia such as bradycardia, asystole, and syncope.

Diagnosis: Diagnosis may be confirmed by blocking the tonsillar and pharyngeal region with topical or local anesthetics. Imaging with a CT scan of the head and a brain MRI should be conducted to rule out pathology related to the nerve compression and possible oropharyngeal carcinoma.

Treatment: Pharmacologic treatment of glossopharyngeal neuralgia is similar to that for TN and may include the use of antiepileptic medications. If medical management fails, then surgical procedures may be considered, such as a microvascular decompression to remove pressure from the glossopharyngeal nerve, radiofrequency thermocoagulation, gamma knife radiosurgery, or rhizotomy.

Atypical Odontalgia (AO)

Atypical Odontalgia is a centralized trigeminal neuropathy often localized in a tooth or tooth area that is frequently misdiagnosed, leading to unnecessary dental treatments in attempts to relieve the pain.

Atypical odontalgia is described as a persistent idiopathic pain that does not fulfill the diagnostic criteria for cranial neuralgias and which is not attributed to another disorder, and can be throbbing and burning in nature.

Management

The pharmacological management of AO may include topical and systemic medications. If the pain is localized to a peripheral origin and the diagnostic block gives an equivocal response but a decrease in pain, a topical medication can be used and a neurosensory stent can be fabricated.

Systemic approaches, such as tricyclic antidepressants, calcium channel blockers (pregabalin and gabapentin), sodium channel blockers (carbamazepine), and antiepileptics such as topiramate, can be used for the management of this condition.

The management of AO is very challenging, and a multidisciplinary approach is necessary, which should include orofacial pain specialists and neurologists in addition to psychiatric and psychological evaluations in order to identify comorbidities with depression and anxiety.

Burning Mouth Syndrome

BMS is defined as a burning painful sensation in the mouth (oral dysesthesia) with normal clinical examination and no obvious organic cause.

BMS is therefore a diagnosis of exclusion.

Evidence suggests that this disorder has a multifactorial cause, with neurologic, psychogenic, and hormonal factors all contributing to the disease.

Prevalence and epidemiology: The prevalence of BMS reported for the general population varies between 0.7% and 15% and seems to depend on the diagnostic criteria used. BMS seems most prevalent in postmenopausal women, although younger women as well as men can also be affected. Most reports suggest a female-to-male ratio of 1:5 to 1:7. Prevalence does seem to increase with age in both male and female subjects.

Etiology: Although the etiology remains mostly unknown, the ICHD-3 beta suggests BMS is a neuropathy. It is commonly accepted that the etiology of BMS is multifactorial and involves the interaction between local and systemic entities.

Local factors: Local factors, such as odontogenic or mucosal disease; mechanical or chemical irritation; hypersensitivity reactions; viral, fungal, or bacterial infection; and xerostomia, can produce oral burning by direct irritation of the tongue and other oral mucosal surfaces.

Systemic factors: Several systemic factors have been suggested as least partially responsible for BMS. Systemic factors to be considered include nutritional and vitamin deficiencies, such as vitamin B_{12}, folic acid, iron, and zinc. Autoimmune, gastrointestinal, and endocrine disorders, such as diabetes and thyroid dysfunction, have been suggested as well. Pharmacotherapeutic agents like angiotensin-converting enzyme inhibitors, including captopril, enalapril, and lisinopril, also deserve consideration.

Clinical features: The clinical presentations of BMS are typically not consistent and vary from patient to patient. The onset of pain may be gradual or sudden, typically with no identifiable precipitating factors. In some cases, however, it can be traced to a precipitating event, such as a dental procedure, trauma, and introduction of a new medication, illness, or stressful life event. At presentation, patients usually complain of chronic pain of 4 months to 6 months duration and describe it as annoying, burning or scalding, tingling, or sometimes itchy or numb.

The pain can be continuous or intermittent and is typically localized to the tongue (67.9%), usually the anterior two-thirds, but may involve other mucosal surfaces, such as the palate, lip, buccal mucosa, and floor of the mouth. The pain tends to present bilaterally and symmetrically more so than unilaterally.

Associated features: In addition to the burning sensation, many patients also complain of dry mouth (xerostomia) and taste alterations. Alterations, such as sour and bitter taste perceived as stronger, sweet tastes perceived as weaker, and salty tastes perceived as weaker or stronger are commonly reported.

Diagnosis: A diagnosis of BMS is considered to be one of exclusion of all secondary factors. A comprehensive medical and dental history, including a complete review of current medications, along with an exhaustive review of systems is essential for establishing a definitive diagnosis. Patients should be queried as to any history of previous upper respiratory tract infections, middle ear disease, or surgery that may have damaged the chorda tympani nerve.

Management strategies: It must be determined if the presentation is primary or secondary. If the complaint seems secondary to an identifiable etiologic factor, treatment of the underlying condition most often alleviates the BMS complaint.

Behavioral Therapies

BMS patients should be educated as to the potentially detrimental effects of parafunctional habits, such as clenching, bruxism, and tongue habits. The use of oral care products should be scrutinized and amended to avoid the use of products that contain alcohol and those that contain flavoring agents or other known oral irritants.

Self-regulatory approaches, such as regular exercise, diaphragmatic breathing, maintaining a proper diet and adequate hydration, and intentional relaxation, have been shown beneficial in reducing chronic pain complaints.

Cognitive behavioral therapy provided by trained clinicians has also proved beneficial in some instances.

Topical Therapies

Several topical therapies have been recommended and used in the management for BMS.

* 1 mg tablet of clonazepam for 3 minutes and then expectorate reduces the pain significantly.
* 0.15% Benzydamine hydrochloride 3 times per day
* Salivary substitutes
* Topical antifungals
* Topical capsaicin (0.025% cream) or rinsing with Tabasco sauce and water (1:2–4 solution).

Systemic Therapies

Systemic agents to consider include:
* α-Lipoic acid, 600 mg per day for 2 months
* Clonazepam, 0.5 mg per day at bedtime
* Gabapentin, 100 mg to 300 mg up to 3 times per day
* Pregabalin, 25 mg to 75 mg up to 3 times per day
* Serotonin/norepinephrine reuptake inhibitor: Sertraline, 50 mg per day; paroxetine, 20 mg per day; or duloxetine 30 mg to 60 mg per day. P. salivary stimulant: Pilocarpine, 5 mg to 10 mg 3 times per day, or cevimeline, 30 mg 3 times per day.
* Tricyclic antidepressant (TCA): Amitriptyline, 25 mg to 100 mg per day at bedtime, or nortriptyline, 10 to 75 mg per day at bedtime.
* Botulinum toxin A injected intradermally (16 total units) into the tongue and lower lip gives relief for 20 weeks.

HEADACHE

Headache affects most people at least occasionally. Headache denotes pain or discomfort from the level of the brows back to the suboccipital region.

Classification of Headache

Primary headache
* It is a condition in which headache is a primary manifestation with no underlying disease.
* It is usually benign and recurrent.

Secondary headache
* It is a condition in which headache is a secondary manifestation of an underlying disease process. It is usually sudden and progressive.

Primary headache disorders can be categorized in three types.
* **Cluster headache:** Pain is in and around one eye.
* **Tension headache:** Pain is like a band squeezing the head.
* **Migraine headache:** Pain, nausea and visual changes are of typical classic form.

Migraine

Prevalence in western countries—10 to 12% in adults.

Migraine is a common primary headache with an additional number of rarer related syndromes. The 2 most common types of migraine headaches are migraine without aura (MWA) and migraine with aura (MA).

MWA is an inherited disorder affecting the young, with an onset before the age of 20 years in about half of the cases. There is up to a twofold increase of MWA among first-degree relatives of patients with MWA and a fourfold increase in MA.

Migraine presentation may be divided into phases and each may occur alone or in combination with each other. The headache phase is identical in MA and MWA.

Phases of Migraine

Prodrome: Premonitory signs and symptoms occurring days or hours before some or all headaches. Nonspecific neurologic/autonomic signs and constitutional symptoms. Tiredness, difficulty in concentration, and stiff neck.

Aura (in MA): Focal neurologic signs or symptoms:
* Visual (flashing lights), sensory (pins and needles), and motor (speech) symptoms.
* Develop over 5 to 20 minutes and last for less than 60 minutes.
* Followed in about 10 minutes by a typical headache.

Headache Phase

Postdrome phase: Depressed, irritable, and tired.

TABLE 12.1: Differential diagnosis of headaches	
Condition	Signs and symptoms
Migraine	Prodromal symptoms—euphoria, depression, irritability, food cravings, constipation, neck stiffness, increased yawning × Aura—visual, sensory, verbal, and/or motor disturbances × Throbbing and pulsatile × Photophobia and phonophobia × Long duration
Cluster headache (subclassification of TAC)	× Orbital and temporal regions × Short-lived × Unilateral × Autonomic symptoms—ptosis, miosis, lacrimation, rhinorrhea × Nasal congestion
Tension-type	Diffuse, dull aching pain × Bilateral × Precipitated by stress and mental tension
Paroxysmal hemicrania (subclassification of TAC)	Unilateral × Shorter-lived than cluster headaches (lasts 2–30 minutes) × Most often in V1 distribution × Orbital, temporal, and frontal regions × Abrupt onset and cessation × Similar autonomic symptoms as cluster headaches
Temporal arteritis	Age >50 years × Localized headache of new onset × Tenderness or decreased pulse of the temporal artery × Erythrocyte sedimentation rate >50
Other TACs	× SUNCT (short-lasting unilateral neuralgiform headache attacks with conjunctival injection and tearing) × SUNA (short-lasting unilateral neuralgiform headache attacks with cranial autonomic symptoms)

Migraine Triggers

× Several factors have been reported as initiators of individual attacks in migraineurs, termed triggers or precipitating factors.
× Anxiety and stress.
× Fatigue, sleeping difficulties.
× Foods and drinks.
× Menstruation.
× Weather changes.
× Smells, smoke, and light.

Differential Diagnosis

× Tension-type headache (TTH)
× Oral/dental pain
× Sinusitis
× Vascular disorders
× Transient ischemic attacks, thrombo-embolic stroke, intracranial hematoma, subarachnoid hemorrhage, and arterial hypertension may cause migraine-like headaches.
× Intracranial tumors, infections and regional trauma may induce migraine-like headaches.
× Some are sudden-onset headaches or are accompanied by atypical neurologic signs and symptoms.

Management

× Non-pharmacologic
× Pharmacologic

Non-pharmacologic treatment

× Sleep
× Diet
× Lifestyle modification

Pharmacologic treatment

Abortive (acute, symptomatic)
× Aim to rapidly relieve headache with no recurrence or side effects.
× Used when fewer than 4 to 8 attacks per month or to supplement prophylactic regimens.

TABLE 12.2: Some of the common abortive treatments for migraine

Class	Drugs	Initial oral dose mg
Analgesics	⚹ Aspirin	500–1000
Combinations	⚹ Aspirin and	500–600
	⚹ Paracetamol and	200–400
	⚹ Caffeine	50–200
	⚹ Paracetamol and	400
	⚹ Codeine	25
Ergot alkaloids	⚹ Dihydroergotamine NS	2
NSAIDs: Selective COX-2 inhibitors	⚹ Nonspecific Naproxen sodium	550–825
	⚹ Ibuprofen	400–800
	⚹ Diclofenac	50–100
	⚹ Rofecoxib	25–50
Triptans (5-HT agonist)	⚹ Sumatriptan	50–100
	⚹ Sumatriptan NS	20 (1 NS metered dose)
	⚹ Sumatriptan SC	6
	⚹ Naratriptan	2.5
	⚹ Eletriptan	40
	⚹ Rizatriptan	10
	⚹ Zolmitriptan	2.5
	⚹ Zolmitriptan NS	2.5 (1 NS metered dose)
	⚹ Frovatriptan	2.5
Opioids	⚹ Butorphanol NS	1–2 metered doses

Nonspecific medication (Table 12.1).
- ⚹ Triptans
  - ▪ Triptans of choice
    - ⚹ Rizatriptan 10 mg consistently provides rapid relief.
    - ⚹ Almotriptan (12.5 mg) has good efficacy and tolerability.
    - ⚹ Eletriptan will provide high efficacy with low recurrence but low tolerability.
    - ⚹ Frovatriptan for the prevention of menstrually related migraine.
- ⚹ Preventive (chronic, prophylactic Table 12.2): Aims to reduce attack frequency, severity, and duration.

FREQUENTLY ASKED QUESTIONS

1. Define and classify orofacial pain. Write in detail about trigeminal neuralgia.
2. Cluster headache.
3. Migraine

TABLE 12.3 : Choice of migraine preventive treatment

Drug	Dose mg	Adverse effects	Contraindication	Relative indications
Propranolol (SR)	80–240	Bradycardia, hypotension fatigue, sleep disturbances dyspepsia, depression	Asthma, depression, cardiac failure, Raynaud disease, diabetes	Hypertension angina
Amitriptyline	10–50	Sedation, weight gain, dry mouth, blurred vision, constipation, urinary retention, postural hypotension	Mania, urinary retention Heart block	Insomnia, anxiety depression, other chronic pains
Sodium valproate	500–1000	Nausea, vomiting, alopecia, tremor, weight gain/loss	Liver disease, bleeding disorder	Mania, epilepsy, anxiety
Topiramate	25–200	Dizziness, confusion, language problems, paresthesias, nausea, anorexia, diplopia	Renal disease, respiratory disorders, glaucoma	Overweight

BIBLIOGRAPHY

1. Okeson JP (2005). Bell's Orofacial Pain: The Clinical Management of Orofacial Pain. (6th edn.), Quintessence Publishing Co. Ltd, New Malden, Surrey.

2. Monheim LM (1983). Monheim's Local Anesthesia and Pain Control in Dental Practice (7th edn.). Mosby, St. Louis.

3. Burket LS, Greenberg MS, Glick M, Ship JA (2008). Burket's Oral Medicine (11th edn.). BC Decker Inc., Hamilton.

4. Obermann M. Treatment options in trigeminal neuralgia. Ther Adv Neurol Disord 2010;3(2):107–115.

5. Katusic S, Williams DB, Beard CM, Bergstralh EJ, Kurland LT. Epidemiology and clinical features of idiopathic trigeminal neuralgia and glossopharyngeal neuralgia: similarities and differences. Rochester, Minnesota, 1945–1984. Neuroepidemiology 1991;10(5–6): 276–281. 90.

6. Olds MJ, Woods CI, Winfield JA. Microvascular decompression in glossopharyngeal neuralgia. Am J Otol. 1995;16(3):326–330.

7. Benoliel, R., Eliav, E. (2013). Primary Headache Disorders. Dental Clinics of North America 57(3), 513–539.

8. Bender SD. Burning mouth syndrome. Dental Clinics 2018 Oct 1;62(4):585–96.

9. Reddy GD, Viswanathan A. Trigeminal and glossopharyngeal neuralgia. Neurologic Clinics 2014 May 1;32(2):539–52.

10. Kumar A, Brennan MT. Differential diagnosis of orofacial pain and temporomandibular disorder. Dental Clinics 2013 Jul 1;57(3):419–28.

Diseases of Tongue

Chapter

13

INTRODUCTION

Tongue is a complex muscular internal organ well encased within the oral cavity and protected from the environment, with dorsal and ventral surfaces.

The tongue is situated in the floor of mouth having oral and pharyngeal part separated by V-shaped sulcus terminalis which end at foramen cecum. It is composed of a tip, body and root. It has dorsal (superior) and ventral (inferior) surface, the dorsal surface is divided by a groove into symmetrical halves by the median sulcus. The dorsal surface has projections/papillae of the mucous membrane which carries taste buds and also imparts characteristic roughness to the anterior two-thirds of the tongue. The tongue mucosa is very thin and highly vascular on the ventral surface of the oral cavity which allows the rapid delivery of medication into the cardiovascular system bypassing the gastrointestinal tract. On the ventral surface of the tongue is a fold of mucous membrane called lingual frenum that binds the tongue to the floor of the mouth at midline. On either sides of the frenum are small prominences on the floor of mouth called sublingual caruncles in which the submandibular and sublingual glands drain into. The bulk of the tongue consists of several extrinsic and intrinsic muscles which perform the several functions of tongue.

The tongue begins to develop in the fourth week of embryogenesis. The anterior two-thirds of the tongue develop from first brachial arch from the fusion of two lateral swellings and a midline swelling tuberculum impar while posterior one-third develops from 3rd and 4th brachial arches. The failure in the normal course of tongue development may lead to various developmental anomalies of tongue.

FUNCTIONS OF TONGUE

- Ingestion
- Suckling
- Swallowing
- Perception—taste, temperature, pain and general sensation
- Phonation
- Respiration
- Jaw development
- Symbolic function, tongue plays a role in physical intimacy and sexuality in human and mammals.

TONGUE EXAMINATION

One should inspect the tongue when it is at rest. The tongue is stabilized and can be gently guided right and left by holding the tongue tip with the gauze to inspect all the surfaces or its right and left lateral borders. The tongue should be examined for variation in size, color, texture, coating, mucosal eruptions, ulcer, and swelling. The papillae, margins of tongue, taste perception, frenal attachment and the movement of the tongue also should be examined.

DISEASES OF TONGUE

Epidemiology

Tongue lesions are quite prevalent; the prevalence of 12.07 to 13.75% was noted in Indian population. The most common tongue conditions are coated tongue, geographic tongue, fissured tongue and depapillated tongue. Tongue lesions are more common in persons who are denture wearers, tobacco users, diabetic, hypertensive and anemic. The diseases of tongue can be congenital or acquired, and can be manifested as depapillation, discoloration, soreness, pain, redness and swelling.

I. *Diseases of tongue can be categorized as follows:*
- **Injury**
  - Physical, chemical and thermal
- **Infections**
  - *Bacterial:* Tuberculosis and scarlet fever
  - *Viral:* Human immunodeficiency virus (HIV) and hairy leukoplakia
  - *Fungal:* Candidiasis
- **Developmental disturbances**
  - Aglossia
  - Ankyloglossia
  - Macroglossia
  - Geographic tongue
  - Fissured tongue
  - Median rhomboid glossitis
  - Hairy tongue
- **Nutritional deficiency**
  - Iron deficiency anemia
  - Pernicious anemia
  - Vitamin deficiency
- **Premalignant**
  - Leukoplakia
  - Oral submucous fibrosis
- **Tumors**
  - Squamous cell carcinoma

- **Immunological**
  - Recurrent aphthous
  - Pemphigus
  - Lichen planus
- **Miscellaneous**
  - Lichenoid reaction
  - Pyogenic granuloma

II. **International Classification of Diseases (10th Revision)**
ICD-10 Category K14

	K14: Diseases of tongue
Erythroplakia (K13.29)	ICD-10K14.0: Glossitis
Focal epithelial hyperplasia (K13.29)	ICD-10K14.1: Geographic tongue
Hairy leukoplakia (K13.3)	ICD-10K14.2: Median rhomboid glossitis
Submucous fibrosis of tongue (K13.5)	ICD-10K14.3: Hypertrophy of tongue papillae
Leukoedema of tongue (K13.29)	ICD-10K14.4: Atrophy of tongue papillae
Leukoplakia of tongue (K13.21)	ICD-10K14.5: Plicated tongue
Macroglossia (congenital) (Q38.2)	ICD-10K14.6: Glossodynia
	ICD-10K14.8: Other diseases of tongue
	ICD-10K14.9: Disease of tongue, unspecified

Aglossia

It is the complete absence of the tongue at birth.

Ankyloglossia (Tongue Tie)

Ankyloglossia (tongue tie) where the lingual frenum attaches the tongue to the floor of the mouth due to the congenital shortness of lingual frenum, it can be partial or complete. It interferes with oral hygiene, speech, feeding, in addition, it may lead to midline mandibular diastema and lingual periodontal defects, hence frenectomy may be indicated.

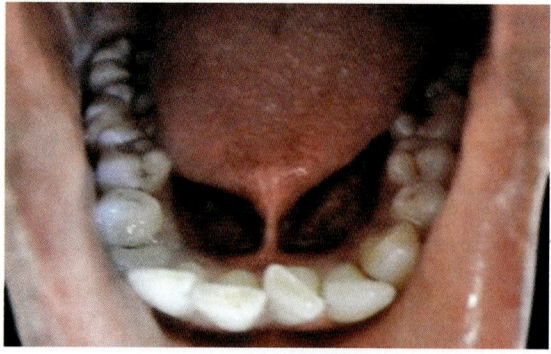

Fig. 13.1: Tongue tie

Hypoglossia/Microglossia

Hypoglossia/microglossia congenitally short or small tongue.

The incomplete development of the tongue is associated with hypoglossia. This rare disease may occur as an isolated disorder or may be one of the manifestations of syndromic condition, e.g. Pierre Robin syndrome, cleft lip and palate. The patient has difficulties in eating and talking.

Macroglossia

Macroglossia an abnormally large tongue. It is characterized by an increase in the size of the tongue. It may be congenital or acquired. The congenital macroglossia is due to overdevelopment of the musculature. It also occurs as a result of a tumor in the tongue such as lymphangioma, hemangioma, inflammatory/allergic processes or as a part of syndrome, e.g. Down syndrome.

Glossoptosis

It is a medical condition and abnormality which involves the downward displacement or retraction of the tongue. It may cause non-fusion of the hard palate leading to cleft palate. It is one of the features of Pierre Robin syndrome and Down syndrome.

Patent Thyroglossal Ducts, Thyroglossal Duct Cyst and Lingual Thyroid

Thyroid gland develops from analage of endothelial cells in the midline of the floor of the pharynx between the first and second branchial arches. The foramen cecum on the dorsum of tongue is the point of attachment of the thyroglossal duct and is formed during the descent of the thyroid diverticulum in embryonic development. Lingual thyroid is mass of the thyroid on the dorsum at foramen cecum which may lead to enlarged tongue and dysphagia.

Cleft, Lobed, Bifurcated and Tetrafurcated Tongues

It is caused by a failure of the lateral lingual swellings to merge partially or completely, the complete cleft tongue is a rare condition. It is the separation of anterior two-thirds of the tongue by deep midline or clefts which may occur in isolation or as a manifestation of syndrome.

Fissured Tongue/Scrotal Tongue

It is presented as numerous small furrow/grooves on the dorsal surface radiating out from a central groove or may form various patterns on the tongue. It is usually painless except in some cases food debris tends to collect in the grooves and produce irritation so patients are advised to keep it clean. It is associated with extrinsic factors such as chronic trauma and vitamin B deficiency, candidiasis, salivary hypofunction. It is commonly associated with Melkersson-Rosenthal syndrome and Down's syndrome. Recently, the various fissure patterns as a tongue print are being studied greatly as a biometric tool for personal identification.

Tongue Coating

The food debris, desquamated epithelial cells and bacteria often form a visible tongue coating. This coating has been identified as a major contributing factor in bad breath which can be managed by brushing the tongue gently with a toothbrush or using special oral hygiene instruments such as tongue scrapers.

Geographic Tongue/Benign Migratory Glossitis

This disease is characterized by red areas in a map-like pattern on the tongue, the irregular patches of depapillation form on the tongue giving the map-like appearance. The classic lesions show the red areas with atrophic filiform papillae and white circinate borders. They are usually seen on the dorsum of the tongue and on the sides of the tongue, but it might also spread to other areas of the mouth. Patients with this condition may also develop burning, soreness or tenderness. Patients with this condition need to avoid eating acidic or spicy foods. There may be an association between certain types of psoriasis (especially pustular psoriasis) and geographic tongue and leukocyte antigen: HLA-Cw6 and HLA-DR5.

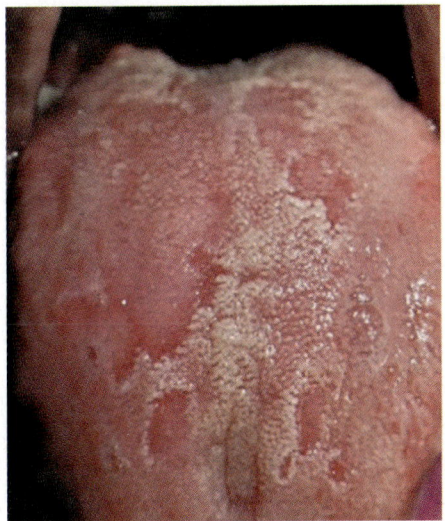

Fig. 13.2: Geographic tongue

Median Rhomboid Glossitis

It appears as a well-demarcated rounded or rhomboid-shaped, raised area in the midline of the tongue dorsum just anterior to the vallate papillae. It is said to be a developmental anomaly resulting from persistence of tuberculum impar due to its failure to retract before the fusion of the lateral halves of the tongue, so that the structure devoid of papillae is interposed between them. The area is devoid of filiform or other papillae. The texture may vary from a reddish, smooth or granular surface to a more lobulated and indurated. It is also linked to the fungal infection due to the demonstration of *Candida* in 90% of cases.

Histologically, it shows the hypoplastic, acanthotic epithelium with elongated rete pegs, subepithelial inflammatory infiltrate, vascular dilatation and fibrosis, and hyalinization of underlying muscle. If symptomatic, it may be treated by surgical excision, cautery and topical and systemic antifungal therapy.

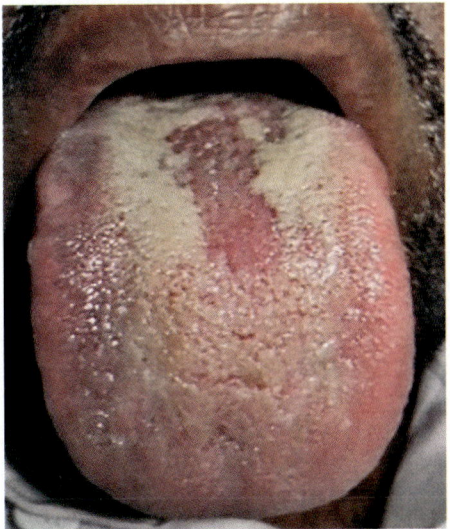

Fig. 13.3: Median rhomboid glossitis

Black Hairy Tongue

It is a condition characterized by hypertrophy or excessive overgrowth of filiform papillae associated with growth of black pigment producing microorganism on the dorsum of tongue. These papillae may continually grow or get worn down over time by daily activities such as eating, brushing, etc. The growing papillae provide favorable environment for the bacteria to grow and lead to darkened or blackened appearance on the tongue. This disease is usually seen in individuals who have poor oral hygiene, heavy smoking habit, antibiotics, psychotropic agents and systemic disturbance, e.g. anemia, hyperacidity, peptic ulcer. It may be asymptomatic or may cause gagging and tickling sensation.

Pigmentations

The extrinsic or intrinsic pigmentations may occur on the tongue.

Exogenous Pigmentation

The exogenous pigmentation involves filiform papillae, the pigmentation of filiform papillae results from microbial growth and metabolic products, food debris, and dyes from candy, beverages and mouth rinses. In addition, the tattooing of lateral margins and ventral surface of tongue result from deposits of amalgam and other metals from lacerations during dental treatment. The medications such as tricyclic antidepressants, zidovudine, doxorubicin, and alpha-methyl dopa are also responsible for exogenous pigmentation.

Endogenous Pigmentation

The endogenous pigmentation of tongue occurs in the following conditions:
× Racial melanin pigmentations, jaundice
× Primary adrenal deficiency (Addison's disease), Peutz-Jeghers syndrome
× Albright's syndrome, acanthosis nigricans
× Neurofibromatosis, hemochromatosis
× For such patients, the tongue evaluation should be done simultaneously.

Oral Hairy Leukoplakia

Oral hairy leukoplakia is a corrugated white lesion that usually occurs on the lateral or ventral surfaces of the tongue in patients with severe immunodeficiency. Epstein-Barr virus (EBV) is implicated as the causative agent in oral hairy leukoplakia. The most common disease associated with oral hairy leukoplakia is HIV infection. Oral hairy leukoplakia is reported in approximately 25% of adults with HIV infection, its prevalence may be higher in patients with acquired immunodeficiency syndrome (AIDS). Oral hairy leukoplakia most commonly involves the lateral borders of the tongue but may extend to the ventral or dorsal surfaces and is usually bilateral. Lesions on the tongue are usually corrugated or frayed appearance or may manifest as a plaque-like lesion.

Histopathologic examination of the epithelium reveals severe hyperparakeratosis with an irregular surface, acanthosis with superficial edema, and numerous virally affected "balloon" cells/koilocytic cells in the spinous layer. The characteristic microscopic feature is the presence of homogeneous viral nuclear inclusions with a residual rim of normal chromatin. The definitive diagnosis can be established by demonstrating the presence of EBV through *in situ* hybridization, electron microscopy, or polymerase chain reaction.

Glossitis

Glossitis is a general term for tongue inflammation which can have various etiologies. It is associated with smoothing of the tongue, discoloration and swelling. It may be transient and chronic. The surface of tongue may appear smooth, red/pale or tongue may swell. There may be tenderness, burning, taste disturbances and difficulty in chewing, speaking and swallowing. This disease can be attributed to various conditions or infections, allergic reaction, genetic predisposition, malnutrition, deficiency of vitamin B or iron, tongue piercing, mechanical irritants, and poor hydration. Some types of glossitis are caused by infections, e.g. median rhomboid glossitis (*Candida* species), "strawberry tongue" (seen in scarlet fever), and syphilitic glossitis (seen in tertiary syphilis). Oral candidiasis can affect the tongue. Risk factors for oral candidiasis include antibiotic and corticosteroid use and immunodeficiency or diabetes mellitus.

The treatment involves elimination of the cause of inflammation, topical medications, e.g. corticosteroids may reduce redness or swelling.

Depapillation of Tongue

Bald tongue of Sandwith is named after scientist Fleming MantSandwith.

It is characterized by a smooth glossy tongue that is often tender, painful caused by complete atrophy of lingual papillae leaving behind an erythematous surface.

The main characteristic features include glossitis, associated with painful, fiery red and enlarged tongue, profused salivation and raw beefy tongue caused mainly by deficiency of niacin/vitamin B_3. The dorsal surface of tongue may be affected completely or in patches associated with pain and erythema.

Bald tongue can be diagnosed by differentiating it from atrophic glossitis, median rhomboidal glossitis, benign migratory glossitis, strawberry tongue.

Causes

Main cause of bald tongue is niacin deficiency which is caused due to alcoholism and digestive system disorder and due to prolonged treatment with isoniazid. Other causes of glossitis include:

1. Iron deficiency anemia mainly caused by blood loss, during gastrointestinal hemorrhage often results in depapillated, atrophic glossitis, giving the tongue bald and shiny appearance, along with pallor lips and tendency towards oral ulceration and cheilosis.

2. Pernicious anemia is usually caused by autoimmune destruction of gastric parietal cells. Parietal cells secrete intrinsic factor, which is required for the absorption of vitamin B_{12}. Vitamin B_{12} deficiency results in megaloblastic anemia and may present as glossitis. The appearance of the tongue in vitamin B_{12} deficiency is described as 'beefy' or 'fiery red and sore'. There may be linear or patchy red lesions.

3. Vitamin B_1 deficiency (thiamine deficiency) can cause glossitis. Vitamin B_2 deficiency can cause glossitis, along with angular cheilitis, cheilosis, peripheral neuropathy and other signs and symptoms. Vitamin B_3 deficiency (pellagra) can cause glossitis. Vitamin B_6 deficiency (pyridoxine deficiency) can cause glossitis, along with angular cheilitis, cheilosis, peripheral neuropathy and seborrheic dermatitis. Folate deficiency (vitamin B_9 deficiency) can cause glossitis, along with macrocytic anemia, thrombocytopenia, leukopenia, diarrhea, fatigue and possibly neurological signs.

4. Bacterial, viral or fungal infections can cause glossitis. *Candida* species are involved in median rhomboid glossitis. *Candida* species also may be involved in creating a more generalized glossitis with erythema, burning, and atrophy, e.g. erythematous candidiasis (e.g. as may occur in HIV/AIDS) may involve the tongue giving glossitis with depapillation.

5. Syphilis is now relatively rare, but the tertiary stage can cause diffuse glossitis and atrophy of lingual papillae, termed "syphilitic glossitis", "luetic glossitis" or "atrophic glossitis of tertiary syphilis". It is caused by *Treponema pallidum* and is a sexually transmitted infection.

Treatment: The goal of treatment is to reduce inflammation. Maintaining good oral hygiene is necessary, including thorough tooth brushing at least twice a day, and flossing at least daily. Corticosteroids such as prednisone may be given to reduce the inflammation of glossitis. For mild cases, topical applications such as a prednisone mouth rinse may be recommended. Antibiotics, antifungal medications, or other antimicrobials may be prescribed if the cause of glossitis is due to infection. Anemia and nutritional deficiencies such as a deficiency in niacin, riboflavin, iron, or vitamin E must be treated, often by dietary changes or other supplements. Avoidance of hot or spicy foods, alcohol, and tobacco is advised to minimize the discomfort.

NUTRITIONAL DEFICIENCIES AND HEMATOLOGIC ABNORMALITIES

The term atrophic glossitis (loss of papillae, redness and painful swelling of the tongue) is used to describe the appearance of the tongue that results from various nutritional deficiencies and hematologic abnormalities. The hunter's glossitis is the term for atrophic glossitis associated with raw, beefy, magenta, bright red tongue.

The redness, loss of papillae, and painful swelling of the tongue are characteristically found in deficiencies of several B vitamins as niacin, riboflavin, pyridoxine, folic acid, and vitamin B_{12}. Similar changes also are associated with iron deficiency. The Plummer-Vinson syndrome/sideropenic anemia manifests as atrophic glossitis, angular cheilitis, generalized atrophic oral mucosa, oral ulcerations, secondary candidiasis, dysphagia and oropharyngeal carcinoma. In many cases, the depapillation of the tongue and atrophic glossitis resolve completely following administration of the appropriate nutritional factor or correction of malabsorption problem.

The medications such as antibiotics, cancer chemotherapeutic agents and anticholinergic agents may also lead to depapillation to cause smooth or bald tongue. Decreased nutritional status of the lingual papillae as a result of vascular changes, chronic xerostomia, chronic candidiasis, diabetes or fibrosis of the submucosal tissues secondary to obliteration of small vessels by an autoimmune process as seen in oral submucous fibrosis, scleroderma, mixed connective tissue disease, and lupus erythematosus may lead to depapillation.

Burning Mouth Syndrome/Glossodynia/Burning Tongue Syndrome

It is characterized by chronic burning sensation of the tongue and other oral mucous membranes in the absence of any identifiable signs or causes. This condition causes burning sensation, loss of taste, and swelling or the feeling of swelling of the tongue. It commonly affects women before or after menopause, the 10 to 20% of the females may be affected. The main cause is not known but it has been commonly associated with medical conditions, e.g. nutritional deficiency.

Traumatic Injuries, Ulcers and Infectious Diseases

Tongue being the central organ in oral cavity is vulnerable for injury from trauma; there can be various reasons for the occurrence of ulcer on tongue. The ulcerations of the tongue result from variety of physical agents and infectious agents. Any jagged, broken cusps or rough surfaces on restorations, biting trauma, oral parafunction/chronic tongue thrusting or sudden blow to jaw may cause ulcerations of the tongue. More chronic ulcers may be seen in patients with uncontrolled grinding and chewing movements as result of *Morsicatio linguarum* or brain damage.

The trauma may be of iatrogenic origin, it may occur while any dental procedures, the fimbriated folds on either side of lingual frenum may get aspirated during dental procedure. The ulcers of the lingual frenum in neonates are due to abrasion of the tongue by lower incisors during suckling, known as Riga's ulcers or Riga-Fede disease.

The vesiculobullous disorders and infectious diseases commonly lead to ulcerations on tongue. Lateral margins and tip of the tongue are frequently involved in severe episodes of recurrent aphthous ulcers and Behçet's syndrome, also the shallow persistent tongue ulcer especially on the posterior ventral surfaces are common in patients with lichen planus. In primary herpes simplex gingivostomatitis, the dorsum, ventral surface and lateral margins of tongue may be ulcerated. Herpes zoster produces a series of ulcers along the anterior third of the tongue unilaterally.

In addition, the ulcerative and proliferative lesions of the tongue occur in a number of chronic granulomatous infections such as tuberculosis, histoplasmosis, blastomycosis, cryptococosis, sporotrichosis, mucormycosis, primary and secondary syphilis, and lymphogranuloma venerum. The multiple pseudomembranous ulcerations of the tongue and palate have been noted with septicemia caused by *Capnocytophaga* species in granulocytopenic patients. The tongue involvement is common in acute necrotizing ulcerative gingivitis; chronic low grade fevers such as scarlet fever, typhoid fever, and *Haemophilus influenzae* B infections. In tertiary syphilis, the characteristic lesion forms on the tongue known as gumma. The soft tissue infections of the tongue frequently reveal *Streptococci* and anaerobes, the Ludwig's angina is characterized by an indurated swelling of the whole floor of the mouth and base of the tongue, which pushes the tongue upward and prevents the patient from closing the mouth. Dysphagia and upper airway obstruction are common complications. Lingual mucosal glands are affected in Sjögren's syndrome and pan sialadenitis. Large cysts of the sublingual glands that often distend the overlying floor of the mouth and displace the tongue are referred to as ranula.

The various nutritional deficiencies, hematological problems and patients with xerostomia frequently show ulcerations on tongue. The solitary eosinophilic ulcer or traumatic granuloma of the tongue sometimes

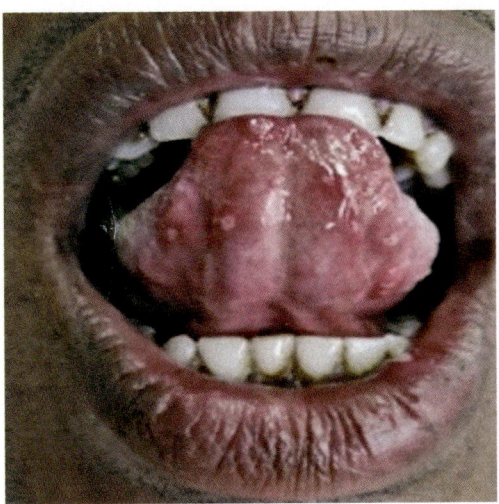

Fig. 13.5: Aphthous ulcers on tongue

mistakenly diagnosed as carcinoma, though it is rapidly developing histologically reveals no evidence of carcinoma and that contains numerous eosinophils. Such ulcers heal spontaneously in 2 to 3 weeks.

Diseases Affecting the Body of the Tongue

In amyloidosis, the amyloid gets deposited in the tongue. The tongue may be diffusely enlarged or is the site of nodular deposits or is unaffected, the enlarged tongue can affect the dentition, chewing, swallowing and speaking. The various neuromuscular disorders of central, peripheral or muscular origin, e.g. hypoglossal nerve weakness, parkinsonism, tardive dyskinesia, various muscular dystrophies and athetosis may produce symptoms of dysphagia, speech chewing problems due to the involvement of tongue. Angioneurotic edema is an acute anaphylactic reaction representing an immediate hypersensitivity response to antigenic stimuli. It manifests as a swelling of the tongue, glottis and laryngeal structures with rapid occlusion of the airway.

The tongue is a frequent site for the oral cancer and many red and white lesions that are considered to have malignant potential. The tongue is common site of oral cavity for

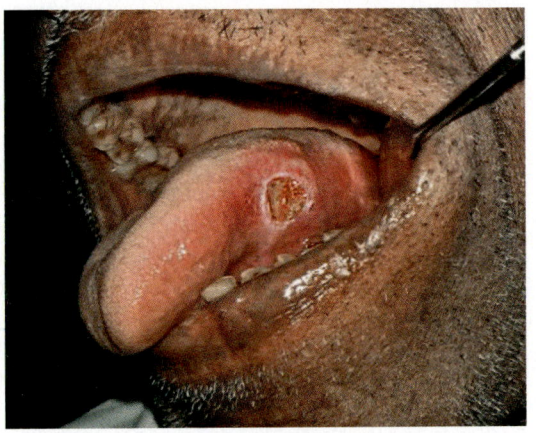

Fig. 13.4: Traumatic ulcer

the involvement by squamous cell carcinoma (SCC); more than 90% malignant tumors of the tongue are SCC. On the tongue, SCC predominantly occurs on lateral borders and ventral surface of tongue. It is manifested in middle and later decades of life (median age 60 years) with male predilection although now it is apparent in younger age group also. It commonly presents as an exophytic growth and an ulcer, the local infiltration and lymphadenopathy are the common features. The etiology is the tobacco consumption, alcohol, chronic dental trauma, it is also been related to syphilis, infection with *C. albicans*, iron deficiency, virus infection. The thorough clinical evaluation is essential for the involvement of oral cavity, base, pharynx and floor and lymph nodes. Chronic ulcer should be biopsied if it does not regress promptly following removal of a suspected irritant.

Treatment depends on TNM staging, the smaller size or early carcinomas are mostly treated by surgical excision or radiation with predictive 5-year survival rate of more than 50%. The advanced carcinoma of the tongue (T3 category) is treated by combined surgical and radiation therapy with 5-year survival rate is 10 to 30%. The advanced stages of node involvement are usually treated by mandibulectomy and radical neck dissection. The prognosis and survival depend upon the degree of local infiltration involving base and the floor, metastasis to submandibular, jugulodigastric and cervical lymph nodes.

The benign tumors of the tongue such as irritation fibromas, tongue papillomas, granular cell myoblastoma, viral-induced keratoacanthoma. These hyperplasias may resemble carcinomas, the presence or absence of cellular atypia separates these hyperplasias from carcinomas.

The tongue lesions occur in the population with significant prevalence. Hence, oral health professionals should be trained enough to evaluate and diagnose the etiology of tongue lesions so that proper treatment can be instilled.

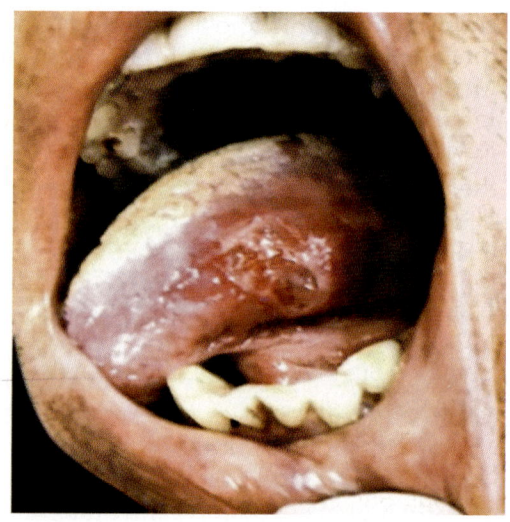

Fig. 13.6: Malignant ulcer involving lateral border of tongue

FREQUENTLY ASKED QUESTIONS

1. Median rhomboid glossitis
2. Depapillation of tongue
3. Geographic tongue

BIBLIOGRAPHY

1. Malcolm A. Lynch, Vernon, J. Brightman, Martin S. Greenberg. Burket's Oral Medicine, Diagnosis and treatment, 8th ed. J. B. Lippincott Company, Philadelphia, 1984.
2. Shafer WG, Hine MK, Levy BM. "A Textbook of Oral Pathology" 1983, 4th ed, WB Saunders Company, Philadelphia.
3. Malcolm A. Lynch, Vernon, J. Brightman, Martin S. Greenberg. Burket's Oral Medicine, Diagnosis and Treatment. 9th ed, J. B. Lippincott Company, Philadelphia 1994; 204–205.
4. B.D. Chaurasia. Human Anatomy. Regional and applied dissection and clinical, Volume 3, Head, neck and brain, Fourth Edition, 2004.
5. Wood NK, Goaz PW. Differential diagnosis of oral and maxillofacial lesions. 5th ed, Harcourt Brace and Company Asia PTE Ltd.
6. Brad W. Neville, Douglas D. Damm, Carl M. Allen, Jerry E. Bouquot: Oral and Maxillofacial Pathology, 2nd ed, 2004.
7. George Laskaris. Pocket Atlas of Oral Diseases, 2nd edition, 2006, Stuttgart, New York.

8. Mahmoud M. Tongue disorders changes in tongue coating Umm Al-Qura University, Makkah, KSA.

9. International Classification of Diseases, 10th Revision.

10. ICD-10 Category K14, ICD-10 Codes for Diseases of tongue.
http//:D201020Codes20Diseases20of20 tongue.html

11. Anuradha Sunil, Jacob Kurien, Archana Mukunda, Ashik Bin Basheer, Deepthi. Common Superficial Tongue Lesions. Indian Journal of Clinical Practice, Vol. 23, No. 9 February 2013.

12. G. Uma Devi, T. Ravi. Disease Diagnosis for Various Signs using Tongue Color Image Segmentation. Aust. J. Basic and Appl. Sci. 9(10): 341–348, 20.

13. Nadkarni N. Tuberculosis of tongue: A case report. Ind J Tub 1997;44:31–3.

14. Mathew Iype E, Pandey M, Mathew A, Thomas G, Sebastian P, Krishnan Nair M. Squamous cell carcinoma of the tongue among young Indian adults. Neoplasia 2001;3(4):273–7.

15. Kojima, K. Clinical studies on the coated tongue. Japanese J Oral Maxillofac Sur, 31, 1985, 1659–1676.

16. Shimizu, T., Ueda T., Sakurai K. New method for evaluation of tongue coating status. J Oral Rehabil, Jun 2007;34(6):442–447. [PubMed] [CrossRef]

17. Bhargava P, Kuldeep CM, Mathur NK. Isolated pemphigus vegetans of the tongue. Indian J Dermatol Venereol Leprol 2001; 67(5):267.

18. Goregen M, Miloglu O, Buyukkurt MC, Caglayan F, Aktas AE. Median rhomboid glossitis: a clinical and microbiological study. Eur J Dent 2011;5(4):367–72.

19. Vañó-Galván S, Jaén P. Black hairy tongue. Cleve Clin J Med 2008;75(12):847–8.

14

Cardiovascular Diseases— Oral Manifestations and Dental Considerations

INTRODUCTION

Cardiovascular diseases (CVD) have now become the most leading cause for mortality worldwide, as well as in India. More than 80% of cardiovascular deaths are predominantly seen in ischemic heart disease and stroke. The age-standardized CVD death rate in India is higher (i.e. 272 per 100,000 population) in comparison to the global burden (i.e. 235 per 100,000 population). Because of the high prevalence of the CVDs and its impact on the overall health of the patient's, the dentist should have a thorough knowledge on oral manifestations and dental considerations for efficient management.

Eliciting History and Clinical Manifestations Amongst Cardiovascular Patients

Cardiovascular history is fundamental for accurate diagnosis and management of the patients. Table 14.1 illustrates assessment criteria for cardiovascular diseases.

CARDIOVASCULAR DISORDERS

Hypertension

Definition: Hypertension is defined as having systolic blood pressure ≥140 mmHg or diastolic blood pressure ≥90 mmHg or as having to use antihypertensive medications.

Etiology and Classification (*refer* to Tables 14.2 and 14.3).

TABLE 14.1: Assessment criteria for cardiovascular diseases

- Past and family history
- Risk factors
- Chest pain
- Shortness of the breath (dyspnea)
- Palpitations
- Dizziness and unsteadiness
- Syncope
- Fatigue
- Bilateral ankle edema
- Discomfort and pain in lower limb
- Cyanosis

TABLE 14.2: Causes of hypertension

Primary hypertension (Idiopathic or essential): Cause unknown in ninety-five percent cases

Secondary hypertension occurs due to secondary causes such as:
- Renal disorders (renal parenchymal disease, renovascular disease, renin-producing tumors, primary sodium retention).
- Endocrine abnormalities (Cushing's syndrome, thyroid disease, primary aldosteronism, pheochromocytoma)
- Aortic coarctation

Contd.

TABLE 14.2: Causes of hypertension *(Contd.)*

- Complications of pregnancy (pre-eclampsia)
- Neurologic diseases × Stress × Alcoholism
- Drug-induced (cyclosporine, tacrolimus, sympathomimetics, steroid hormone, COX-1 and COX-2 inhibitors)

Malignant hypertension
- Systolic BP ≥240 mmHg and diastolic BP ≥ 120 mmHg
- It is associated with organ damage (eyes, kidneys, brain, lungs are affected).

White coat hypertension: Elevated BP in clinical setting/ hospital but not when ambulatory/ home.

TABLE 14.3:

Blood pressure classification	Systolic BP (mmHg)	Diastolic BP (mmHg)
Optimal	<120	<80
Normal	<130	<85
Prehypertension	120–139	80–89
Hypertension		
Stage 1 (mild)	140–159	90–99
Stage 2 (moderate)	160–179	100–109
Stage 3 (severe)	≥180	≥110
Isolated systolic hypertension	≥140	<90

Clinical Manifestations

Generally asymptomatic for many years

Type	Clinical manifestation
Early symptoms	Occipital headache, vision changes, ringing ears, dizziness, weakness, nose bleeding, odontalgia
Signs	Visual changes, enlarged left side of heart, deteriorated renal function are complications of arteriosclerosis
Chronic hypertension	Encephalopathy, a cerebrovascular accident, coronary artery disease, angina pectoris, myocardial infarction, congestive heart failure, aortic aneurysms, hematuria and proteinuria.
Malignant hypertension	Severe kidney damage.

Oral Manifestations

Oral manifestations are a result of antihypertensive medications or occur when target organ disease is present.

TABLE 14.4: Oral adverse effects of antihypertensive medications

Side effects	Drugs
Dry mouth	Diuretics, ACE inhibitors, central acting adrenergic inhibitors.
Lichenoid reaction	Furosemide, labetalol, methyldopa, propranolol and thiazides.
Loss of taste, dry mouth, angioedema	ACE inhibitors
Gingival enlargement, dry mouth, altered taste	Calcium channel blockers
Dry mouth, taste changes, parotid pain	Central acting drugs
Dry mouth, angioedema, sinusitis, taste loss	Angiotensin II antagonists
Lupus-like facial rash	Hydralazine, nifedipine, verapamil, diltiazem.

- Excessive bleeding after surgical procedure may be a complication of severe hypertension.

Diagnosis

Periodic measurement of blood pressure (BP) can be recorded using sphygmomanometer. The patient should be at rest and relaxed.

Measurement of Blood Pressure (BP)

The direct intra-arterial measurement with a catheter is considered a standard measurement tool of BP. Since its an invasive procedure, some indirect methods have been commonly used to assess BP like palpatory and auscultatory methods. The pressure cuff of a sphygmomanometer is wrapped around the arm of the patient an inch above the ante-cubital fossa.

- **Palpatory method:** Palpate for the radial pulse with three fingers (index, middle and ring finger) on the radial artery. Now, inflate the cuff slowly (10 mmHg/sec) in increments, until no longer the radial pulse felt. The cuff inflated further until the pressure is 30 mmHg higher. Deflate the cuff slowly (5 mmHg/sec), the first pulsatile trill appears will be systolic pressure and, the disappearance of the trill is the diastolic BP.

× **Auscultatory method:** Brachial pulse is palpated at the anticubital fossa, followed by placement of the diaphragm of the stethoscope over the artery. In this method the cuff is inflated to a level 30 mmHg above systolic pressure as determined by palpatory method. The cuff is gradually deflated 5 mmHg; arterial pulse (Korotkoff sounds) appears which is the systolic BP, then the sounds totally disappear. The total disappearance of sounds is diastolic BP.

At least two or three separate readings provide the most accurate assessment of BP.

Management

× Treatment depends on stage of disease
× Patients with mild and moderate hypertension should be managed non-pharmacologically:
  ▪ They are advised to restrict salt intake, fatty foods
  ▪ Weight control
  ▪ Avoid smoking
  ▪ Restricting alcohol and caffeine
  ▪ Regular exercise
× Antihypertensive medications advised for other stages of hypertension
× In patients with secondary hypertension, treat the primary cause.

Antihypertensive Medications

TABLE 14.5: Antihypertensive medications

Direct-acting vasodilators: Nitroglycerin, hydralazine, minoxidil, sodium nitroprusside, diazoxide.

Angiotensin II receptor blocker: Losartan, candesartan, valsartan, irbesartan

Diuretics
× Thiazides: Hydrochlorothiazide, chlorthalidone
× High ceiling: Furosemide
× K+ sparing: Spironolactone, amiloride

ACE inhibitors: Captopril, enalopril, lisinopril, perindopril, ramipril, fosinopril

Calcium channel blockers: Verapamil, dlltiazem, nifedipine, felodipine, amlodipine, nitrendipine, lacipine

β-adrenergic blockers: Propranolol, metoprolol, atenolol

β + α-adrenergic blockers: Labetolol, carvedilol

α-adrenergic blockers: Prazosin, terazosin, doxazosin, phentalamine, phenoxybenzamine

Central sympatholytics: Clonidine, methyldopa

Dental Considerations

× Patient assessment is important prior dental treatment in terms of medical history, drug history, controlled or uncontrolled hypertension.
× Elicit history for presence of end organ disease or on antihypertensive medication.
× Schedule short appointments for patients who receive dental treatment.
× Ensure adequate anesthesia to reduce anxiety and pain as it may induce dysrhythmias.
× Prior anesthesia ensure syringe aspiration to prevent the entry of epinephrine into blood vessels.
× Epinephrine in local anesthesia (LA) not contraindicated unless systolic BP is above 200 mmHg and/or diastolic BP 115 mmHg.
× LA with epinephrine in large doses should be avoided in patients with non-selective beta blockers.
× Gingival retraction cords containing epinephrine should be avoided.
× Concentrations of epinephrine greater than 1:100,000 are avoided as it carries a higher risk, and New York Heart Association recommends not more than 0.04 mg of epinephrine with heart disease.
× A substitution to epinephrine is levonordefrin at concentration of 1:20,000.

- Patients with history of combined multiple antihypertensive medications are more difficult to manage than on patients with one or two medications.
- Record blood pressure prior initiating any dental treatment.

The guidelines for BP monitoring:
- Recheck every two years for patients with BP <120/80 mmHg
- Every year for patients with BP 120–139/80–89 mmHg
- Every visit for patients with BP >140–90 mmHg
- Every visit for patients with underlying systemic disease with BP >135–85 mmHg
- Every visit with established hypertension

Modifications of dental treatment in patients with elevated BP
- *Asymptomatic:* If no history of target organ disease and BP <159/99 mmHg, patient can be treated without any modifications in a dental outpatient setting.
- *Asymptomatic:* If BP 160–179/100–109 mmHg and no history of target organ disease, dental treatment depends on risk assessment of an individual.
- If BP >180/110 mmHg, no history of target organ damage, then no elective dental care should be performed.
- Medically compromised patients with end organ disease and uncontrolled diabetes mellitus, no elective treatment until BP is controlled.
- Dentist should be aware of drug interactions with antihypertensive medication and their side effects, i.e. orthostatic hypotension is a major side effect in patients taking antihypertensive medications.

Ischemic or Coronary Heart Disease

The decreased oxygen supply to heart for long-term leads to ischemic heart disease.

Causes

Atherosclerosis	Aortic stenosis
Hypertension	Congenital heart disease
Aneurysm	Thrombus formation

◆ Angina Pectoris

Angina pectoris is an ischemic heart disease that occurs secondary to atherosclerosis in the walls of the arteries, leading to stenosis and reduced blood flow to heart. It is characterized by paroxysmal thoracic pain due to deprivation in oxygen to the myocardium. The pain occurs when cardiac work and oxygen demand exceed the supply of oxygen. It is precipitated by increased physical exercise, emotional stress, cold weather, smoking.

Clinical Features

Age	Occur in older individuals
Chest pain	Classically described as a sense of choking, tightness, heaviness, compression of the chest
Levine's sign	Patients make a fist over the location of pain on chest
Radiation of pain	Shoulders, arm, fingers, neck, mandible and sometimes teeth

Management

1. Control risk factors such as smoking, hypertension, fatty foods and strenuous exercise.
2. Pharmacologic mode of management
   a. *Nitrates:* These are first line of drugs—it has a vasodilation property, can be administered sublingually at the dose of 0.3–0.6 mg.
   b. *Beta-adrenergic blockers:* These are second line therapy when nitrates fail to respond. It improves myocardial oxygen consumption by inhibiting the sympathetic nervous system.
   c. *Calcium channel blockers:* These medications prevent calcium entry to the myocardium, thereby preventing contraction, and also relax smooth vessels of blood vessels, thereby dilating the coronary artery and thus increases oxygen supply.

Flowchart 14.1: Variants of angina

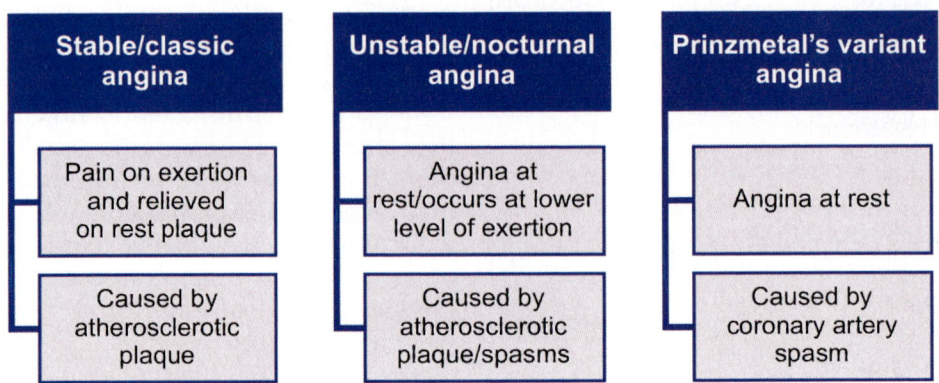

3. Other modalities when pharmacotherapy fails:
   a. Coronary angiography
   b. Coronary artery bypass grafting (CABG)
   c. Percutaneous transluminal coronary angioplasty (PTCA)

Anticoagulants such as aspirin are commonly prescribed following CABG and PTCA.

Oral Manifestations

- Pain in jaws and teeth
- Occasionally burning sensation in the tongue and hard palate
- Concurrent chest pain and orofacial pain
- Orofacial manifestations secondary to antianginal medications are as follows:
  - Nitroglycerin administration has a side effect of burning sensation at the site of placement and headache due to rapid vasodilatation property.
  - Calcium channel blockers cause gingival enlargement.

Dental Considerations

- Schedule short mid-morning appointments to reduce stress
- Employ good sedation techniques that are not cardio depressing
- Use of epinephrine at the dose of 0.04 mg
- Avoid epinephrine impregnated gingival cord

- Encourage use of alternative vasoconstrictors such as phenylephrine (1:2,500); levonordefrin (1:20,000).
- Availability of nitroglycerine, oxygen and emergency equipment readily available. Antibiotic prophylaxis prior dental treatment in patients with coronary bypass operation.

Management of angina attack on the dental chair:
- Dentist should discontinue the dental treatment immediately.
- Place patient in the supine position and ensure good airway.
- Administer sublingual nitroglycerin
- Monitor vital signs
- If clinical signs of cyanosis is evident, supplement oxygen therapy, followed by 2nd tablet of sublingual nitrates, if ineffective an amylnitrite ampule is broken and held under patients nose to enhance vasodilatation. No relief even after 10 minutes, a third tablet of nitroglycerin is administered. Even after 3 tablets, symptoms are unresolved, suspect myocardial infarction that warrants medical emergency.

◈ Myocardial Infarction (MI)

It is the severe form of coronary artery disease; it occurs if an angina attack persists longer than 30 minutes. Acute MI is an irreversible ischemic event that produces an area of myocardial necrosis.

TABLE 14.6: Myocardial infarction: Causes and clinical features

Causes	Clinical features of MI
× Coronary atherosclerosis × Thrombosis × Vasospasm × Increased myocardial demand × Coronary artery occlusion	× Substernal pain × Palpitations, dizziness, vomiting × Shortness of breath, cough × Patient becomes pale, vital signs are unstable, increased BP, weak thready/absent pulse

Oral Manifestations and Dental Considerations

× The oral manifestations are similar to angina pectoris but with greater severity in pain.
× Physician consent is mandatory prior to any dental treatment as these patients are on anticoagulants in order to prevent thromboembolic event.
× Defer dental treatment with recent MI within 6 months
× Provide effective local anesthesia
× Premedication with antianxiety drugs
× Schedule appointments either in late mornings or early noon.
× Elective procedures, especially that require general anesthesia should be avoided at least for the first 4 weeks following MI, as there is increased risk of re-infarction.

Management of MI in Dental Office

× Monitor vital signs every 5 minutes
× Provide oxygen therapy
× Give analgesic nitrous oxide at the rate of 5 L/min to calm the patient and limit the release of catecholamines, which might trigger arrhythmias
× Perform resuscitative procedure
× Administer 2 mg of intravenous morphine for pain relief
× Availability of emergency drugs such as atropine, lidocaine, phenylephrine readily available.

Infective Endocarditis and Associated Disease

◆ Rheumatic Fever (RF)

× RF is an autoimmune inflammatory condition that follows infection caused by group A beta-hemolytic streptococci.
× RF precedes with pharyngitis and sore throat.

Clinical Features

Major manifestations	Minor manifestations
Carditis	Arthralgia
Chorea	Fever
Erythema marginatum	Abnormal C reactive protein
Polyarthritis	Previous RF of rheumatic heart disease
Subcutaneous nodules	Characteristic ECG recording

Oral Manifestations

× Oropharyngitis
× Increased oral temperature
× Edematous and erythematous soft palate
× Tonsillar ulcerations
× Skin rashes (erythema marginatum)
× Gingiva is usually spared

Dental Considerations

× Physician consent prior any dental treatment
× Risk of developing infective endocarditis (IE), hence treatment and precautions similar to IE.
× Avoid general anesthesia

◆ Rheumatic Heart Disease

It is an autoimmune, non-suppurative disease of the heart that occurs subsequent to acute rheumatic fever.

Clinical findings: Heart murmur, tachycardia, arrhythmias may be present.

Oral manifestations and dental considerations:

* Oropharyngitis and increased oral temperature
* Progressive disease leads to congestive heart disease produces distended neck veins and bluish color over skin.
* Prescribe antibiotic prophylaxis prior dental treatment.

◆ Infective Endocarditis (IE) (Table 14.7)

Etiopathogenesis

Flowchart 14.2

IE is a cardiac infection preceded by bacteremia and fungemia

Microbes enter circulation from mouth, GIT, genitourinary tract

These microorganisms adhere to damaged heart valves, indwelling catheter, shunts

This produces turbulent blood flow and provide suitable environment for colonization of microorganisms and cardiac damage

Cardiac damage is through microbial proliferation and cardiac tissue destruction, microbial vegetations into circulation and production of immune complexes

TABLE 14.7: Infective endocarditis

IE based on clinical presentation	Organisms
Sub-acute IE	Alpha-hemolytic Streptococcus: *Streptococcus viridians*
Acute IE	*Staphylococcus aureus*
Chronic IE	*Streptococcus faecalis*

Clinical Findings

Age	Affects older individuals
Symptoms	Low-grade fever, malaise, lethargy, weight loss, joint pains, dyspnea, orthopnea, hematuria, café-au-lait pigmentation on skin.
Signs	Anemia, heart murmur, vasculitis, evidence of sublingual hemorrhages, petechial hemorrhages, Osler's nodes, Roth's spots, Janeway's lesions, Splenomegaly

Oral Manifestations and Dental Considerations (Table 14.8)

* Pallor mucous membrane and facial skin
* Mucosal petechiae that do not blanch under pressure
* Followed by purpuric lesions

TABLE 14.8: Oral manifestations and dental considerations

Dental procedures, which require antibiotic prophylaxis	Procedures, which do not require antibiotic coverage
Periodontal probing and sub-gingival procedures, which elicits bleeding	Exfoliation of primary teeth
Extractions	Making of impressions
Surgical procedures	Non-surgical procedures that do not induce bleeding
Operative procedure requiring manipulation beyond the apex	Taking radiographs
Raising mucogingival flaps/ periodontal surgeries	Removal of orthodontic bands and brackets
Implant placement	Adjustment and placement orthodontic brackets
Administering LA	
Sialography	
Wedge placement, rubber dam and matrix band placement	

TABLE 14.9: Therapeutic regimens for a dental procedure

Situation	Agent	Adult	Children
Oral	Amoxicillin	2 gm	50 mg/kg
Unable to take oral medication	Ampicillin or cephazolin or ceftriaxone	2 gm IM* or IV# 1 gm IM or IV	50 mg/kg IM or IV 50 mg/kg IM or IV
Allergic to penicillins or ampicillin—oral	Cephalexin^{Φδ} or clindamycin or azithromycin or clarithromycin	2 gm 600 mg 500 mg	50 mg/kg 20 mg/kg 15 mg/kg
Allergic to penicillins or ampicillin and unable to take oral medication	Cephazolin or ceftriaxone^{δ} or clindamycin	1 gm IM or IV 600 mg IM or IV	50 mg/kg IM or IV 20 mg/kg IM or IV

*IM: Intramuscular; #IV: Intravenous
^{Φ} or other first or second-generation oral cephalosporins in equivalent adult or pediatric dosage
^{δ} Cephalosporins should not be used in an individual with a history of anaphylaxis, angioedema, or urticaria with penicillins and ampicillin.

Cardiac diseases that require antibiotic prophylaxis for dental treatment

✕ Prosthetic heart valve	✕ History of IE
✕ Congenital heart disease	✕ Heart transplantation

Congenital Heart Disease

It is the most common heart disease amongst children.

Classification

Flowchart 14.3 describes classification of congenital heart disease.

Flowchart 14.3: Classification of congenital heart disease

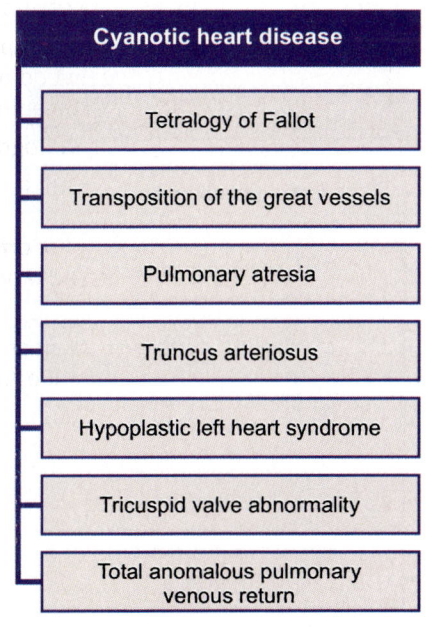
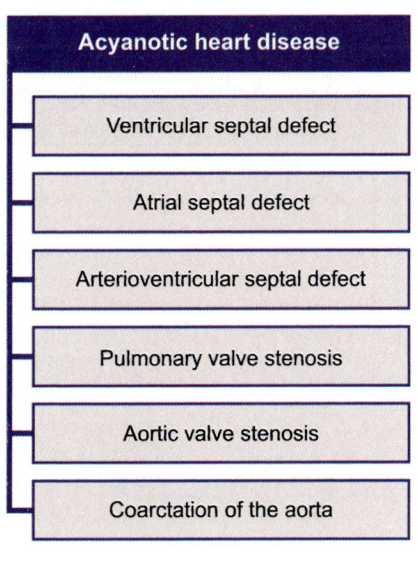

Cyanotic heart disease
- Tetralogy of Fallot
- Transposition of the great vessels
- Pulmonary atresia
- Truncus arteriosus
- Hypoplastic left heart syndrome
- Tricuspid valve abnormality
- Total anomalous pulmonary venous return

Acyanotic heart disease
- Ventricular septal defect
- Atrial septal defect
- Arterioventricular septal defect
- Pulmonary valve stenosis
- Aortic valve stenosis
- Coarctation of the aorta

Oral Manifestations and Dental Considerations

* Cyanosis of mucosa, lips and auricles of ear
* Cleft palate
* Midline abnormalities
* Growth anomalies of primary teeth
* Delayed eruption of both primary and permanent teeth
* Hypoplastic enamel
* Increased incidence of dental decay
* Antibiotic prophylaxis to prevent infective endocarditis prior dental treatment.
* Bleeding tendencies due to platelet dysfunction and excessive fibrinolytic activity.

Heart Failure (Congestive Heart Failure)

Heart failure is a clinical syndrome where the heart muscle fails to contract adequately resulting in inadequate cardiac output and reduced oxygenated blood supply to end organs. Failure of heart can be either left-sided or right-sided.

Causes

Flowchart 14.4 describes causes of heart failure.

Clinical Findings

Manifestations in left-sided heart failure	Manifestations in right-sided heart failure
Symptoms are related to pulmonary edema	Symptoms are related to congestion of blood both systemically and in the portal hypertension
Tachycardia	Hepatomegaly
Fatigue on exertion	Distended neck veins
Dyspnea	Fullness in abdomen
Cough	

Oral Manifestations

* Infections
* *Bleeding tendencies:* Petechiae, ecchymosis
* Drug-related xerostomia
* Lichenoid mucosal lesions
* Distension of neck veins (external jugular vein)

Dental Considerations

* Obtain medical consultation prior initiating dental treatment
* Administration of prophylactic antibiotics

Flowchart 14.4: Causes of heart failure

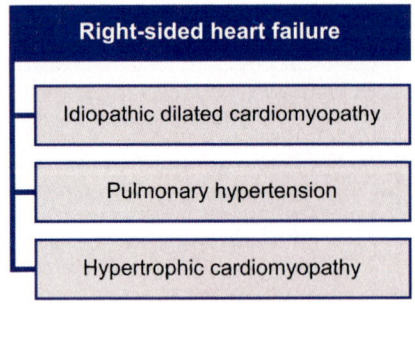

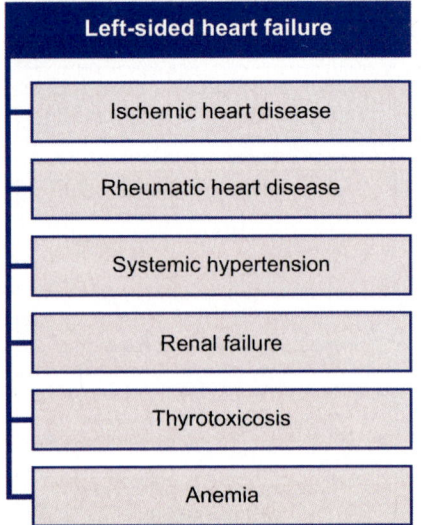

- Defer dental care for 6 months of recent MI
- Monitor blood levels of digitalis for evaluation of digitalis toxicity and may cause vomiting and nausea
- Monitor vital signs
- Prefer upright dental chair position as supine position of patient may precipitate pulmonary complications and cause dyspnea
- Avoid respiratory depressant medication during treatment
- Advise complete blood count prior any surgical procedures
- Elective surgery with patients under general anesthesia is relatively contraindicated because of cardiac–depressant effect of volatile anesthesia
- NSAIDs other than aspirin should be avoided in patients with ACE inhibitors, as there is risk of kidney damage.
- Schedule appointment in late morning as there is peak endogenous epinephrine at early morning
- Use of electromechanical toothbrushes for effective cleaning of teeth
- Use of hemostatic agents over the extraction sites.

FREQUENTLY ASKED QUESTIONS

1. Oral manifestations/dental considerations of cardiovascular diseases.
2. Angina pectoris
3. Discuss the prophylactic regimen for SABE.

BIBLIOGRAPHY

1. Prabhakaran D, Jeemon P, Roy A. Cardiovascular Diseases in India: Current Epidemiology and Future Directions. Circulation 2016:19;133(16):1605–20.
2. Greenberg MS, Glick M, Ship JA. Burket's Oral Medicine. 11th ed. BC Decker Inc. 2008. p.77–106.
3. Greenberg MS, Glick M, Ship JA. Burket's Oral Medicine. 12th ed. Jaypee Brothers Medical Publishers, Pvt. Ltd. 2015. p.91–122.
4. Greenberg MS, Glick M, Ship JA. Burket's Oral Medicine. 10th ed. BC Decker Inc. 2008. p.85–125.
5. Bricker SL, Langlais RP, Miller CS. Oral Diagnosis, Oral Medicine and Treatment Planning. 2nd Ed. BC Decker Inc. 2002.
6. Glynn M, Drake WM. Hutchinson's Clinical Methods. 24th Ed. Elsevier, 2014.
7. Walker BR, Colledge NR, Ralston SH, Penman ID. Davidson's Principles and Practice of Medicine, International Edition, 22nd Ed. S Chand, 2014.

Respiratory Disorder— Oral Manifestations and Dental Considerations

INTRODUCTION

Patients with respiratory disorders have an increased risk of morbidity on a dental chair due to reduced pulmonary function, medications that they take, drug interactions and risk of disease transmission. Thus, there is a need for understanding clinical manifestations, diagnosis, oral manifestations, oral health considerations and management.

Functions of the Lung

Ventilatory function	Non-ventilatory function
Gaseous exchange: It involves exchange of carbon dioxide and oxygen gases between the circulating blood and air in the alveolus	Defense against noxious atmospheric substance
Oxygen supply to end organs	Conversion of angiotensin I to angiotensin II, which is the potent vasoconstrictor by endothelial cells of the lung.
	Metabolism of bradykinin, serotonin and some prostaglandins

Medical History and System Review

× Breathing difficulties
× Frequent upper respiratory infections
× Cough (productive or nonproductive)
× Hoarseness, dyspnea, production of sputum, hemoptysis, wheeze, chest pain.
× Abnormalities in size and shape of the lung
  ▪ Barrel-shaped chest—find in asthma and emphysema
  ▪ Pigeon chest find in asthma of early childhood
  ▪ Flattening of upper anterior chest in fibrosis of lung
  ▪ Distended veins on chest and jugular veins—superior vene cava obstruction and portal hypertension.

CLASSIFICATION OF RESPIRATORY DISEASES

Table 15.1 provides classification of respiratory diseases.

TABLE 15.1: Classification of respiratory diseases

Upper respiratory infections
× The common cold
× Sinusitis
× Pharyngitis and tonsillitis
× Laryngitis

Contd.

TABLE 15.1: Classification of respiratory diseases (*Contd.*)

Lower respiratory disorders
* Asthma
* Chronic obstructive pulmonary disease
  + Chronic bronchitis
  + Emphysema
* Pulmonary foreign bodies
* Pneumonitis
* Granulomatous lung disease
  + Tuberculosis
  + Sarcoidosis

Occupational lung disease
* Pneumoconiosis

Other diseases affecting the respiratory tract
* Histoplasmosis
* Wegener's granulomatosis
* Midline granuloma
* Cystic fibrosis

Upper Respiratory Infections

◈ The Common Cold (Acute Rhinitis, Coryza)

Description

* It is the most common infection of upper respiratory tract caused by group of viruses
* Common cold lasts for 5–7 days.

Etiology

* Rhinovirus, coxsackie virus A21, respiratory syncytial virus, parainfluenza virus
* The mode of spread is through aerosol droplets, hand to hand and body to body contact.

Clinical Features

* Rhinorrhea (nasal discharge)
* Nasal congestion
* Often precedes sore throat
* Associated with other symptoms such as headache, cough, fever, myalgia.

Treatment

* **Antihistamines:** These medications reduce nasal secretion

* **Sympathomimetic amines (phenyl propanolamine):** These medications relieve nasal congestion
* **Symptomatic therapy:** These medications include analgesics, antipyretics and fluid intake to treat myalgias, fever and dehydration respectively.
* **Antibiotics:** These medications have no role in treating common cold until secondarily infected with bacterias.

◈ Sinusitis

Description

* It is the inflammation of sinus secondary to bacteria or viral infections.
* It could be a sequelae of common cold
* Infective organisms causing sinusitis: *Streptococcus pyogenes*, *Staphylococcus aureus*, and *Haemophilus influenzae* are the most common organism among children.

Clinical Features

* Severe pain localized to the region of sinus involved
* This can be accompanied with headache, fever, malaise
* Edema and erythematous areas over the malar eminence
* Referred pain in the maxillary teeth (especially in premolars and molars) may seek for dental treatment
* Morning headache is the common symptom that disappears gradually during day because of the upright position
* Postnasal discharge.

Diagnosis

* It is based on history
* Transillumination test: It usually appears dull
* Increased pain on firm pressure over the sinus
* Radiographic evaluation (intraoral periapical radiographs, occlusal films and paranasal view)
* Computed tomography

Treatment

- Sinusitis cannot be differentiated as viral of bacterial, therefore, first line of medication irrespective of causative organism would be antibiotics along with sympathomimetic medication.
- If found no relief on medication, surgical drainage can be performed.

◈ Pharyngitis and Tonsillitis

Description

Inflammation of mucosa and lymphoid tissue in pharynx is termed pharyngitis and tonsillitis respectively.

Etiology

Infection from herpes simplex virus, infectious mononucleosis, group A beta hemolytic streptococci and rarely diphtheria.

Clinical Features

- Sore throat, dysphagia, may be associated with common cold
- Extreme pain, swelling, dysphagia in case of peritonsillar abscess, which is the serious illness because of possible extension of infection to the deeper structures.

Diagnosis

- Throat culture to differentiate viral and bacterial pharyngitis
- Differential white cell count and mononucleosis antibody tests.

Treatment

- If it is due to viral etiology, treat symptomatically such as analgesics, decongestants and antihistamines
- If it is because of bacterial origin, it should be treated with beta-lactam antibiotics
- Among children, amoxicillin is the choice of drug if *H. influenzae* is the etiologic agent.

Oral Manifestations and Dental Considerations in Upper Respiratory Diseases

- Multiple oral ulcerations are the most common feature of respiratory diseases. Erythema multiforme and acute ulcerative gingivitis are noted as late manifestation.
- **Herpangina:** Multiple painful ulcers often preceded by vesicles involving posterior pharynx. The gingiva remains unaffected.
- The anatomic relation of maxillary premolars and molars are in close relation with maxillary sinus, maxillary sinusitis can cause pain resembling the tooth pain. The associated teeth may be tender on percussion and feel elongated.
- Radiographs of the sinuses (panoramic and water's view) show a cloudy antrum, generalized thickening of mucosal lining, a fluid level and often polyps.
- Periapical abscess of maxillary premolars and molars occasionally open into the maxillary sinus. The infected tooth may produce foul smelling, nasal discharge and halitosis, whereas sinusitis produces headache-like pain without bad odor. Pain aggravation on bending head forward suggests sinusitis.
- The paresthesia of the sinus region may indicate malignant growth in the sinus.
- During extraction the root stump can be forced into the maxillary sinus, this event should be reported to the patient and an oral surgeon should attempt to remove the root piece.
- Following the removal of the root piece near the maxillary sinus, there is impaired healing and results in an exophytic tissue growth, which tends to bleed.
- Radicular cyst of maxillary premolars and molars when secondarily infected encroached on sinus; it is been misdiagnosed as acute sinusitis and treated inappropriately. Suitable investigations are required for correct management.

Lower Respiratory Tract Infections

◈ Asthma

Description

- It is a respiratory disorder associated with hyperactivity of airway that produces recurrent bronchial smooth muscle contraction, inflammation and swelling of bronchial smooth muscle resulting in narrowing of airways.
- There is hypersecretion of thick mucosa results in sputum plugging with subsequent increased airway resistance to expiration, and the lungs become hyperinflated.

Etiology

- Allergens, upper respiratory tract infections, exercise, cold air
- Medications such as salicylates, NSAIDs, cholinergic medication and beta-adrenergic blocking agents
- Chemicals, tobacco smoke, anxiety, stress and nervousness, atopy
- It can have a significant hereditary contribution.

Classification

Table 15.2 provides classification of asthma.

Clinical Features

Asthma can be acute, intermittent or chronic

Clinical type	Clinical features
Acute	- The asthmatic attacks last for a few minutes and resolve spontaneously with drugs - The symptoms include wheezing, cough, chest tightness, dyspnea and flushy
Intermittent	- If the individuals present with symptoms for less than 5 days/month is considered as intermittent
Chronic	- Individuals with symptoms for more than 5 days/month
Status asthmaticus/ acute severe asthma	- Is an medical emergency - The condition persists despite the therapy and individuals fail to respond

TABLE 15.2: Classification of asthma		
Category	Etiology	Mechanism

Extrinsic asthma	Caused due to allergens such as pollens, dust, house mites and animal danders	- When IgE combines with mast cells, there is release of vasoactive substances (histamine, leukotriene, prostaglandins, bradykinins, platelet-activating factor (PAF).
		  ◆ IgE + mast cells → vasoactive substances
		  ◆ Histamine → causes bronchoconstriction and increased vascular permeability
		  ◆ Leukotrienes → increased migration of leukocytes to airway space and cause increased tissue edema
		  ◆ PAF → it increases plasma leakage into airway space

Intrinsic asthma	Non-allergic stimuli	- Vagal mediated bronchospasm
Exercise-induced asthma	Bronchoconstriction due to increased physical activity	- Thermal changes produce mucosal irritation and trigger symptoms
Drug-induced (aspirin-induced or triad asthmatics)	Medications-induced asthma. For example: Ibuprofen, aspirin, beta adrenoreceptor blockers, tartrazine sulfites in food preservatives and local anesthesia	- The blockage of cyclo-oxygenase pathway by medications causes accumulation of leukotrienes through lipoxygenase pathway that causes bronchial spasm.
Infectious asthma	Bacteria, virus, Mycoplasma	- Infectious agents cause bronchial inflammation.

Diagnosis

- It is based on history
- Symptom of asthma tends to worsen at night and in early morning hours
- Allergens can trigger attacks
- Radiographic evaluation reveals increased anteroposterior chest diameter
- Spirometry shows reduced forced expiratory volume
- Allergen skin test can help determine the substances that cause allergic reaction in an individual
- Sputum smears are performed to evaluate for eosinophilia.

Management

Medication	Description
Bronchodilators (albuterol, terbutaline, epinephrine, metaproterenol)	It causes bronchodilation and smooth muscle relaxation, thereby reducing the resistance to airway Epinephrine is the drug of choice for severe asthma attack
Methylxanthines (theophylline, aminophylline)	Chronic asthma can be managed by this group of medications Bronchial smooth muscle relaxation by blocking adenosine receptors and inhibition of forms of cyclic AMP.
Corticosteroids (prednisone, beclomethasone)	Advised in refractory cases of asthmatics It reduces inflammatory response and prevents formation of mast cell mediators
Inhibitory of mast cell release (cromolyn sodium)	Prophylactic medication that protects against allergic/exercise-induced asthma
Anticholinergics (ipratropium bromide)	It inhibits the vagal reflex, thus preventing bronchoconstriction and mucous secretion

Oral Manifestations and Dental Considerations

- Pseudomembranous candidiasis in chronic asthmatic patients on steroid inhalers. Lozenge or liquid form of nystatin can be used for 2 weeks to treat these patients.
- Dental products such as toothpaste, fissure sealants, tooth enamel dust, methyl methacrylate can exacerbate asthma.
- Chronic asthmatics with severe airway obstruction can cause mouth breathing and dolichocephalic face form.
- Decreased salivary flow due to prolonged use of beta-2 agonists, this increases the incidence of dental caries, calculus deposition, gingivitis, periodontitis, change in oral microflora.
- Fluoride supplements can be used as a preventive and prophylactic measure
- Regular oral rinse following the use of inhalers
- Administer prophylactic steroids for individuals who are on long-term systemic steroids to avoid adrenal suppression
- Avoid anxiety, supplement with anxiolytics to reduce anxious patients
- Barbiturates and narcotics should be avoided in asthmatics as it may cause bronchoconstriction
- Schedule appointments late morning to reduce the risk of asthmatic attack
- Accessibility for oxygen and bronchodilators during exacerbations of asthma
- Sulfite in local anesthesia can exacerbate the asthma in susceptible cases
- Recommend and prescribe acetaminophen instead of aspirin
- Discontinue dental procedure during acute asthma attack, position the patient in a comfortable position, accessibility to beta-2 agonists and oxygen therapy. If no improvement noted, administer 1:1000 epinephrine subcutaneously.

◈ Chronic Obstructive Pulmonary Disease (COPD)

Description

It is a chronic inflammatory disease of lungs that causes limitation or obstruction of airflow.

Two major diseases include:
- Chronic bronchitis
- Emphysema

☛ Chronic Bronchitis

Description
- It is a chronic inflammatory condition affecting the bronchoalveolar epithelium for at least 3 months for more than two years.

Pathogenesis
- There is increased mucin secretion associated with ciliary dysfunction
- Airway limitation, diminished gaseous exchange
- Chronic hypercarbia (increased levels of carbon dioxide in blood due to diminished gaseous exchange)
- Hypoxemia
- Secondary bacterial infection (particularly *Streptococcus pneumoniae, Haemophilus influenzae*)
- As a sequence the condition may lead to pulmonary hypertension, respiratory failure and eventually cor pulmonale (i.e. right heart failure secondary to chronic pulmonary obstruction)
- Constituents in tobacco cause several changes in the morphology and function of respiratory system (Table 15.3):

Clinical Features
- Productive cough, wheezing, shortness of breath, exertional dyspnea
- Reduced forced expiratory rate
- Liver enlargement due to congestion
- Ascitis and peripheral edema, pulmonary hypertension, cor pulmonale
- Chronic bronchitis patient shows characteristic presentation termed blue bloaters (patient appears blue and overweight).

TABLE 15.3: Tobacco product and its effects	
Tobacco product	*Effects*
Tobacco smoke	Increase in number of goblet cells because of hyperplasia and metaplasia
Acrolein	Impaired ciliary and macrophage function
Nitrogen dioxide	Toxic damage to respiratory epithelium
Hydrogen cyanide	Functional impairment of respiratory enzymes that are required for respiratory metabolism
Carbon monoxide	Reduction in oxygen carrying capacity of red blood cells by combining with hemoglobin to form carboxy-hemoglobin
Polycyclic hydrocarbons	These are the known carcinogens

Treatment
- There is no cure for chronic bronchitis
- Patients advised to stop smoking
- Expectorants (guaifenesin) prescribed in patients with excessive sputum production
- Bronchodilators (theophylline and selective beta-2 agonists) to relax smooth muscles of bronchioles
- Corticosteroids in refractory cases
- Antibiotics to treat the secondary lung infections
- Diuretics in patients with severe bronchitis and right-sided heart failure.

Oral manifestation and dental considerations
- Patients with habit of smoking may show tobacco-associated oral lesions and oral potentially malignant disorders (e.g. smokers melanosis, nicotina stomatitis, leukoplakia, erythroplakia, non-healing ulcer or malignancy)
- Patients with poor oral hygiene present with gingival and periodontal diseases
- Patient is seated in an upright position while peforming dental treatment to prevent breathing difficulties caused in supine position.

- Anticholinergics and antihistamines are avoided as they dry the respiratory mucosa and increase mucous thickness.
- Respiratory depressants such as barbiturates and narcotics should be avoided.
- Patients on long-term steroid therapy may require additional dosage to prevent adrenal suppression.

☞ Emphysema (means air in tissues)

Description: It is an obstructive lung disease that causes damage to the alveolar sac.

Etiopathogenesis

- Tobacco smoke and environmental pollutants are the major contributing factors for emphysema
- It can also be preceded by chronic bronchitis
- It may be due to hereditary deficiency of alpha-1 antitrypsin
- Smokers have increase number of neutrophils and macrophages in their alveoli
- Smoking stimulates release of elastase and enhances its activity in macrophages.
- Smoking inhibits alpha-1 antitrypsin.
- Tobacco smoke contains reactive oxygen species with inactivation of anti-proteases.
- This results in enlargement and dilatation of acini, collapse of terminal bronchioles and loss of elastic recoil, causing alveolar destruction and diminished gaseous exchange due to the collapsed alveoli, finally overinflated lung tissue and poorly oxygenated blood.

Clinical Features

- Barrel chest, dyspnea
- Patients are described as pink puffers (because they find difficulty in catching breath and their skin appears pink)
- Easy fatigability, exertional dyspnea, weight loss, non-productive cough, tachypnea, increased use of accessory respiratory muscles (i.e. intercostal and supraclavicular muscles)
- Expiratory wheeze, respiratory acidosis, hypoxemia, pulmonary hypertension, peripheral edema, cor pulmonale and congestive heart failure.

Diagnosis

- Diagnosed by clinical features, laboratory diagnosis and radiologic investigation
- Hyperinflation of lungs
- Increased retrosternal air space, flat diaphragm, lung parenchymal damage
- Decreased pO_2 and relatively normal pCO_2
- Biopsy confirms disease

Oral manifestations and dental considerations

- Tobacco-induced oral lesions as discussed in chronic bronchitis
- These patients have mouth breathing, results in xerostomia that results in increased incidence of dental caries, gingival and periodontal diseases and change in oral microflora.
- Avoid respiratory depressants, general anesthesia, bilateral inferior alveolar nerve block, anticholinergics and rubber dam placement.
- Position patient in upright position to improve patients ability to ventilate.

Occupational Lung Disorders

◈ Pneumoconiosis

Description

It is a chronic pulmonary disease caused due to occupational hazard, due to inhalation of mineral or organic dusts such as asbestos, coal dust and silica.

Pathogenesis

The alveolar macrophages engulf the foreign particles and expire, thereby releasing lysosomal enzymes that destroy lung parenchyme, that eventually leads to fibrosis.

Clinical Features

- Initially patient presents with non-productive cough, dyspnea and progress to productive cough and right-sided heart failure.
- **Silicosis:** Produced by inhalation of crystalline silica particles or silicon dioxide. It occurs due to exposure to mining,

quarrying, sandblasting, grinding and polishing ceramics.

- **Asbestosis:** Caused due to inhalation of asbestos fibers and dusts, the use of production of asbestos is in insulation, floor tile and friction and fire proofing materials.
- **Coal miners lung (black lung):** Caused due to long-term inhalation of coal dust.

Oral Manifestations and Dental Considerations

- Deposition of silica gritty particles in the oral cavity.
- Teeth abrasion
- A bite guard can be provided as preventive measure.

Other Diseases Affecting the Respiratory Tract

◈ Cystic Fibrosis

Description

- It is an inherited life-threatening disorder damaging lungs and digestive system, characterized by numerous mutations in gene that encodes the cystic fibrosis transmembrane conductance regulator.
- The body produces thick and sticky mucous that blocks the lungs and obstruct pancreas.

Clinical Features

- Affects young children.
- Pulmonary manifestation—cough, recurrent infections of lower respiratory tract, bronchospasm, tachypnea, clubbing and bronchiectasis

- Digestive malfunction—meconium ileus, fatty tools, the digestive problems result in malnutrition and affect growth.
- There is an increased risk of diabetes and osteoporosis.

Oral Health Manifestations and Considerations

- Patients have history of mouth breathing, change in morphology of face, increased incidence of dental caries, missing teeth, increased deposition of teeth, gingivitis and periodontal diseases.
- Patients advised meticulous oral hygiene.
  Tuberculosis is discussed in infectious diseases.

FREQUENTLY ASKED QUESTIONS

1. Oral manifestations/dental considerations of respiratory disorders.
2. Describe sinusitis.

BIBLIOGRAPHY

1. Greenberg MS, Glick M, Ship JA. Burket's Oral Medicine. 11th ed. BC Decker Inc. 2008. p.77–106.
2. Greenberg MS, Glick M, Ship JA. Burket's Oral Medicine. 12th ed. Jaypee Brothers Medical Publishers Pvt. Ltd. 2015. p.91–122.
3. Greenberg MS, Glick M, Ship JA. Burket's Oral Medicine. 10th ed. BC Decker Inc. 2008. p. 85–125.
4. Bricker SL, Langlais RP, Miller CS. Oral Diagnosis, Oral Medicine and Treatment Planning. 2nd Ed. BC Decker Inc. 2002.
5. Silverman, Eversole, Truelove. Essentials of Oral Medicine. 1st ed. BC Decker Inc. 2002. p.84–100.

Gastrointestinal Diseases— Oral Manifestations and Dental Considerations

INTRODUCTION

The gastrointestinal (GI) system encompasses oral cavity, pharynx, esophagus, stomach, small and large intestine, rectum. In addition, liver, biliary system and pancreas play an important role in performing various physiologic functions. The oral health practitioners should be aware of oral manifestations and dental considerations in GI diseases.

Classification

1. **Oral-related GI disorders**
   - Eating disorder: Anorexia and bulimia
   - Xerostomia
   - Ptyalism
2. **Upper GI disease**
   - Gastroesophageal reflux disease (GERD)
   - Hiatal hernia
3. **Diseases of the lower GIT**
   - Disorders of stomach
   - Disorders of intestines
   - Inflammatory bowel disease
     - Crohn's disease
     - Ulcerative colitis
   - Peptic ulcer (hypersecretion disorder)
   - Antibiotic-induced diarrhea and pseudomembranous enterocolitis
4. **Disease of hepatobiliary system**
   - Jaundice
   - Hepatitis
   - Liver cirrhosis
   - Drug-induced hepatotoxicity
5. **GI syndromes**
   - Gardener's syndrome
   - Plummer-Vinson syndrome
   - Cowden's syndrome

Eating Disorders

A. **Anorexia:** It is a condition, in which individuals have extreme loss of appetite, probably because of fear of becoming fat. In spite of being underweight, individuals consume less food and are thin and malnourished.

B. **Bulimia:** Bulimia means OX-hunger. In this condition individuals eat abnormally. It occurs when one eats considerably large quantity of food (binge) over a short period of time, then induces oneself to vomit (purge); or uses excessively laxatives or diuretics to avoid weight gain. These individuals cannot resist eating, they engage in bingeing and purging at least twice a week for 3 months. They have excessive concern with the body shape and weight.

Clinical Features

Anorexia develops in young adolescence between 14–18 years of age and bulimia in early twenties. Both conditions are psychiatric disorders with physical complication.

Anorexic patients have no body fat, have protruding bones, bradycardia, leukopenia, and absence of menstruation (amenorrhea) among women.

Bulimic patients have hypokalemia and metabolic alkalosis due to vomiting and use of excessive laxatives.

Oral Manifestations and Dental Considerations

- Erosion of enamel on lingual surfaces of maxillary anteriors
- Mandibular incisors are usually spared by tongue
- Dentinal hypersensitivity due to erosion— prescription of desensitizing agents and restoring the teeth depending on the severity of the lesions
- Parotid gland enlargement because of starving
- Erythematous pharyngeal mucosa due to starving
- Psychological counselling and good nutritional food intake

Xerostomia and ptyalism are discussed in detail in salivary gland disorders.

UPPER GI DISEASES

1. Gastroesophageal Reflux Disease (GERD)

- It is the most common disease of the upper GIT
- It is the condition with regurgitation of gastric contents (chyme) from stomach into the esophagus.

Clinical Features

- In early onset, patients may be asymptomatic, as disease progresses endoscopic examination shows surface abnormalities.
- Heartburn, chest pain, esophageal ulcerations, esophagitis, stricture, dysphagia and dysplasia may be noted.
- *Barrett's esophagus:* It is a variant of GERD, wherein the squamous lining of esophagus is replaced with the columnar epithelium.

These patients have reported to have an increase in incidence of adenocarcinoma.

Management

◈ Medical Management

- *Weight loss:* It will reduce the pressure difference between the abdomen and the thorax, thereby reduces reflux
- Cessation of smoking
- Reducing fatty meal, this reduces the gastric emptying time and speeds up the digestion process
- Frequent small meals
- Avoid sleeping immediately after meals
- Elevation of head on bed that will empty the esophagus and prevents the symptoms
- H2 blocker antagonists to reduce the heart burn and regurgitation
- Proton pump inhibitors heal erosive and ulcerative esophagus
- *Promotility drugs (Cisapride):* These drugs increase the lower esophageal sphincter that reduces the acid reflux, decrease heart burn at night.

◈ Surgical

- Indicated when all therapies in medical management fails
- Antireflux operations are performed to correct the functional and anatomical abnormalities of GERD.

Oral Manifestations and Dental Considerations

- Dysguesia, dental erosion/pulpitis, dentinal hypersensitivity, atrophy and erythematous oral mucosa due to chronic exposure of acid
- Dysguesia can be managed with mild baking soda mouth rinse
- Depending on severity of dental erosions—mild erosive cases can be treated with topical fluoride application, advanced erosive areas involving dentin can be restored, involving pulp can be endodontically treated.

* Individuals on H2 blockers (cimetidine) will experience toxic reactions to intravascular injections of lidocaine
* Cimetidine interacts with antifungal agent (ketoconazole) and prevents its absorption.
* H2 blockers in elderly individuals have shown CNS side effects such as confusion, delirium, and seizures.

2. Hiatal Hernia

* The hiatus is a narrow opening in the gastroesophageal junction, which permits esophagus through the diaphragm to the stomach.

Normal

* When the hiatus is weakened or enlarged due to various factors such as hereditary, obesity, exercising (weightlifting), or chronic straining while passing stools.
* The stomach herniates into the chest cavity through the enlarged or weakened hole resulting in hiatal hernia.

Types

1. *Sliding hiatal hernia:* The most common type, the gastroesophageal junction and superior portion of the stomach slide above the diaphragm.
2. *Rolling hiatal hernia:* The gastroesophageal junction is at normal location but the superior portion of the stomach herniates above the diaphragm.
3. *Complicated hiatal hernia:* Almost the entire stomach moves into the chest.

Clinical Features

* Infants with hiatal hernia regurgitate blood stained food and have difficulty in breathing and swallowing
* Adults have acid reflux into the esophagus, causes esophageal erosions, bleeding, and inflammation of esophageal lining producing scarring resulting in narrowing. This causes dysphagia, bloating, heartburn on bending forward or lying down

* The pain spreads to jaw and down to the arms similar to the angina attack

Diagnosis

Diagnosis is by barium meal, endoscopy.

Management

◈ In Infants

The defect may be self-corrected, but precautionary measures such as head raised position while sleeping and administering of thicker consistency foods.

◈ In Adults

A. **Conservative management**
* Avoid activity that increases abdominal pressure such as abdominal exercises, tight belts
* Sleeping in head elevated position, which will reduce the symptom
* H2 blockers reduce the production of gastric acids from the parietal cells
* Frequent small meals
* Light supper with nothing consumed 2–3 hours before bedtime
* Foods that increase the reflux of acids should be avoided that include alcohol, nicotine, caffeine, chocolate, fatty foods, peppermint, etc.

B. **Surgical management**
* Indicated only when medical management fails
* Laparoscopic surgical corrections can be made.

Oral Health Considerations

* It is similar to GERD
* If the patients are treated with anticholinergic medications that cause xerostomia, then prescribe artificial saliva, alcohol-free mouthwashes and advise increased fluid intake
* Tooth cavities as a sequelae of xerostomia can be restored

DISEASES OF LOWER GIT

1. Disorders of Stomach

Cells in stomach and its function:

Cell type in stomach	Secretion	Function
Parietal cell	˟ Hydrochloric acid ˟ Intrinsic factor	˟ Digestion of food ˟ Killing of swallowed bacteria ˟ Required for absorption of vitamin B$_{12}$
Chief cells	Pepsinogen	Digestion of proteins
G cells	Gastrin	Potent stimulator of HCl, pepsin, casein
Mucous cells	Mucous	Coat and lubricate the stomach to propel the chyme

The disorders that affect the secretion or production of cells in the stomach impairs the physiological functions.

2. Peptic Ulcer Disease

◈ Gastric Ulcers

˟ It is the benign ulcerative condition of the epithelial lining of the stomach
˟ It can be a gastric ulcer in stomach and duodenal ulcer in duodenum

Pathogenesis

˟ Ulcers are due to imbalance in defense mechanism such as mucous production and HCl production, bicarbonate secretion and mucosal resistance.
˟ *Helicobacter pylori* (*H. pylori*) plays an important role in development of an ulcer
˟ *H. pylori* causes hyperacidity, gastritis and reduced mucosal resistance that lead to ulcer formation.

˟ Incidence of duodenal ulcers increases in cigarette smokers, patients with chronic renal disease and in alcoholics.

Clinical Features

˟ Burning epigastric pain that radiates to back especially during the empty stomach or 2–3 hours after a meal, and during middle of the night
˟ 3–8% of gastric ulcers represent malignant ulceration.

Management

˟ **Antacids:** H2 blockers and proton pump inhibitors can be prescribed.

◈ Duodenal Ulcers

Causes

˟ *H. pylori* infection, NSAIDs, stress, glucocorticoids, parathyroid disease, malignant carcinoid, cirrhosis, Zollinger- Ellison disease, polycythemia vera, and chronic lung disease.

Clinical Features

˟ Epigastric pain, burning and gnawing sensation associated with nausea and vomiting when the stomach is empty
˟ Blood loss in stool and vomit, may lead to iron deficiency anemia
˟ Patients with duodenal ulcer awaken at night and have intense urge to eat because indigestion of food rapidly provides relief
˟ Life-threatening complication such as hemorrhage, perforation and obstruction can occur.

◈ Zollinger-Ellison Syndrome

˟ Caused by gastrinoma of pancreas, causes multiple ulcers and diarrhea
˟ There is elevated levels of serum gastrin, and HCl.

Lab Diagnosis

˟ Anemia, leukocytosis, examination of stool, serum calcium test due to associated hyperparathyroidism.

Management

- Drugs that eradicate *H. pylori* (if the organism is evidenced)
- Antacids: H2 blockers, proton pump inhibitors
- Anticholinergic medication to reduce the production of acid from gastric mucosa.

Oral Health Considerations

- Oral manifestations of peptic ulcers are rare
- The manifestations may be due to anemia from GI bleeding or persistent regurgitation of gastric acid that leads to dental erosion
- Vascular malformations on the lip
- Avoid medications that exacerbate ulcerations such as aspirin and other NSAIDs
- Intake of antibiotics such as erythromycin and tetracycline may decrease their absorption.
- Xerostomic patients having denture should be advised denture adhesives and artificial saliva that aid in retention of denture
- Increased risk of dental caries due to hyposalivation
- Cimetidine and ranitidine prescribed in duodenal ulcers may be associated with thrombocytopenia and compete with antibiotics or antifungal medications.

3. Inflammatory Bowel Disease

As the name suggests it is the inflammation of large and small intestines.

It comprises
- Ulcerative colitis
- Crohn's disease

◈ Ulcerative Colitis

It is the ulceration affecting entire large intestine.

The etiology for the disease is not established, possible has bacterial, viral, immunologic or psychological role, or it could be due to autoimmune reaction with sensitization and destruction of the colonic mucosa.

Clinical Features

- Rectal bleeding
- Severe nocturnal diarrhea
- Erythema nodosum, i.e. red swollen nodules on thighs and legs
- Episcleritis, uveitis, corneal ulcers and retinitis cause pain and photophobia
- Liver disease and underlying anemia (hypochromic anemia) due to blood loss
- Electrolytic imbalance, hypoalbuminemia, low magnesium and potassium occur because of diarrhea.

Management

- Sulfasalazine is commonly used in ulcerative colitis
- Corticosteroids and corticotropin are used in patients who do not respond to sulfasalazine
- Other immunosuppressive medication such as azathioprine, cyclosporine and mercaptopurine can be used
- Surgical intervention when traditional medical therapy fails.

Oral Manifestations and Oral Health Considerations

- Delayed healing and increased risk of infection are sequelae of anemia
- Minor or major type aphthous ulcers
- **Pyoderma gangrenosum:** Occur as deep ulcer that may involve tonsillar pillar
- **Pyostomatitis vegetans:** Purulent inflammation of oral cavity characterized by deep tissue vegetations or proliferative lesions that may ulcerate and suppurates. These lesions are due to circulating immunocomplexes induced by antigens that are derived from gut lumen or damages colonic mucosa.
- **Hairy leukoplakia:** The presence of this lesion may be the marker of immunosuppression, the reason may be the use of immunosuppressive medication by these individuals.
- These patients are on regular glucocorticoids, consider the side effects of medication, such as hypertension,

hyperglycemia, osteoporosis, adrenal suppression, bone fracture. Careful seating of patients during dental treatment to avoid vertebral compression.

- Corticosteroids undergo metabolism in liver, liver function tests are required to elicit any changes in functions of liver that may affect the treatment.
- Because of impaired vitamin B_{12} absorption investigate for complete blood count
- Because of malabsorption of vitamin K, there may be defective synthesis of vitamin K dependent clotting factors (II, VII, IX, X), investigate for bleeding time, international normalized ratio.

◆ Crohn's Disease (Regional Enteritis)

- It is a chronic granulomatous disease of unknown origin and produces inflammation of small and large intestine
- Ileum is the most common site

Types

- *Non-perforating form:* The disease that tends to recur slowly
- *Perforating form:* The disease that tends to recur rapidly

Clinical Features

- It involves both genders, middle aged women are most commonly affected
- Disease shows familial tendency
- Diffuse ulceration of intestinal mucosa
- Hyperplasia of lymphoid tissue
- Fibrosis and muscular hypertrophy leading to constrictures
- Fever, abdominal pain accompanied with loose stools
- Reduced absorption of nutrients such as calcium, iron, folate, vitamin B_{12}, bile salts, fat, protein, etc.
- Patients have electrolytic imbalance, anemia, leukocytosis

Features that differentiate Crohn's disease from ulcerative colitis
Crohn's disease has following characteristics:
  1. Involvement of small intestine

  2. Rectum is spared
  3. Appearance of fissures or sinus tract
  4. Formation of sarcoid-like granuloma

Oral Manifestations

- Recurrent aphthous ulcerations
- Chronic stomatitis
- Anemia (pallor, glossitis, angular cheilitis)
- Lip swelling
- Pyostomatitis vegetans
- Cobblestone mucosal architecture
- Granulomatous changes of salivary glands, which is the hallmark of Crohn's disease
- Inflammation of salivary gland duct
- Oral epithelial tags and folds
- Gingivitis
- Candidiasis
- Lichenoid mucosal reactions
- Biopsy of ulcers shows granulomatous inflammations.

Oral Health Considerations

- Anti-inflammatory and sulfa medications used to manage Crohn's disease are associated with risk of lichenoid reaction
- Increased incidence of infections such as dental caries, bacterial and fungal infections
- Topical steroids can be administered for infections, inflammations or granulomatous lesions
- Any surgical intervention requires following lab investigations:
  - CBC, hematocrit values, hemoglobin level, platelet count, prothrombin time/INR/partial thromboplastin time and other liver function test and estimation of blood glucose level.

4. Antibiotic-induced Diarrhea and Psueodomembranous Enterocolitis

- Antibiotics-induced diarrhea occurs due to alteration in colonic microflora because of chronic use of antibiotics, which result in diarrhea, e.g. clindamycin, ampicillin, cephalosporins.
- Pseudomembranous enterocolitis is formation of thick mucosal exudate that

has appearance of membrane induced by antibiotics. *Clostridium difficile* that produces cytopathic toxins is involved in pathogenesis of pseudomembranous enterocolitis.

DISEASES OF HEPATOBILIARY SYSTEM

- Hepatobiliary system comprises liver, biliary tract and pancreas that aid in digestion
- Liver is the major organ that contributes for many catabolic and detoxifying actions.
- Following are the functions of liver:
  - Heme excretion
  - Store glycogen
  - On depletion of glycogen storage, liver gluconeogenesis form amino acids
  - Lipids are metabolized in the liver to form cholesterol
  - Synthesis of clotting factors I, II, V, VII, IX, X of which II, VII, IX, X are vitamin K dependent clotting factors
  - Metabolism of drugs by cytochrome P-450 occurs in hepatocyte
  - First pass metabolism of oral medication occurs in liver
  - Liver inactivates action of insulin, aldosterone, antidiuretic hormone, oestrogen and androgen.

Liver dysfunction can cause multiple systemic diseases, one of which is jaundice that can lead to liver failure and cirrhosis.

Jaundice

- It is accumulation and circulation of excess bilirubin in the tissue. There is yellowish discoloration of skin and mucous membrane and in sclera of the eye.
- Jaundice occur when total bilirubin level >3 mg/dl.

◈ Hemolytic Jaundice

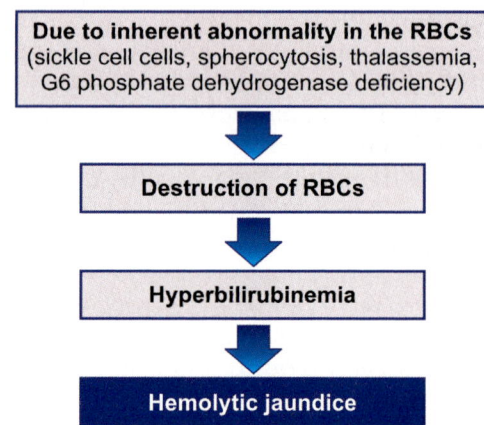

◈ Obstructive Jaundice (Cholestasis)

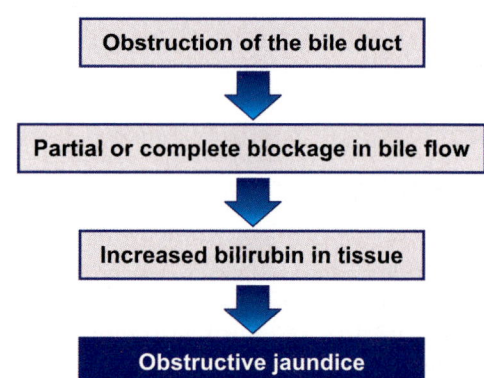

◈ Hepatocellular Jaundice

Caused by hepatitis and cirrhosis

Oral Manifestations

- Petechiae
- Ecchymosis
- Yellowish discoloration of mucosa
- Manifestations of anemia such as angular cheilitis, pallor, glossitis
- Sweet ketone breath (it is indicative of liver gluconeogenesis)

Type	Description
Hemolytic jaundice	Excessive production of bilirubin due to hemolysis of RBCs
Obstructive jaundice	Obstruction of biliary tree therefore prevention of excretion of bilirubin
Hepatocellular jaundice	Occurs due to liver parenchymal disease

Oral Health Considerations

- Risk of bleeding due to defective synthesis of clotting factors and vitamin malabsorption
- Secondary infections due to anemia
- Investigate for liver function test

Hepatitis

It is the inflammation of hepatocytes in liver

Etiology: Physical, chemical, parasitic, bacterial, viral agents are the cause for hepatitis

◈ Viral Hepatitis

Hepatitis A, hepatits B, hepatitis non-A, non-B, hepatitis C, delta hepatitis, hepatitis E.

◈ Alcoholic Hepatitis

- It is a toxin-induced liver disease, that causes cirrhosis and fulminant hepatic failure
- This condition is caused by excessive use of alcohol, which causes direct cellular toxicity of acetaldehyde.

Oral Health Considerations

- Jaundice
- Intraoral petechiae and ecchymosis
- Gingival bleeding
- Manifestations of malnutrition such as vitamin deficiency and anemia (angular cheilitis, pallor, glossitis)
- Sweet ketone breath
- Elective dental treatment is deferred in patients who have ingested large amount of alcohol
- Investigate for liver function tests to provide necessary dental treatment.

Cirrhosis

- It is a condition characterized by fatty infiltration, necrosis, fibrosis that reduce hepatocytes, thus the metabolic, synthesis and excretory functions are impaired.

Etiology: Alcohol abuse, biliary obstruction, viral infection, toxins, congestive cardiac failure, hemochromatosis, immune mediated injury.

Oral manifestations: Poor oral hygiene, calculus, dental caries, periodontal disease, xerostomia, fungal infections, bilateral sialadenosis, precancerous lesions such as erythroplakia and ulcerations of oral mucosa, gingival and mucosal bleeding, anemia.

Oral health considerations

- Evaluate for bleeding disorders
- Investigate for liver function tests.
- Obtain CBC, PT<APTT, AST, aspartate transaminase (APT) and alanine amino-transferase (ALT)
- Hemorrhagic procedures should be deferred until physician consent
- Avoid general anesthesia halothane that potentiates liver damage
- Avoid hepatotoxic medication (aceta-minophen)

FREQUENTLY ASKED QUESTIONS

1. Discuss the oral manifestations and dental considerations of inflammatory bowel disease.
2. Oral manifestations and dental considerations of GI diseases.

BIBLIOGRAPHY

1. Hall, John E., Arthur C. Guyton. Guyton and Hall. Textbook of Medical Physiology. 13th ed. Philadelphia, PA: Saunders Elsevier, 2016.
2. Greenberg MS, Glick M, Ship JA. Burket's Oral Medicine. 11th ed. BC Decker Inc. 2008. p.77–106.
3. Greenberg MS, Glick M, Ship JA. Burket's Oral Medicine. 12th ed. Jaypee Brothers Medical Publishers Pvt. Ltd. 2015. p.91–122.
4. Greenberg MS, Glick M, Ship JA. Burket's Oral Medicine. 10th ed. BC Decker Inc. 2008. p. 85–125.
5. Bricker SL, Langlais RP, Miller CS. Oral diagnosis, Oral Medicine and Treatment Planning. 2nd Ed. BC Decker Inc. 2002.
6. Silverman, Eversole, Truelove. Essentials of Oral medicine. 1st ed. BC Decker Inc. 2002.p.84–100.

Renal Diseases— Oral Manifestations and Dental Considerations

Chapter

17

INTRODUCTION

Kidneys are the vital organs situated in the peritoneum that maintains internal homeostasis by regulating fluid electrolyte, acid–base balance and purifies blood by removing toxic substances. Nephrons are the functional unit of kidneys. Kidneys remove toxic and waste products from blood and excrete approximately 1.5 to 2.5 L of urine in a day.

Functions of Kidney

- **Regulatory function:** Acid–base and fluid electrolyte balance
- **Excretory function:** Removes metabolic waste products such as urea, creatinine, uric acids, excretion of urine, and removes drug metabolites from blood
- **Non-excretory/endocrine function:** Secretes renin (has an important role in regulation of BP), synthesis active form of vitamin D (promotes hydroxylation of 25(OH)D to 1,25(OH)$_2$D, which is an active form) and erythropoietin (production of red blood cells).

Classification of Renal Diseases

1. **Based on onset**
   - Acute
   - Chronic

2. **Based on location of nephron destruction**
   - Acute
     - Pre-renal failure
     - Renal/intrinsic failure
     - Post-renal failure
   - Chronic
     - Pre-renal failure
     - Renal/intrinsic failure
     - Post-renal failure

3. **Based on disorders of hydrogen ion concentration and electrolytes**

Diagnosis in Renal Disease

1. **Serum chemistry:** Changes in internal body homeostasis are reflected in serum chemistry. Serum creatinine and blood urea nitrogen (BUN) are important markers of GFR.

Parameter	Normal range
GFR	100–150 ml
Creatinine clearance	85–125 ml/min
Serum creatinine	0.6–1.2 mg/dl
Blood urea nitrogen	8–18 mg/dl
Serum calcium	8.5–10.5 mg/dl
Serum phosphate	2.5–4.5 mg/dl
Serum potassium	3.8–5 mEq/l

2. **Urine analysis:** Urine analysis includes detection of protein (proteinuria), blood (hematuria) in urine, specific gravity

or osmolality of urine and microscopic examination. Proteinuria and hematuria are the important markers for kidney disease.

3. **Creatinine clearance test:** This test helps to determine whether the kidneys are functioning normally. Specifically, the creatinine clearance test gauges the rate at which a creatinine is "cleared" from the blood by the kidneys. It is done on urine sample collected for 24 hours.

4. **IV pyelography:** Radiologic examination of kidney with IV contrast medium injection, this test cannot be used for low GFR that prevents the excretion of dye.

5. **Renal ultrasonography:** It distinguishes solid tumors from fluid-filled cysts.

6. **CT and MRI:** The application of CT is limited for imaging in kidneys, but both imaging modalities are helpful in detection of retroperitoneal masses.

7. **Biopsy:** Nephrologists usually perform percutaneous needle biopsy guided by USG.

Renal Failure

Acute Renal Failure (ARF)

* Decline in kidney function over a period of days to weeks that leads to severe azotemia (abnormal accumulation of nitrogenous products in blood).
* It mainly occurs in hospital admitted patients due to medications, surgery, pregnancy related complications, and trauma can result in ARF.

The causes for ARF can be categorized into three categories as given in Table 17.1.

Chronic Renal Failure (CRF)

National Kidney Foundation—kidney disease has termed CRF as either of the following:

1. The presence of kidney damage for >3 months with structural and functional abnormalities of kidneys associated with or without reduction in GFR, which manifests as pathological abnormalities or other markers of kidney damage such as abnormalities in the composition of blood or urine.

TABLE 17.1: Causes for ARF

Condition	Pre-renal failure	Renal/intrinsic	Post-renal failure
Description	Compromised renal function without injury to kidney	Damage within kidneys	The conditions that obstruct the flow of urine at any level of urinary tract and subsequent reduction in glomerular filtration rate (GFR)
Cause	✗ Volume depletion ✗ Cardiovascular diseases that result in decreased cardiac output ✗ Changes in fluid volume distribution such as in burns and sepsis	1. Glomerular disease: Glomerulo-nephritis is immune mediated damage to kidneys 2. Vascular disease: Obstruction of renal artery by thrombus 3. Tubulointerstitial disease: It includes interstitial nephritis, acute tubular necrosis	Prostatic enlargement (could be benign or malignant neoplasm) Cervical malignancy
Clinical presentation	Azotemia	✗ Hypertension, proteinuria, hematuria ✗ Red blood cells, sudden severe lower back pain, oliguria	Total anuria or polyuria

2. The GFR is <600 cc/min/1.73 m² for >3 months with or without signs of kidney damage

Clinical staging of chronic kidney disease

Stage	GFR cc/min	Manifestation
1	>90	Normal kidney function, may have proteinuria, hematuria
2	60–90	Reduced kidney function, may have proteinuria, hematuria
3	30–60	Anemia
4	15–30	Patient should be medically prepared for dialysis
5	<15	Long-term chronic dialysis

Etiology of CRF: The most common causes of CRF or end stage renal disease (ESRD)/uremic syndrome are (Table 17.2):
× Glomerulonephritis
× Nephrotic syndrome
× Pyelonephritis
× Hypertensive nephrosclerosis
× Connective tissue disorders
× Polycystic kidney disease
× Metabolic disorders
× Interstitial nephritis
× Obstructive uropathy

Clinical manifestations of CRF/uremic syndrome/ESRD: Renal disease affects various multi-organ systems with the following manifestations (Table 17.3):

TABLE 17.2: Causes of CRF		
S. no	Diseases that cause CRF	Characteristics
1.	Glomerulo-nephritis (GN)	× GN is immunologic in origin × Often associated with infectious agents such as Streptococcus, Staphylococcus, Pneumococcus × Sudden in onset, patients have hypertension, proteinuria

2.	Nephrotic Syndrome	× It is a clinical state characterized by increased glomerular membrane permeability resulting in:
		  ✦ Proteinuria
		  ✦ Edema
		  ✦ Hypoalbuminemia
		  ✦ Hypercholestremia
		× Clinically patients present with edema of lower extremities and in periorbital region, lethargy, tiredness, muscle wastage
		× Hypertension, nitrogen imbalance, hypercoagulation, loss of proteins (albumin binding proteins, and immunoglobulins).
		× Urine may appear frothy
		× Muerke's lines: These are transverse white bands on fingernails in chronic hypoalbuminemia patients

3.	Pyelo-nephritis	× Caused by pyogenic infection in kidney with *E. coli* × Patients have generalized sepsis, bacterial endocarditis, and staphylococcal septicemia
4.	Hypertensive nephro-sclerosis	× Vascular or glomerulus lesion that causes hypertension without renal failure is referred to as hypertensive nephrosclerosis. × Hypertension is the leading cause of CRF—the heart; brain, eyes and kidneys are the target organs of hypertension.

Contd.

TABLE 17.2: Causes of CRF *(Contd.)*

S. no	Diseases that cause CRF	Characteristics
5.	Connective tissue disorders	✷ Systemic lupus erythematosis, rheumatic arthritis, progressive systemic sclerosis have shown clinical evidence of renal involvement. There may be progressive sclerosis of vasculature of kidney
6.	Polycystic renal disease	Is an autosomal dominant inheritance Associated with hematuria, abdominal pain, recurrent urinary tract infection, and hypertension.
7.	Metabolic disorders	Diabetes mellitus (DM), amyloidosis, gout primary hyperparathyroidism are the most common causes of CRF Diabetic nephropathy refers to various changes that affect the structure and function of kidneys in presence of DM. The disease progresses stagewise beginning with early functional changes, followed by structural changes, and progresses to nephropathy, advances to progressive renal failure and finally azotemia resulting in ESRD.
8.	Toxic nephro-pathy	The kidney is the route of excretion of many foreign substances, and medications when exposed to the nephrotoxic medications and chemicals, they damage kidney.

TABLE 17.3: Renal disease and its manifestations

System	Manifestations
Gastro-intestinal	Nausea, vomiting, anorexia, ammo-niacal taste and smell, stomatitis, parotitis, esophagitis, gastritis
Neuro-muscular	Headache, peripheral neuropathy, paralysis, myoclonic jerks, seizures
Hemato-logic immuno-logic	Normocytic and normochromic anemia, coagulation defect, increased susceptibility to infection, decreased erythropoiesis
Cardio-vascular	Hypertension, congestive heart failure, arrhythmias
Endocrine-metabolic	Renal osteodystrophy, secondary hyperparathyroidism, impaired growth and development
Dermato-logic	Pallor, hyperpigmentation, ecchy-mosis, uremic frost, pruritis
Biochemical disturbance	Metabolic acidosis results in anorexia, lethargy, nausea, Kussmaul's breathing

Renal Osteodystrophy (Renal Rickets)

It is skeletal changes as a result of chronic kidney disease.

Pathogenesis

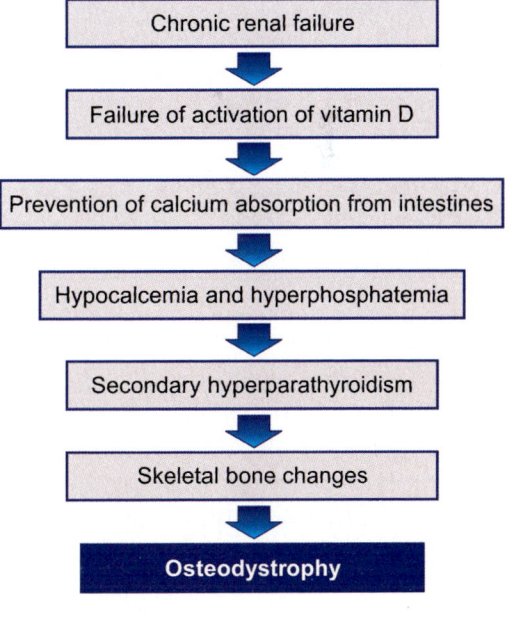

Radiographic Features

✷ Generalized loss of bone density
✷ Thinning of bony cortices
✷ Brown's tumor secondary to hyper-parathyroidism

- Increased jaw size in dialysis patients due to widened marrow spaces
- Hypoplasia and hypocalcification of teeth
- Loss of lamina dura
- Osteoporosis circumscripta (well-defined radiolucency in skull)
- Ground glass appearance
- Central giant cell lesion
- Socket sclerosis (calcified healing in extraction socket)
- Metastatic calcifications of falx cerebri

Oral Manifestations

Dry mouth	Hyposalivation
Enlarged salivary glands	Retrograde parotitis
Uremic stomatitis	Uremic odor
Poor taste sensation, ammonia like taste and smell	Metallic taste
Enamel hypoplasia	Extrinsic and intrinsic stains on teeth
Malocclusion	Pale mucosa
Petechie and ecchymosis	Prolonged bleeding
Gingival bleeding	Candida infections
Dysesthesia of lips and tongue area as consequence of neuritis secondary to metabolic acidosis	Low caries rate, calculi formation
Peripheral giant cell lesion	

Uremic Stomatitis

- It is a rare lesion affecting oral cavity in undiagnosed CRF patients.
- It is sequelae of formation of ammonia due to hydrolysis of urea in saliva by the urease enzyme. The ammonium compounds cause chemical injury and irritation to mucosa. It occurs when concentration of urea exceeds 30 mmol/l.

Clinically there are two types of uremic stomatitis:
- **Type I:** Localized or generalized erythema of oral mucosa with thick pseudo-membranous exudate, which does not leave ulcerated base on its removal.

- **Type II:** Leaves ulceration on pseudo-membrane removal.

Both types are associated with pain, halitosis, xerostomia, gingival bleeding, dysgeusia, secondary candida infection, and anemia due to underlying kidney disease.

Management of CRF

Management of CRF can be divided in two categories:
- Conservative therapy
- Renal replacement therapy

Conservative Therapy

- **Regulation of dietary proteins:** Patients are restricted for protein intake
- Limiting phosphate containing foods to prevent hyperphosphatemia
- Maintain blood pressure
- Maintain adequate hemoglobin level by substituting erythropoietin stimulating factor
- Cessation of smoking
- **Administering statins:** Lipid lowering medications
- Access for dialysis when blood creatinine level increases (> 4 mg/dl or GFR- <20 ml/min)

Renal Replacement Therapy

- **Dialysis:** It removes the nitrogenous and toxic products from blood by means of a hemodialyzer system (artificial kidney) in end stage renal disease when GFR is <20 ml/min.
- The two methods of dialysis are:
  - *Hemodialysis:* Vascular access in arms or legs is used for hemodialysis, performed 3 times per week
  - *Peritoneal dialysis:* Access to the body is achieved through catheter placed in peritoneal cavity of the abdomen, performed every 8–12 hours, 5 to 7 days a week.
- **Kidney transplantation:** It indicated for irreversible kidney damage. Patients are usually on immunosuppressive medication, hence more prone for secondary infections and exposed to the side effects of medications.

Dental Considerations

Oral health management in patients with kidney disease can be considered in two groups:

× In patients with acute renal failure
× In patients with chronic renal failure/end stage renal disease

In patients with acute renal failure:

× Elective dental care in individuals with ARF is deferred as individuals have accumulated toxic products.

In patients with chronic renal failure

× Individuals with CRF are unable to perform the normal kidney functions, therefore, oral health practitioners should be aware of various complications during dental treatment
× Excessive bleeding and anemia should be suspected in individuals with CRF
  ▪ Local hemostatic agent such as DDAVP (1-Deamino-8-D arginine vasopressin) should be considered to stop bleeding, which is effective for shorter duration
  ▪ Longer hemostasis can be attained with DDAVP conjugated with estrogen
  ▪ Tranexamic acid (an antifibrinolytic agent) can be used to control post-operative bleeding
  ▪ Local hemostatic aids such as microfibrillar collagen and oxidized regenerated cellulose can be used
× Obtain platelet count and complete blood count to manage bleeding and assess anemic conditions
× Patient undergoing dialysis will be heparinized, therefore, elective dental and oral surgical procedures should be scheduled on non-dialysis days, as this is the time where blood is free of toxins.
× Avoid tying cuff to the arm of vascular access for dialysis to measure blood pressure, avoid both intramuscular and intravenous injections to the arm; do not use the access site as an injection site
× Avoid longer sitting in patients with access site in the leg
× Patients with CRF are more prone for infections; therefore, meticulous oral hygiene, maintenance of good oral hygiene, use of antifungal and antimicrobial oral rinse may reduce dental infections.
× Prophylactic antibiotic regimen can be administered as these individuals are more prone for bacterial endocarditis.
× Hemodialysis patients receive blood transfusion, these patients are more prone for blood borne diseases such as hepatitis B, HIV and even tuberculosis
× Avoid excessive stress to prevent elevation of blood pressure, as these individuals are known hypertensive
× Avoid nephrotoxic medications such as phenacetin, ketorolac, aspirin, NSAIDs, tetracycline, carbenicillin, cephalosporins, aminoglycosides, steroids, etc. Instead alternative medications such as acetaminophen, barbiturates, penicillin, and narcotics can be used with caution.

FREQUENTLY ASKED QUESTIONS

1. Oral manifestations/dental considerations of renal diseases.

BIBLIOGRAPHY

1. Hall, John E., and Arthur C. Guyton. Guyton and Hall Textbook of Medical Physiology. 13th ed. Philadelphia, PA: Saunders Elsevier, 2016.
2. Greenberg MS, Glick M, Ship JA. Burket's Oral Medicine. 11th ed. BC Decker Inc 2008. p.77–106.
3. Greenberg MS, Glick M, Ship JA. Burket's Oral Medicine. 12th ed. Jaypee Brothers Medical Publishers Ltd. 2015. p.91–122.
4. Greenberg MS, Glick M, Ship JA. Burket's Oral Medicine. 10th ed. BC Decker Inc 2008. p.85–125.
5. Bricker SL, Langlais RP, Miller CS. Oral diagnosis Oral Medicine and Treatment Planning. 2nd Ed. BC Decker Inc 2002.
6. White, Stuart C., and M. J. Pharoah. Oral Radiology: Principles and Interpretation. 6th ed. St. Louis, Mo: Mosby/Elsevier, 2009.p.454–461.
7. Silverman, Eversole, Truelove. Essentials of Oral medicine. 1st ed. BC Decker Inc 2002.p.84–100.

Diabetes Mellitus and Endocrine Disorders— Oral Manifestations and Dental Considerations

INTRODUCTION

Endocrine system is the collection of various glands that produce hormones, which are released directly into the blood stream. The hormones are specific chemical messengers as they transfer information from one group of cells to another, or act on specific tissue or organ. The hormones are proteins, polypeptides, steroids or derivatives of amino acids. These hormones play a key role in metabolism and regulation of all physiologic functions of the body. The overactivity of hormones is prevented by negative feedback mechanism. The various endocrine glands in our body are pituitary, thyroid, parathyroid, thymus, pancreas, adrenal, pineal, ovaries and testes.

TABLE 18.1: Terminologies with description

Terminology	Description
Endocrine glands	These are ductless glands that release their secretion directly into blood that act on target cells located at distant sites
Exocrine glands	These glands have ducts that secrete on epithelial surface
Neuro-endocrine	Hormones secreted by neurons into circulation that act on distant sites

Contd.

Terminology	Description
Paracrine	Hormones secreted by cells into extracellular fluid that affect neighboring/ different cells
Autocrine	Hormones secreted by cells into extracellular fluid that affect same cells

Endocrine Glands, Hormones and Functions (Table 18.2)

Endocrine disorders can be due to
- Hypofunction (under production of hormone)
- Hyperfunction (excessive production of hormones)
- Hormone resistance (target organs are resistant to the hormonal effects in spite of optimal production of hormones)

Diabetes Mellitus (DM)

DM is a chronic metabolic or genetic disorder characterized by relative or absolute lack of insulin that results in elevated glucose levels and produces disturbances in carbohydrate, lipid and protein metabolism.

TABLE 18.2: Endocrine glands, hormones and functions

Endocrine glands	Hormone secreted	Major function
Hypothalamus	✗ Thyrotropin-releasing hormone (TRH)	✗ Stimulates secretion of TSH and prolactin
	✗ Corticotropin-releasing hormone (CRH)	✗ Release of ACTH
	✗ Growth hormone–releasing hormone (GHRH)	✗ Causes release of growth hormone peptide
	✗ Growth hormone inhibitory hormone (GHIH) (somatostatin)	✗ Inhibits release of growth hormone peptide
	✗ Gonadotropin-releasing hormone (GnRH)	✗ Causes release of luteinizing hormone and follicle stimulating hormone
	✗ Dopamine or prolactin-inhibiting factor (PIF)	✗ Inhibits release of prolactin
Pituitary gland		
Anterior lobe hormones (adeno-hypophysis)	✗ Adrenocorticotropic hormone (ACTH)	✗ Secretion of cortisol ✗ Regulation of androgen production
	✗ Thyroid stimulating hormone (TSH)	✗ T3 and T4 are associated with metabolism of all parts of the body (carbohydrate and protein metabolism, synthesis and degradation of triglycerides and cholesterol) ✗ Stimulate contraction of heart and heart rate ✗ Maturation of central nervous system
	✗ Prolactin	✗ Regulates lactation
	✗ Luteinizing hormone (LH)	✗ Ovulation in female ✗ Estrogen and progesterone synthesis in ovaries ✗ Testosterone formation in male
	✗ Follicle stimulating hormone (FSH)	✗ Development of ovaries ✗ Maturation of testes
	✗ Growth hormone (GH)	✗ Skeletal development, growth and protein synthesis
	✗ Melanocyte stimulating hormone	✗ Melanin pigmentation
	✗ Beta-endorphin	✗ Endogenous opiates released after exposure to painful stimulus
Posterior lobe hormones (Neurohypophysis)	✗ Antidiuretic hormone (ADH)/ Vasopressin	✗ Regulates plasma osmolality ✗ Conserves water by reabsorption of water by kidneys ✗ Decreases urinary output by acting on distal renal tubule ✗ Causes vasoconstriction and increases blood pressure
	✗ Oxytocin	✗ Stimulates the contraction of the uterus during pregnancy ✗ Promote milk secretion and ejection from the lactating breast

Contd.

TABLE 18.2: Endocrine glands, hormones and functions (*Contd.*)

Endocrine glands	Hormone secreted	Major function
Thyroid gland	⤬ Thyroxine (T4) and triiodothyronine (T3) ⤬ Calcitonin	⤬ Increases body metabolic rate ⤬ Increases bone calcium absorption and reduces extracellular calcium levels
Parathyroid gland	⤬ Parathyroid hormone (PTH)	⤬ Regulates serum calcium levels by absorbing calcium from gut, kidneys and release of calcium from bones
Adrenal cortex	⤬ Cortisol ⤬ Aldosterone	⤬ Controls various metabolic functions involving proteins, carbohydrates and fat ⤬ Anti-inflammatory effects ⤬ Increases sodium absorption, potassium secretion, hydrogen ion secretion
Adrenal medulla	⤬ Epinephrine and nor-epinephrine	⤬ Sympathetic stimulation
Pancreas	⤬ Insulin from β cells ⤬ Glucagon from α cells	⤬ Controls carbohydrate metabolism by promoting entry of glucose into cells and reduces blood glucose levels ⤬ Increases blood sugar level by promoting synthesis and release of glucose from liver
Testes	⤬ Testosterone	⤬ Develops male reproductive system and secondary male sexual characteristics
Ovaries	⤬ Estrogens ⤬ Progesterone	⤬ Promotes development of females reproductive system, female breasts, secondary sexual characteristics of female ⤬ Promotes uterine secretion
Pineal gland	⤬ Melatonin	⤬ Regulates biological rhythm that controls sleep and wake cycle.
Thymus	⤬ Thymosin	⤬ Development of immune system
Kidney	⤬ Renin ⤬ 1,25- dihydroxy-cholecalciferol ⤬ Erythropoietin	⤬ Converts angiotensinogen to angiotensin I ⤬ Increases intestinal absorption of calcium and bone mineralization ⤬ Increases erythrocyte production
Heart	⤬ Atrial natriuretic peptide (ANP)	⤬ Reduces blood pressure and increases sodium excretion from kidneys
Stomach	⤬ Gastrin	⤬ Secretion of hydrochloric acid from parietal cells
Small intestine	⤬ Secretin ⤬ Cholecystokinin (CCK)	⤬ Stimulates pancreatic acinar cells to release of bicarbonate and water ⤬ Stimulates gallbladder cells and release of pancreatic enzymes release
Adipocytes	⤬ Leptin	⤬ Inhibits appetite and promotes thermogenesis

Classification

I. Formerly DM was classified based on:
   a. Age at onset
   b. Type of therapy
II. According to American Diabetes Association (Table 18.3).

Blood Glucose Regulation

Flowchart 18.1 provides blood glucose regulation.

Pathophysiology

Type 1 Diabetes Mellitus (Fig. 18.2)

* In response to stress, cortisol secretion is increased in Type 1 diabetic patients that cause breakdown of proteins and loss of nitrogen in the urine.
* Fat breakdown into fatty acids and glycerol. The glycerol is converted to glucose for cellular use.
* Fatty acids are further reduced to ketone bodies (acetone and beta hydroxyl butyric acid), its accumulation in blood results diabetic ketoacidosis.
* Ultimately results in coma and death

Type 2 Diabetes Mellitus

* Most common type (85%)
* Etiology is multifactorial with environmental and lifestyle factors (obesity) superimposed on genetic predilection
* Type 2 DM is a result of:
  * Peripheral resistance of insulin
  * Increased production of glucose by liver
  * Impaired insulin secretion from beta cells of pancreas
* In response to high glucose levels, there is increased secretion of insulin (hyperinsulinemia) from pancreas
* Unlike the patients with Type 1, Type 2 DM patients are generally resistant to diabetic ketoacidosis because of sufficient production of pancreatic insulin, which prevents ketone formation.
* Ketoacidosis in Type 2 DM is usually due to physiologic stress.

Gestational DM

* DM occur during pregnancy is gestational DM
* Pregnant women develop either Type 1 or 2 DM

TABLE 18.3: Classification of diabetes mellitus according to American Diabetes Association

Type	Former nomenclature	Etiology
Type 1	✕ Juvenile diabetes ✕ Insulin dependent diabetes mellitus (IDDM) ✕ Type I	✕ Autoimmune destruction of beta cells ✕ Immune mediated ✕ Idiopathic cause
Type 2	✕ Adult onset diabetes ✕ Non-insulin dependent diabetes mellitus (NIDDM)	✕ Insulin resistance in peripheral tissue ✕ Relative insulin deficiency
Other specific types of DM	✕ Genetic defects of beta cell function ✕ Genetic defects in insulin action ✕ Disease of exocrine pancrease ✕ Endocrinopathies such as hyperthyroidism ✕ Drugs or chemical induced ✕ Exogenous steroids ✕ Infections ✕ Chronic alcohol intake ✕ Immune mediated diabetes ✕ Genetic syndromes (Down's syndrome, Klinefelter syndrome, etc)	
Gestational diabetes	✕ Glucose intolerance amongst pregnant women	

Flowchart 18.1: Blood glucose regulation

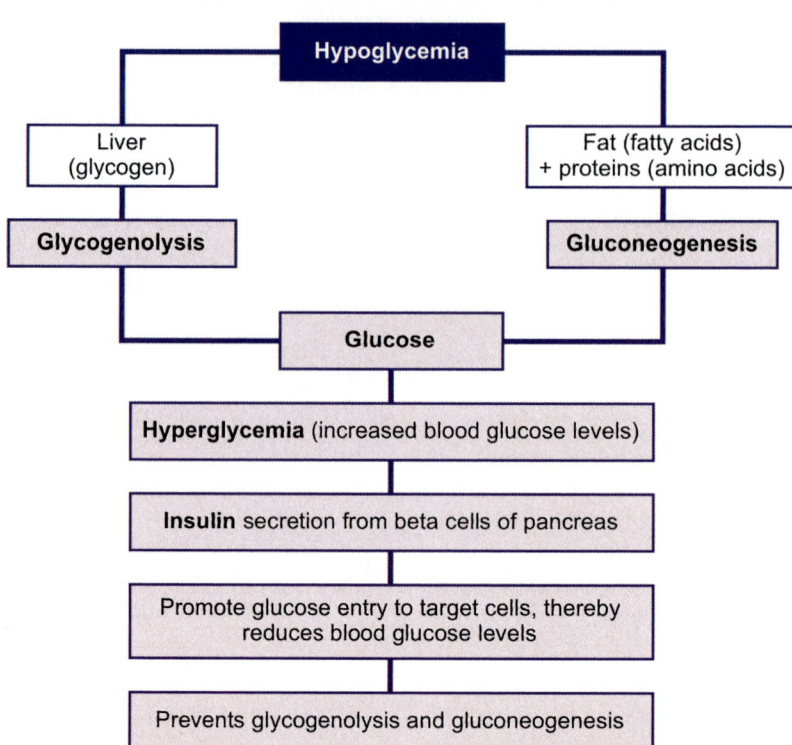

- It is usually associated with increased insulin resistance
- It is seen in older women, overweight women, women of minority ethnic group
- Hormones that increase blood sugar levels—glucagon, growth hormone, epinephrine, thyroid hormone, and corticosteroids. Only hormone that reduces blood glucose levels is insulin.

General characteristics of Type 1 and Type 2 DM are shown in Table 18.4.

Characteristics	Type 1	Type 2
Incidence	5%	85%
Clinical	Abrupt onset	Gradual in onset
Age	Less than 20 years of age	More than 40 years of age
Weight	Thin/loss of weight	Obese
Endogenous insulin	Absent	Low, normal, or high levels
Islet cell antibodies	Present	Absent
Ketoacidosis	Common	Less common
Genetic susceptibility	HLA-D linked	No HLA association
Pathogenesis	Autoimmunity/immune mediated destruction of pancreatic beta cells	Insulin resistance by peripheral tissues

TABLE 18.4: General characteristics of Type 1 and Type 2 DM

Flowchart 18.2: Type 1 diabetes mellitus

```
                    Cell
                     ↓
            No glucose uptake
                     ↓
   Lack of insulin secretion from beta cells of pancreas
                     ↓
      Due to autoimmune destruction of beta cells
  and idiopathic cause—the destruction of beta cells
              is not understood
                     ↓
              Hyperglycemia
                     ↓
      Exceeds renal threshold (>200 mg/dl)
                     ↓
                Glycosuria
                     ↓
             Osmotic diuresis
                     ↓
            Polyuria, nocturia
                     ↓
      Polyuria with vascular osmolarity
                     ↓
       Stimulates osmoreceptors in brain
                     ↓
        Polydipsia (excessive thirst)
                     ↓
  Lack of metabolism of ingested nutrients/lack
          of entry of glucose into cells
                     ↓
         Lead to glucose starved cells
                     ↓
       Hunger, malnutrition, weight loss
                     ↓
        Polyphagia (increased food intake)
```

Clinical Features

TABLE 18.5: Clinical features of type 1 DM and type 2 DM

Type 1 DM	Type 2 DM
Polydipsia	Visual changes
Polyuria	Weight loss/gain
Polyphagia	Postural hypotension
Weight loss	Nocturnal urination
Visual impairment	Loss of sensation
Bed wetting	Paresthesia
Thirst/dry mouth	Pruritis
Headache	Impotence
Irritability	
Ketoacidosis	
Chronic skin infections	
Periodontal diseases	

Oral Manifestations

TABLE 18.6

Oral dysesthesia	Dental caries, increased dental plaque, gingivitis, periodontitis, periodontal abscess
Burning mouth	Increased glucose level in gingival crevicular fluid
Delayed wound healing	Sialadenitis (especially of parotid gland)
Increased susceptibility for infection	Neuropathy
Candida infection (acute pseudomembranous candidiasis of tongue, buccal mucosa and gingiva)	Antral mucormycosis is a serious complication amongst immuno-compromized individuals with diabetes.
Xerostomia, antidiabetic medication induced salivary hypofunction	Dental caries, increased dental plaque, gingivitis, periodontitis, periodontal abscess
Mucosal ulcerations	Increased glucose level in gingival crevicular fluid
Sialadenitis (especially of parotid gland)	

Diagnosis (Table 18.7)

* Glycosylated hemoglobin assay will determine blood glucose status over 30–90 days, there are two different glycosylated hemoglobin A1 (HbA1) test and hemoglobin A1c (HbA1c).

Normal HbA1 value	8%
Normal HbA1c value	6–6.5%
Glycosylated hemoglobin level HbA1c	Clinical interpretation
4–6%	Normal
Less than 7.5%	Good diabetes control
7–9%	Moderate diabetes control
>9%	Poor diabetes control

* Glycosylated hemoglobin assay is used to monitor glycemic control in patients already diagnosed as having diabetes.
* HbA1c value of more than 8% suggests change in management protocol
* *Fructosamine test* is used to determine long-term glucose control analysis. The normal range is 2–2.8 mmol/l
* *Glucometers* are self-screening tools regularly used at home and even used as chair side investigation for measurement of blood glucose levels.

Complications

DM affects multiple organ systems affecting micro and macro vasculature (Table 18.8).

Management

* The overall goal of medical management is prevention of diabetic complications and achieving blood glucose levels

TABLE 18.8

Organ involved	Associated complication
Cardio-vascular system	* Atherosclerotic plaque in major and minor vessels leading to peripheral vascular disease * Coronary artery disease * Cerebrovascular disease * Gangrenous foot * Ischemic ulcers
Kidneys	* Nephropathy　* Renal failure
Nervous system	* Peripheral neuropathy * Cranial neuropathy * Changes in cardiac rate, rhythm, dysfunction * Postural hypotension * Gastrointestinal neuropathy * Impotence
Skin and oral mucosa	* Unusual infections and delayed wound healing
Eyes	* Retinopathy, cataracts, blindness
Teeth and surrounding structures	* Gingivitis and periodontal diseases

* Proper diet, lifestyle modification, weight reduction, prevention of smoking and alcoholism and adequate exercise are important in management of DM.

Oral Hypoglycemic Agents

Medication	Generic name
Sulfonylureas	
First generation	Chlorpropamide Tolbutamide Tolazamide Acetohexamide

Contd.

TABLE 18.7: Diagnostic criteria for diabetes mellitus			
	Normal	Impaired fasting glucose	Diabetes mellitus
Fasting glucose	<110 mg/dl	110–126 mg/dl	≥126 mg/dl
2 hours post-prandial plasma glucose	<140 mg/dl	140–200 mg/dl	≥200 mg/dl
Oral glucose tolerance test			Plasma glucose at 2 hours ≥200 mg/dl

Medication	Generic name
Second generation	Glyburide Glipizide Glimepiride
Biguanides	Metformin
Thiazolidinediones	Rosiglitazone Pioglitazone
Alpha-glucosidase inhibitors	Acarbose
Meglitinide	Repaglinide Nateglinide

Insulin Preparations

Insulin type	Time of onset (hour)	Duration (hour)
Fast-acting insulins		
× Lispro	15 min	<5
× Insulin injection (regular)	30–60 min	6–8
× Prompt insulin zinc suspension	1–2	12–16
Intermediate-acting insulins		
× Isophane insulin suspension	1–2	18–28
× Insulin zinc suspension	1–3	18–28
Long-acting insulin		
× Protamine zinc insulin suspension	4–8	36
× Extended insulin zinc suspension	4–8	20–36

Dental Management

Dental management of patients can be performed under three categories:

A. Diagnosis of unsuspected diabetes
B. Management of oral condition in diabetic patients
C. Managing dental emergencies in diabetic patients

A. **Diagnosis of unsuspected diabetes**
   × Recognize signs and symptoms of diabetes as mentioned earlier
   × Elicit proper medical history, concomitant systemic disease, drug history
   × Use of glucometer as a chair side screening tool to assess blood glucose levels

B. **Management of oral condition in diabetic patients**
   × Monitor blood glucose level with glucometer in dental office
   × Antibiotic prophylaxis is mandatory for patients with high HbA1c level (>11–12%)
   × Carbohydrates (candies, table sugar, juice or soda) should be kept readily available to prevent hypoglycemic event
   × Determine the type of diabetes, treatment, level of control and presence of diabetes-associated complications (e.g. hypertension, cardiovascular diseases, renal insufficiency require BP monitoring and modification of anticoagulant drugs such as aspirin, NSAIDs).
   × Obtain medical consultation prior any dental procedure if blood glucose levels is below 60 mg/dl
   × Schedule dental appointments either before or after periods of insulin activity, this reduces the risk of hypoglycemia
   × Ensure patient has consumed regular meal before and after periods of insulin activity, this reduces the risk of hypoglycemia.
   × Ensure adequate pain control and stress reduction as this may cause endogenous production of epinephrine and cortisol secretion, epinephrine is not contraindicated in these individuals as this will provide adequate dental anesthesia
   × Candidiasis is the most prevalent oral infection in DM patients, sugar-free topical antifungal agents are advised for 7–10 days, if treatment is unsuccessful, then switch to systemic antifungal agents.
   × Avoid nephrotoxic antiviral medications such as acyclovir, famicyclovir, valacyclovir in patients with renal insufficiency having herpes simplex viral infection.

- Burning mouth in diabetic individuals can be managed by amitriptyline.
- Well-controlled DM patient may not require antibiotic prophylaxis during surgical procedures, whereas prophylactic antibiotics to be considered in poorly controlled DM.
- Corticosteroids used for treating various oral lesions should be used cautiously with patient's physician consultation especially with systemic steroids, which require dose modifications of DM drugs.

C. **Managing dental emergencies in diabetic patients:** Diabetic emergency in dental office may be
  - Hypoglycemic (most common)
  - Hyperglycemic (less likely to occur in dental office)

Management of hypoglycemia in dental office
- Recognize the signs and symptoms of hypoglycemia, this includes:
  - Confusion, irritability, sweating, tremor, anxiety, dizziness, tingling or numbness, tachycardia, severe hypoglycemia result in seizure or loss of consciousness
- Monitor blood glucose level with a glucometer
- If glucometers are unavailable, the condition should be treated as a hypoglycemic episode

Management of hyperglycemia in dental office
- The symptoms are similar to hypoglycemia
- Monitor blood glucose levels with glucometer
- If glucometer is unavailable, treat the episode as a hypoglycemic event as individuals are more prone for severe adverse effects of hypoglycemia and manage as stated earlier, even in doubt a little sugar may not be detrimental even if the patient is hyperglycemic.
- Opening airway, administering oxygen, monitor the vital signs and transport patients to hospital for further medical management.

TABLE 18.9: Management of hypoglycemia in the dental office

Patient condition	Management
Conscious patient and able to take food by mouth	- Give 15 g oral carbohydrate - 125–175 ml fruit juice or soda - 3–4 tablespoon of sugar - Hard candy
Patient is unable to consume food by mouth and intravenous line is available	- Give 50% dextrose solution or - 1 mg glucagon
Patient is neither able to take food by mouth nor intravenous line available	- Give 1 mg glucagon subcutaneously or intramuscularly at almost any body site

Pituitary Gland Disorders

Hypersecretion of growth hormone (GH)	Gigantism	Excessive production of growth hormone occurs before epiphyseal closure
	Acromegaly	Excessive production of growth hormone occurs after epiphyseal closure
Hyposecretion of GH	Dwarfism	

Gigantism and Acromegaly

GH affects the entire body that results in enhanced growth of connective tissue, cartilage and bone. The new growth enlarges craniofacial skeleton, increased metabolic effects cause increased protein synthesis, lipolysis, gluconeogenesis, glycogenolysis.

Etiology

Pituitary adenomas

Clinical Features

- Well-proportionate individual who is usually tall, but physically weak

- The liver, spleen, kidneys and other internal organs are enlarged
- Diabetes mellitus, hypertension, cardiomegaly, congestive heart failure, abnormal electrolyte filtration, osteoporosis, visual disturbances are associated systemic diseases
- Enlargement of nose and frontal bossing
- Soft tissue edema leads to increase in shoe, hat, glove and ring sizes
- Headache, muscle pain, muscle weakness
- Coarsening of skin as the subcutaneous tissues increase in size

Oral Manifestations

- Thick lips, macrocephaly, macrognathia, disproportionate mandibular growth with prognathic mandible, generalized spacing, anterior open bite, malocclusion, tooth migration
- Macroglossia, hypertrophy of pharyngeal and laryngeal tissues producing hoarseness in voice, stridor, dyspnea, patient susceptible for sleep apnea.

Radiographic Features

- Enlarged sella turcica
- Enlarged paranasal sinuses
- Widened carpel joint spaces
- Thickened cranium with exaggerated muscle and ridge attachments
- Enlargement of the mandible, excessive condylar growth and height of ascending ramus
- Hypercementosis
- Enlarged pulp chambers

Dental Management

- Patients with hyperpituitarism may have underlying systemic disease (hypertension, cardiomegaly, heart failure, insulin resistance, diabetes mellitus Type 2, hepatomegaly, goiter), dentist should be aware of underlying systemic disease
- General practitioners should be aware of complications and dental treatment should be performed with physician consultation.

Dwarfism (Hypopituitarism)

Hypofunction of pituitary gland to secrete GH results in dwarfism.

Etiology

Craniopharyngioma, trauma, infarction, infection, radiotherapy and idiopathic disorders.

Clinical Features

- Large head, short muscular arms
- Low levels of ACTH lead to hypoadrenalism with complaints of weakness and signs of hypertension
- Lack of secretion of thyroid results in secondary hypothyroidism that produces weakness, hypotension, cold intolerance, mental illness, bradycardia, delayed sexual development, amenorrhea, hypogonadism.
- Reduced mandibular size
- Microdontia
- Small dental arch that contributes to crowding and malocclusion
- Hypofunction of salivary glands results in salivary hypofunction, that contributes to increased oral infection.

Radiographic Features

- Delayed exfoliation of primary teeth
- Delayed eruption of permanent teeth
- Absent third molars
- Small mandible which results in crowding and malocclusion

Dental Consideration

- Fluoride treatment for early management of dental caries
- Early orthodontic evaluation to correct malocclusion
- Hypopituitarism with hypoadrenalism require supplemental corticosteroids.

Disorders of Posterior Pituitary (ADH)

Disorder	Description	Signs and symptoms
Diabetes insipidus	Decreased production of ADH	× Kidneys are unable to retain water × Symptoms include polyuria (>3 L/d), polydipsia, hypernatremia × Water deprivation test is used for diagnosis
Syndrome of inappropriate ADH (SIADH)	Excessive production of ADH	× Hyponatremia, altered mental status that lead to seizures and death if undetected, stroke, infection, trauma and hemorrhage

Adrenal Gland Disorders—Cushing's Syndrome (Hyperadrenocortism)

Cushing's syndrome is caused by excessive production of cortisol by adrenal cortex.

Clinical Features

- × Fluid retention, hypertension
- × Glycosuria, hyperglycemia, increased tendency for diabetes
- × Hypokalemia, hypernatremia
- × Central obesity, moon face, buffalo hump, purple striae over the abdomen
- × Skeletal muscle weakness, thin skin, thin limbs and fingers
- × Osteoporosis, back pain
- × Hirsutism, virilism
- × Thromboembolism, amenorrhea
- × Psychological disturbances.

Oral Manifestations

- × Enlarged and swollen gingiva that bleeds readily
- × More prone for bacterial and fungal infections such as periodontal and candida infections.

Dental Considerations

- × Individuals on long-term use of glucocorticoids have tendency to bleed and bruise easily
- × Impaired wound healing and delayed scar formation
- × Individuals are more prone for infection as they are immunocompromised, therefore, these individuals should be on prophylactic antibiotics
- × Individuals are more prone for candida infection as oral microflora is altered.

Addison's Disease (Adrenal insufficiency/ Hypoadrenocorticism)

Glucocorticoids and mineralocorticoids secretion is reduced due to hypofunction of adrenal glands.

Clinical Features

- × Muscle weakness, lethargy and fatigue
- × Nausea, vomiting, loss of appetite and weight
- × Hypoglycemia, dehydration and postural dizziness
- × Hypotension, cardiac arrhythmias and cardiovascular collapse from electrolyte imbalance
- × Irregular menstrual cycle amongst women
- × Loss of body hair because of decreased androgens
- × The feedback loop from adrenal gland to pituitary gland fails in response to decreased production of cortisol and increased secretion of ACTH in blood, this in turn stimulates melanocytic stimulating hormone, which causes increased melanin pigmentation of skin and mucosa.

Oral Manifestations and Dental Considerations

- × Diffuse melanin pigmentation involving buccal mucosa, tongue and gingiva
- × Acute adrenal insufficiency as a sequela of steroid deficiency causes increased risk of infection and stress induced complication

- There is significant risk amongst individuals who regularly take steroids for 2 weeks continuously, individuals are at moderate risk of adrenal suppression who receive steroid on alternate days
- Patients on topical steroids have found no significant risk for adrenal suppression.
- The individuals with adrenal suppression have reduced ability to withstand stress of dental treatment and thus requires increased steroid dosage prior dental treatment for extensive surgical procedure
- These individuals should be managed with reduced stress with short morning appointments, use of anxiolytic agents such as nitrous oxide, oxygen, postponement of extensive procedure and deferral of oral surgical procedure.
- In case of dental emergency in patients with adrenal insufficiency should be administered 100 mg hydrocortisone intra-muscularly prior the dental procedure. The following day, twice the normal equivalent dose should be prescribed if pain or infection persists. Dose is tapered by halving the dose daily once for next 5 days.

Disorder of Adrenal Medulla (Pheochromocytoma)

The condition occurs due to excessive secretion of catecholamine's (epinephrine and norepinephrine) by adrenal medulla.

Clinical Features

- Hypertension, tachycardia, palpitations
- Headache, sweating, tremor, hyperglycemia

Oral Manifestations and Dental Considerations

- Individuals with persistent headache should be evaluated by dentists to rule out myofacial pain dysfunction syndrome
- Pheochromocytoma with multiple endocrine neoplasia IIb, there may be multiple neuromas in oral cavity (tongue, buccal mucosa), high narrow arched palate and maxillary anterior protrusion.

Parathyroid Gland Disorders

Parathyroid glands are situated in pairs posterior to thyroid gland. It secretes parathormone (PTH) that maintains plasma concentration of ionized calcium (Flowchart 18.3).

Flowchart 18.3: Type 1 diabetes mellitus

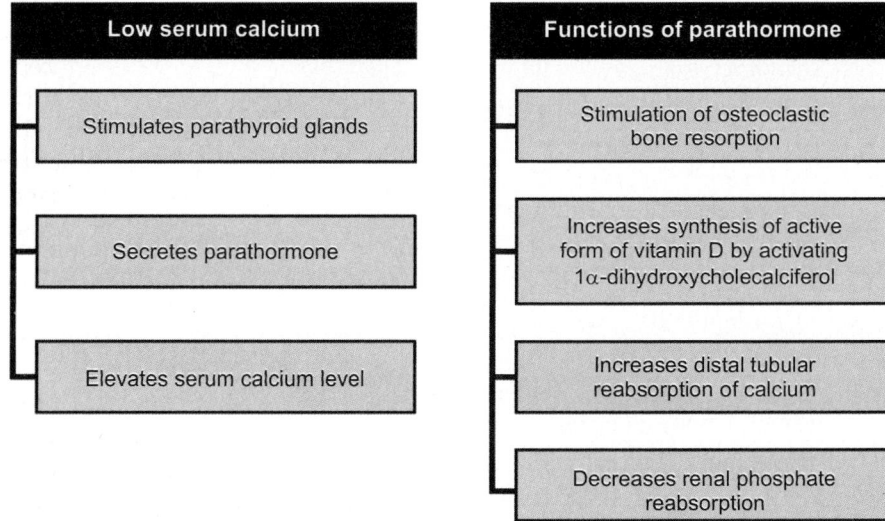

Functions of ionized calcium:
- It is essential for neuromuscular excitability
- Bone and tooth development
- Maintain membrane integrity
- Cell communication
- Cell adhesion
- Play an important role in blood clotting

Calcitonin, a hormone secreted by thyroid gland, reduces serum calcium level and the functions are exactly opposite to PTH.

Disorders of Parathyroid Hormone

Hyperparathyroidism (hypersecretion of parathormone)

Type	Etiology
Primary hyper-parathyroidism	- Caused by neoplasia of parathyroid glands
Secondary hyper-parathyroidism	- Caused secondary to chronic renal disease - In individuals undergoing chronic renal dialysis - Vitamin D deficiency (osteo-malacia, rickets)
Ectopic (psuedohyper-parathyroidism)	- Caused due to ectopic malig-nant tumors of lungs, breast, liver, pancreas, kidneys)

Clinical Features

Women of age 30–60 years are most commonly affected.

System	Symptom and sign
Cardiovascular problems	Cardiac arrhythmias, excita-bility, hypertension
Gastrointestinal disorders	Pain in abdomen, peptic ulcera-tions, pancreatitis, constipation
Neuromuscular disorders	Mental confusion, lethargy, drowsiness, stupor
Disorders of eye	Deposition of calcium in cornea, calcinosis
Genitourinary disorders	Polyurea, polydipsia, kidney stones, kidney damage
Bone	Bone pain, pathologic fractures, hypercalcemia, osteopenia

Oral Manifestations

- Vague jaw pain
- Loosen teeth and drifting of teeth
- Pulp stones, root resorption
- Soft tissue calcifications of salivary glands (sialolithiasis)
- Skeletal muscle weakness.

Radiographic Features

General radiographic manifestations
- Subtle erosions in the sub-periosteal surface of phalanges of hands
- Generalized demineralization of skeletal tissues
- **Osteitis fibrosa cystica:** Localized demineralization of bone due to osteoclastic activity
- **Brown's tumors:** These are radiolucent lesions that occur in the late stage of the disease, could be central or peripheral
- Pathological calcifications in soft tissues
- Thinning of cortex of the calvarium and loss of central (diploic) trabeculation.

Radiographic Appearance in Jaws

- Cortical thinning of inferior border of mandible, mandibular canal and maxillary sinuses
- **Osteoporosis of jaws:** Overall reduction in bone density in jaws
- Ground glass appearance
- **Brown's tumor:** Commonly observed in jaws and facial bones. It usually resembles central giant cell granuloma radiographically and histologically. The basal metabolic tests and serum biochemistry for calcium, phosphorus and alkaline phosphatase should be evaluated along with biopsy of the lesion. If the calcium, alkaline phosphatase levels are increased and reduction in phosphor is noted, Brown's tumor secondary to hyperparathyroidism should be considered.
- *Loss of lamina dura:* It may be localized or generalized depending on the severity of disease or may show partial or complete loss around the teeth.

× Presence of lytic bone cysts in jaws
× Pulp calcifications

Hypoparathyroidism

Hyposecretion of parathormone from parathyroid glands resulting in decreased serum calcium (hypocalcemia) and increased phosphor (hyperphosphatemia).

Etiology

× Accidental removal/damage to parathyroid gland during thyroidectomy
× DiGeorge syndrome (congenital absence of parathyroid glands)
× Hypomagnesaemia
× Radiation therapy.

Clinical Features

× Increased neuromuscular excitability (tetany), therefore, spasmic muscular contraction
× Numbness and tingling in the extremities
× **Chvostek's sign:** Spasm of the facial muscle particularly the lips and alae of the nose on tapping the facial nerve at the point of origin (anterior to tragus of the ear)
× **Trousseau's sign:** Carpal spasm (spasm in hand) after inflating cuff during measurement of blood pressure
× Memory loss, seizures, nail deformities
× Candidiasis, cataract development

Oral Manifestations and Dental Considerations

× Mucocutaneous candidiasis
× Circumoral paresthesia is the first symptom of hypoparathyroidism.

If the hypoparathyroidism occurs before tooth development, following changes are noted:
× Abnormal eruption pattern during tooth development
× Enamel hypoplasia and poorly mineralized dentin
× Malformed teeth, anodontia, short blunt root apices, elongated pulp chambers, pulp stones in primary and permanent teeth, impacted teeth, mandibular tori

If the hypoparathyroidism occurs after tooth development, there are no abnormalities noticed.

Thyroid Gland Disorders

Table 18.10 provides thyroid gland disorders.

Regulation of Thyroid Hormone

Refer to Flowchart 18.4.

Disorders of Thyroid Gland

Table 18.11 provides disorders of thyroid gland.

TABLE 18.10: Thyroid gland disorders		
Thyroid gland	*Hormone*	*Function*
Follicular cells	Triiodothyronine (T3) Tetraiodothyronine, (Thyroxine T4)	× Increases metabolic rate × Enhances oxygen consumption × Lowers cholesterol level × Increases epinephrine secretion × Stimulates growth × Promotes protein, carbohydrate and lipid metabolism
Parafollicular C cells	Calcitonin	× Reduces plasma calcium levels by affecting bone and kidney
T3 (10%) and T4 (90%) are the hormones secreted by follicular cells of thyroid gland, T3 is the active hormone that binds to the thyroid hormone receptor, which bring about physiologic changes, on requirement T4, is converted to T3. These hormones exist either in free or bound with protein (thyroglobulin).		

Flowchart 18.4: Regulation of thyroid hormone

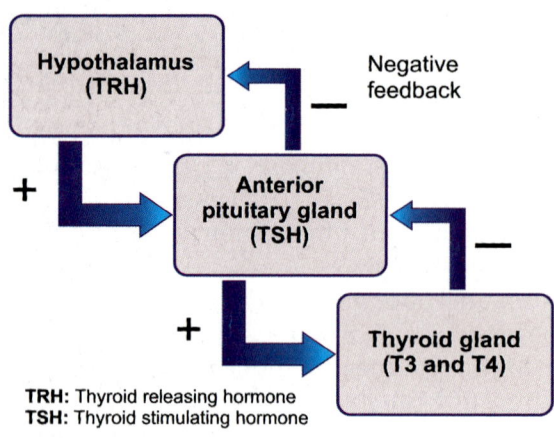

TRH: Thyroid releasing hormone
TSH: Thyroid stimulating hormone

Hyperthyroidism

Clinical Features

* The thyroid gland is enlarged, palpable, overlying skin is warm, systolic bruit on palpation
* Patients are thin, nervous, emotionally instable, irritable

* Weight loss in spite of increased appetite
* Heat intolerance, sweating
* Tremors, muscle weakness
* Palpitations, tachycardia
* Menstrual changes
* Exophthalmos
* Clubbing of fingers and toes

Oral Manifestations

* Premature loss of primary teeth
* Early eruption of secondary teeth
* Enlarged tongue
* Lingual thyroid tissue
* Difficulty in swallowing
* Increased susceptibility of patients for dental caries and periodontal disease

Dental Considerations

* Agranulocytosis and leukopenia are the side effects of antithyroid medications (propylthiouracil), thus these patients are more prone for infections, increased incidence of sialolith formation and increased anticoagulant effects of warfarin

TABLE 18.11: Disorders of thyroid gland

Disease	Characteristics	Causes
Goiter	Hypersecretion of thyroid hormones	× Graves disease (diffuse toxic goiter) × Toxic multinodular goiter × Toxic uninodular goiter × Hashimoto's thyroiditis (hypothyroid state) × Endemic goiter (caused due to dietary deficiency of iodine)
Hyperthyroidism (thyrotoxicosis) Graves disease	Increased secretion of T3 and T4	× Hyperactive thyroid nodule × Toxic adenoma × Toxic multinodular goiter × Jod-Basedow disease
Hypothyroidism	Deficiency of circulating thyroid hormone	× Destruction of thyroid gland × Dysfunction of hypothalamus pituitary axis × Hashimoto's thyroiditis (autoimmune disorder involving lymphocytic infiltration of the gland)
Cretinism	Reduction/deficiency of thyroid hormone in children and infants	× Congenital absence of gland, hypoplasia, thyroid dysplasia, fibrous replacement
Myxedema	Reduction/deficiency of thyroid hormone in adults	× Surgical excision of the thyroid gland × Radiation therapy × Atrophy of anterior pituitary gland × Hashimoto's disease

- Practitioners should be cautious while prescribing aspirin, as this may increase the circulating T4 leading to thyrotoxicosis
- NSAIDs can decrease effect of blockers
- The use of epinephrine and other sympathomimetics needs special precaution in patients with non-selective blockers
- Hyperthyroid patients are more susceptible for CVS diseases, which include atrial dysarrhythmias, tachycardia, hypertension
- Local hemostatic measures required to control bleeding during dental treatment
- Epinephrine is contraindicated in patients with thyroid storm and elective dental procedures can be deferred.

Radiographic features: Generalized loss of bone density in some areas of edentulous alveolar bone.

Diagnosis: Suppressed or reduced TSH level is the most sensitive test for hyperthyroidism

Treatment
- β-blockers for tachycardia
- Antithyroid medications
- Radioactive ^{131}I
- Surgery

Hypothyroidism

The conditions associated with hypothyroidism are cretinism (in infants and children) and myxedema (in adults)

Cretinism	Myxedema
Clinical features	
Mental retardation	Puffy face
Hypothermia	Dull facial expression
Feeding difficulties in infants	Non-pitting edema
Retarded physical growth	Weight gain
Hypertelorism	Queen Anne's sign (non-pitting edema of eyelids with loss of eyebrows on lateral third)
Broad face	Bradycardia

Cretinism	Myxedema
Delayed fontanelle closure	Cold intolerance
Stout neck	Cold skin
Protruded abdomen	Constipation
Constipation	
Bradycardia	
Oral manifestations	
Enlarged tongue and gingiva	Rampant caries
Open mouth with mouth breathing	Delay in eruption of primary and secondary teeth, therefore, malocclusion
Gingivitis	Slurred speech
Radiographic Features	
Delayed closure of epiphyses and skull sutures	Thinning of lamina dura
Delayed eruption	Relatively small jaws
Short roots	In adults: Periodontal disease, loss of teeth, spacing between teeth due to enlarged tongue, external root resorption.
Dental considerations	
Hypothyroid patients are lethargic and have diminished respiratory rate therefore increased risk of aspiration of dental materials	
Hypothyroid patients on anticoagulants will have a risk of bleeding, hence estimation of PT, PTT and INR is recommended prior any dental treatment	
Prophylactic antibiotics for compromised cardiac patients	
Narcotic analgesics should be limited as it may cause CNS depression	
These individuals have deposition of mucopolysaccharides which prevent constriction of small vessels	

Contd.

Contd.

Cretinism	Myxedema
× Excessive bleeding following trauma, which can be prevented by local pressure application and hemostyptics	
× Delayed wound healing due to decreased metabolic activity in fibroblasts and stressful situation such as surgery or trauma may precipitate the condition	
Treatment	
× Thyroid hormone replacement therapy (levothyroxine sodium)	

FREQUENTLY ASKED QUESTIONS

1. Describe the etiopathogenesis, clinical features, diagnosis and oral manifestations of diabetes mellitus.
2. Explain radiographic features of hyperparathyroidism.
3. Oral manifestations of endocrine disorders.
4. Write a short note on oral hypoglycemics.
5. Explain blood glucose regulation.
6. Explain pituitary gland disorders.
7. Discuss adrenal gland disorders.
8. Describe hyperthyroidism.

BIBLIOGRAPHY

1. Silverman, Eversole, Truelove. Essentials of Oral medicine. 1st ed. BC Decker Inc 2002.p.84–100.
2. Hall, John E., and Arthur C. Guyton. Guyton and Hall Textbook of Medical Physiology. 13th ed. Philadelphia, PA: Saunders Elsevier, 2016.
3. Greenberg MS, Glick M, Ship JA. Burket's Oral Medicine. 11th ed. BC Decker Inc 2008. p.77–106.
4. Greenberg MS, Glick M, Ship JA. Burket's Oral Medicine. 12th ed. Jaypee Brothers Medical Publishers Pvt. Ltd. 2015. p.91–122.
5. Greenberg MS, Glick M, Ship JA. Burket's Oral Medicine. 10th ed. BC Decker Inc 2008. p.85–125.
6. Bricker SL, Langlais RP, Miller CS. Oral Diagnosis, Oral Medicine and Treatment Planning. 2nd Ed. BC Decker Inc 2002.
7. Walker BR, Colledge NR, Ralston SH, Penman ID. Davidson's Principles and Practice of Medicine, International Edition, 22nd Ed., S. Chand 2014.
8. White, Stuart C., and M. J. Pharoah. Oral Radiology: Principles and Interpretation. 6th ed. St. Louis, Mo: Mosby/Elsevier, 2009.p.454–461.

Red Blood Cell Disorders—Oral Manifestations and Dental Considerations

INTRODUCTION

Blood is the fluid connective tissue that predominantly contains water containing both the cellular elements (red blood cells, white blood cells, and platelets), and extracellular elements (plasma—a mixture of water and proteins). The plasma proteins are albumin, globulin, and fibrinogen, and other dissolved solutes such as glucose, lipids, electrolytes, and dissolved gases.

The primary function of blood is to deliver oxygen and nutrients to and remove wastes from body cells, in addition, includes defense, distribution of heat, and maintenance of homeostasis. Blood constitutes approximately 8 percent of adult body weight. In an adult male the average blood is about 5 to 6 liters of blood; average of 4–5 liters in females. The pH of the blood is 7.4, it is also slightly alkaline, and its temperature is slightly higher than normal body temperature. There is wide array of hematological disorders that show various oral manifestations that can be identified by an oral physician.

Hemopoiesis

Schematic representation of hemopoiesis: The primitive stem cells in the bone marrow is pluripotent in nature, they differentiate as lymphopoietic and hematopoietic series. The hemopoiesis is self-regulatory process and there is a constant check system for formation/elimination from the system. Blood cells are formed on demand and eliminated whenever required. The demand for production of cells is infection, immune challenges, hemorrhage, hypoxia (Flowchart 19.1).

The lifespan of various types of blood cells is as follows:

Cells	Life span	Site of destruction
Erythrocytes	120 days	Reticuloendothelial system (more than 50% are destructed in spleen, and remaining is destroyed in liver, bone marrow, mononuclear phagocyte system).
Neutrophils	6 hours to 3 days	Apoptosis
Platelets	5–10 days	Spleen and phagocytosis by macrophages.

Before understanding the disorders of RBC, we should understand the normal blood parameters (Table 19.1).

Flowchart 19.1: Hemopoiesis

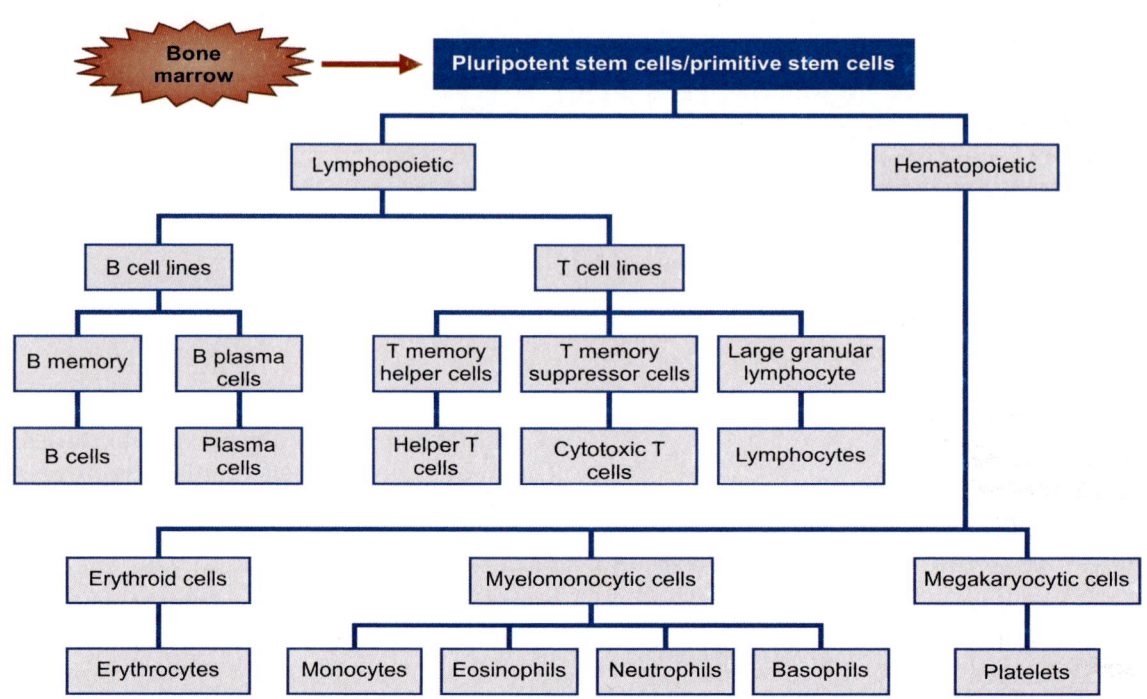

TABLE 19.1: Red cell indices				
Parameter	Men	Women	Increased	Decreased
RBC count ($\times 10^{12}$/litre)	4.4–6.1	4.2–5.4	✗ Erythrocytosis ✗ Polycythemia	✗ Anemia
RBC indices			✗ Macrocytosis	✗ Microcytosis
Hemoglobin (g/dl)	13–18	11.5–16.5	✗ Erythrocytosis ✗ Polycythemia	✗ Anemia
Hematocrit (packed cell volume)	0.40–0.54	0.37–0.47	✗ Erythrocytosis ✗ Polycythemia	✗ Anemia
Mean corpuscular volume (MCV) (fl)	75–99	75–99	✗ Vitamin B_{12} and folate deficiency	✗ Iron deficiency anemia ✗ Thalassemia
Mean corpuscular hemoglobin (MCH) (pg)	27–31	27–31	✗ Hyperchromia	✗ Hypochromic anemia
Mean corpuscular hemoglobin concentration (MCHC) (g/dl)	32–36	32–36	✗ Hyperchromia	✗ Hypochromic anemia

TABLE 19.2: Conditions affecting RBC counts	
Increased levels of red blood cell	Decreased levels of red blood cell
Erythrocytosis	Anemia (Classification described in Table 19.3)
Polycythemia vera	
Fluid loss due to dehydration, diuretics, diarrhea, burns	

Red Blood Cell Disorders (Table 19.2)

Erythrocytosis

Definition: It is a condition that describes an increase in circulating RBCs and raised hematocrit in blood.

Causes: Tissue hypoxia, congenital heart disease, high altitude, post-renal transplantation.

Types

* Relative erythrocytosis
* Absolute erythrocytosis
* Idiopathic erythrocytosis

Polycythemia Vera

Polycythemia means "too many cells in blood". First described by Vasquez in 1892.

Description: It is a chronic myeloproliferative disease, with an abnormal increase in the number of red blood cells in the peripheral blood, usually with an increased hemoglobin level.

Types

* Primary polycythemia or polycythemia rubra vera
* Secondary polycythemia
* Relative polycythemia

Clinical Manifestations

* More common in men
* Occurs in middle age or later
* Present as diffusely reddened or flushed skin
* Pruritis
* Tender splenomegaly, gastrointestinal pain
* Mucosal cyanoses, acrocyanosis
* Bleeding tendencies
* Headache, dizziness, weakness, lassitude, tinnitus, visual disturbances
* Mental confusion, slurring of speech, inability to concentrate
* Gas pains, belching, peptic ulcers, hemorrhage from varices
* Plethoric color of the skin in polycythemia

Oral Manifestations

* Deep purplish red hue of oral mucosa
* Tongue and gingiva are most commonly affected
* Swollen and engorged gingivae that bleed upon slightest provocation
* Submucosal petechiae, ecchymosis and hematomas
* Glossitis
* Gingival bleeding

Diagnosis: Elevated RBC mass, normal oxygen saturation, palpable splenomegaly

Treatment

* Phlebotomy (to remove RBCs) and myelosuppressive chemotherapy are the cornerstones of therapy
* The goal of phlebotomy is to maintain normal red cell mass and blood volume, with a target hematocrit of less than 45% for men, and less than 42% for women.
* Hydroxyurea is a principal myelo-suppressive agent in high-risk patients
* Current recommendations for treatment of young patients primarily rely on phlebotomy because the thrombosis is far less likely to occur in children and the long-term risks of leukemia over a longer life span are increased.
* *Secondary polycythemia:* Phlebotomy is used for symptomatic hyperviscosity. The goal is to treat the underlying cause of polycythemia.

Dental Considerations

* Control of hemorrhage after oral surgical procedures
* Significant bleeding requires platelet transfusion, ε-aminocaproic acid, and tranexamic acid
* Control blood counts by phlebotomy or drug therapy.

Anemia (Table 19.3)

Iron Deficiency Anemia

Definition: It is defined as a reduction in total body iron, that is required for hemoglobin synthesis.

TABLE 19.3: Classification of anemia

A. **Pathophysiologic**
I. Anemia due to blood loss
- Acute post-hemorrhagic anemia
- Chronic blood loss
II. Anemia due to impaired red cell production
    a. Cytoplasmic maturation defect
    - Deficient haem synthesis
    - Iron deficiency anemia
    - Deficient globin synthesis
    - Thalassaemic syndromes
    b. Nuclear maturation defects
    - Vitamin B_{12} and/or folic acid deficiency
    - Megaloblastic anemia
    c. Defect in stem cell proliferation and differentiation
    - Aplastic anemia
    - Pure red cell aplasia
    d. Anemia of chronic disorders
    e. Bone marrow infiltration
    f. Congenital anemia
III. Anemia due to increased red cell destruction
- Hemolytic anemia
    A. Extrinsic (extracorpuscular) red cell abnormalities
    B. Intrinsic (intracorpuscular) red cell abnormalities

B. **Morphologic**
I. Microcytic hypochromic, e.g. iron deficiency anemia, thalassaemia, sideroblastic anemia and anemia of chronic disease
II. Normocytic normochromic, e.g. anemia due to acute blood loss, anemia of chronic disease
III. Macrocytic normochromic, e.g. megaloblastic/pernicious anemia
IV. Spherocytosis: Hereditary spherocytosis, autoimmune hemolytic anemia

C. **Hematopoietic stem cell proliferation and differentiation abnormality**
- Aplastic anemia
- Pure red cell aplasia

D. **Bone marrow failure due to systemic diseases (anemia of chronic disorders)**
- Anemia of inflammation/infection, disseminated malignancy
- Anemia in renal disease
- Anemia due to endocrine and nutritional deficiency
- Anemia in liver disease

Contd.

TABLE 19.3: Classification of anemia (*Contd.*)

E. **Bone marrow infiltration**
- Leukemia
- Lymphoma
- Myelosclerosis
- Multiple myeloma

F. **Congenital anemia**
- Sideroblatic anemia
- Congenital dyserythropoietic anemia

Causes

- Inadequate intake and increased demand during gestation/pregnancy/and lactating mother.
- Reduced absorption due to gastrectomy, malabsorption, excessive use of antacids
- Most common in women due to blood loss during menstruation.

Clinical Manifestations

- Weakness, fatigue, lemon-tinted pallor of the skin, lips, mucous membranes and sclera, dyspnea on exertion, palpitations, numbness and tingling in fingers and toes, bone pain.
- Older patients may develop angina and congestive cardiac failure
- Brittle nails with spooning (koilonychia) and cracking and splitting of nail beds, palmar crease rubor.

Oral Manifestations

- Plummer-Vinson syndrome/Paterson-Brown Kelly syndrome/sideropenic dysphagia

Atrophic glossitis/ bald tongue	Stomatitis
Mucosal pallor	*Angular stomatitis* (painful fissures at the corners of the mouth) and *cheilosis* (dry scaling of the lips and corners of the mouth)
Migratory glossitis	Oral candidiasis
Recurrent aphthous stomatitis	Glossodynia
Recurrent oral ulcers	Burning mouth

- First described by Plummer in 1914 and Vinson in 1922.

The main features include
- The classic triad of esophageal web, iron deficiency anemia, and dysphagia
- Other features are migratory glossitis, koilonychia, and growth in postcricoid area
- Plummer-Vinson syndrome is associated with increased risk of squamous cell carcinoma of pharynx and oesophagus.

Diagnosis
- The peripheral smear shows microcytic hypochromic anemia
- Low serum iron, low transferrin saturation, and low ferritin
- The low serum ferritin <25 mcg/L level is the diagnostic feature of iron deficiency anemia

Treatment
- **Oral iron supplementation:** Ferrous sulphate 325 mg orally for three times daily for 3 months
- Failure of oral therapy or hemoglobin less than 6 gm% than parenteral iron dextran/ iron gluconate/ iron sucrose is given

Dental considerations
- If the hemoglobin is less than 8 g/dl, avoid general anesthesia
- Poor wound healing in anemic patients
- Narcotics should be limited in severe anemic individuals
- Dentists should be aware of increased risk for ischemic heart diseases.

Pernicious Anemia/Megaloblastic Anemia

Description: Pernicious anemia is the form of megaloblastic anemia caused due to deficiency of vitamin B_{12}, which is an extrinsic factor. This is due to atrophy of gastric mucosa and subsequent lack of intrinsic factor. Vitamin B_{12} and folic acid are needed for the maturation of RBCs in the bone marrow; and intrinsic factor is required for absorption of vitamin B_{12}.

Causes
- Reduced intake or absorption of vitamin B_{12} or folic acid
- Deficiency due to gastrectomy, tropical sprue, alcoholism, scleroderma and drugs such as colchicine.
- Autoimmunity causes self-destruction of intrinsic factor/ gastric parietal cells
- Folic acid deficiency is seen in chronic alcoholics, drug users and vegetarians with reduced intake of leafy vegetables.

Clinical Manifestations
- Generalized weakness, anorexia, abdominal pain, weight loss, shortness of breath, yellowish pigmentation
- Neurological abnormalities in vitamin B_{12} deficiency, tingling of the extremities is presented even before appreciating features of anemia, cerebral disturbances due to memory loss, irritability, depression (There are no neurological abnormalities in folic acid deficiency as in pernicious)

Oral Manifestations
- Hunter's glossitis or Moller's glossitis
- **Glossodynia:** Painful tongue
- **Glossopyrosis:** Burning sensation of lingual mucosa
- **Disguesia:** Distortion of the sense of taste.
- Persistent or recurrent stomatitis
- Oral mucosa becomes intolerant to dentures
- **Hunter's glossitis:** Inflamed tongue, 'Beefy red' in color, small and shallow ulcers may develop, gradual atrophy of papillae, ultimately results in smooth or 'bald' tongue.

Diagnosis
- **Schilling test:** Demonstrates vitamin B_{12} deficiency
- Achlorhydria
- Antibodies to intrinsic factor/parietal cells
- Peripheral smear shows macrocytic normochromic anemia
- Mean corpuscular volume is increased
- Decreased folic acid

Treatment

* High dose of oral supplementation of 1000–2000 mcg daily for 2 weeks, followed by 1000 mcg for maintenance
* Parenteral vitamin B_{12} injections once in a month

Dental considerations

* Patients with pernicious anemia should be given diphenhydramine elixir for symptomatic relief, so that individuals can take food by mouth
* Surgical procedures should be deferred until the anemia and thrombocytopenia are medically controlled, otherwise, bleeding could be a problem.
* Folate deficiency due to alcoholism leads to bleeding problems because of inhibition of liver coagulant precursors, therefore, obtain bleeding profiles prior any dental procedure.

Hemolytic Anemia

Description: Hemolytic anemia results from excessive destruction of red blood cells

Causes

* **Extracorpuscular defect**
  * Autoimmune hemolytic disease
  * Overwhelming infections or toxins
  * Rh factor incompatibility
* **Intracorpuscular defects**
  * Hereditary spherocytosis
  * Glucose-6 phosphate deficiency
  * Sickle cell anemia
  * Thalassemia
* **Congenital hemolytic anemia**
  * Membrane defects (hereditary spherocytosis)
  * Enzyme deficiency (G-6-PD deficiency and pyruvate kinase deficiency)
  * Disorders of hemoglobin (sickle cell anemia and thalassemia)

Clinical Manifestations

* Acute back pain
* Free hemoglobin in plasma and urine
* Renal failure

* Fatigue, loss of stamina
* Breathlessness, tachycardia, jaundice and hemoglobinuria
* Splenomegaly

Oral Manifestations

* Pallor/yellowish discoloration of oral mucosa
* Paresthesia of mucosa
* Hyperplastic marrow spaces in mandible, maxilla and facial bone

Hemoglobinopathies

Description

* Hemoglobinopathies occur due to point mutations and deletions in globin genes that cause changes in amino acid that causes defective synthesis of globin protein, resulting in abnormal hemoglobin
* Sickle cell anemia and thalassemia are considered as hemoglobinopathies. The qualitative defect in globin chain synthesis occurs in sickle cell anemia, whereas thalassemia is due to quantitative defect.

Sickle Cell Anemia

Description

* It occurs due to qualitative defect in globin chain, i.e. glutamic acid is replaced by valine
* It is an autosomal recessive disorder
* Due to structural variation in globin chain synthesis, hemoglobin is susceptible for low oxygen tension, low temperature or decreased pH; this leads to sickling of cell that leads to stasis, vascular obstruction, and hemolysis of the red cells.

Types

* Sickle cell trait (heterozygous)—one of the beta chains is abnormal
* Sickle cell trait (homozygous)—both the beta chains are abnormal

Clinical Manifestations

* Impaired growth and development

- Most susceptible for infections
- Delayed sexual maturity
- End organ damage due to vascular obstruction
- Splenic fibrosis
- Jaundice

Oral Manifestations

- Pallor
- Osteomyelitis due to compromised blood supply
- Impaired healing
- Delayed eruption
- Step ladder trabeculae on radiographs
- Hyperplasia and widening of marrow spaces
- Thickening of diploe with hair on end appearance on lateral skull radiographs

Diagnosis

- Peripheral smear shows normocytic normochromic cells
- Decreased hemoglobin and abnormal hemoglobin on electrophoresis

Treatment

- Children born with sickle cell disease will undergo close observation by the pediatrician and will require management by a hematologist to assure they remain healthy.
- 1 mg folic acid supplement daily for life.
- Penicillin for first 5 years of age in children as they are more prone for infections due to immature immune system.
- Blood transfusion in severe anemia and bone marrow transplantation.

Thalassemia

Description: Congenital hemoglobinopathies due to reduced rate of production of one more of globin chains (either alpha or beta) in hemoglobin molecule.

Types

- **Alpha thalassemia:** Alpha chain is deficient in hemoglobin molecule

- **Beta thalassemia:** Beta chain is deficient in hemoglobin molecule
  - *Beta thalassemia minor:* The individuals are heterozygous for beta chains
  - *Beta thalassemia major/Cooley's anemia:* The individuals are homozygous for beta chains.

Clinical Manifestations

- Clinical features are similar to sickle cell anemia
- Retarded growth and development
- Ashen grey skin color due to pallor and jaundice
- Cardiomegaly, splenomegaly, hepatomegaly.

Oral Manifestations

- Malocclusion, spacing, and occlusal abnormalities
- Sialadenitis of parotid gland due to deposition of iron
- Discolored primary and permanent teeth
- Chipmunk facies—prominent premaxilla
- Short roots with thin lamina dura
- Generalized rarefaction of alveolar bone, enlarged marrow spaces and coarse trabeculation
- Hair on end appearance on skull
- Thickened diploe
- Rib—within-a-rib appearance: A long linear density within or overlapping the medullary space of the rib and running parallel to its long axis.
- Poorly defined cortices of skull

Diagnosis

- Peripheral smear shows normocytic normochromic cells
- Similar to sickle cell anemia

Treatment

- Multiple blood transfusion for amongst thalassemia major individuals
- Folic acid supplements
- Splenectomy

Dental Considerations

* Prophylactic antibiotic prior dental treatment
* Risk of hepatitis due to blood transfusion
* Poor wound healing
* Surgical correction for facial deformities

Aplastic Anemia

Description: It is a rare but life-threatening blood dyscrasia associated with pancytopenia and bone marrow aplasia.

Types

* Acquired (drugs, viruses, chemicals, toxins and radiation)
* Inherited
* Idiopathic

Clinical Manifestations

* Sudden onset of bleeding due to thrombocytopenia—increased bruising, purpura and petechiae , epistaxis, gingival bleeding
* Fever and more prone for infection—particularly neutropenia
* Fatigue, malaise, chest pain, shortness of breath.

Oral Manifestations

* Oral bleeding
* Prone for infections especially candidiasis and viral infection
* Gingival hyperplasia and spontaneous gingival bleeding
* Herpetic lesions

Treatment

* Blood transfusion
* Immunosuppressive medication is effective in restoring blood cell production
* Prophylactic antibiotics—broad spectrum antibiotics, antifungal therapy.

FREQUENTLY ASKED QUESTIONS

1. Discuss the etiology, clinical features, oral manifestations, diagnosis and management of iron deficiency anemia.
2. Write a short note on Plummer-Vinson syndrome.
3. Oral manifestations and dental considerations of anemia.
4. Discuss hemoglobinopathies.
5. Discuss the etiology, clinical features, oral manifestations, diagnosis and management of pernicious anemia.

BIBLIOGRAPHY

1. Hall, John E., and Arthur C. Guyton. Guyton and Hall Textbook of Medical Physiology. 13th ed. Philadelphia, PA: Saunders Elsevier, 2016.
2. Greenberg MS, Glick M, Ship JA. Burket's Oral Medicine. 10th ed. BC Decker Inc 2008. p.85–125.
3. Greenberg MS, Glick M, Ship JA. Burket's Oral Medicine. 11th ed. BC Decker Inc 2008. p.77–106.
4. Greenberg MS, Glick M, Ship JA. Burket's Oral Medicine. 12th ed. Jaypee Brothers Medical Publishers (P) Ltd. 2015. p.91–122.
5. Bricker SL, Langlais RP, Miller CS. Oral Diagnosis, Oral Medicine and Treatment Planning. 2nd Ed. BC Decker Inc 2002.
6. Walker BR, Colledge NR, Ralston SH, Penman ID. Davidson's Principles and Practice of Medicine, International Edition, 22nd Ed., S. Chand 2014.
7. White, Stuart C., and M. J. Pharoah. Oral Radiology: Principles and Interpretation. 6th ed. St. Louis, Mo: Mosby/Elsevier, 2009 pp. 454.
8. Shafer, Hine and Levy. Shafer's Textbook of Oral Pathology, sixth edition. Diseases of Blood and Blood Forming Organs. Elsevier Publications 2009 pp. 754–796.
9. Harsh Mohan. Textbook of Pathology. 6th ed. Jaypee Brothers Medical Publications 2010. pp 284–324.

White Blood Cell Disorders— Oral Manifestations and Dental Considerations

INTRODUCTION

White blood cells (WBCs) are nucleated cells classified as granulocytes (neutrophils, eosinophils, and basophils) and agranulocytes (B and T lymphocytes, monocytes and macrophages), or either by their cell lineage (myeloid and lymphoid cells). Their normal range of WBCs in blood is between 4000 and 11,000 per microliter. The WBCs originate from pluripotent stem cells, and colony-forming unit. The most abundant granulocyte is the neutrophil.

The functions of the WBCs are shown in Table 20.1.

Classification of WBC Disorder

Can be broadly classified as quantitative and qualitative disorders:

× **Quantitative disorder:** In this disorder, the cells appear normal, but present in abnormal quantities either in excess or deficient.
× **Qualitative disorder:** In this disorder, abnormal cells appear in circulation due to extrinsic or intrinsic abnormalities (Table 20.2).

QUANTITATIVE LEUKOCYTIC DISORDERS

Granulocytosis

It can be either neutrophilia, eosinophilia, basophilia.

TABLE 20.1: Functions of WBCs

WBC type	Normal range	Function
Neutrophils	41–78%	Phagocytosis of the bacteria
Basophils	0–2%	They contain heparin that prevents blood from clotting, also contains vasodilator histamine that promotes blood flow to tissues.
Eosinophil's	0–4%	Defense against multicellular parasites and anti-inflammatory
T and B lymphocytes	23–44%	Cellular and humoral immunity
Monocytes	0–7%	Phagocytosis, antigen presentation, and cytokine production

× **Definition:** Abnormally increased number of cells (>11,000/µL) and absolute neutrophil count >7,700/µL.
× **Abnormal increase** in number of neutrophils (neutrophilia), increase in eosinophils (eosinophilia), increase in basophils (basophilia).
× **Causes:** Bacterial infection, stress, smoking, pregnancy, burns, acute myocardial infarction, acute gout, acute glomerulonephritis, rheumatic fever,

TABLE 20.2: WBC disorders

Quantitative disorders	Granulocytosis Agranulocytosis
Qualitative disorders	*Defects in adhesion* × Leukocyte adhesion deficiency (Type 1, 2, and 3) *Defects in phagocyte activation* × Hyperimmunoglobulin E (Job's syndrome) × Chronic granulomatous disease × Chédiak-Higashi syndrome *Granulocyte disorder* × Myeloperoxidase deficiency × Chédiak-Higashi syndrome × Chronic granulomatous disease
Neoplastic disorders	× Leukemia × Lymphoma × Multiple myeloma

strenuous exercises and myeloproliferative disorders.

Agranulocytosis (Neutropenia and Granulocytopenia)

Definition: Agranulocytosis is reduced quantity of granulocytes.

Causes

× Impaired production is the main cause
  ▪ It is due to severe vitamin B_{12} deficiency/ bone marrow replacement resulting from malignant infiltration
  ▪ Increased utilization due to the acute phase of infections/autoimmune diseases
× Mild (1000–2000 cells/μL) to moderate neutropenia (500–1000 cells/μL)
  ▪ Is due to Epstein-Barr virus infection or respiratory syncytial virus
  ▪ Drug-induced such as antineoplastics alkylating agents, antimetabolites antibiotics (chloramphenicol, sulfonamides, penicillins), anticonvulsants (carbamazepine), antithyroid agents, mercurial diuretics, and phenothiazines.
  ▪ Autoimmune disorders such as rheumatoid arthritis, Felty's syndrome,

lupus erythematosis, Wegener's granulomatosis.
× Severe form (less than 500 cells/μL)

Oral Health Considerations

× Ulcerations and necrotizing lesions on gingiva, floor of the mouth, buccal mucosa, pharynx
× The ulcers lack the surrounding inflammation and are characterized by foul smell and necrosis
  The distinct form of agranulocytosis is the cyclic neutropenia.

Cyclic Neutropenia

× It is autosomal dominant disorder due to mutations in the gene for neutrophil elastase
× It is a rare disorder characterized by periodic failure of stem cells in bone marrow, resulting in repetitive episodes of fever, mouth ulcers, and infections due to neutropenia.
× The individuals present with cyclical episodes of neutropenia, with a regular 21 days interval, neutropenia persists for 3–5 days characterized by infections.

Clinical Features

× Fever, stomatitis, pharyngitis, skin abscess, lymphadenopathy
× History of repeated infections of ear and respiratory infections
× The severe consequences of neutropenia are gangrene, bacteremia, septic shock.

Oral Manifestations

× Recurrent aphthous ulcers, recurrent gingivitis and periodontitis
× Ulcers lack surrounding inflammation/ red inflammatory border and are characterized by necrosis.

Treatment

× Administration of hematopoietic growth factors such as granulocyte colony stimulating factor.

Chronic Neutropenia

Definition: A low absolute neutrophil count for more than 6 months.

Classification

- Congenital neutropenia (also called Kostmann's syndrome)
- Acquired
- Idiopathic (it is the predominant type)

Etiology: Kostmann's syndrome is caused due to mutations in variety of genes (ELANE, HAX1, and GF11 genes).

Clinical Features

- Deep tissue infections, lung and liver abscesses, severe skin infections
- Infants are chronically ill after birth with anemia, thrombocytopenia
- The bone marrow shows promyelocytic maturation arrest.

Oral Manifestations

- Recurrent gingivitis and periodontitis in early childhood
- Premature primary tooth loss

Treatment: Administration of granulocyte colony stimulating factor

Diseases of Agranulocytes

Agranulocytes include T and B lymphocytes, monocytes that constitute of about 20–40% of WBCs.

Lymphocytes facilitate cellular and humoral immunity.

The diseases of agranulocytes are shown in Table 20.3.

QUALITATIVE DISORDERS

Lazy Leukocyte Syndrome

Definition: It is caused by loss of chemotactic function of neutrophils.

Description: Marrow contains normal number of matured neutrophils, but patients have severe neutropenia because the cells are unable to migrate from the marrow to peripheral blood.

Clinical Features and Oral Manifestations

- Individuals are more prone for infections as neutrophils fail to migrate at the site of inflammation.
- Becomes apparent at the age of 1–2 years when infectious complications begin.
- Gingivitis, stomatitis, otitis media and bronchitis
- Total leukocyte count <100–200 mm

Treatment

- The management of patients with the lazy leukocyte syndrome does not present major difficulties since appropriate antibiotic therapy is generally effective although less promptly than in hematologically normal subjects.

TABLE 20.3: Lymphocyte disorders

	Lymphocytopenia	Lymphocytosis
Definition	✗ A decrease in number of lymphocytes <1,000 cells µL in blood	✗ An increase in number of lymphocytes
Causes	✗ Iatrogenic ✗ Infections (bacterial, viral, fungal, parasitic) ✗ Systemic diseases (systemic lupus erythematosis, rheumatoid arthritis, Sjögren's syndrome), lymphoma, sarcoidosis, renal failure, aplastic anemia, Cushing's syndrome) ✗ Others (malnutritions, stress)	✗ Viral infections (Epstein-Barr virus, cytomegalovirus, HIV, pertussis) ✗ Lymphoproliferative disorders (acute and chronic lymphocytic leukemia)
Treatment	✗ Treat the underlying disease	

× The treatment of major infectious episodes as well as the prevention of recurrences include the well-known measures common to other granulocyte function disorders.
× Oral prophylaxis
× Oral rinses for stomatitis—chlorhexidine.

Chédiak-Higashi Syndrome

Description

× Chédiak-Higashi syndrome (CHS) was described by Beguez Cesar in 1943, Steinbrinck in 1948, Chédiak in 1952, and Higashi in 1954.
× It is a rare childhood autosomal recessive disorder that affects multiple systems of the body.

Clinical Features

× Individuals exhibit hypo-pigmentation of the skin, eyes, and hair
× Prolonged bleeding times; easy bruisability
× Recurrent infections
× Abnormal natural killer cell function
× Peripheral neuropathy
× Most patients who do not undergo bone marrow transplantation die of a lymphoproliferative syndrome, although some patients with Chédiak-Higashi syndrome have a relatively milder clinical course of the disease.

Leukemia

Definition: It is the disordered differentiation and malignant proliferation of hematopoietic tissue that displaces normal blood forming elements of the bone marrow.

Classification

× Based on cell type
  • Lymphoid
  • Myeloid
× Based on degree of maturity
  • Mature cells
  • Immature cells
× Based on clinical course
  • Acute
  • Chronic

Broadly classified as:
1. Acute lymphoblastic/lymphoid leukemia
2. Chronic lymphoblastic/lymphoid leukemia
3. Acute myelocytic/myeloid leukemia
4. Chronic myelocytic/myeloid leukemia
   Characteristics of acute and chronic lymphoid leukemia shown in Table 20.4.

Clinical Features

These are shown in Table 20.5.

TABLE 20.4: Features of leukoplakia		
Features	*Acute lymphoid leukemia*	*Chronic lymphoid leukemia*
Age of occurrence	× Most common amongst children × Can involve about 15% adults	× 15–39 years of age
Gender predilection	× Male predominance	× Male predominance
Male to female ratio	3:2	2:1
Classification	× L1—has small lymphoblast cells predominantly affect children × L2: Mixed blast cells and occur in adults × L3: Uniform large blast cells which resemble Burkitt's lymphoma and are associated with worst prognosis	× M1, M2, M3: Predominantly has granulocytes × M4, M5—proliferation of monocytes × M6—presence of erythrocytes components × M7—presence of megakaryocytes components
Prognosis	× Favorable prognosis of all leukemias	× Most aggressive disease amongst men

TABLE 20.5: Different features of leukoplakia	
Acute leukemia	Chronic leukemia

× Due to replacement of normal cells by leukemic cells the following manifestations are noted-
  ✦ Anemia
  ✦ Neutropenia
  ✦ Thrombocytopenia
  ✦ Hepatosplenomegaly
  ✦ Back pain and pain in abdomen, bone and joint
  ✦ CNS abnormalities.
	× The symptoms are generally milder than acute leukemia
	× Due to leukemic cell infiltrates-
	  ✦ Anemia
	  ✦ Skin pallor
	  ✦ Shortness in breadth
	  ✦ Petechiae and ecchymosis on skin due to thrombocytopenia

× Night sweats, fever, weight loss, lethargy, weakness, individuals are more prone for infections	× Night sweats, fever, weight loss, lethargy, weakness, anorexia, individuals are more prone for infections
× Cervical lymphadenopathy and enlargement of Waldeyer's ring are due to lymphoid expansion	× Chronic myeloid leukemic (CML) patients always have abdominal full due to splenomegaly, hepatomegaly
× Life-threatening bacterial, fungal and viral infections due to splenomegaly and granulocytopenia	× CML patients have increased serum vitamin B_{12} due to overproduction of transcobalamin by granulocytes
× CNS manifestations such as palsies, vomiting and headache. These manifestations are more severe with acute lymphocytic leukemia	× Individuals are more prone for infections due to reduced immunoglobulins
Chloroma: The localized accumulation of leukemic cells in gingiva, neck, head. The chloroma turns to green on exposure to sunlight.	

Oral Manifestations

× Gingival enlargement is the most common finding in AML
× Chemotherapy induced mucositis is most common finding amongst individuals undergoing treatment
× Infections such as herpes simplex viral infection and candidiasis due to neutropenia
× Odontalgia due to leukemic cell infiltrates
× Ulecration in palate
× Gingivitis and gingival bleeding
× Petechiae and ecchymosis of hard and soft palate, tongue and tonsils
× Graft-versus-host disease when individuals undergo allogenic hematopoietic stem cell transplantation
× Salivary gland enlargement due to leukemic cell infiltrate.

Radiographic Features

× Loss of lamina dura
× Displacement of teeth
× Loss of the crypt outline around the unerupted teeth
× Widened PDL space and abnormal marrow spaces in the bone
× Periodontal destructions
× Increased mobility
× Protrusion of teeth
× Rarefying osteitis
× Chloroma within the jaw bone

Diagnosis

× **For acute leukemia**
  ▪ Increased WBC count of more than 1,00,000 cells/mm³
  ▪ Decreased platelet count below 1,00,000 cells/mm³

× **For chronic leukemia**
  ▪ Increased WBC count
  ▪ Bone marrow aspirate shows increased cellularity and Philadelphia chromosome

Treatment

Chemotherapy to reduce the blood count, decrease lymphadenopathy, and splenomegaly
× Chemotherapy is achieved in the following phases:
  ▪ *First phase (induction phase):* Causes initial killing of tumor cells and act as cytotoxic agent
  ▪ *Second phase (consolidation phase):* Killing of remaining cells
  ▪ *Third phase (remission phase):* It is maintenance treatment to prevent leukemic cell proliferation.

Dental Considerations

× In pre-induction phase thorough clinical and radiographic examination should be performed
× Debridement and fluoride application is completed
× In the induction phase patients are neutropenic and are highly susceptible for infections; therefore should maintain meticulous oral hygiene by total elimination of plaque
× Oral care with 0.12% chlorhexidine gluconate and nystatin
× During maintenance phase and remission phase of therapy, routine dental care is provided.
× Use of topical antimicrobials that may reduce the systemic infections
× Topical anesthetic and analgesics can be used to reduce pain
× Cytoprotective agents such as palifermin (keratinocytic growth factor) is used to reduce the severity and duration of mucositis
× Emergency dental care are infrequent, if the granulocyte count is below 2000 cells/ ml, antibiotics is must

× Absorbable gelatin sponges with topical thrombin and microfibrillar collagen can be placed to control bleeding.

Lymphoma

Definition

× These are the solid neoplastic growth of lymphoid cells that arise in reticulo-endothelial and lymphoid tissue and can spread to distant lymphoid tissues such as liver, spleen, and bone marrow.
× Lymphoma frequently originates in the lymph nodes but can arise extranodularly.
× Extranodular lymphomas have more benign course.

Classification

× Hodgkin's lymphoma
× Non-Hodgkin's lymphoma
× Burkitt's lymphoma

Hodgkin's Lymphoma (HL)

× It is a malignant disorder originating in the lymphoid tissue
× It constitutes of about 10% of lymphomas
WHO classification of Hodgkin's lymphoma (HL)
× The major subtypes of HL are
  ▪ Classic (characterized by presence of Reed-Sternberg cells)
  ▪ Nodular
× The four subtypes are:
  ▪ Nodular sclerosis [60–80%]
  ▪ Mixed cellularity [15–30%]
  ▪ Lymphocyte depletion [<1%], and
  ▪ Lymphocyte-rich [5%]

Clinical Features

× It has bimodal age distribution (first being at age thirty and second being after the age of 55)
× Frequently occurs in men
× Patients complain of pain in chest, cough, dyspnea if mediastinal lymph nodes are involved
× Night sweats, fever, weight loss

- Generalized pruritis, pain in the involve lymph node
- Waldeyer's ring is commonly involved in Hodgkin's lymphoma

Staging System

Ann-Arbor staging classification—the Cotswolds staging system of HL
Stage
I. Involvement of one lymph node region or lymphoid structure (e.g. spleen, thymus, or Waldeyer's ring)
II. Involvement of two or more lymph node regions on the same side of the diaphragm

III. Involvement of lymph node regions on both sides of the diaphragm
  1. Splenic hilar, coeliac, or portal nodes
  2. Para-aortic, iliac, or mesenteric nodes

IV. Involvement of extranodal sites other than one contiguous or proximal extranodal site
Modifying features
A No symptoms
B Fever, drenching night sweats, loss of >10% body weight over 6 months
X Bulky disease (mediastinal mass >1/3 of thoracic diameter or any nodal mass >10 cm in diameter)
E Involvement of one contiguous or proximal extranodal site
Source: Reproduced from Burket's 12th edition.

Treatment

Treatment is based on the following:
- The histology of the disease
- The anatomical stage
- Presence of prognostic features

Stagewise management of HL
- **Early stage disease:** Combination chemotherapy followed by involved field radiation therapy (IFRT)
- **Advanced stage:** Longer course of chemotherapy often without radiation therapy
- **Refractory cases**
  - High dose chemotherapy followed by stem cell transplant
  - Patients who fail to respond to the above therapy: Brentuximab vedotin, an anti-CD-30 antibody conjugated to an antimicrotubule drug.

Oral Health Considerations

- Chemotherapy-induced oral mucositis, oral ulcerations, candida infections
- Damage to the salivary glands if it is in the field of radiation therapy
- Topical varnish and fluoride application for prevention of caries
- Osteoradionecrosis is rare that is limited to the lower border and angle of mandible.

Non-Hodgkin's Lymphoma (NHL)

- NHL is the malignant disease of lymphoid system highly heterogenous both histologically and clinically.
- It is a lymphoproliferative disorder that is multicentric in cell origin and is usually multifocal when detected.
- NHL is associated with systemic diseases such as Sjögren's syndrome, celiac disease, and rheumatoid arthritis
- Approximately 85% to 90% of NHL cases arise from B cells, e.g.
  - Burkitt lymphoma,
  - Chronic lymphocytic leukemia/small cell lymphoma
  - Diffuse large B-cell lymphoma,
  - Follicular lymphoma,
  - Mantle cell lymphoma
- The remaining arise from T cells, e.g.
  - Mycosis fungoides,
  - Anaplastic large cell lymphoma,
  - Precursor T-lymphoblastic lymphoma

Etiology

- **Infectious agents:** Epstein-Barr virus, human T cell leukemia type I virus, hepatitis C virus, *Helicobacter pylori* infection
- **Environmental factors**
  - Chemicals, e.g. pesticides, herbicides, hair dye, etc.
  - Chemotherapy
  - Radiation exposure
- **Immunodeficiency states:** AIDS, celiac disease

* **Chronic inflammation:** Sjögren's syndrome, Hashimoto thyroiditis

Clinical and Oral Manifestations

* Painless lymphadenopathy that is rubbery in consistency, mobile, and rarely matted
* Abdominal pain, vomiting, gastrointestinal obstruction are the common abdominal complaints
* Rapid nodal growth may impair lymphatic drainage, resulting in lymphedema, pain, paresthesia and skin infiltrations
* Thoracic involvement may cause pleural effusions, ascites, and dyspnea
* Bone marrow infiltrations can cause destructive lesions in bone, pathological fractures, anemia
* Splenomegaly
* Hypogammaglobulinemia and opportunistic infections are frequent
* Oral involvement is rare, it can cause gingival and mucosal swelling
* Destruction of jaw bone, tooth ache
* Nerve invasion can cause paresthesia or anesthesia
* Non-healing mucosal ulceration

Clinical difference between HL and NHL

Clinical differences between Hodgkin's lymphoma and non-Hodgkin's lymphoma are shown in Table 20.6.

Treatment

NHL is a radiosensitive tumor, radiotherapy is of choice for all the subtypes:

NHL type	Behavior	Treatment
Indolent lymphoma	Grade I or low grade type	Radiotherapy
Aggressive lymphoma	Grade II or high grade lymphoma	Radiotherapy is used after or to consolidate chemotherapy and for palliative treatment

The "staging," or evaluation of extent of disease, for both HL and NHL are similar, discussed in the section of HL.

Burkitt's Lymphoma (BL)

It is the most aggressive and common types of childhood NHL. It starts in the abdomen and spreads to other organs including brain. In African children, it often involves facial bones and associated with Epstein-Barr virus.

Types

* African (endemic) BL
* Sporadic (non-endemic/American) BL
* Subset of aggressive lymphoma (immunodeficiency related)

TABLE 20.6: Lymphomas		
	Hodgkin's lymphoma	*Non-Hodgkin's lymphoma*
Age	* Bimodal age distribution * 1st peak: 15–34 years * 2nd peak: Over 50 years	* Increased with advanced age
Appearance	* Localized involvement of lymph node or contiguous lymph node involvement	* Widespread involvement of lymph nodes
Involvement site	* Extranodal involvement uncommon	* Extra nodal involvement common
Spread of disease	* Orderly spread by contiguity	* Non-contiguous spread
Location	* Frequently involves the cervical chain giving the bull-neck appearance	* Frequently involves hard and soft palate—Waldeyer's ring
Fever type	* Pel-Ebstein fever	* Non-specific fever

Clinical and Oral Manifestations

Burkitt's lymphoma is shown in Table 20.7.

Oral Manifestations

- Jaw tumors that are clinically evident that results in tooth mobility and pain, intraoral swelling of the mandible and maxilla, and anterior open bite.

Radiographic Features

- Resorption of alveolar bone
- Loss of lamina dura
- Enlargement of tooth follicles
- Destruction of cortex of the tooth crypts
- Displacement of tooth and tooth buds by enlarging tumor resulting in teeth floating in air appearance
- Sunray appearance

Management

- Aggressive chemotherapy is used to cure BL. The most commonly used chemotherapeutic agents are cytarabine, cyclophosphamide, methotrexate, doxorubicin, vincristine, and etoposide.

Multiple Myeloma

Definition

- It is the malignant neoplasm of plasma cells (derived from B cells)

- It is most common malignancy of bone in adults.

Clinical Features

- Age of occurrence: 35–70 years
- Commonly affects men
- Patient complains of fatigue, bone pain, pathologic fractures, osteopenia, weight loss, anemia, usually complain of low back pain
- Secondary features include amyloidosis, hypercalcemia, Bence Jones proteins in patient's urine, which causes urine to be foamy
- Focal osteolytic bone lesions

Oral Manifestations

- Tooth pain, mobility of teeth, swelling, hemorrhage, paresthesia, dysesthesia
- Macroglossia, gingival and soft tissue enlargement due to amyloid deposition
- Pallor, petechiae, ecchymosis, and increased bleeding tendency.

Radiographic Features

- Mandible is most commonly affected than maxilla, punched-out radiolucency in the bones without corticated margins, asymptomatic osteolytic lesions, sunray appearance.
- Generalized bone rarefactions and osteoporotic changes as disease advances.

TABLE 20.7: Burkitt's lymphoma	
Type	Clinical features
Endemic BL	- Occurs most commonly in African children age of occurrence 4–7 years - Male to female ratio—2:1 - Caused by Epstein-Barr virus - Primarily involves the facial bone and jaws - Extranodal sites are kidneys, gasterointestinal tract, ovaries, breast - Rarely occurs in the United States
Sporadic BL	- Uncommon form of NHL - Affects older adult patients (age >40 years) - Illeocecal area in the abdomen is the most common site of involvement - Other features are pleural effusion, ascites, involvement of lymph nodes, Waldeyer's ring, ovaries, breast, kidneys.
Immunodeficiency related BL	- Manifestations are secondary to immunosuppressive drugs used to prevent transplant rejection

Treatment

- Chemotherapy with radiation therapy for painful bony lesions
- Combination of cyclophosphamide/melphalan with prednisolone is often used

Dental considerations

- Dental treatment is complicated by anemia, infections, hemorrhagic tendency, renal failure and use of corticosteroids.
- Bleeding tendency due to thrombocytopenia

FREQUENTLY ASKED QUESTIONS

1. Write a short note on cyclic neutropenia, agranulocytopenia.
2. Discuss the classification, clinical features, oral manifestations, diagnosis and management of leukemia.
3. Describe lymphoma.
4. Discuss multiple myeloma.

BIBLIOGRAPHY

1. Hall, John E., and Arthur C. Guyton. Guyton and Hall Textbook of Medical Physiology. 13th ed. Philadelphia, PA: Saunders Elsevier, 2016.
2. Greenberg MS, Glick M, Ship JA. Burket's Oral Medicine. 10th ed. BC Decker Inc 2008. p.438–452.
3. Greenberg MS, Glick M, Ship JA. Burket's Oral Medicine. 11th ed. BC Decker Inc 2008. p.395–410.
4. Greenberg MS, Glick M, Ship JA. Burket's Oral Medicine. 12th ed. Jaypee Brothers Medical Publishers (P) Ltd. 2015. p.441–462.
5. Bricker SL, Langlais RP, Miller CS. Oral diagnosis Oral Medicine and Treatment Planning. 2nd Ed. BC Decker Inc 2002.
6. Walker BR, Colledge NR, Ralston SH, Penman ID. Davidson's Principles and Practice of Medicine, International Edition 22nd Ed. S. Chand 2014.
7. White, Stuart C., and M. J. Pharoah. Oral Radiology: Principles and Interpretation. 7th ed. St. Louis, Mo: Mosby/Elsevier, 2009 pp.444–450.
8. Shafers, Hine and Levy. Shafer's Textbook of Oral pathology sixth edition. Diseases of Blood and blood forming organs. Elsevier Publications 2009 pp. 754–796.
9. Harsh Mohan Textbook of Pathology. 6th ed. Jaypee Brothers Medical Publications 2010. pp 284–324.

HIV Infection and Acquired Immune Deficiency Syndrome (AIDS)

AIDS or acquired immune deficiency syndrome is caused by human immuno-deficiency virus (HIV). HIV is a type of retrovirus with nucleic acid in the form of RNA and during replication this RNA changes into DNA. Its shape is round and 80–100 nm in diameter. It comprises four elements—genome, matrix, capsid, envelope. It is originated between 1960s and 1970s, where humans were infected with it from chimpanzee.

Etiology and Spread

There exist two recognized types of HIV: HIV-1 and HIV-2. Both the types have similar modes of transmission, and can cause immunosuppression or AIDS. This virus attack on the immune system, especially the CD4 T-lymphocytes (CD4 cells). Once infected, the virus gradually and silently suppresses the host's defense mechanisms, resulting in opportunistic infections and even cancers. Differentiated CD4 cells have an essential role in the activation of cell-mediated and humoral immune systems. Various causes and modes of spread for HIV are as follows.

Causes

People transmit HIV in body fluids, including blood, semen, vaginal secretions, anal fluids and breast milk.

Spread

* Anal or vaginal intercourse with a person who has HIV
* Sharing equipment for injectable banned drugs, hormones, and steroids with a person who has HIV
* A pregnant woman with HIV infection who has recently given birth might transfer the disease to her child during pregnancy, childbirth, or breastfeeding.
* Through blood transfusions and during blood donations.

REVISED CLASSIFICATION SYSTEM FOR HIV-1993 BY CDC2

The CDCs proposed classification system for HIV infection: Divides HIV infected patients into three laboratory categories and three clinical categories.

Clinical Category A

Conditions

* Asymptomatic HIV infection
* Persistent generalized lymphadenopathy
* Acute (primary) HIV infection with accompanying illness or history of acute HIV infection
* Conditions listed in categories B and C must not have occurred.

Clinical Category B

Symptomatic conditions in an HIV-infected adolescent or adult that are not included among conditions listed in clinical category C and that meet at least one of the following criteria:

a. The conditions are attributed to HIV infection or are indicative of a defect in cell-mediated immunity or

b. The conditions are considered by physicians to have a clinical course or to require management that is complicated by HIV infection.

Examples of, but not limited to, the following conditions:

× Bacillary angiomatosis
× Candidiasis, oropharyngeal (thrush)
× Candidiasis, vulvovaginal; persistent, frequent, or poorly responsive to therapy
× Cervical dysplasia (moderate or severe)/ cervical carcinoma *in situ*
× Constitutional symptoms, such as fever (38.5°C) or diarrhea lasting greater than 1 month
× Oral hairy leukoplakia
× Herpes zoster (shingles) involving at least two distinct episodes or more than one dermatome
× Idiopathic thrombocytopenic purpura
× Listeriosis
× Pelvic inflammatory disease, particularly if complicated by tubo-ovarian abscess
× Peripheral neuropathy

Clinical Category C

Conditions

× Candidiasis of bronchi, trachea, or lungs
× Candidiasis, esophageal
× Cervical cancer, invasive
× Coccidioidomycosis, disseminated or extrapulmonary
× Cryptococcosis, extrapulmonary
× Cryptosporidiosis, chronic intestinal (greater than 1 month's duration)
× Cytomegalovirus disease (other than liver, spleen, or nodes)

× Cytomegalovirus retinitis (with loss of vision)
× Encephalopathy, HIV related
× Herpes simplex: Chronic ulcer(s) (greater than 1 month's duration) or bronchitis, pneumonitis, or esophagitis
× Histoplasmosis, disseminated or extrapulmonary
× Isosporiasis, chronic intestinal (greater than 1 month's duration)
× Kaposi's sarcoma
× Lymphoma, Burkitt's (or equivalent term)
× Lymphoma, immunoblastic (or equivalent term)
× Lymphoma, primary, of brain
× *Mycobacterium avium* complex or *M. kansasii*, disseminated or extrapulmonary
× *Mycobacterium tuberculosis*, any site (pulmonary or extrapulmonary)
× Mycobacterium, other species or unidentified species, disseminated or extrapulmonary
× *Pneumocystis carinii* pneumonia
× Pneumonia, recurrent
× Progressive multifocal leukoencephalopathy
× Salmonella septicemia, recurrent
× Toxoplasmosis of brain
× Wasting syndrome due to HIV

Laboratory Categories

Category 1: A CD4+ lymphocyte count of more than 500 cells/mm^3

Category 2: A CD4+ lymphocyte count from 200 through 499 cells/mm^3

Category 3: A CD4+ lymphocyte count below 200 cells/mm^3.

Clinical Features

The early symptoms of HIV infection may include: Fever, chills, joint pain muscle aches, sore throat, sweats particularly at night, enlarged glands, a red rash tiredness, weakness unintentional weight loss, thrush.

Flu-like symptoms {acute retroviral syndrome} can be seen within a month or two, but not in all patients (when CD4 count falls below 200 cells/mm³). These symptoms usually disappear within a couple of weeks {2–6 weeks}, and a person may be asymptomatic (CD4 cell count up to or above 500 cells/mm³)for many years. This period can last for five to seven years or longer in adults and two to five years or longer in children born with HIV. If patient is not on medication, HIV weakens the ability to fight infection which leads to late stage or stage 3 (CD4 cell count <50 cells/mm³).

Symptoms of late-stage HIV infection may include: Blurred vision, diarrhoea, which are usually persistent, chronic dry cough, a fever of over 100 °F (37 °C) lasting for weeks, night sweats, permanent tiredness, shortness of breath or dyspnea, swollen glands lasting for weeks, unintentional weight loss,white spots on the tongue or mouth.There are many opportunistic infections found in HIV patients (Table 21.1).

Investigation

HIV infection is confirmed by correct laboratory testing. Western blot analysis is standard confirmatory test. This is highly sensitive and specific, with low false-positive rates.

But, many cases of recent HIV infection may be missed because it takes several weeks to develop antibody response. As a concern, other testing methods have been developed and approved by the Food and Drug Administration (FDA). Currently, there are four rapid HIV tests that have been approved by the FDA. Two of these rapid HIV tests (OraQuick and Multispot) are able to screen for both HIV-1 and HIV-2, whereas the other two tests (Reveal and Uni-Gold Recombigen) only screen for HIV-1 (Table 21.1).

Treatment

The initial task is to identify the state of current infection (acute or chronic) and it consists of a complete medical history, physical examination, and laboratory evaluation. Treatment of HIV has now become simpler and cheaper because of availability of fixed dose combinations and low cost generic drugs. There are many classes of antiretroviral drugs with many new additions to manage and prevent drug resistant mutations and it completely depends upon CD4+ count and viral load. Treatment is suggested when count goes below 200 cells/mm³. It is based on targeting the opportunistic infections associated with immunosuppression and the HIV itself. These are:

1. Fusion inhibitors
2. Nucleoside reverse transcriptase inhibitors (NRTIs)

S. no	Headings	Tests	
TABLE 21.1: Investigations for HIV/AIDS			
1.	Specific	ELISA	
2.	Antibodies based tests	1. Screening: ELISA, Rapid test	2. Supplemental or confirmatory test a. Western Blot . b. Immunofluorescent assay c. Radioimmuno precipitation assay
3.	Other tests	a. P24 Antigen detection b. Polymerase chain reaction test c. Culture d. Plasma /viral load e. Alternative to classical test: Saliva and urine test	

3. Non-nucleoside reverse transcriptase inhibitors (NNRTIs), and

4. Protease inhibitors (PIs).

WHO guidelines for ART initiation have also changed recently based on the evidence of benefits of early ART initiation in terms of providing healthier life to HIV infected patients. Guidelines for ART in paediatric age group have also been revised recently.

Recently wide range of NRTIs drugs which include abacavir (ABC), didanosine (ddI), emtricitabine (FTC), lamivudine (3TC), stavudine (d4T), tenofovir disoproxil fumarate (TDF), zalcitabine (ddC), and zidovudine (AZT, ZDV) are used. It binds near the catalytic site of reverse transcriptase and inhibits a crucial step in the transcription of the RNA genome into a double-stranded retroviral DNA.

The treatment of HIV infection requires combination therapy known as highly active antiretroviral therapy (HAART).

Oral Health Considerations

Each patient must be assessed individually. Initial priorities to treat the patient are:
1. Alleviate pain
2. Restore function
3. Prevent further disease
4. Consider esthetic results

Pain is the most common cause for which patient visits a dentist. Before reaching the diagnosis, detailed history, vital sign and cardiovascular history and other history should be taken. HIV-infected patients will require care either for their routine dental treatment or oral conditions associated with their underlying disease. Prior to initiating therapy, the dental practitioners should check for patient's immune status, medication profile, CD4+ count, neutrophil count, and platelet count.

1. For pulpits dentist should do the needful restoration and if it is not restorable then plan extraction. Before extraction antibiotics should be given to the patients. In case of abscess it is necessary to differentiate its origin between periodontal and periapical and frame the treatment accordingly.

2. Treatment of NUG/NUP involves mechanical debridement to eliminate microbial accumulations with scaling of gross deposits followed by meticulous scaling and root planing, oral hygiene instruction, chemotherapeutic agents and frequent recall visits. In addition to antibiotics and antifungal agents, twice daily home use of a 0.12% chlorhexidine oral rinse is recommended for preventing and controlling plaque formation and to reduce the development of gingivitis.

3. Periodontal lesions that fail to respond to correctional therapy must be evaluated further, usually by biopsy for a definitive diagnosis. Teeth with a poor prognosis may be maintained instead of extracted if a patient is deemed a poor candidate for tooth replacement.

4. "Dry socket" (localized osteitis), is common complication with an extraction which occurs in 3–4% of all extractions among the general population. Studies to date suggest that this complication rate is similar in the HIV positive group. Wisely use of aseptic and atraumatic surgical techniques is essential to minimize the introduction of pathogens into a surgical wound and to reduce postoperative complications. Also use of a prophylactic, intra-alveolar socket medicament after surgery may prevent delayed healing in patients with HIV.

5. Orthodontic treatment is considered in early stages and it is contraindicated in late stage. In some cases, orthodontic treatment may be modified for the HIV patients. Specific modalities can be chosen that avoid stress on teeth. Combination of different appliance therapy are used to reduce length of time and to provide faster results. Combined restorative and orthodontic treatments are another available alternative.

6. Oral lesion like ulcers and opportunistic infections should be treated as an

emergency by routine management. It can be treated either topical or systemic administration of drugs on the basis of severity and extent of infection. Fluconazole 750 mg tablet and gel for 14 days are widely used in treatment of oropharyngeal candidiasis.

For oral candidiasis topical application of clotrimazole used as an oral troche 10 mg. One troche should be dissolved in mouth for 15–20 mins for 5 times a day and dose for systemic clotrimazole drug is 200 mg. Maintenance phase is necessary as the patient's HIV status progresses.

In case of deep mycosis, the role of the dental practitioner is to instruct the patient for regular home care to optimize oral hygiene.

7. For viral infections acyclovir and valaciclovir are used. Acyclovir resistant herpes ulcerations are usually treated with foscarnet. Herpes zoster is treated with acyclovir 800 mg five times daily for 10 days with added symptomatic treatment (3,4).

Precaution for patients: When patients are on ART, chance of major complications is reduced so the goal of the therapy is to improve oral hygiene and function, manage HIV-associated oral lesions and drug-induced oral side effects and improve quality of his or her life. Patients with low platelet counts are at high risk for increased bleeding and should be managed accordingly. Hemoglobin below 7g/dl requires conservative dental treatment.

Precaution for dentist: The most important part in these cases is infection control, it plays a vital role in health safety of both patients and doctors as well as assistants. Proper method of sterilization and use of personal protection measures like immunization, clothing, hand gloves, eyewear, face shield are recommended.

FREQUENTLY ASKED QUESTIONS

1. Oral manifestations/dental considerations of HIV.

BIBLIOGRAPHY

1. David Fajardo-Ortiz, Malaquias Lopez-Cervantes, Luis Duran, Michel Dumontier, Miguel Lara, Hector Ochoa, Victor M. Castano. The emergence and evolution of the research fronts in HIV/AIDS research. PLOSONE 12(5): e0178293.https://doi.org/10.1371/journal. pone.0178293

2. Kam KM, Wong KH, Li PC, Lee SS, Leung WL, Kwok MY. Proposed CD4(+) T-cell criteria for staging human immunodeficiency virus-infected Chinese adults. Clin Immunol Immunopathol 1998;89:11–22

3. Book chapter: Burkitt; Oral Medicine, 9th edition. J.B Lippincott Co 301–321.

4. HIV and AIDS in dental practice.1st edition, Thomson Press Ltd.

Neuromuscular Disorders

INTRODUCTION

Neuromuscular disorder literally means caused due to muscle impairment because of pathology in the associated nerves.

These neuromuscular disorders have a collective lifetime prevalence rate of 3% to 5% which makes their encounter common with the dental practitioner.

These disorders affect the dentition, soft tissues and the occlusion and hence we should be aware of their oral manifestations, dental management and treatment.

History Taking for Neuromuscular Disorders

1. While obtaining the medical history, the clinician should attempt to define onset and course of the illness as well as the distribution of symptoms.
2. The course of the disease may be chronic and progressive, monophasic, or relapsing.
3. The patients presenting symptoms are dependent upon the muscle groups that are predominantly affected. Early manifestation of proximal lower extremities weakness is progressive difficulty climbing stairs and in arising from a chair, commode, or the floor.
4. A patient with neck weakness will often complain of difficulty lifting their head off a pillow. Further, sudden braking or accelerating in a car can cause the head to jerk back and forth. Involvement of cranial muscles may result in ptosis, diplopia, dysarthria, or difficulty chewing and swallowing.
5. The examiner should ask about the presence of extreme fluctuations in strength during the day or associated with physical activities. Such fluctuations in strength are more typical of neuromuscular junction disorders.
6. Observant patients may also detect a progressive loss of muscle bulk about various aspects of their body, particularly involving the anterior thigh, shoulder, and occasionally face and small intrinsic hand muscles.
7. Alternatively, some muscle groups may be noted to be enlarged. Some disorders are associated with fasciculations, myalgias, cramps, stiffness or myotonia, periodic paralysis, and myoglobinuria. If these symptoms are not offered by the patient, their presence should be inquired by the clinician.
8. It is important to inquire about sensory symptoms. Patients may complain of feeling "numb," but this word has different meanings for different people. If not offered by the patient, the examiner should specifically ask the patient about the presence or absence of sensory loss or tingling, prickly, or burning pain.

9. The pain associated with these disorders is typically described as a deep, aching discomfort in the muscles and is seldom severe enough to warrant analgesics. Usually the pain is diffuse rather than localized and is not tender.
10. The past medical history of patients should be addressed because various medical diseases are associated with neuromuscular disorders. For example, inflammatory myopathies may be seen in patients with connective tissue disease; concurrent autoimmune disorders may be present in patients with myasthenia gravis.
11. A careful family history is also vitally important in attempting to define the possible mode of inheritance or degree of genetic penetrance. When a hereditary disorder is suspected, it is valuable to examine affected family members.
12. In patients with progressive weakness, a history regarding possible toxin exposures is important. These exposures may come from the work or home environment or from medications. Such toxins can result in damage of the peripheral nerves, neuromuscular junction, or muscle. The severity of the clinical manifestations often depends upon the type of toxin as well as the dose and duration.

Clinical History in Neuromuscular Diseases

- Weakness
  - Anatomic distribution/pattern of weakness and focal wasting or hypertrophy of muscle groups (arms versus legs, proximal versus distal, symmetric versus asymmetric)
  - Myopathies have weakness that is usually proximal greater than distal with rare exception
- *Course of weakness:* Acute onset (days to weak)
  - Chronic (month to year)
  - Episodic

- Is the weakness getting worse, staying the same, or getting better?
- Ascertain the rate of progression (days, weeks, months or years)
- Fatigue or lack of indurance
- Muscle cramp or stiffness
- Lack of sensory loss
- *Gait characteristics:* Toe walking, excessive, lordosis, Trendelenburg or gluteus maximus, lurch, etc.
- Functional difficulties
  - Ambulatory distances
  - Frequency of falls
  - Transition from the floor to standing
  - Problems of climbing stairs
  - Problems in dressing
  - Problems in reaching overhead
  - Difficulty lifting
  - Running ability, problems in physical education and recreational or athletics performance
- Onset age (neonatal , childhood, teen, adult (20–60 yrs) or geriatric)
- Identify factors which worsen or help primary symptoms
- History of recent illness (e.g. recent viral illness, respiratory difficulties, pneumonia, pulmonary infection)
- Pain
- Feeding difficulties, dysphagia , nutritional status and body composition
- Cardiac symptoms (dizziness, syncope, chest pain , orthopnia, cardiac complaints with exertion)
- Pulmonary symptoms (breathing difficulties, sleep disturbances, morning headache)
- Anesthetic history (e.g. malignant hyperthermia)
- History regarding child's acquisition of developmental milestones
  - Ascertain when the child was able to control his or her head, sit independently, crawl, stand with or without support, walk with and without support, gain fine motor prehension and acquire bimanual skill (bringing objects to midline, transfer of objects)

- History regarding language acquisition, mental development and school performance
- History regarding pregnancy and neonatal period
  - Quality of fetal movement, pregnancy complication, perinatal complication, evidence of fatal distress, respiratory difficulties in the recovery room, need for resuscitation or ventilation problems in early infancy, infantile hypotonia, weak cry, poor feeding.

This chapter focuses on the most common neuromuscular disorder affecting the orofacial region and their management, pertaining to oral physicians.

- CVD
- Multiple sclerosis
- Parkinsonism
- Huntington's disease
- Seizure disorders
- Bell's palsy
- Myasthenia gravis

1. Cerebrovascular Disease or CVA or Stroke

Refers to disorders that cause damage to cerebral blood vessels due to impaired cerebral circulation.

Etiology

A. It is caused due to sudden impairment in central leading to death or focal neurologic deficit.
B. Strokes result from:
  - Hypertension
  - Trauma
  - Substance abuse
  - Aneurysmal rupture
C. 85% strokes result from ischemia due to atherosclerotic disease, thromboembolic event, occlusion of cerebral vessels.

Clinical Features

It depends on the size and location of the affected brain region. Common signs and symptoms are:

- Sensory and motor deficit

- Paresis in eye movements
- Visual defects
- Sudden headache
- Dizziness
- Nausea
- Seizures
- Impaired memory

Diagnosis

1. Stroke should be considered whenever a patient experiences the aforementioned clinical features.
2. Other diagnostic methods are MRI brain, non-contrast CT scan
3. Lab investigations include complete blood count, urinalysis, coagulation profile and when indicated blood culture, ECG and lumbar puncture.

Treatment

1. Management of acute stroke includes medical therapy to reduce bleeding or thromboembolic occlusion.
2. Thrombolysis with intravenous tissue plasminogen activator (TPA) from 3–4.5 hours after stroke onset.

Oral Health Considerations

1. Following stroke patients may experience oral problems like masticatory and facial muscle paralysis, impaired taste sensation, diminished gag reflex and dysphagic which need to be managed according to the presenting complaint.
2. Maintenance of oral hygiene replacement of missing teeth should be done.
3. Blood pressure should be monitored to prevent stroke and history should be taken about previous episode of stroke.
4. Patients with a history of stroke are usually using aspirin and warfarin, hence use of NSAIDs may increase the risk of bleeding and their long-term use may reduce the protective effect of aspirin.
5. Stress reduction during dental visits should be done for which pre-operative inhalation N_2O-O_2 or oral anxiolytic can be used.

6. Local anesthesia containing epinephrine can be used in stroke patients but should be used judiciously.

2. Multiple Sclerosis

It is a relapsing remitting autoimmune inflammatory demyelinating disease of the CNS.

Etiology

1. It can be caused secondary to trauma.
2. Though the exact cause of MS is unknown, genetic susceptibility clearly exists.
3. It is mostly an autoimmune reaction in which major histocompatibility complex (MHC) on chromosome 6p21 has been identified.
4. Infections agents like Epstein-Barr virus and human herpesvirus 6 are also implicated in the pathogenesis of MS.

Clinical Features

1. Age of onset of MS is typically between 20–45 years.
2. It is more common among women than men (2:1 ratio).
3. Clinical features of MS depend upon the area of the CNS involved and frequently affected areas include optic chiasma, brainstem, cerebellum and spinal cord.
4. The sudden onset of optic neuritis without any other CNS signs or symptoms could be the first symptom of MS.
5. Diplopia, blurring, nystagmus are also commonly seen.
6. Limb weakness is characteristic of MS and can be manifest as loss of strength, fatigue or gait problems.
7. Ataxia may affect the head and neck of MS patients and may cause cerebellar dysarthria.
8. These patients often show sensory impairment including paresthesia and hyperesthesia.
9. These patients often show sensory impairement including paresthesia and hyperesthesia.

Diagnosis

1. MS lesions are called 'plaques' which are characterised by perivenular cuffing with inflammatory mononuclear cells, which are seen in the white matter and periventricular area of the CNS.
2. These plaques are visible as hypertense and hypotense areas on T2 and T1 weighted images respectively, suggestive of chronic and active lesions which are diagnostic of MS.
3. Other advanced imaging techniques that are being evaluated for diagnosis of MS are diffusion sensor imaging, magnetization transfer imaging, proton magnetic resonance spectroscopy and functional MRI.

Treatment

1. Glucocorticoids can be used to manage both initial attacks and acute exacerbation of MS.
2. Intravenous methylprednisolone is administered at a dose between 500–1000 mg per day for 3–5 days
3. Disease modifying agents include injectable (interferon) IFN-beta/a, IFN-beta/b, and glatiramer acetate.
4. Nitroxantrone (novantrone) is a chemotherapeutic agent administered intravenously that is effective in reducing neurologic disability.
5. Some other common agents used for management of MS are anticonvulsants, benzodiazepines, tricyclic antidepressants, smooth muscle relaxant, anticholinergic agents and analgesics.

Oral Health Considerations

1. MS patients can present with trigeminal neuralgia (TN) with possible absence of trigger zones and continuous low intensity pain which should be managed similar to typical TN.
2. Patients may present with neuropathy of the maxillary (V2) and mandibular branch (V3) of the trigeminal nerve which may result in burning, tingling or reduced sensation.

3. Neuropathy of the mental nerve can cause numbness of the lower lip and chin.
4. Facial weakness and paralysis may be seen in MS patient.
5. Dysarthria may be seen as scanning speech in these patients.
6. Elective dental treatment should be avoided in MS patients during acute exacerbation.
7. These patients may require dental treatment in operating room under general anesthesia.
8. Patients relatives or nurse should be appraised about the importance of daily home care of oral hygiene.

3. Parkinsonism

It is a neurodegenerative disorder characterized by rigidity, tremors, bradykinesis and impaired postural reflex.

Etiology

1. In idiopathic parkinsonism, there is dopamine depletion due to degeneration of the dopaminergic higrostriatal system in the brainstem.
2. This leads to an imbalance of dopamine and acetylcholine which are neurotransmitters that are normally present in the corpus striatum.
3. Symptoms similar to parkinsonism may also be induced by drugs that cause a reduction of dopamine in the brain, the most common drugs being phenothiazine derivatives.
4. Although, a definite etiology has not been established, the most likely explanation is that the disease results from a combination of accelerated aging, genetic predisposition, exposure to toxins and abnormality in oxidative mechanisms.

Clinical Features

1. It affects people older than 50 years of age.
2. The 4 cardinal motor signs of parkinsonism are resting tremors, rigidity or stiffness, bradykinesia and postural instability or impaired balance and coordination.

3. 50% of patients with this develop dementia, depression, anxiety, apathy and irritability.
4. Anatomic dysfunction can cause orthostatic hypotension, constipation, urinary frequency and urgency and abnormal sweating.

Diagnosis of Parkinsonism

1. The diagnosis is based on the health history, neurologic examination and response to levodopa therapy.
2. Differentiating classic parkinsonism from a variety of parkinsonian syndromes characterized by motor decline and dementia can be challenging.
3. Anatomic and functional brain imaging, CSF evaluation can be useful to exclude other diagnosis.

Treatment

1. Dopamine replacement therapy using levodopa combined with carbidopa remains the initial gold standard.
2. Anticholinergics such as scopolamine may help control tremor and rigidity.
3. Dopamine agonists such as bromocriptine, pergolide, pramipexole alone or in combination with levodopa may control parkinsonism.
4. Rivastigmine, a cholinesterase inhibitor, is effective in treating parkinsonism dementia.
5. Clozapine is effective for treating parkinsonism psychosis.
6. Exercise has demonstrated significant benefit in physical conditioning, gait, balance, leg strength and walking speed.

Oral Health Considerations

1. Patients experience increased salivation and drooling, making maintenance of dry field difficult for some dental procedures.
2. Angular cheilitis is common in these patients.
3. Use of anticholinergic drugs causes xerostomia which leads to damage to teeth

and PDL and also difficulty in retaining dentures, mucosal ulcerations, denture sores, increased chance of bacterial and fungal infections.

4. Patient loses facial expressions and has slow speech that is soft and fading.
5. Tremor of the head, lips and tongue is common.
6. These patients require periodontal recall every 4–6 months owing to poor oral hygiene.
7. Enameloplasty or mouth guard is required to prevent injury to the tongue due to tardive dyskinesis.
8. Salivary substitutes and topical fluoride application are necessary in patients with xerostomia.
9. During dental procedures, chair should be positioned at 45 degree to limit muscle rigidity and breathing difficulties.
10. Appointments should be short and relaxing with nitrous oxide sedation which helps reduce stress and prevalence of tremors.

4. Huntington's Disease

Etiology

It is hereditary degenerative disease of the central nervous system characterized by chorea (involuntary movements) and dementia.

Clinical Features

1. The earliest manifestation of this disease consists of depression and irritability coupled with slowing of cognition.
2. There are subtle changes in coordinated and minor choreiform movements appear.
3. There could be progressive nonsensing of choreic movements that are observed in the face, tongue and head.
4. In advanced cases, the hyperkinesis becomes aggravated and movement can become violent, with difficulty in speech and swallowing.

Diagnosis

1. The diagnosis is based on neurological, neuropsychological and psychiatric evaluation.
2. MRI or contrast enhanced CT scan of brain can be done to reveal structural changes at particular sites in the brain.
3. Genetic testing is a confirmatory test for this disease.

Treatment

1. There is no cure for Huntington's disease, progression cannot be halted and treatment is purely symptomatic.
2. Treatment is usually involving blocking of dopamine receptors such as haloperidol and phenothiazines, which temporarily reduce the hyperkinesis and the behavioural disturbances.

Oral Health Considerations

1. Dysphagia and choreic movements of the face and the tongue will make dental treatment quite challenging.
2. Sedation with diazepam can be considered.
3. Whenever possible, dentures for such patients should be avoided because of the danger of fracture or its accidental swallowing.

5. Seizure Disorders

Seizures are paroxysmal disorders of cerebral function characterized by an attack involving changes in the state of consciousness, motor activity or sensory phenomenon.

Etiology

1. Isolated, nonrecurrent, generalized seizures among adults are caused by metabolic disturbances, toxins, drug effects, hypotension, hypoglycemia, uremia, encephalopathy drug overdoses and drug withdrawal.
2. Cerebrovascular disease may account for approximately 50% of new cases of epilepsy in patients older than 65 years.

3. Other etiologies for epilepsy include degenerative CNS disease, developmental disabilities and familial/genetic factors.

Clinical Features

There are seven types of seizures:

a. **Grand mal**
   1. It is most common type of seizure which can occur alone or with other types.
   2. This seizure begins with aura in which patient experiences epigastric discomfort or hallucinations of heating, vision or smell.
   3. It is followed by the tonic phase in seconds by unconsciousness, cry and tonic muscle spasm.
   4. The tonic phase is followed by the clonic phase composed of convulsive jerky movements, incontinence and tongue biting.
   5. Jaw is clamped shut and there is foaming at the mouth.

b. **Petit mal**
   1. These seizures occur exclusively in children and frequently disappear during second decade of life.
   2. The patient loses his consciousness, but will continue his normal activity immediately after the seizure.

c. **Psychomotor**
   1. During the seizure, the patient exhibits purposeless movements and bizzare behaviour.
   2. Patient may wander about aimlessly or may exhibit violent behaviour during the seizure.

d. **Jacksonian**
   1. The seizure begins with clonic movements of a distal portion of extremities or the face.
   2. The convulsive movements spread to the limbs, become generalized and cause loss of consciousness.

Diagnosis

1. History and physical examination are critical to diagnose a seizure.

2. Complete neurologic examination is essential which includes the testing of cranial nerve function, assessment of mental status and testing of motor function.
3. Blood studies like complete blood count, electrolytes, glucose, magnesium, calcium are done to identify any metabolic cause of seizure.
4. All the patients should undergo MRI and CT scan for detection of any pathology in the brain responsible for seizures.
5. An EEG (electroencephalogram) is an important tool for classifying seizure disorder.

Treatment

A. **Immediate management during seizure**
   1. The patient should be moved away from danger like fire, water or sharp objects.
   2. After convulsion seizes, the patient should be positioned supine with legs slightly elevated.
   3. Basic life support should be given if indicated.
   4. If convulsion continues for more than 5 minutes urgent medical help should be summoned.
   5. Intravenous anticonvulsant like diazepam should be given.

B. **Pharmacologic management**
   1. Lamotrigine, carbamazepine and phenytoin are indicated for the treatment for partial seizures.
   2. Valproic acid is indicated for the treatment of generalized tonic—clonic seizures.

Oral Health Considerations

1. These patients have high rate of physical injuries, including dental and facial trauma.
2. Hence, precipitation of seizures during dental treatment should be avoided by reducing psychologic stress. Inhalation sedation with nitrous oxide (up to 20%) and oxygen is highly recommended.

3. Phenytoin-induced gingival hyperplasia is commonly seen in anterior labial surfaces of the maxillary and mandibular gingiva. Maintenance of oral hygiene by chlorhexidine mouthwash can reduce the inflammation or surgical reduction can be done if recession.
4. Patients taking AEDs (antiepileptic drugs) have marked bone marrow suppression which causes increased chances of infection and prolonged bleeding. Hence, a complete blood count should be done prior to any dental treatment.
5. Aspirin and other NSAIDs should be avoided in patients taking valproic acid and it can possibly cause increased bleeding.

6. Bell's Palsy

It is also called facial paralysis or seventh nerve paralysis.

Etiology

1. The exact etiology is not known but viral infection like herpes simplex affecting the facial nerve causes inflammation and hence paralysis of the nerve.
2. Other causes like trauma during dental extraction, surgical procedures like parotidectomy, tumors of the cranial base, parapharyngeal space and infratemporal fossa can lead to seventh nerve palsy.

Clinical Features

1. Bell's palsy begins with slight pain around one ear, followed by an abrupt paralysis of the muscles on that side of the face.
2. The eye on the affected side stays open, corner of the mouth drops, and there is drooling.
3. As a result of masseter weakens, food is retained in both the upper and lower buccal and labial fold.
4. The face becomes expressionless and the creases of the forehead are flattened.
5. Due to impaired blinking, corneal ulcerations from foreign bodies can occur.

6. Involvement of the chorda tympani nerve leads to loss of taste perception on the anterior two-thirds of the tongue and reduced salivary secretion.

Diagnosis

1. A thorough history taking and physical examination helps in diagnosing Bell's palsy and the extent of the weakness of the facial muscles.
2. Blood tests to detect viral or bacterial infection can diagnose the etiology for Bell's palsy.
3. MRI or CT scan can be advised to rule out any pathology in the brain.

Treatment

1. Spontaneous improvement is generally seen within 6 months in most cases.
2. Combination of acyclovir 400 mg 5 times daily with prednisolone (40–60 mg daily) for a week is believed to be more effective than steroid alone.
3. Supportive measures like protecting the eye with eye patches, artificial tear substitutes should be given.
4. Injection of botulinum toxin has shown to be effective in treating this disease.
5. Physiotherapy can be advised for the muscles of face.

Oral Health Considerations

1. Patient has dropping corner of mouth due to which there is drooling of saliva. Hence dental treatment becomes difficult.
2. There may be for oral hygiene due to retention of food in the upper and lower buccal and labial folds due to weakness of buccinator.
3. Patient experiences difficulty in speech and mastication.

7. Myasthenia Gravis

Etiology

1. It is a chronic neuromuscular disease caused by autoimmune destruction of the skeletal neuromuscular junction

resulting in impaired neurotransmission and muscle weakness

2. In this condition, autoantibodies are produced to the acetylcholine receptors on the motor end plates of muscles, thus binding of acetylcholine is blocked, muscle activation is inhibited.

3. The most common autoantibody is anti-acetylcholine receptor (AChR) and less commonly a muscle specific receptor tyrosine kinase (MUSK).

Clinical Features

1. Patients with ocular symptoms like diplopia and/or ptosis.

2. Oropharyngeal, facial and masticatory muscle weakness is common and results in dysphagia, asymmetry and dysarthria.

TABLE 22.1: Guidelines for oral healthcare of patients with neuromuscular disease

Medical consultation	Stress reduction/ anxiolytic guidelines	Chair position guidelines	Analgesia guidelines
✗ It should be summoned when patient's status, severity and level of control is uncertain.	✗ A rapport should be established to reduce stress and anxiety.	✗ Local anesthesia can be safely used in patients with seizure disorder.	✗ NSAIDs can be used safely in majority of patients with neurologic disease
✗ Patient who has not seen a physician within last year	✗ The type of steroid taken, dose and duration of treatment should be ascertained.	✗ Intraoral anesthetics should be administered slowly following aspiration	✗ Major concern is bleeding tenderness which is most prevalent in patients with cerebrovascular disease who take anticoagulants.
✗ Corticosteroids have been taken within last 12 months	✗ Patient should obtain proper rest the night before treatment and should reduce work on the day of treatment.	✗ In patients with impaired mental capacity, lip biting after LA administration is a common post-operative problem.	✗ Respiratory depressant narcotics should be used with caution in patients with neurologic respiratory difficulties
✗ Medications and dosage are not well known by the patient	✗ Appointment should be in the morning and kept short		
✗ Need for additional medication or change in medication during dental treatment	✗ Benzodiazepines, which have minor CNS depressant activity, are the sedative/anxiolytic drugs of choice.		
✗ There are plans for stressful or complex oral surgical procedures.			
✗ Iatrogenic problem arises from dental treatment, e.g. Bell's palsy that persists more than 6 hours after dental injection.			

TABLE 22.2: Guidelines for oral healthcare of patients with neuromuscular disease

Antibiotic guidelines	Airway maintenance and gaseous administration	Drug effects and interactions guidelines	Infection control guidelines
Culture and sensitivity testing should be done whenever oral infection is present.	Rubber dam is recommended for routine operative procedures in patients with neurologic disease especially in patients with drooling saliva.	Valproic acid inhibits platelet aggregation and can produce palatal petechiae and abnormal bleeding.	Antibiotic prophylaxis and oral antibiotic rinses should be used when the patient is severely immunocompromised.
Oral penicillin can be used safely as long as the patient is not hypertensive to it.	Nitrous oxide therapy is an excellent anxiolytic.	Carbamazepine depresses bone marrow leading to bleeding tenderness and increased incidence of oral infections.	Contact with blood, saliva and aerosol should be minimized.
Broad spectrum antibiotics should be prescribed with caution in epileptic women who use oral contraceptives.		Primidone and phenobarbital cause atexia and drowsiness. Additional sedatives and respiratory depressants should be avoided.	Routine aseptic protocol should be followed.
In patients with myasthenia gravis, aminoglycosides who have a neuromuscular blocking effect, should be avoided.		Patient with history corticosteroid therapy may have adrenal suppression. Consultation with the physician is mandatory	

3. In severe cases, respiratory difficulty arises.
4. Patient's tongue may be supple and flaccid with bilateral groves on the dorsal surface due to atrophy of tongue musculature.
5. Palatal muscles may be affected causing patient to have difficulty in elevating soft palate.

Diagnosis

1. The clinical examination and history are highly suggestive of myasthenia gravis.
2. Diagnosis is confirmed by a variety of bedside, electrophysiological and immunological tests.
3. The most commonly used immunological test to establish a diagnosis of myasthenia gravis quantifies serum anti-AChR, with a reported sensitivity of 85%.

Treatment

1. Anticholinesterase drugs such as neostigmine and pyridostigmine bromide increase acetylcholine availability and receptor binding and provide symptomatic benefit.
2. Plasma exchange and high-dose intravenous immunoglobulin can rapidly and temporarily reduce circulating antibodies.
3. Autoantibody production can be reduced using corticosteroids and non-steroid immune suppressants.

Oral Health Considerations

1. Patient may have difficulty with prolonged mouth opening and swallowing.
2. Aspiration risks can be high and can be reduced by adequate suction, the use

of rubber dam and avoiding bilateral mandibular anaesthetic block.

3. The patient may be at risk for respiratory crisis due to overmedication.
4. Drugs that may affect the neuromuscular junction such as narcotics, tranquilizers and barbiturates should be avoided.
5. Certain antibiotics like tetracycline, streptomycin, sulphonamides and clindamycin can affect neuromuscular activity and should be avoided.

Guidelines for Oral Healthcare of Patients with Neuromuscular Disease

See Table 22.1.

BIBLIOGRAPHY

1. Greenberg M., Glick M. Burket's Oral Medicine Diagnosis and Treatment. 10th edition: BC Decker Inc; Elsevier; 2003.
2. Greenberg M., Brightman V. Burket's Oral Medicine Diagnosis and Treatment. 9th edition: Lippincott.
3. Wood N., Goaz P. Differential diagnosis of Oral and Maxillofacial Lesions. 5th edition. Elsevier; 2007.

Forensic Odontology

Forensic odontology is a specialized field of dentistry that deals with legal aspects. In other words, it is the application of dental science to Law. It is derived from Latin 'Forum' meaning 'Court of Law' where legal matters were debated during the Roman era. FDI defines forensic odontology as that branch of dentistry that in the interest of justice deals with the proper handling and examination of dental evidence and with the proper evaluation and presentation of dental findings.

Though the permanent tooth develops in the first two decades of life, they harbor a lot of information in the hard tissues. Forensic odontologists are highly experienced trained individuals whose job is to extract this information and use it for identification of unknown remains. Apart from its use in identification, teeth are also used as weapons and in some fortunate circumstances leave the information of the biter. Analysis of bite marks is the second major responsibility of a forensic odontologist. Forensic odontologists have also been known to assist archeologists and anthropologists in determining the ethnicity and building up a picture about the lifestyle and diet of a population. In addition, acting as an expert witness in the court of law is a legal duty of a forensic odontologist.

In the latter part of this century forensic odontology has evolved by leaps and bounds by incorporating dental anatomy, histology, radiography, pathology and dental materials

HISTORY OF FORENSIC ODONTOLOGY

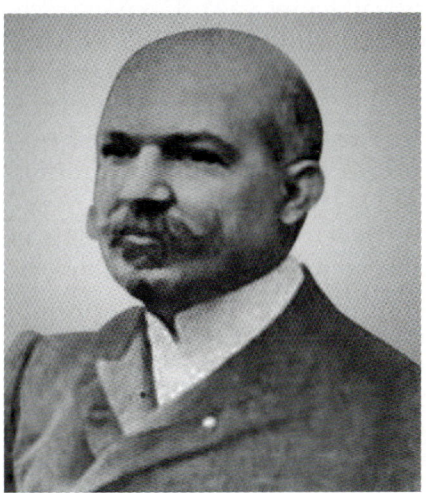

Fig. 23.1: Dr. Oscar Amoedo: Father of Forensic Odonotology

Historically some cases of identification have been reported far back as 49AD. It has been said that Nero's mistress was satisfied that the decapitated head was of Nero's wife since she could recognize the anterior tooth.

Folklore attributes the first use of bitemark identification to King William the conqueror in 1066 AD who had a habit of sealing his envelopes with sealing wax with his teeth marks on them. His mal-aligned anterior teeth allowed the substantiation of the authencity of his documents.

Dr Oscar Amoedo is regarded as the Father of Forensic Odontology. His notes made from observations during mass disasters served as the first textbook of forensic odontology termed 'L'art Dentaire en Medicine Legale'. The techniques used in forensic odontology have evolved with the evolution of mankind. During the American Revolution Paul Revere a young dentist helped identify war causalities by their dental work.

After the first dental identification in a mass disaster during the charity bazaar fire of Paris in 1897, dental identification has been used during various mass fatalities including the Thai Tsunami in 2006 and the terrorist attack of 9/11. DNA extracts from the toothbrushes of the victims were used in identification of some victims during 9/11 and 87% Thai Tsunami victims were identified using their dental records.

Forensic odontology officially entered the Indian subcontinent in 1998, but its presence was felt way before that. Raja Jaichand of Kannuj was identified by his false teeth. In fact the late prime minister Mr. Rajiv Gandhi was assassinated in a terrorist attack in 1991, and was identified by his dentition.

METHODS OF IDENTIFICATION

Reason why identification is required:
1. Legal and humanitarian reasons
2. Settlement of property and insurance
3. Facilitate remarriage of a surviving spouse
4. Last rites according to relevant religious and cultural customs.

Dental Identification

◈ Identification of an Individual

Comparative Identification

When the deceased's identity is suspected scientific methods are employed to confirm the identity by comparison of the antemortem and postmortem records of the individual.

A postmortem dental record is prepared by careful examination, charting and written description of all the dental structures including radiographs and additional supportive records like casts and photographs. Antemortem and postmortem radiographs can be marked using a rubber dam punch to avoid confusion. Once post-mortem record is complete, a thorough comparison is made with the antemortem records. Features that are noticed during comparison include tooth morphology, dental restorations, and pathologies. Similarities and discrepancies are noted during comparison. The discrepancies can be explainable or non-explainable. An explainable discrepancy is when the point of discordance can be explained using the time gap between the antemortem and postmortem records.

An example of an explainable discrepancy is the presence of an intact tooth antemortem but a restored or an extraction space postmortem. Similarly extension of a filling from antemortem to postmortem can be explained.

A person with multiple dental restorations and unusal features like a mesiodens or a rotated incisor has a better likelihood of being easily identified as compared to someone who has no dental treatment done. As concluded by Acharya and Taylor unlike 12 points of concordance that fingerprints need, a single point of concordance is sufficient to establish an identity but the uniqueness of the feature has to be considered as well as the circumstances of the case.

Once an identity is established, it has to be legally documented in the form of a detailed report and conclusion is based on facts. The explainable discrepancies and significance of similarities have to be mentioned and either of the following conclusions can be drawn:
a. **Positive identification:** Indicates the antemortem and postmortem dental

data match each other. The identity can be proven "beyond reasonable doubt".

b. **Probable identification:** There is a high level of concordance between the two sets of data but may lack radiographic support. There is a consistency in data but due to the lack of quality, the identity cannot be confirmed.

c. **Possible identification:** The postmortem and antemortem data correspond but the information that is available is insufficient.

d. **Excludes identification:** There is inconsistency in postmortem and antemortem data. The data contains unexplainable differences which indicates a negative result.

e. **Insufficient information:** The available postmortem and antemortem information is minimal or insufficient to draw conclusions on the identity of the deceased.

Dental records : A dental record has subjective and objective record of the patient and the dentist is in possession of it. Whenever possible the original records should be examined. Such records may be in the form of photographs, radiographs, casts or dental charts. Frequently people visits multiple dentists, hence all the chronologically relevant contents should be noted on the composite Interpol antemortem form.

Reconstructive Identification

The purpose of reconstructive identification is to narrow down the search for the deceased individual. It helps to generate a profile of a person whose identity is unknown. Information about the deceased person's race, age, gender, socioeconomic status, occupation, and various other parameters can be determined by reconstructive identification. The skull can help identify the gender and the race to some extent. Skull along with the rest of the bones can aid in determining gender with an accuracy of 98%. Along with the shape and form of skull, other features like cusp of carabelli, shovel-shaped

incisors, 3–4 cuspal premolars all aid in determination of race.

For adults age can be estimated by examining the development of teeth and comparing the teeth to an atlas of tooth development proposed by various authors like Schour and Massler, Demirijian and so on. The age can be estimated using the development stages of a tooth uptil their eruption. Gustafson used the regressive changes of the dentition like attrition, secondary dentin formation, cemental apposition, loss of periodontal attachment and transparent dentin to determine age.

Age estimation: Age can be estimated by
a. Histological methods
b. Radiographical methods
c. Eruption

Age estimation is required for an aborted fetus, a homicide victim, severely mutilated mass disaster victim, or living person who requires age estimation. Age estimation of a living person is required if birth certificate is not available or if the records are suspected. Quite a few times a request is made to help determine whether the child has attained an age of criminal responsibility.

Age estimation in Neonates: Histological methods is the more sensitive technique. Early mineralization can be detected up to 12 weeks before it is visible on a radiograph. Although radiographic interpretation has an advantage that it is non-mutilating. The incremental lines can be taken into consideration. The neonatal line is present on the developing deciduous teeth and the first permanent molar. The presence of neonatal line indicates a live birth but the absence is not an indication of a stillbirth since the neonatal line takes 3 weeks to form after birth.

Calcification of deciduous teeth begin at 12–14 weeks IU, whereas calcification of the first molar starts at the age of 6 months.The dry weight of the mineralized tooth cusps can also be measured. Stack mentions that the combined weight of the teeth in a child at 6 months IU is about 60 mg, 0.5 gm in a newborn and 1.8 gm at 6 months after birth.

Age estimation in juveniles/adolescents:

Unless there is enough of evidence and antemortem data to support the findings, age estimation should be used as an important parameter in identification rather than a definitive parameter. While writing the conclusion it should be mentioned that "the findings are consistent with a person of that age." The atlas for age estimation gives an age range for a particular range of development. Atlas has to be customized for different populations since growth variations exist for different population groups due to the difference in genetic and environmental factors. Following are the common dental development atlas.

Schour and Massler's Atlas

It describes 20 chronological stages of tooth development starting from 5 months IU until 21 years of age.

Advantages: Both deciduous and developing dentitions are shown and it includes root development and eruption sequence for deciduous teeth. The figures are to 1:1 scale and hence it becomes easy to directly compare with radiographs.

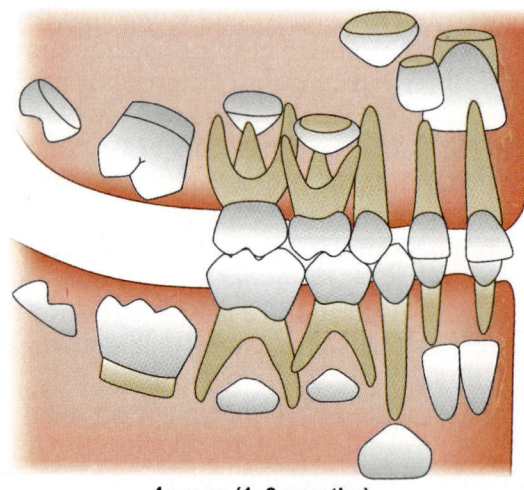

4 years (1–9 months)

Fig. 23.2: Schour and Massler's pictorial presentation of teeth development

Disadvantages : No separate charts for males and females. The mean ages correspond well to males than to females.

Uberlaker modified the original chart and the modified altas should be used since it is more accurate.

Demirjian's Atlas

Eight stages of dental development are shown on the atlas. Each stage of mineralization is given a score which provides an estimate of dental maturity on the scale of 0 to 10. Data obtained from the regression graph indicate that the differences between males and females are not significant until the age of 5 years. A formula for an Indian population was developed by Acharya which is as follows:

Males: Age = 27.4351 − (0.0097 × S2) + (0.000089 × S3)

Females: Age = 23.7288 − (0.0088 × S2) + (0.000085 × S3)

Advantages: Missing teeth from one side can be substituted by those of the opposite side. There is a detailed description accompanying the atlas and it is simple to use.

Disadvantages: Consider only mandibular teeth and does not include the developing third molar (Fig. 23.3).

Third Molar Development

After 14 years of age once the 2nd molar is erupted, the 3rd molar is the only tooth of significance, even if the third molar has not erupted yet, its calcification should be investigated. The eruption of the third molar definitely places the age of the individual at approximately 18 years of age, though the absence of the third molar is not an indication that the individual is below 18 years of age. In many countries including India 18 years is considered the age where the individual can be tried as an adult and not considered a juvenile anymore. The juvenile justice amendment bill states that a juvenile who has committed a crime cannot be sentenced to death or life imprisonment in prison. Due

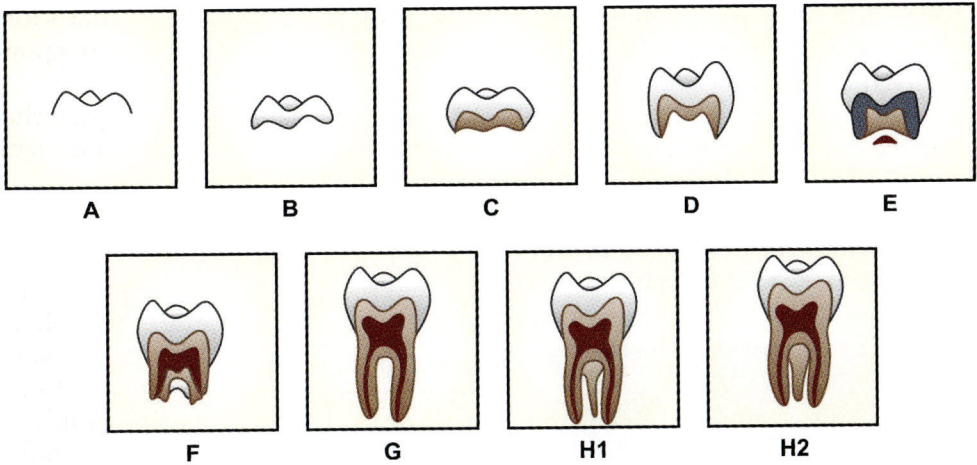

Fig. 23.3: Demirjian's method

to this law the third molar in spite of having an erratic calcification and eruption timing is still considered vital since it is the only tooth undergoing calcification.

Eruption Timing

Eruption is regarded the least accepted method for dental age assessment. This is because eruption of teeth is known to be affected by dietary, climatic, racial and geographical variation. The deciduous teeth help estimate age from 6 to 33 months and permanent teeth help estimate age from 6 to 25 years. The advantage of this method is that it does not require any special equipment, expertise and is very economical.

Age Estimation in Adults

Gustafson's method: Gustafson evaluated ground sections of teeth for 6 parameters. These 6 physiological parameters which included attrition, loss of periodontal attachment, secondary dentin deposition, sclerotic or transparent dentin formation, root resorption and cemental apposition were measured and given a score from 0 to 3. The above parameters were chosen since they showed age related changes. Transparent or sclerotic dentin and secondary dentin formation have the most correlation with age, and the former can be used independently

to estimate age as well. The drawback of this method is that it is subjective. Johanson modified it and introduced 6 scores instead of 3 with an interval of 0.5. This decreased the subjectivity of the method.

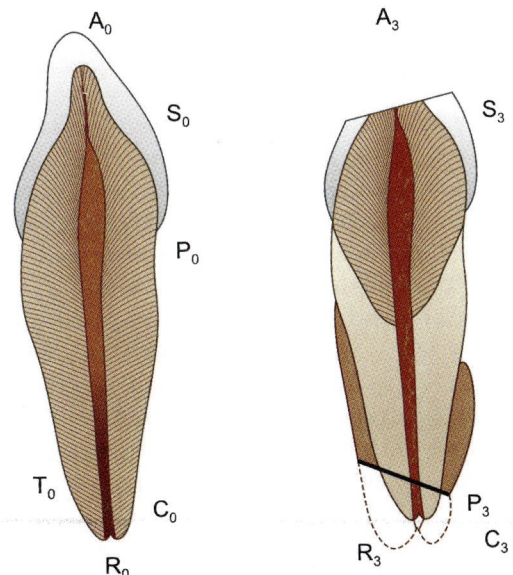

Fig. 23.4: Gustafson's variable and the first and last grades given by Johanson

Bang and Ramm's method: Transparent dentin or sclerotic dentin measurement is a relatively accurate and easy method to estimate age. Root dentin becomes transparent during the third decade of life starting from the apical region and progressing coronally as age advances. It is least affected by external stimuli and so more accurate. The diameter of the dentinal tubules decreases as a result of intra-tubular calcification. It appears dark in reflected light and light in transmitted light, translucency is measured either on intact extracted teeth or ground sections of teeth although the latter gives a better clarity.

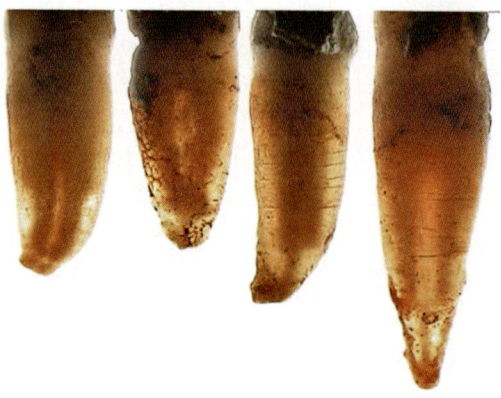

Fig. 23.5: Transparent or sclerotic dentin

Age estimation using tooth–pulp ratio: The area of the pulp chamber and root canal and the tooth area of canine is measured and their ratio is known as pulp to tooth area ratio. As age advances the area of pulp chamber and root canal reduces. A ratio is calculated to compensate for image magnification on radiographs and the angulation between X-ray beam and film. Population-based formulae are better, the formulae based on the Indian population predict age more accurately as compared to the formulae given by Cameriere.

Report writing in age estimation: A report is a formal document. The method used for age estimation should be mentioned in the report as well. More than one age estimation method should be used to arrive at a more accurate result. The validity of the method on the local population should be mentioned. Age should be always been mentioned as an approximate age and it is never a definite number.

Gender determination: Out of the three major parameters in dental profiling determination of gender is second important parameter. Morphology or skull and mandible, tooth measurements and analysis of dental DNA can be used to determine gender.

Morphology of skull and mandible: A number of features of skull and mandible are used to determine gender. Skull along with the rest of the skeleton can help achieve an accuracy of 98%. The reliability increases after puberty. According to William and Rogers, an ensemble of 6 traits, including mastoid process, supra-orbital ridge, size and architecture of skull, extension of the zygomatic arch beyond the external auditory canal, nasal aperature and gonial angle of the mandible can help achieve an accuracy of 94%.

Tooth measurements: The buccolingual and mesiodistal dimensions of teeth can be used to determine gender. This is especially used in children where skeletal secondary sexual characteristics have not yet developed.

Race determination: The diversity of humans is a result of combination of genetic and environmental factors including geographical location. Traditionally the human species around the world are classified into three races, viz Caucasoid, Mongoloid and Negroid. This traditional classification has been disregarded by anthropologists. Scott and Turner divided humans based on geographical origin and this classification is the current accepted classification. This diversity is seen in the human dentition as well as characterized by anthropologist, thus making it convenient to identify an individual's population origin based on the dentition.

The non-mentric morphological trait is one of the means of identifying population origin. Their presence or absence of such traits is evaluated. More than 30 nonmetric traits which include cusp of Carabelli, winging, four cuspal mandibular molars, three cuspal mandibular premolars and shoveling. Both high and low incidences of these traits should be considered. Due to overlap of these traits in different populations, more than 2–3 non-metric traits should be considered which drawing conclusions about a particular population.

Determination of occupation/habits/socioeconomic status: In addition to the three major parameters, the findings on teeth, such as erosion, stains can help determine the occupation of the individual as well as any habits the individual possesses like drinking excessive carbonated drinks, anorexia. Stains on the teeth indicates if the individual drinks a lot of tea/coffee, chews pan, tobacco. The notching of incisors suggests habitual placement of nails or bobby pins like carpenters and tailors do respectively. The presence or absence of dental treatment as well as the quality and quantity of treatment indicate the financial status of the individual.

Identification in Edentulous Individuals

In edentulous individuals labeled dentures or the uniqueness of the denture material can be used to narrow down the search for the identity of the deceased. Presence of Kevlar fibres in the denture has been used to help establish the identity of the individual. Denture marking or labeling is particularly useful during mass fatality incidents.

DNA in Dental Identification

Dental identification essentially needs dental records, but in the absence of dental records DNA proves vital. Since dental tissues are resilient to environmental changes, teeth are considered to be an excellent source of DNA. Polymerase chain reaction causes amplification of DNA at pre-selected sites, so DNA retrieved from a root canal treated tooth is useful. DNA has been used for identification at mass disaster sites as well. DNA from the deceased is matched with an antemortem sample obtained from toothbrush, hairbrush, blood, or any other personal belongings. Mitochondrial DNA is better cause of its maternal inheritance and high copy number. The maternal inheritance allows the DNA to be matched with the parents and siblings of the deceased.

Cheiloscopy and Palatalscopy

The wrinkles and grooves on the labial mucosa form a characteristic pattern called 'Lip Prints', the study of which is referred to as cheiloscopy. Lip prints were first described by Fisher in 1902. Edmond Locard, the French criminologist and the pioneer of forensic science, had first suggested the use of lip prints as evidence. Quite a few times lip prints are invisible; these latent lip prints are lifted using aluminium powder and magnetic powder. The oil produced by the sebaceous glands at the edges of the lips are responsible for the latent lip prints. The usefulness of the uniqueness of lip prints in identification is established but their sustainability to age changes and trauma has yet to be determined.

Palatal rugae are irregular asymmetric ridges that run laterally from the incisive papilla and the anterior part of the mid-palatine raphe. The study of palatine rugae is called rugoscopy. Palatal rugoscopy was first proposed in 1932 by Trobo Hermisa and are useful in identifying the edentulous. The rugae pattern on the deceased's maxilla can be compared to the pattern of ridges on old dentures or even to plaster models that may be available with the treating dentist. Subsequent studies on palatal rugae as a method of identification have concluded that it is difficult to formulate a universally accepted classification of palatal rugae and is more valuable as a method of comparative identification rather than determining the predipondence of a certain kind in males or females. The classification suggested by Lysell is the most commonly quoted one.

- Primary rugae (>5 mm)
- Secondary rugae (3–5 mm)
- Fragmentary rugae (2<3 mm)

Rugae less than 2 mm is not taken into consideration.

Thomas and Kotze further catergorized rugae into branched, unified, cross-linked, annular and papillary. They suggested further that as long as the technique used to compare the rugae is accurate, one need not conform to a particular classification. Ohtani et al added that the more complex the rugae pattern, greater is the tendency for non-identification.

Mass Disasters and Mass Fatalities

Webster's dictionary describes a disaster as a sudden calamitous event producing great material damage, loss of life and mental stress. Disasters can be man-made or natural. When a death of 12 or more persons occurs in a single episode, it is accepted as a mass disaster. Natural disasters are even more enormous sometimes because man cannot control nature's fury.

While managing a mass disaster priority should be given to the survivors. All efforts should be carried out to save the life of the injured person first. The area should be cordoned off with rope or tape and no outsiders should be allowed within the perimeter.

Norway was probably the first country to develop a model of investigation procedure in a mass disaster and included a dentist as well in the team.

A mass disaster is of two types:
1. *Open disaster:* Where there is no manifesto of the deceased, e.g. terrorist attack
2. *Closed disaster:* Where there is a manifesto of the deceased, e.g. plane accident

Identification in a mass fatality or a closed disaster is essentially the same as in comparative identification of an individual except the circumstances in which it is carried out is more complex due to the emotional and physical nature of the situation. Lack of standardization of dental records, poor working conditions, psychological stress, decomposition, dismemberment of human remains at the site of disaster all compounds

the complexity of the situation and in turn affects the identification process. There could also be political and jurisdictional issues that may have to be addressed.

Forensic odontologists are a part of the identification team that may also include forensic pathologist, fingerprint experts, and biotechnologist as well. In addition to a forensic odontologist, general dentists and dental auxillaries should also be included considering the vast nature of the destruction. Each team member should be aware of the protocol and procedures to be followed. Tasks may vary from taking radiographs to making notes. According to the INTERPOL's disaster victim identification guide, the odontology section should be divided into three subsections, namely antemortem unit, postmortem unit and the comparison and identification unit.

Antemortem Unit

The most important requirement is to obtain a work area specific to the dental team, and the most important purpose is to obtain antemortem records of the individuals missing or believed to be involved in the disaster and dispatch the dental record to the postmortem unit. More than one dentist is required for the antemortem unit. It is the duty of the dentist to provide written records, radiographs and study models to the antemortem unit. Once the dental records are collected, a composite chart is prepared on the INTERPOL antemortem form which is yellow in color. Majority of times, the dentist fails to undertake a full mouth charting when the patient first attends and only indicates work done by one dentist. The aim of the antemortem unit is to obtain as much data as possible about as much victims as possible in as short a time as possible.

Postmortem Unit

Before postmortem charting, personal effects are removed, fingerprints, radiographs and photographs are taken and then the jaws are resected. A portable dental radiography apparatus can be installed at the temporary mortuary with proper precaution for radiation hazard. The dentists work in pairs, one of them examining the oral cavity and the other carrying out the charting. The charting is done on an INTERPOL postmortem form which is pink in color. If the jaws are removed they should be immediately tagged with a waterproof label with the body number mentioned, bagged and tagged. In mass disasters there may be maxillofacial injuries and teeth and jaws go missing. In such cases the missing parts should be searched for, recovered and labelled. If the portions are not recovered, then the missing parts should be marked as "lost postmortem". Composite restorations cause a problem because they are not easily detected. After the charting is done the jaws have to be repatriated.

Antemortem and Postmortem Comparison Unit

Each antemortem record is compared to the most likely postmortem file spread out on a table. If the postmortem records do not provide any useful information, we move on to the next most likely record. Computer programmes like CAMPI have been used but a computer never carries out an identification, the final identification is always carried out manually. A computer just reduces the number of records to be compared. Consultation should be carried out with other teams such as DNA, fingerprinting, etc. As a positive identification is established, the antemortem and postmortem records should be stapled together. As time progresses the number of positive dental identification will grow and the supply of incoming

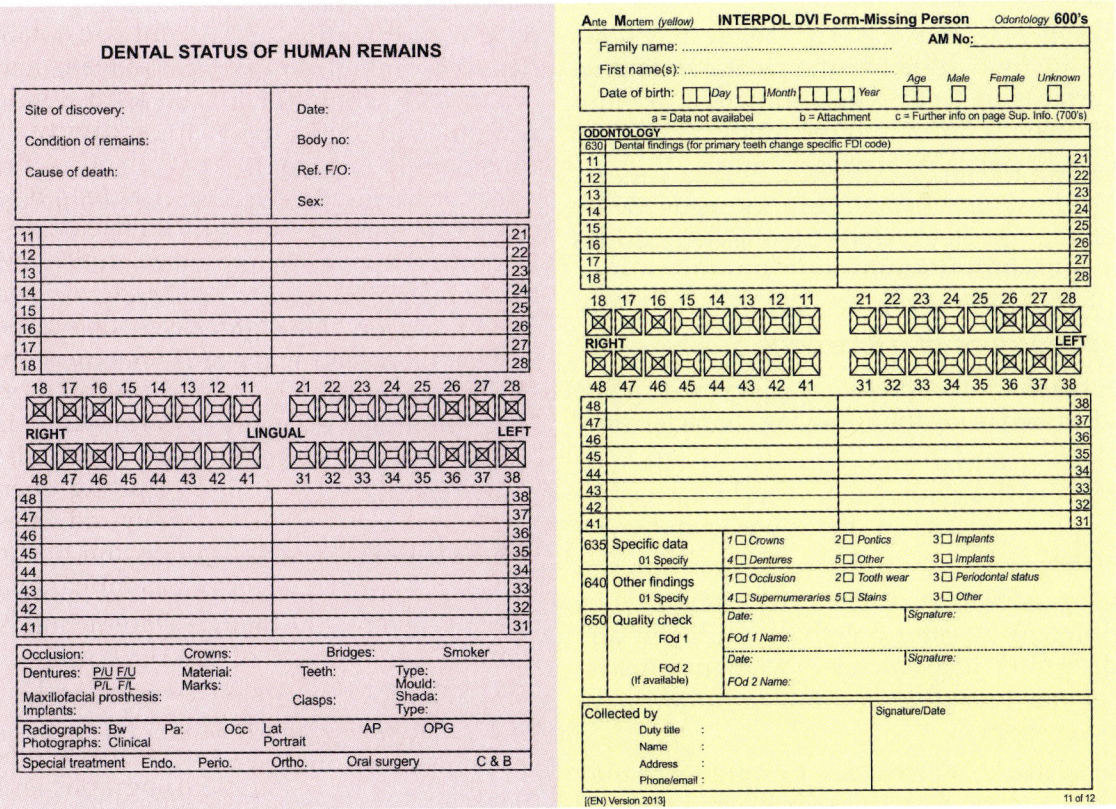

Fig. 23.6: INTERPOL antemortem yellow form and postmortem pink form

antemortem records will reduce. The left over unidentified victims cause problems and take a lot of time. According to the guide provided by INTERPOL, success of a disaster identification depends on the co-operation of different identification teams.

Bitemarks

McDonald has defined bitemarks as "a mark caused by the teeth either alone or in combination with other mouth parts". It can caused by humans or animals and can be made on inanimate objects as well. Biting is considered a primitive weapon.

Classification

McDonald's classification

Tooth pressure marks: Marks produced by direct application of pressure by teeth. It shows indentation of incisal or occlusal surfaces.

Tongue pressure marks: The tongue may press on the rigid areas like the palatal or lingual surfaces of teeth when sufficient amount of tissue is taken into the mouth. This may cause a central area of ecchymosis.

Tooth scrape marks: Marks caused by scrapping of teeth along the object. It exhibits as abrasions or scratches.

Appearance of a Bitemark

A bitemark is actually an injury and can be identified using the following characteristics:

Gross characteristics: Circular or elliptical mark with a central area of ecchymosis. The elliptical mark is due to the upper and lower arches.

Class characteristics: The marks produced by different classes of teeth are different and distinctive. Incisors create rectangular marks, canines triangular and molars spherical or point shaped.

Individual characteristics: Certain teeth may show unique characteristics like rotation and fractures.

Bitemark Investigation

Preliminary questions: Drinnan and Melton as well as Sweet have suggested preliminary questions to aid in the investigation of the bitemark:
1. Is the injury a bitemark?
2. If it is a bitemark, is it human or animal?
3. Is the bitemark by an adult or a child?
4. Are there any unique characteristics that can help analyze the bitemark?
5. Can these characteristics be compared to the teeth of the subject?

Evidence Collection from the Victim

In the event that a bitemark case comes to the dentist directly the law enforcement authority has to be informed. Studies have shown that there is a probability of transmission of HIV, hepatitis B, and syphilis from the bite to the victim, so due care has to be taken especially when there is a break in the dermis. The victim's name, age, gender, date of examination, and name of examiner has to be noted. In case the bite mark is on an area where there is a possibility of self-inflection, then the vicitim can also be considered as a suspect.

According to Brown, visual examination has to be carried out before the autopsy is done. During visual examination the following points have to be noted.
1. Orientation of the bitemark
2. Color, size and shape of the bitemark
3. Type of injury
4. Contour and elasticity of the bite site
5. Differences between upper and lower arches

Photography

Pictures should be taken as soon as the case presents itself to the dentist since the injury changes color because of healing. Both color and black and white pictures are to be taken.

Orientation photograph: It depicts the location of the bitemark on the body.

Close-up photograph: The ABFO scale no. 2 is a rigid reference scale. It is placed on the bitemark in one plane and a photograph is taken. The scale should not obstruct the view of the bitemark on the photograph. A second close-up photograph can be taken to depict that no part of the bitemark is obstructed by the scale.

The camera is positioned such that its long axis is perpendicular to the bitemark to reduce distortion. If the bitemark is on a curved surface like the forearm and the upper and lower arches of the bitemark are far apart, then separate photographs of each arch should be taken. According to Brown, if the victim is alive then photographs can be repeated every few hours to record the color changes due to healing.

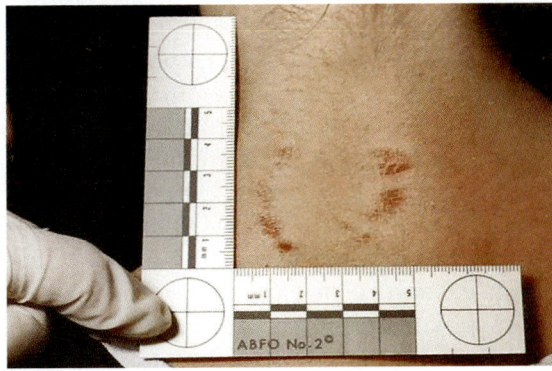

Fig. 23.7: Correct position of ABFO scale no. 2

Saliva Swab

The saliva left behind on a bitemark can be swabbed for DNA. The site of injury should not be washed before swabbing. If the bite mark is made through clothes, then the clothes should be swabbed for salivary DNA. A cotton swab moistened with distill water should be swabbed for DNA. Swabbing should always be done from the centre of the injury to the periphery in circular motions. There are two schools of thought, one which says that the swab should be air dried, bagged labeled and then stored in the fridge and the other which says that the swab should be placed in a plastic bag and labeled and then stored. The former has a disadvantage of contamination and the later of degradation of DNA and bacterial growth.

Impression

Impressions can be made only when tooth indentations exist. Impressions are made using Vinyl Poly siloxane and can be reinforced with dental stone or impression compound to prevent dimension change. In case of suspected self-inflected bites impressions of the victims dentition should also be taken.

Evidence Collection from the Suspect

A warrant (court order), a signed and witness informed consent are needed before collection of evidence. Infection protocol. The following evidence have to be procured from the suspect

1. Photographs of the suspect teeth in occlusion and in open bite.
2. Impressions of the maxillary and mandibular teeth.
3. Saliva swabs

Evidence has to be stored in well-labeled boxes or bags. The labels should include case number date, times, place as well as witness present during evidence collection. A 'chain of custody' should be maintained. Every individual that handles the evidence after collection signs and puts a date/time stamp on it.

Bitemark Analysis and Comparison

Factors to be considered during bitemark analysis include movement on the part of the victim, the elasticity of the area bitten, movement of the perpetrator and distortion during photography. Due to these variables majority of the bitemarks cannot be analyzed. It is erroneous to forcefully analyse and compare such bitemarks. Measurements such as intercanine distance are obtained once the canines are identified. These measurements are then compared to the model of the dentition of the suspect.

Bitemark analysis and comparison are two different concepts. Bitemark analysis is conducted as a part of a medicolegal autopsy. It provides information that when shown to the criminal justice system can dramatically influence the outcome.

Analysis should be carried out before introducing any suspect to prevent bias. It involves answering basic questions. Answers to these questions produce a large amount of information which along with other non-dental evidence can be valuable to the prosecution or the defense.

Bitemark comparison, on the other hand, is the comparison of a human bitemark to a suspect, dentition using various methods such as dental models and overlays. This is usually done to eliminate the suspect from a pool of perpetrators.

Direct method: Authors such as Ciapparelli and Hughes advocate the direct method of comparison where the suspect's dental models are placed directly over the photograph of the bitemark.

Indirect method: The incisal and occlusal surfaces of the teeth are traced onto clear acetate paper and superimposed onto bitemark photographs that are of 1:1 scale. The lifesize image is taken to minimize distortation. Authors Johansen and Bowers have suggested the use of adobe Photoshop® instead over transparent overlays with the incisal and occlusal edges.

Conclusions in Bitemark Analysis

Definite biter: There is enough of evidence to indicate that the bitemark is produced by the suspect beyond reasonable doubt.

Probable biter: Some degree of specificity is present due to significant number of matching points.

Possible biter: The bitemark and the suspect's dentition are consistent although there are not significant number of matching points to be absolutely certain.

Not the biter: There is no consistency between the bite mark and the suspects teeth.

Due to the confusion between bite mark comparison and bitemark analysis, there is a possibility that the information from bitemark analysis could also be lost if bite mark evidence is disallowed.

Forensic Radiology

The first civil case in which X-rays were accepted in US court took place in Denver. The earliest case of an identification on an unknown decent made through comparisons of sinuses in skull radiographs was published in 1926.

The antemortem radiographs are evaluated for quality, type of radiograph and the time period of when it must have been taken. It is possible to fix sub-optimal radiographs but it would depend on the situation when the comparison is required as in the case of mass disasters fixing the radiograph is not of prime importance. The postmortem specimen is evaluated and it is exposed such that it duplicates the areas of interest seen in the antemortem films. It is difficult to re-create the antemortem film geometry on postmortem films. It may require a number of attempts. Because of the complex nature of exposing radiographs, more postmortem radiographs are taken than the bare minimum necessary. The films are then marked as AM or PM. Points of concordance and disconcordance are noted.

Dental treatment carried out on the ante-mortem and postmortem radiographs is considered for comparison. In the absence of dental intervention, less common but static anatomical features are used as concordant points.

Sometimes despite a number of attempts, it is not possible to duplicate radiographs of the maxilla during postmortem because of the X-ray beam angulation of the antemortem dental films.

Facial bones are difficult to use for radio-graphical identification because of their anatomical complexity and overlapping structures. Frontal sinuses are used for comparison instead. The radiographic view most commonly used to demonstrate it is Water's view. The first radiographic comparison of paranasal sinuses was carried out by Culbert and Law.

Bite wing photographs are easily performed as compared to periapical radiographs.

Width and length of the maxillary sinus are measured in computer tomography scans with the application of software.

CONCLUSION

Dental identification is based on unique individual characteristics of the dentition and dental restoration, the resilience of dental tissues, the regressive changes in teeth.

FREQUENTLY ASKED QUESTIONS

1. Write a note on bitemark analysis.
2. Write a note on Demirjian's method.
3. Write a note on age estimation in juveniles.

BIBLIOGRAPHY

1. Patel J, Singh HP, Paresh M, Verma. Forensic Odontology in the era of computer and technology. IJMDS; January 2013; 2(1): 59–64.
2. C Priyadarshini, Manjunath P, Puranik, SR Uma. Dental Age Estimation Methods: A Review International Journal of Advanced Health Sciences 2015; 1 (12): 19–25.
3. BR Chandra Shekar, CVK Reddy. Role of dentist in person identification. Indian J Dent Res 2009; 20(3): 356–60.
4. Preeti Sharma, Susmita Saxena, Vanita Rathod. Comparative reliability of cheiloscopy and palatoscopy in human identification. Indian J Dent Res 2009; 20(4): 453–57.
5. Jyotsna Seth, Anubha Agarwal, Himanshu Aeran, Yogeshwari Krishnan. Dental Age Estimation in Children and Adolescents. Indian Journal of Dental Sciences 2018; 10 (4):248–51.
6. Kuldeep Singh, R.K.Gorea, Vipin Bharti. Age estimation from eruption of permanent teeth. JIAFM 2005; 27 (4):231–35.
7. A K Srivastava, Amit Kumar, Abhishek Kumar, Ankita Srivastav. Mass Disaster: Identification of Victims with Special Emphasis on Dental Evidences. J Indian Acad Forensic Med 2015; 37(2):190–95.
8. Javier Ata-Ali, Fadi Ata-Ali. Forensic dentistry in human identification: A review of the literature J Clin Exp Dent 2014;6(2): 162–7.
9. Thorakkal Shamim. Forensic Odontology. Journal of the College of Physicians and Surgeons—Pakistan. JCPSP 2010; 20(1) : 1–2
10. Niveditha Thampan, R. Janani, R. Ramya, R. Bharanidharan, A. Ramesh Kumar, K. Rajkumar. Antemortem dental records versus individual identification. Journal of Forensic Dental Sciences 2018; 10 (3): 158–64.
11. Nadeem Jeddy, Shivani Ravi and T. Radhika. Current trends in Forensic Odontology. Journal of forensic dental sciences 2018; 9(3): 115–19
12. Acharya AB, Sivapathasundharam B. Forensic Odontology. In: Rajendran R, Sivapatha-sundharam B. Eds. Shafer's Textbook of Oral Pathology. Fifth Edn. Elsevier: New Delhi; 2006. p. 1199–227.

Geriatric and Oral Health

INTRODUCTION

Geriatrics is the branch of medicine that treats all health issues related to the aging patients, including the clinical problems of senescence and senility. This chapter focuses on geriatric changes present in oral cavity which may co-exist all manifested separately.

Physiology of Aging

It is generally believed that the physiological systems deteriorate with advancing age. Theoretically process of aging is simply the death of cells.

Progressive age changes are characterized in the following categories.

- Gradual tissue desiccation.
- Gradual retardation of cell division, capacity of cell growth, and tissue repair including reduced capacity to produce immune bodies.
- Gradual retardation in the rate of tissue oxidation (lowering of the basal metabolic rate).
- Cellular atrophy, degeneration, increased cell pigmentation, and fatty infiltration.
- Gradual decrease in tissue elasticity and degenerative changes in the elastic connective tissue.
- Decreased speed, strength, and endurance of skeletal "neuromuscular reactions".
- Decreased strength of skeletal muscle.

- Progressive degeneration and atrophy of the nervous system.

Following are the different oral changes seen with aging:

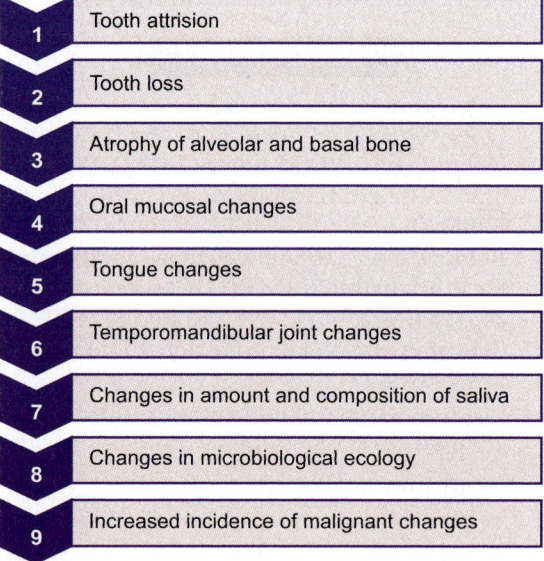

1. Tooth attrision
2. Tooth loss
3. Atrophy of alveolar and basal bone
4. Oral mucosal changes
5. Tongue changes
6. Temporomandibular joint changes
7. Changes in amount and composition of saliva
8. Changes in microbiological ecology
9. Increased incidence of malignant changes

Changes in Teeth with Aging

The gradual changes taking place in the dental tissues after teeth are fully formed are referred to as age changes. The teeth change in form and color with age. The tooth form is affected by wear and attrision.

1. **Changes in enamel:**
   - All changes in the enamel are based on ion exchange mechanisms. It

is generally accepted that enamel becomes less permeable and possibly more brittle with age.

- Some acquired properties of surface enamel are slowly built up during life, such as the fluoride content. These changes in the surface content may therefore be considered age changes.

2. Changes in cementum

- Cementum may be resorbed and new cementum may form both locally in resorption defects or more generally over the roots, especially in the apical half, to compensate for tooth wear during function.
- The composition of cementum has also been reported to change with age, for example, the fluoride and magnesium content.
- The most characteristic age change in cementum is the gradual increase in thickness cementum deposition occurs throughout life.
- The total width of cementum almost triples between the age of 10 to 75 years.

3. Changes in dentine: The two age dependent changes take place in dentine:

- Continued growth referred to as physiological secondary dentine formation and gradual obturation of the dentinal tubules, referred to as dentine sclerosis.
- These processes occur concomitantly, but they are independent.
- The formation of secondary dentine reduces the pulp chamber. This reduction in size does not affect the pulp chamber evenly, and it varies for different types of teeth.

4. Changes in pulp

- The dental pulp in teeth from old individuals differ from that in younger teeth by having more fibers and fewer cells.
- The blood supply apparently decreases with age; at least, the number of arteries entering the apical foramen does.

- The number of branches of blood vessels was markedly reduced with age, including the branching in subodontoblastic region.
- Increased number of pulp stones is seen in pulp with increasingly age but it also has been considered as pathological changes.

5. Tooth attrision

- With age, enamel and dentine undergo certain sclerotic changes following increased mineralization and deposition of trace elements.
- In spite of this increased hardness (and brittleness) the every day use of a natural dentition causes progressive tooth attrision.

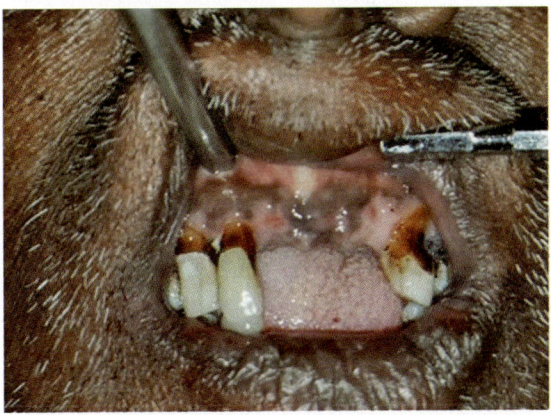

Fig. 24.1: Severe gingival recession and cervical abrasion

6. Root surface caries

- Root surface caries result from an age-related conditions that develop on cementum following gingival recession.
- These lesions appear as well-defined and discolored defects on cementum or at the cementum-enamel junction
- The prevalence of untreated root surface caries has been reported as 22% in an older population.
- Other factors that predispose elderly individuals to root surface caries are a poor diet (with frequent sugar consumption), salivary gland hypofunction, insufficient fluoride

exposure, gingival recession, oral-facial motor deficits, poor oral hygiene, and decreased access to regular dental treatment.

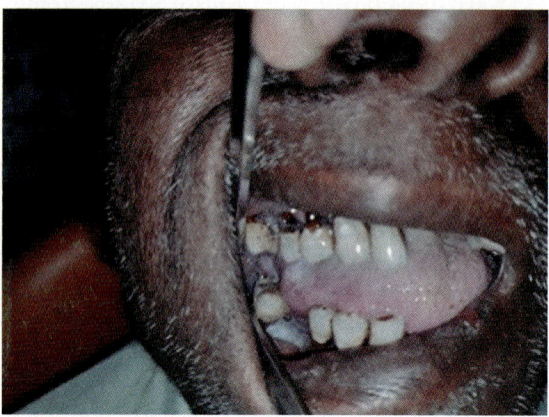

Fig. 24.2: Root caries

7. Tooth loss

- Successive tooth loss, which can lead to the complete edentulous state, is the most conspicuous change in the stomatognathic system in the elderly of the civilized world.
- The picture of the toothless old individual with hollow cheeks, retracted lips, strongly prominent chin, hanging nose and collapsed bite is classical.
- Caries and periodontitis account for more than 90% of tooth extractions.

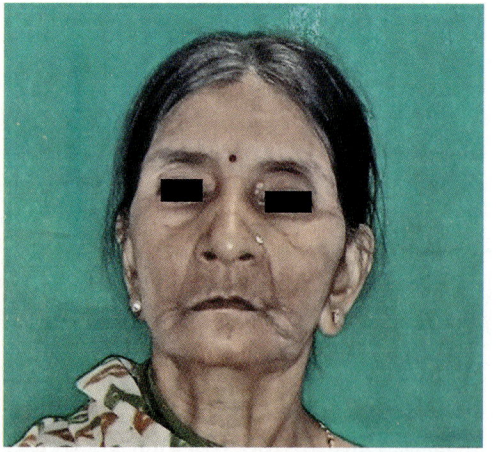

Fig. 24.3: Toothless old individual with hollow cheeks, retracted lips, prominent chin.

Changes in Periodontal Tissues with Aging

Decrease in number of fibroblast has been reported with increasing age.

With aging collagen fiber becomes more stable, showing increased thermal stability, insolubility and mechanical strength.

- Gingivitis is much more likely to develop in older patients because of oral and systemic factors.
- Dental plaque, gingival bleeding, and calculus accumulations develop as a result of softer diets, reduced oral motor activity, and salivary gland hypofunction.
- Gingival recession, root caries, tooth furcation involvement, and tooth drifting and mobility increase the likelihood of developing gingivitis.
- Gingival hyperplasia has been associated with the use of phenytoin, cyclosporine, and calcium channel blockers.
- Diabetes, even when well controlled, is associated with rapid periodontal breakdown.

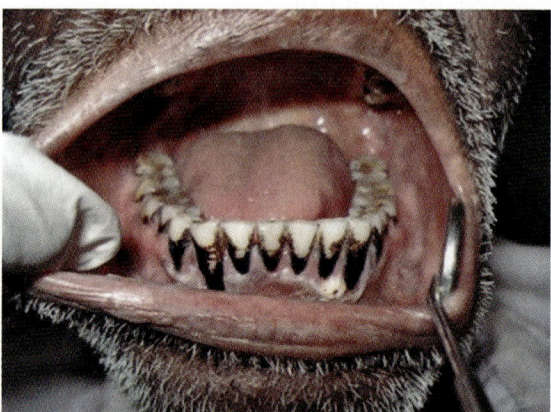

Fig. 24.4: Gingival recession and stains on teeth due to habit

Changes in Bone with Aging

- Compact or cortical bone.
- Spongy or trabecular or cancellous bone.

Effect of Aging

- Thinning of cortical bone
- Increase in porosity
- Loss of trabecular

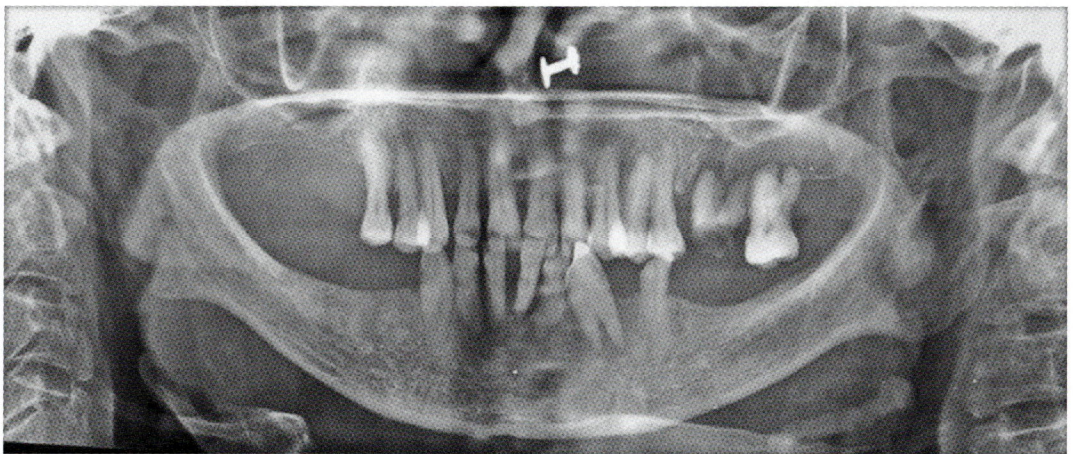

Fig. 24.5: Generalized alveolar bone loss

* Cellular atrophy
* Sclerosis

With aging, changes in bone composition have also been observed that alter the volumetric proportions of adipose tissue, hematopoietic tissue, trabecular bone and osteoid, the unmineralized newly formed matrix, decreases by 3 fold by age 20, then remains constant.

The volume of hematopoietic tissue is also highest in the young, decreasing by 50 to 60% by age 40. Adipose tissue volume increases throughout life, with the most marked increase occurring between the ages of 40 and 60 years. Bone volume declines by 30% or more after age 60.

Osteopenia is a condition of low bone mass and osteoporosis is a disease in which low bone mass is associated with fractures. Both the conditions are common in old age but difficult to diagnoses. Osteoporosis is regarded as being more frequent and advanced in elderly females than elderly males.

Changes in Oral Mucosa with Aging

As a result of the metabolic changes in the elderly person, including a shift in water balance the oral mucous membranes may become atrophic and friable taking on a shiny wax-like appearance.

The gingivae also show these changes together with a loss of stippling.

The progressive thinning of the epithelial layer occurs in combination with a decrease in the elastic properties of connective tissue. Clinically these effects add up to a reduction in resiliency of those tissues which may be subjected to pressure.

In addition, the decrease in surface capillaries and consequent reduced blood supply delay micronutrition and impairs the capacity to regenerate.

As a result of the above disturbances, the aging mucosa is more sensitive to external influence. It can be easily damaged by coarse food or ill-fitting appliances and its healing capacity is markedly slower than mature mucosa.

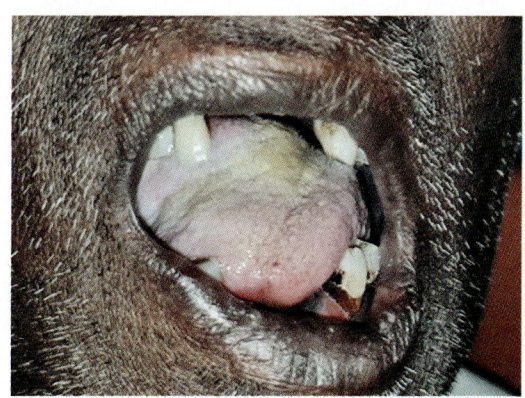

Fig. 24.6: Coatings on tongue mucosa

Oral Mucosal Diseases

Oral vesiculobullous diseases in older adults include lichen planus, pemphigus vulgaris, and cicatricial pemphigoid.

Lichenoid mucosal lesions can also be caused by a variety of medications commonly prescribed in older patients (e.g., acyclovir, gold salts, methyl-dopa, and thiazide diuretics).

- Pemphigus vulgaris is a potentially serious autoimmune vesiculobullous disorder that usually affects individuals in their fifth and sixth decades.
- Cicatricial pemphigoid is another immunologically mediated disorder; it affects primarily older women.
- Persistent low-grade irritation by an ill-fitting denture can induce a hyperplastic reaction, leading to the formation of an epulis fissuratum.
- Nutritional and hematologic deficiencies that are common in older adults can predispose to recurrent ulcers.
- Oral cancer is the most significant oral mucosal disease in older adults.
- Incidence rates increase with age; over 95% of all oral cancers occur in individuals aged 45 years.

Nutritional Deficiencies

Nutritional deficiencies are often associated with changes in the mucosa of the aging mouth. Most characteristics are the smooth, atrophic tongue and angular cheilitis. Abnormal taste sensations and burning sensations are also common and probably due to progressing atrophy of taste buds hastened by concomitant dehydration, iron deficiency and frequently through vitamin B complex deficiencies.

Tongue Disorders

Tongue is a most valuable source of diagnostic information. Changes in appearance, sensation and movement are not infrequent in the elderly. The more common complaints are outlined below.

Atropic Glossitis

Essentially it is reflection of nutritional failure originating from reduced intake or malabsorption, and is particularly associated with deficiencies of the vitamin B complex.

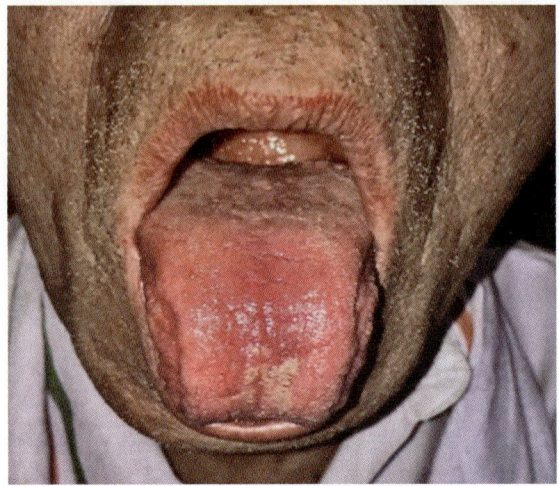

Fig. 24.7: Atrophy of tongue mucosa

Furred Tongue

- Fur is formed continuously and is normally removed by food and saliva.
- With reduction of salivary flow and poor oral hygiene the keratin accumulates on the surface of the filiform papillae.
- This then provides a good environment for accumulation of bacteria, debris and coloring substances.

Fissured Tongue

- It is often regarded as a result of long standing glossitis and scarring and is irreversible.
- The fissures are rather deep and tend to collect cellular and food debris and microbiological flora.
- As a result the adjoining areas of the tongue often show inflammation.

Glossopyrosis

- Is a very common symptom amongst elderly people. A variety of causes may be responsible.

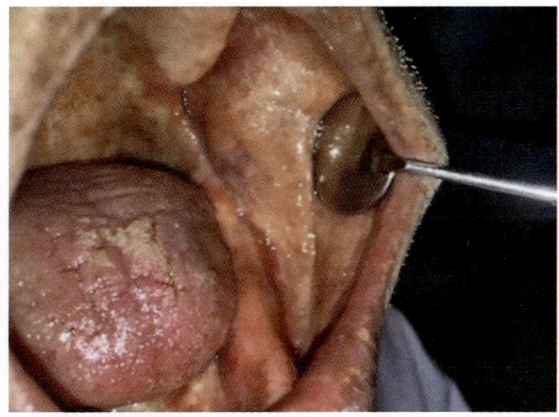

Fig. 24.8: Fissured tongue

× Such sensation on mucous membrane could be a result of a minimal cerebral vascular accident (especially if there is a history of hypertension) dizziness or unexplained syncope.

× Where clinical changes in the tongue can be recorded, the symptoms may be associated with local irritation nutritional deficiencies or systemic disease such as diabetes, pernicious anemia or the Plummer-Vinson syndrome.

× In the absence of clinical signs psychological pressures and tensions may be suspected.

Temporomandibular Joint Disorders with Aging

In old people generally the range of mandibular movements is basically undisturbed and usually the temporomandibular joint functions well. This might be due partly to the fact that although they are stress bearing, it is only a limited degree. Those who are edentulous have some change as opposed to the people with some natural teeth.

Joint Dislocation

The danger of subluxation of the temporomandibular joint as a result of even simple dental procedure is increased in the older person. For example, a complaint of altered function and discomfort following pressure on the mandible must be investigated both clinically and radiographically.

Degenerative Joint Disease

Amongst the elderly there is an incidence of up to 27% to 50% of structural changes in the joint. Degenerative joint disease undoubtedly increases in the older age groups. The radiographical changes that are associated with this form of arthritis are marginal erosions, seen as discontinuance in the cortical layer of the joint surfaces.

× Osteophytic depositions especially in the anterior part of the condyle head.

× Osteoporosis.

× Sclerosis of joint surfaces.

× Reduced distance between joint surfaces

× Abrasion of articular fossa and the condylar head.

× Degeneration and partial destruction of the articular disc and exposure of bony structure.

× Adhesions between joint capsule can also be seen. All these changes may be attributed to a combination of aging changes and stress above the physiological limits.

× In severe degenerative joint disease clinical symptoms:
  - Pain and tenderness of the joint
  - Clicking and crepitations on movement
  - Reduced mobility of the joint is not a common presentation.

Rheumatoid Arthritis

Rheumatoid arthritis is a systemic disease with special affinity to collagen and, therefore, to connective tissue and bone. It is justifiable to assume that at least half of such patients have or will have temporomandibular joint disturbances of a progressive type. The changes in the temporomandibular joint resulting from rheumatoid arthritis appear to go parallel with the disease in other parts of the body.

It is not a disorder mainly of old age as the onset usually comes in the age period of 25–50 years. However, with increasing age it becomes more marked with an increased frequency in the elderly.

Salivary Gland Disorders with Aging

Salivary flow reduces due to intake of medications like antihypertensive, antiparkinsonian drugs, antihistaminic drugs, antipsychotic drugs.

Salivary Gland Atrophy

Consequences
* Diminished functions like mastication
* Digestive problems
* Poor retention of dentures
* Interference with patient's ability to wear dentures.
* Susceptibility of mucosa to frictional irritation from denture movement

No reduction in salivary output from the parotid gland, whereas that of submandibular gland is reduced.

Submandibular gland: 45% of total output.

Changes in composition
* Ptyalin—decreased
* Mucin—increases

Physical changes
* Viscous ropy
* Plaque formation and growth of cariogenic bacteria.
* Salivary gland dysfunction

Extraoral manifestations of salivary gland dysfunction include
* Candidiasis in the labial commissures.
* Dry cracked lips.
* Parotid or submandibular gland enlargement
* With associated pain and suppuration may indicate infection or ductal obstructions.

Infectious Diseases with Aging

Due to numerous age and disease-related changes in the oral and systemic immune systems, older adults are more susceptible to developing opportunistic oral infections.

Viral, fungal, and bacterial organisms invade, infect, and become latent in the hard and soft tissues of the oropharyngeal region, predisposing the person to disseminated systemic infections.

Viral Infections

The most common oral viral infections come from the herpes family
* Herpes simplex virus [HSV] and
* Varicella-zoster virus [VZV]

Fungal infection

The most frequent oral fungal infection in older adults is caused by *Candida albicans*.

The predisposing factors are
* Removable dental prostheses poor oral or denture hygiene.
* Endocrine disorders (e.g. diabetes).
* Underlying immunosuppression.
* Nutritional deficiencies.
* Salivary gland hypofunction.
* Medications (e.g., antibiotics, corticosteroids, *immunosuppressants*, and cytotoxic agents) have all been associated with oral fungal infections
* The loss of vertical dimension, as well as drooling problems secondary to cerebrovascular accidents, creates a moist environment in the labial commissures that also favors yeast infection.

Bacterial Infection

The bacteria that cause the most common infections are those associated with:
* *New and recurrent dental caries: Streptococcus mutans* and Lactobacillus
* *Periodontal diseases: Porphyromonas gingivalis* and *Treponema denticola*
* *Acute and chronic salivary infections: Staphylococcus aureus* and *Streptococcus viridans*.

Disorders of Taste Sensation with Aging

Taste sensation tends to be less intensive in the elderly person particularly with regards to sweet and salty foods.

Parageusia may be due to age changes in the papillary structure of the tongue.

In the elderly the circumvallate papillae tend to become more prominent with a result that bitter tastes can become highly disagreeable.

BIBLIOGRAPHY

1. Greenberg, Glick, Chapter 24, Geriatrics. Burket Textbook Of Oral Medicine, 10th edition.
2. David B. Ferguson. Chapter 14 The Ageing Mouth Textbook of Oral Biosciences.
3. Major M. Ash Jr. Chapter 7 Aging, Retrogressive Changes and Dysfunction Text Book of Oral Pathology, 6th edition.
4. Dental management of the medically compromised patient, 6th edition, little falace, page no 526–541.
5. Yolanda Ann Slaughter. Oral Diagnosis for the Geriatric Population: Current Status and Future Prospects J. Dental Clinics of North America 49(2005) 445–461.
6. Elisa M.Ghezzi, Jonathan A. Systemic Diseases and Their Treatment in the Elderly: Impact on Oral Health J Public Health Dent 2000;60(4):289–96.
7. Donald R. Morse. Age related changes of the dental pulp complex and their relationship to systemic aging, Oral surg oral med oral pathol 1991; 72:721–45.
8. Fransson C. Berglundh T, Lindhe. The effect of age on the development of gingivitis J Clin Periodontol 1996; 23:379–385.
9. Margareta Persson, Tor Osterberg. Influence of Parkinson's disease on oral health Acta Odontol Scand 1992; 50: 37–42.
10. Angus WG Wall Jimy G. Steele. Oral health and nutrition in older people, Journal of Public Health Dentistry 2000; 60 (4):304–7.
11. Michael I. MacEntee. Oral care for successful Aging in Long-term Care Journal of Public Health Dentistry 2000; 60 (4):326–29.
12. Ejvind, Budtz Jorgensen. Prosthodontics for the elderly, diagnosis and treatment. 1st edition.

Oral Radiology

Radiation Physics

INTRODUCTION

WC Roentgen on 18th Nov. 1895, discovered X-rays and their property to penetrate human tissues. He called them X-rays as their nature was unknown initially. X-rays consist of 'wave packets' of energy. Each packet is called a photon and is equivalent to one quantum of energy. The X-ray beam is made up of millions of photons.

Radiation physics deals with production and interaction of X-rays (with tissues). To understand this, atomic physics forms the base which further guides about radiations and their interaction with matter.

Atomic Structure

Atom is formed by proton, neutron and electron. Protons and neutrons are called nucleons and form the nucleus.

Atomic number (Z) is the number of protons and number of electrons (N) in an atom.

Atomic mass number (A) = Z + N

IONIZATION

When the number of electrons in an atom is equal to the number of protons in the nucleus, the atom is electrically neutral. When atom looses an electron, nucleus becomes positive ion and free electron becomes a negative

ion. This ion pair (+ve and –ve) formation is called ionization.

To ionize an atom, sufficient energy is required to overcome the electrostatic force of binding electrons to the nucleus. Tightly bound electrons require the energy of X-rays or high energy particles to remove them from their shells.

Non-ionizing radiations do not have sufficient energy to remove bound electrons from their orbitals. For example, visible light, infrared, microwave radiation.

Radiation is a transmission of energy through space and matter. Particulate and electromagnetic are the forms of radiation (Fig. 25.1).

1. Particulate Radiation (PR)

The capacity of this radiation to ionize the matter depends on mass, velocity and charge of particles. The rate of loss of energy from a particle as it moves along its track through matter or tissue is called linear energy transfer (LET) .

LET is directly proportional to physical size and charge of particle and inversely proportional to velocity.

Particular radiations transmit kinetic energy by fast moving particles—beta and gamma.

Four types of particulate radiations are encountered in radiation physics, those are

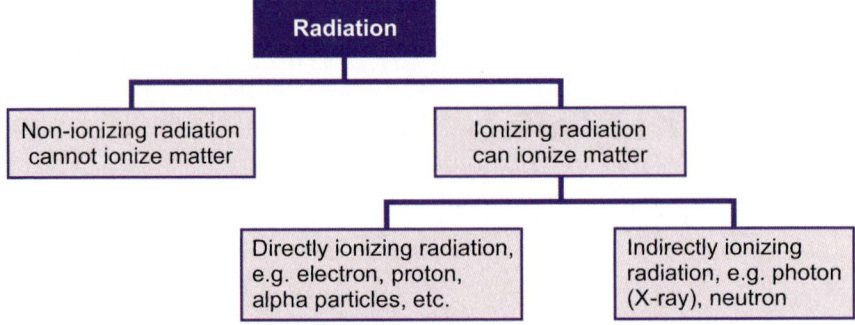

Fig. 25.1: Interaction of radiations with matter

electrons, alpha particles, proton particles, and protons.

Electrons can be further classified as beta particles which are fast moving particles emitted from nucleus of atom. Cathode rays are also considered as streams of high speed electrons that originate in X-ray tube.

Alpha particles are emitted from the nuclei of heavy metals. As they have double positive charge and heavy mass, they can densely ionize matter through which they pass. This property allows these particles to quickly transfer their energy and penetrate only a few micrometers of body tissue.

Protons: When a neutron decays, it splits to give β particle, a proton and a neutrino. β particles are similar in behavior as electrons. β particles can penetrate the matter to a greater depth than alpha particles (maximum 1.5 cm). Due to this low penetration power, β particles are used as therapeutic measure for a few skin cancers.

2. Electromagnetic Radiation (ER)

It is the movement of energy through space in the form of electric and magnetic fields. ER uses both particle and a wave to move through matter, hence it is said that it works on dualistic theory, i.e. wave theory and quantum theory.

Wave theory: This theory results due to propagation of ER in the medium as wave (not resembling wave of water), such wave is a combination of electric and magnetic fields placed at right angle to one another and oscillate perpendicular to the direction of motion. All electromagnetic waves travel at the velocity of light (3.0×10^8 m/sec.) in vacuum.

Quantum theory: This theory is based on photons, which are small bundles of ER. Each photon has no mass or weight, but has specific amount of energy and travels at speed of light. The unit of photon energy is eV or ER. When passes through matter, the intensity of these radiations can be reduced, also called attenuation and the energy is transferred to that matter, i.e. absorption. Some energy during this propagation can get deflected from actual path taking new direction is called scattering.

ER follows inverse square law.

PRODUCTION OF X-RAYS

In a X-ray tube, electrons travel from the cathode to the anode. When these high speed electrons interact with target electrons, their energy is converted to 99% as heat and 1% as X-rays. This process of X-ray production can occur by formation of bremsstrahlung and characteristic radiation, also called spectrum.

Bremsstrahlung or braking radiation or continuous spectrum: The X-ray photons emitted by the rapid deceleration of the high speed electrons are called braking radiation (braking the speed of electrons).

The energy is resultant photon and is equal to the amount of energy lost by bombarding electron. A wide range of spectrum of photon energies is produced and so called continuous spectrum. Small deflections produce low energy photons which have less penetrating power. They do not contribute to the useful X-ray beam. The removal of low energy photons from the beam is filtration.

Characteristic radiation/spectrum: X-ray beam has fewer fractions of photons generated as characteristic radiation.

After ionization of tungsten atom by electron, the orbiting tungsten electrons rearrange themselves for fixing the atom to neutral state.

This process involves moving of electron from one shell to another which results in emission of X-ray photon with specific energies.

The X-ray photons emitted from the target are described as characteristic of tungsten atom and form the characteristic spectrum/radiation (Fig. 25.2).

X-RAY MACHINE

To make a radiographic image X-ray machine produces X-rays that pass through the patient tissues and strike on the image receptors or film. Most commonly used X-ray machine is wall-mounted unit (Fig. 25.3). The component parts of wall-mounted machine are:

- X-ray tube head
- Cylinder
- Extension arm
- Ready light
- Separate control panel.

X-ray Tube Head

The tube head consists of heavy metal housing containing X-ray tube which has an anode and cathode situated within and evacuated glass envelope. Energy from some of the electrons is converted into X-rays when electrons stream from filament of cathode to the target in the anode. A power supply is necessary to heat cathode to generate electrons and establish a high voltage potential between anode and cathode (Fig. 25.4).

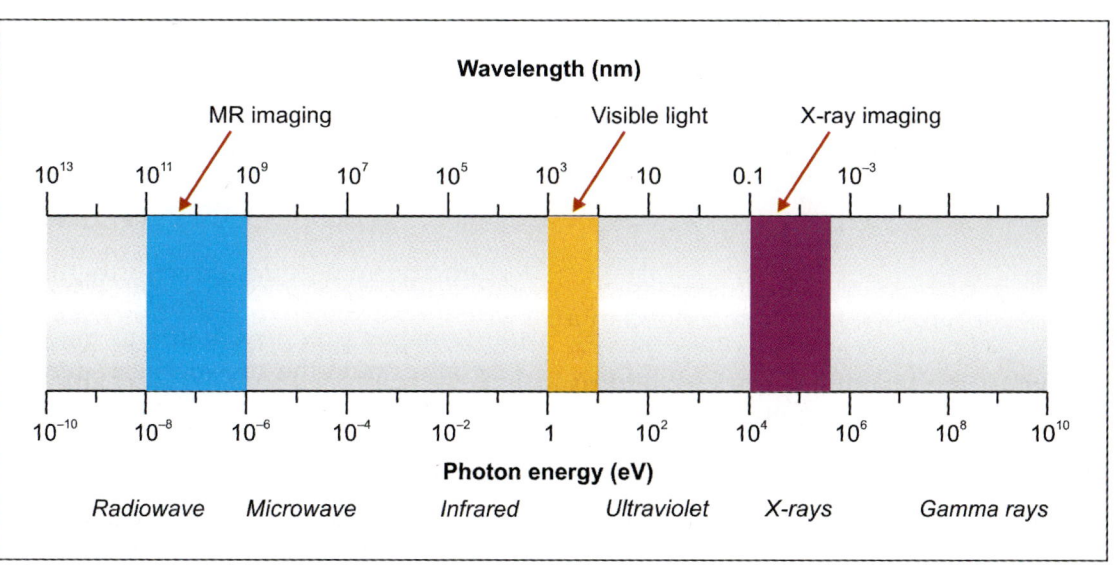

Fig. 25.2: Electromagnetic spectrum

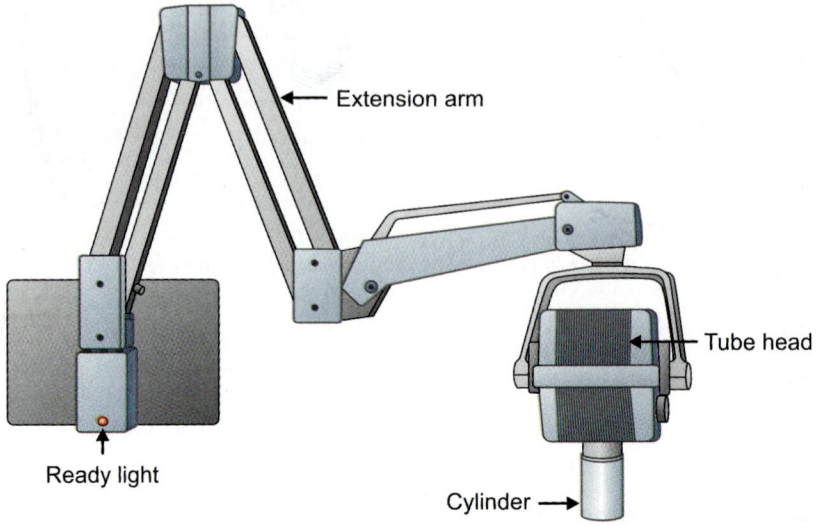

Fig. 25.3: X-ray machine

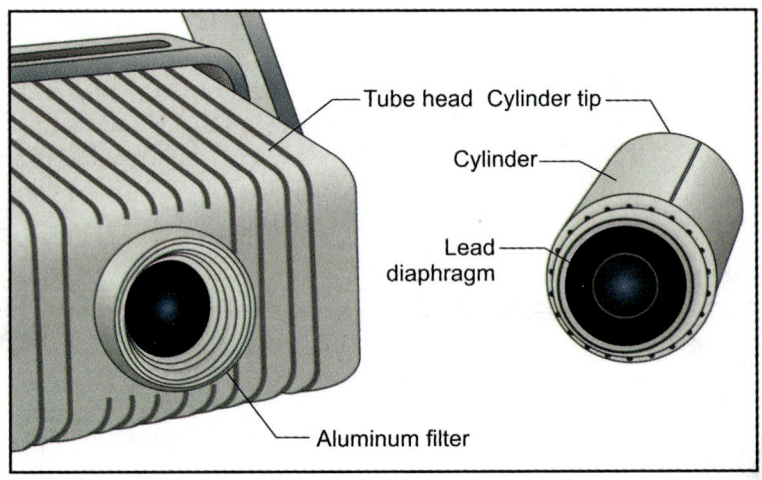

Fig. 25.4: X-ray tube head

Anode

Purpose of tungsten target embedded in a copper stem in an X-ray tube **(Fig. 25.5)** is to convert the kinetic energy of colliding electrons into X-ray photons. Tungsten is a target element having several characteristics such as:

- High atomic no. 74 (most efficient in producing X-rays)
- High melting point (3422°C) (as heat is generated at the anode)
- High thermal conductivity (to readily dissipate its heat to copper stem)
- Low vapor pressure (helps to maintain the vacuum in the tube at high operating temperature)

Cathode

It consists of filament and focusing cup. Filament made of tungsten wire is the source of electron within the X-ray tube **(Fig. 25.5)**. Filament is mounted between two stiff

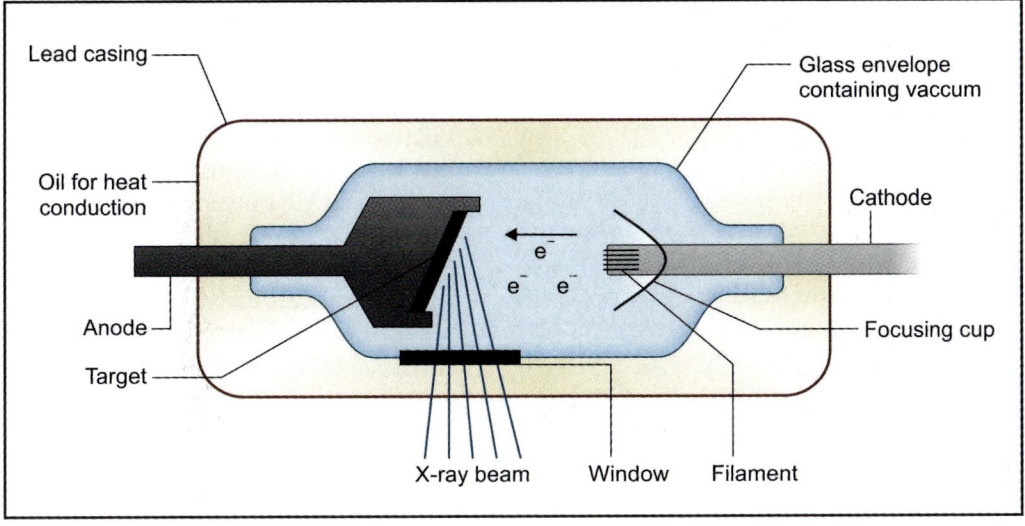

Fig. 25.5: X-ray tube

support wires that carry electric current. Filament is heated through current supplied, to emit electrons at a rate proportional to the temperature of the filament. Filament lies in focusing cup. Focusing cup is a negatively charged concave reflector made up of molybdenum. The shape of focusing cup is parabolic which electrostatically focuses the electrons emitted by the filament into a narrow beam directed at a small rectangular area on anode called focal spot. Vacuum prevents oxidation or 'burnout' of the filament.

Sharpness of the image increases as the focal spot decreases, but heat generated per unit target area increases as the focal spot decreases. Target is placed at an angle to electron beam. Target is inclined at 20° to central ray. Effective focal spot is 1 mm × 1 mm and actual focal spot is 1 mm × 3 mm.

Apparent size of focal spot seen from position perpendicular to electron beam is smaller than actual focal spot size (line focus principle).

POWER SUPPLY

Functions

1. To heat X-ray tube filament by providing a low voltage current.

2. To accelerate electrons from the cathode to the focal spot on the anode by generating a high potential difference.

Tube Current

The tube current is the flow of electrons through the tube that is from the cathode to the anode. Beyond the anode, this current is carried through the power supply back to the cathode.

Tube Voltage

As the tube voltage increases, the speed of electrons moving towards anode increases. X-rays are produced at the target with greater efficiency when the voltage applied across the tube is high.

Timer

The electronic timer controls the length of time that high voltage is applied to the tube and the time during which tube current flows and X-rays are produced. The number of pulses divided by 60 (the frequency of power sources) gives the exposure time in seconds. A setting of 30 pulses means that there will be 30 pulses of radiations equivalent to a 0.5 sec exposure.

Tube Rating and Duty Cycle

At the anode, heat is build-up which is measured in heat units (HU)

$$HU = kVp \times mA \times Seconds$$

where, kVp is tube voltage.

Each X-ray machine comes with a tube rating chart that describes the longest exposure time tube can be energized for a range of voltages and tube current values without risk of damage to the target from overheating. The frequency with which exposure can be made without overheating the anode is *duty cycle*. A typical duty cycle is 1:60 , meaning that one could make 0.25 sec exposure every 15 seconds.

Factors Controlling X-ray Beam

1. The quality of X-ray beam depends on exposure parameters; like exposure rate, tube current (mA), tube voltage (kVp), exposure time and shape and intensify of beam.
    * *Tube current:* The quantity of radiation produced by X-ray tube is directly proportional to the tube current (mA) and the time. It is expressed as mAs, i.e. product of tube current and exposure time.
    * As long as the product of current and time remains the same, any variation in them will not affect the quantity of radiation.
2. **Tube voltage:** Potential difference between the cathode and anode can be fixed by increasing the tube voltage. This uses the energy of each electron reaching the target. It also uses number of photons generated, their mean and maximal energy. Higher the kVp, higher is the energy of X-ray beam and greater the penetration power. Beam quality depends upon energy of X-ray beam.
3. **Exposure time:** By varying the exposure time, both the duration of exposure and number of photons generated vary.
Routinely practiced exposure parameters for dental radiology are: kVp 65–70, 8–10 mA and time will depend upon the site of examination.
Advanced machines provide panels with adjustment functions.
4. Filtration is the process of absorption of the long wavelength (low energy) X-rays by a sheet of material called filter. The reason for using filter is to remove the low energy (long wavelength) X-rays. A filter is an absorbing material (generally aluminum) placed in the path of the X-ray beam to remove a low energy (long wavelength) X-rays and decrease patient radiation dose.
5. Collimator is a metallic barrier with an opening in the center and serves to limit the size and shape of the useful X-ray beam reaching the patient. This will not only reduce dose, but may also improve image quality. This is generally done with a lead diaphragm (collimator) within the tube head or at the end of a lead lined cylinder. Decreasing the size of the X-ray beam to the minimum size needed to image the area of interest is an obvious means of reducing the dose to patients.
6. Inverse square law: The intensity of an X-ray beam depends on the distance of the measuring device from the focal spot. For a given beam the intensity is inversely proportional to the square of the distance from the source.

$$\frac{I_1}{I_2} = \frac{(D_2)^2}{(D_1)^2}$$

I—intensity, D—distance.

(For example: Dose of 10 Gy is measured at a distance of 20 m, a dose of 8 Gy will be found at 2 m and so on)

This decrease in intensity is due to spreading or widening of the beam when it leaves the source. Thus, changing the distance between X-ray tube and patient has significant effect on beam intensity.

This law suggests the use of appropriate exposure parameters and distance between X-ray tube and patient. Variation in distance between film and tooth needs corresponding modification of kVp and mA to get accurate resultant image.

Interaction of X-ray with Matter at the Atomic Level

When X-ray beam passes through patient, it interacts with all hard and soft tissues of body. Either these X-ray photons are attenuated or get scattered. The frequency of these interactions varies according to the type of tissue exposed. This variation in interaction allows radiologist to differentiate between enamel, dentin, bone and other soft tissues.

Initially, it was thought that there are a few main interactions of X-rays, depending on the energy of incoming photon, like unmodified or pure scatter, photoelectric scatter or pure absorption, Compton effect or scatter and absorption and pair production or pure absorption (Fig. 25.6).

But the current concept describes these types of beam attenuation of dental X-ray beam as coherent scattering, photoelectric absorption and Compton scattering. 9% of primary photons pass through tissues without interactions.

Coherent Scattering

Other name: Classical, elastic or Thompson scattering.

Interaction: This scattering involves low energy incident photon relatively low binding energy. Such photons may not get absorbed but scattered without loss of energy. The incident photon can allow momentary vibration of electron with which it interacts. This vibration of electron further releases energy in the form of another X-ray photon.

% of interactions: 7

Effects on image: Negligible in producing fog (in resultant image)

Photoelectric Effect

Other name: Pure absorption.

Interaction: On this interaction X-ray photon interacts with a bound inner shell electron of the tissue atom. The tightly bound inner shell electron is ejected with considerable energy

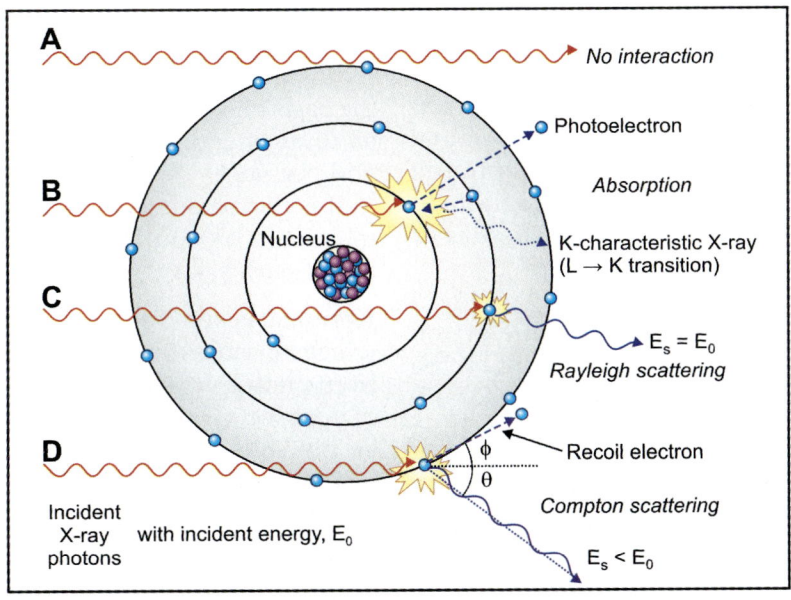

Fig. 25.6: Interaction of X-rays at atomic level

and undergoes further interactions. The first X-ray photon disappears, depositing all its energy. So, this is called pure absorption.

The vacancy created in inner shell is filled by outer shell electrons (process of dropping from one shell to another). Stability of atom is finally achieved by the capture of a free electron to return the atom to its neutral state.

The overall result of this interaction is ionization of the tissues.

(Hard tissues has much greater photo-electric interaction than soft tissues due to high atomic number.)

% of interactions: 27

Effect on image: Do not cause fogging of film. Due to difference in photoelectric absorption in different tissues, there is identified difference in optical density of the image.

Compton Effect

Other name: Scattering and absorption.

Interaction: The incoming X-ray photon interacts with a loosely bound or free outer shell electron of the tissue atom. The outer shell electron gets ejected with loss of some energy of the incoming photon. The ejected electron further undergoes into ionizing interaction.

The remaining energy of incoming photon is deflected or scattered from its original path as scattered photon. This photon can undergo photoelectric interaction or Compton interactions within the tissues or may escape from the tissues.

In this interaction energy of incident photon is higher than outer shell electron but this interaction is not dependent on the atomic number (Z) of tissues. Therefore, it provides very little diagnostic information as it cannot differentiate between atomic number of different tissues. High energy scattered photons produce forward scatter. Low energy scattered produce back scatter and can degrade image which can be prevented by using grids.

% of interaction: 57.

Effect on image: These scatterings darken the image, carrying no useful information.

Compton scattering depends on number of free electrons irrespective of type of tissues. So the structure with high number of electrons will have more Compton interactions, e.g. bone.

Dosimetry

Determining the quantity of radiation exposure or dose delivered to human body is called dosimetry. Monitoring and measuring radiation dose is necessary for personnel. There are various sources of ionizing radiations including dental operatory (dental X-ray). This effect on body can be measured by knowing a few important terms and formulae.

The important terms in dosimetry are:
- Dose
- Exposure
- Kerma
- Absorbed dose
- Equivalent dose
- Effective dose
- Radioactivity

Dose: It is the amount of energy absorbed per unit of mass at a site of interest.

Exposure: It is the measure of radiation on the basis of its ability to produce ionization in air under standard conditions of temperature and pressure.

It is the amount of charge per mass of air measured as coulomb/kg (initially called Roentgen).

Kerma: It is kinetic energy released in matter which measures the kinetic energy transferred from photons to electrons, expressed in units of dose, i.e. Gray/Gy. Kerma values made in air are called air kerma. An exposure of 1R or 1 coulomb/kg results in a tissue kerma of about 0.01 Gy.

Absorbed dose: It is the measure of the amount of energy absorbed from the radiation beam per unit mass of tissue. It varies with type and energy of radiation and the matter absorbing it.

Equivalent dose: It is a measure which allows comparison of biologic effects of different types of radiation on different tissues. (For example, alpha particles penetrate only few millimeters in tissue and get absorbed, whereas X-ray penetrates more and lose some of their energy getting partially absorbed.)

This relative biologic effectiveness of different types of radiation is called the radiation weighing (WR) factor.

For X-rays, gamma rays and beta particles WR is 1

For alpha particles WR is 20.

Effective dose: It is used to denote the total effective dose received by a population, from a particular source of radiation. It is used to estimate the risk in humans, e.g. exposure of mandible can be used to calculate the equivalent whole body dose (effective dose of body). This allows comparing the risk from exposure to one part of body to the risk of other.

Radioactivity: The measurement of radioactivity (A) describes the decay rate of a sample of radioactive material (Table 25.1).

Monitoring and measuring of radiation dose is possible with the help of certain devices which are routinely practiced in dentistry. They are:

1. Film badges
2. Thermoluminescent dosimeters (TLD)
3. Ionization chamber.

▶ **1. Film Badge**

It is made of plastic frame containing different metal filters and a small radiographic film. This assembly reacts to radiation exposure. This badge can be hanged to clothes (usually at the level of reproductive organs) for 1–3 months before processing.

These badges are personal monitoring devices.

Advantages

1. It can measure the type of radiation encountered.
2. It provides a permanent record of dose received.
3. It is simple, sturdy and inexpensive to use.

Disadvantages

1. It cannot provide immediate indication of exposure.
2. Badges may undergo filter loss due to which there can be error in measuring radiation dose.
3. Processing of badges itself can give errors in reading the dose.

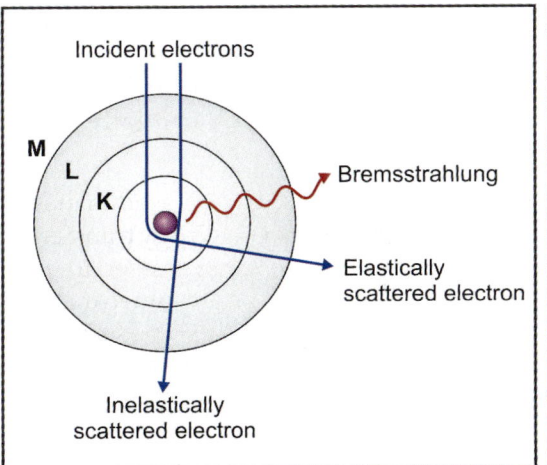

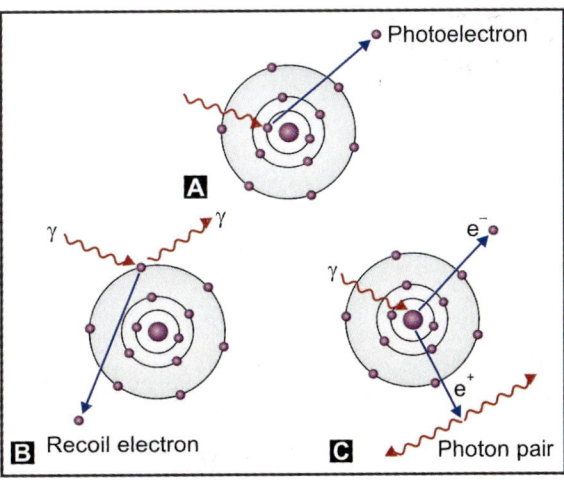

Fig. 25.7: Various interactions of photoelectron in an atom

▶ 2. Thermoluminescent Dosimeters (TLD)

TLDs are used as personal monitoring devices to measure whole body or the extremities dose received. These dose meters contain lithium fluoride (LiF), which absorbs radiation and releases the energy in the form of light when heated (Fig. 25.8).

The intensity of the emitted light is proportional to the radiation energy absorbed. These monitors consist of plastic case (with lithium fluoride plate inside) and worn similarly as film badge for 1–3 months.

Advantages

1. Measurements are used easily by automated devices.
2. Readings are rapidly obtained.
3. Suitable for a wide variety of dose measurements.
4. The lithium fluoride is re-usable.

Disadvantages

1. It cannot provide permanent record as read-out is destructive.
2. It provides limited information on the type and energy of the radiation.
3. It is comparatively expensive.
4. Badges need to be sent to specific centers (Bhabha) to obtain readings.

▶ 3. Ionization Chambers

They are used for personal monitoring also called thimble chambers. They are used by physicists usually to measure radiation

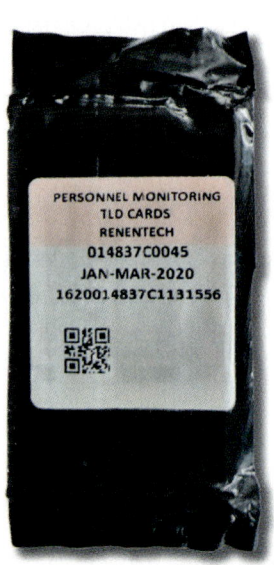
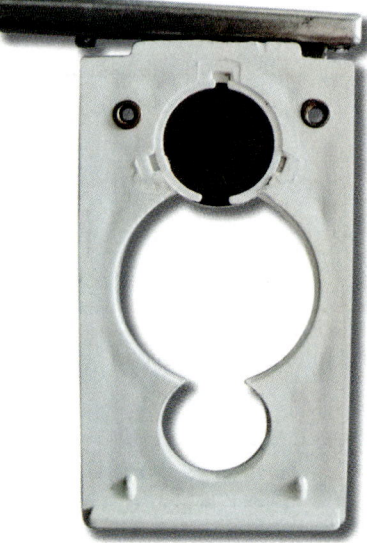
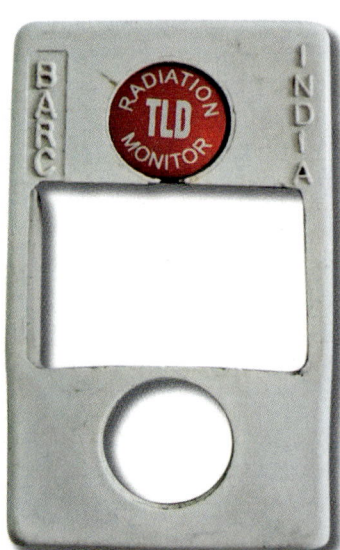

Fig. 25.8: TLD badge

TABLE 25.1: Summary of radiation quantities and units			
Quantity	SI unit	Traditional unit	Conversion
Exposure	Coulomb/kilogram (C/kg)	Roentgen (R)	1 C/kg = 3876 R
Absorbed dose	Gray (Gy)	Rad	1 Gy = 100 rad
Equivalent dose	Sievert (Sv)	Rem	1 Sv = 100 rem
Effective dose	Sievert (Sv)	--	--
Radioactivity	Becquerel (Bq)	Curie (Ci)	1 Bq = 2.7 × 10^{11} Ci

exposure. In these closed chambers, radiation leads to ionization of the air molecules which result in a measurable discharge that is used for direct readings (of exposure).

1. Draw a well-labeled diagram of X-ray tube and mention functions of its parts.
2. Write a note on types of radiation.
3. Write a note on factors controlling X-ray beam.
4. Write a note on inverse square law.
5. Write a note on types of scattering.
6. Write a note on dosimetry.

BIBLIOGRAPHY

1. Whaites E. Essentials of Dental Radiography and Radiology, 4th edition. Spain: Churchill Livingstone Elsevier; 2007.
2. White S., Pharoah Medicine Oral Radiology. Principles and Interpretation, 6th edition. Elsevier Inc; 2011.
3. White S., Pharoah Medicine Oral Radiology. Principles and Interpretation. 5th edition. Mushy; 2004.
4. Goaz P. wwtes. Oral Radiology Principles and Interpretation. 2nd edition: BI Publishers; 1998.
5. Whaites E. Essentials of Dental Radiography and Radiology 2nd edition. Churchill Livingstone; 1997.
6. Langland O, Langlais R, Preece J. Principles of Dental imaging. 2nd edition. Lippincott Williams and Wilkins; 2002.
7. Langland O, Langlais R. Principles of Dental Imaging 1st edition. Lippincott Williams and Wilkins; 1997.
8. Wood N, Goaz P. Differential diagnosis of Oral and maxillofacial lesions. 5th edition: Elsevier; 2007.
9. Karjodkar F. Textbook of Dental and maxillofacial Radiology. 2nd edition: Jaypee Brothers Medical Publishers; 2009.

Radiation Biology

The subject of radiation biology deals with the effects of ionizing radiation on living systems. During the passage through living matter, radiation loses energy by interaction with atoms and molecules of the matter, thereby causing ionization and excitation. The ultimate effect is the alteration of the living cells resulting in modification of biologic molecules within seconds to hours. The molecular changes may lead to alterations in cells and organisms that persist for hours, decades and possibly even generations. These changes may result in injury or death. The initial interaction between ionizing radiation and matter occurs at the level of the electron within the first 10^{-13} second after exposure.

Direct or Target Action Theory

It is the effect which occurs when the energy of a photon or secondary electron ionizes biological macromolecules. This states that the changes occur due to:

a. Absorption of energy by biological molecules.
b. Transfer of energy between unstable intermediate molecules.
c. Formation of stable damaged molecules by disassociation or cross-linking.

The resultant molecules differ structurally from the original molecule, hence the consequence is a biological change in the irradiated organism.

In direct effects, biologic molecules (RH, where R is the molecule and H is a hydrogen atom) absorb energy from ionizing radiation and form unstable free radicals which occur in less than 10^{-10} second after interaction with a photon.

Free radicals are extremely reactive and have very short life, quickly reforming into stable configurations. They play a dominant role in producing molecular changes in biologic molecules.

Free radical production:
$$RH + X\text{-radiation } R^* + H^+ + e^-$$
$$\text{Dissociation: } R^* \longrightarrow X + Y^*$$
$$\text{Cross-linking: } R^* + S^* \longrightarrow RS$$

The altered biologic molecules differ structurally and functionally from the original molecules, the consequence is a biologic change in the irradiated organism. Approximately, one-third of the biologic effects of X-ray exposure results from direct effects. Direct effects are the most common outcome for particulate radiation such as neutrons and particles.

Specific targets within the cell, probably the DNA or RNA in the nucleus, take a direct hit from incoming X-ray photon, or high energy electron, which breaks the relatively weak bonds between the nucleic acids. It depends on factors like:

a. The type and number of nucleic acid bonds those are broken.
b. The intensity and type of radiation.
c. The time between exposures.
d. The ability of the cell to repair the damage.

The subsequent effect includes

× Abnormal replication.
× Cell death.
× Only temporary changes—the DNA being repaired successfully before further cell division.
× If the radiation affects somatic cells, the effect on the DNA could result in radiation-induced malignancy.
× If the damage is to reproductive stem cells, radiation-induced congenital abnormalities can be noticed.

Radiolysis of Water

Water is the predominant molecule in biologic systems (about 70% by weight), it frequently participates in the interactions between X-ray photons and biologic molecules. A complex series of chemical changes occurs in water after exposure to ionizing radiation. Collectively these reactions result in the radiolysis of water.

$$\text{Photon} + H_2O \longrightarrow H^* + OH^*$$

Although the radiolysis of water is complex, on balance water is largely converted to hydrogen and hydroxyl free radicals. When dissolved oxygen is present in irradiated water, hydroperoxyl free radicals may also be formed.

$$H^* + O_2 \longrightarrow HO_2$$

Hydroperoxyl free radicals contribute to the formation of hydrogen peroxide in tissues:

$$HO_2 + H^* \longrightarrow H_2O_2$$

$$HO_2^* + HO_2^* \longrightarrow O_2 + H_2O_2$$

Both peroxyl radicals and hydrogen peroxide are oxidizing agents and primary toxins produced in the tissues by ionizing radiation (Fig. 26.1).

Indirect Effects

Water is a predominant molecule of the biological system. When the photon is absorbed by the water molecule, it is ionized and releases free radicals which further interact and produce changes in the biologic molecule, this effect is termed 'indirect'. The interaction of hydrogen and hydroxyl free radicals with organic molecules results in the formation of organic free radicals. About two-thirds of radiation-induced biologic damage result from indirect effects. Such reactions may involve the removal of hydrogen:

$$RH + OH^* \longrightarrow R^* + H_2O$$

$$RH + H^* \longrightarrow R^* + H$$

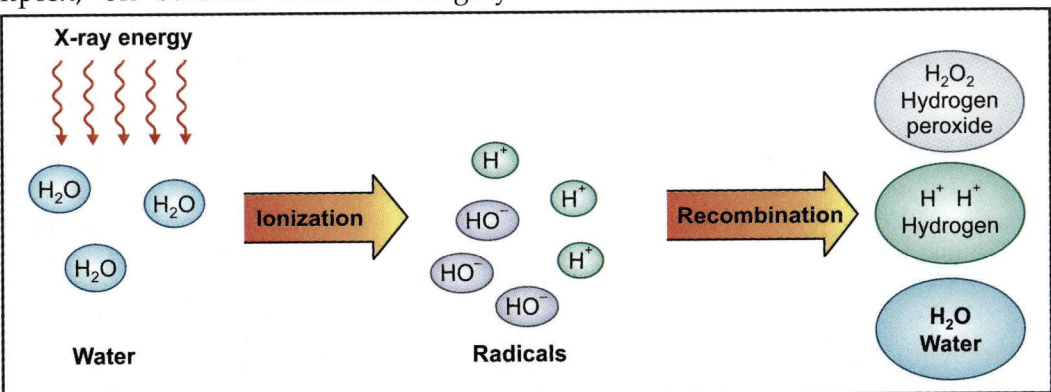

Fig. 26.1: Radiolysis of water and formation of free radicals when H_2O is irradiated, and formation of hydrogen peroxide molecule

Organic free radicals are unstable and transform into stable, altered molecules. They have different chemical and biologic properties from the original molecules. Both direct and indirect effects are completed within 10^{-5} second.

Effect on biological molecules: The changes in deoxyribonucleic acid include damage to a cell's deoxyribonucleic acid (DNA); it is the primary cause of radiation-induced cell death, heritable (genetic) mutations, cancer formation (carcinogenesis). Radiation-induced change protein, lipids, and carbohydrates after low or moderate doses (up to 10 Gy) of radiation do not contribute to radiation effects (Fig. 26.2).

Radiation produces a number of different types of alteration DNA, including the following:

1. Breakage of one or both DNA strands
2. Cross-linking of DNA strands within the helix to other DNA strands or to proteins
3. Change or loss of a base
4. Disruption of hydrogen bonds between DNA strands
5. Proteins: Denaturation, inter and intramolecular cross-linking
6. Enzymes get inactivated leading to failure in conversion of substrate to product.
7. Breakage of DNA strands.
8. Cross-linking of DNA strands.

Deterministic effect: It is an effect in which the severity of the response is proportional to the dose. For example, oral changes after radiation therapy. These effects usually cause cell killing, and may occur in all people when the dose is large enough.

Effect on intracellular structures: The effects of radiation on intracellular structures result from radiation-induced changes in their

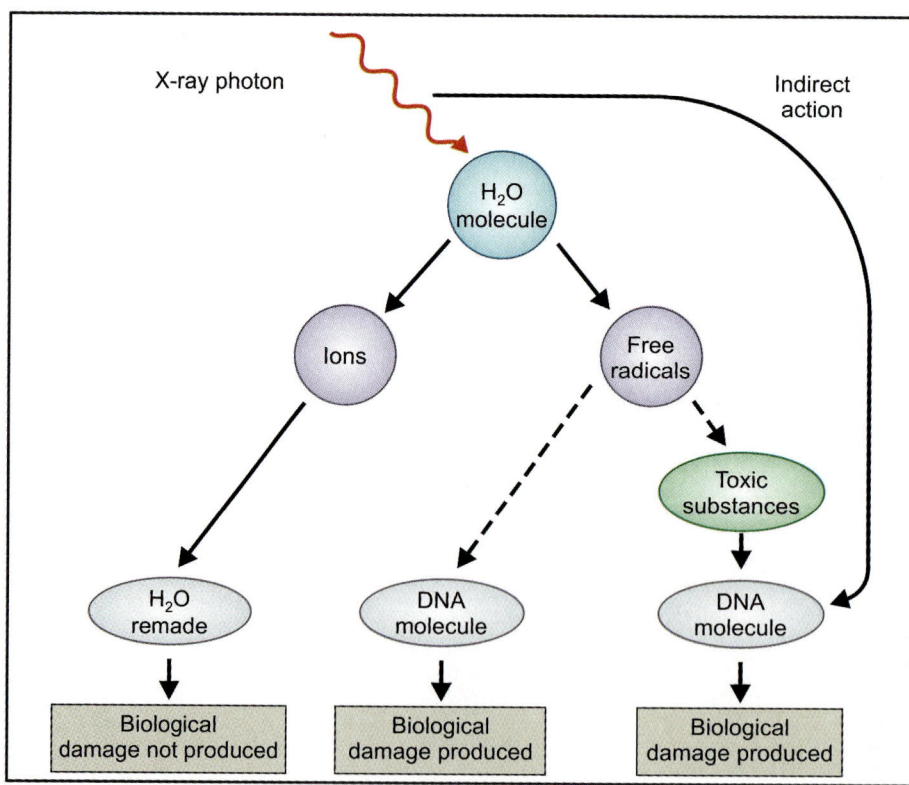

Fig. 26.2: Indirect effects: The action of DNA by free radicals or toxic products of free radicals is called indirect action

macromolecules. These changes manifest initially as structural and functional changes in cellular organelles. The changes may cause cell death.

Nucleus: A wide variety of radio-biologic data indicates that the nucleus is more radiosensitive than cytoplasm, especially in dividing cells. The sensitive site in the nucleus is the DNA within chromosomes.

Chromosome aberrations: Chromosomes serve as useful markers for radiation injury. Chromosome aberrations are observed in irradiated cells at the time of mitosis, when the DNA condenses to form chromosomes. The type of damage that may be observed depends on the stage of the cell in the cell cycle at the time of irradiation, completion of a subsequent mitosis. Chromosome aberrations have been detected in peripheral blood lymphocytes of patients exposed to medical diagnostic procedures. The frequency of aberrations is generally proportional to the radiation dose received (Fig. 26.3).

Effect on cell replication: Radiation is especially damaging to rapidly dividing cell systems, such as skin and intestinal mucosa and hematopoietic tissues. Irradiation of such cell populations will cause a reduction in size of the irradiated tissue as a result of mitotic delay (inhibition of progression of the cells through the cell cycle) and cell death.

The three mechanisms of reproductive death are DNA damage, bystander effect, and apoptosis.

Deoxyribonucleic acid damage: Cell death is caused by damage to DNA, which in turn causes chromosome aberrations. It is the rate of cell replication in various tissues, and thus the rate of reproductive death, that accounts for the radiosensitivity of tissues.

Bystander effect: Cells that are damaged by radiation release into their immediate environment molecules that kill nearby cells. This bystander effect has been demonstrated for both particles and X-rays and causes chromosome aberrations, cell killing, gene mutations and carcinogenesis.

Apoptosis: Apoptosis, also known as programmed cell death, occurs during normal embryogenesis. Apoptosis is particularly common in hemopoietic and lymphoid tissues.

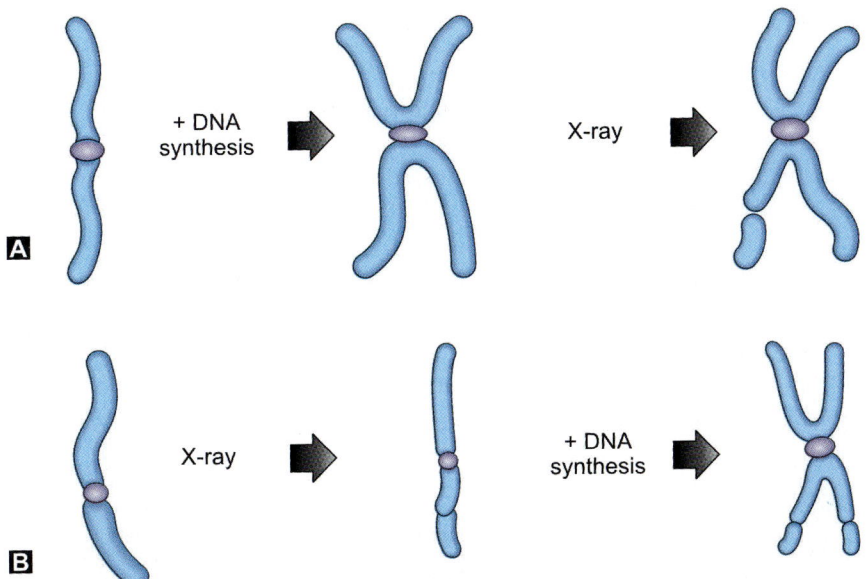

Fig. 26.3: A. After DNA synthesis the irradiated cell results in a single-arm (chromated) aberration, **B.** Before DNA synthesis, the irradiated cell results in a double-arm (chromosome) aberration

Cell recovery: Cell recovery from DNA damage and the bystander effect involves enzymatic repair of single-strand breaks of DNA. Because of this repair, a higher total dose is required to achieve a given degree of cell killing when multiple fractions are used (e.g. in radiation therapy).

Stochastic effect: It is that effect for which the probability of the occurrence of a change, rather than its severity is dose dependent. For example, radiation-induced cancer, greater exposure of a person or population to radiation increases the probability of the cancer but not its severity.

A comparison of deterministic and stochastic effects is mentioned in Table 26.1.

Acute exposure: It occurs when a large dose of radiation is absorbed in a short period of time, e.g. nuclear accident. The most important are the radiation-induced cancers. It is believed that radiation causes cancer by modifying the DNA. The most commonly found cancers are:

a. Thyroid cancer
b. Oesophageal cancer
c. Brain and nervous system cancers
d. Salivary gland cancers
e. Cancer of other organs, like skin, paranasal sinuses and bone marrow
f. Leukaemia

Other late somatic changes: Growth and development is retarded, mental retardation, cataract and genetic damage.

Short-term effects: These effects of radiation on a tissue are determined primarily by the sensitivity of its parenchymal cells. If continuously proliferating cells are irradiated, e.g. bone marrow, oral mucous membrane, the effect of irradiation becomes apparent (highly radiosensitive) (Table 26.2). Tissues composed of cells that rarely or never divide (low radio-sensitivity) over a short term.

Casarett has divided mammalian cells into five categories of radiosensitivity on the basis of histologic observations of early cell death.

× **Vegetative intermitotic cells:** These are most radiosensitive.
× **Differentiating intermitotic cells:** These are less radiosensitive.
× **Multipotential connective tissue cells:** These have intermediate radiosensitivity.
× **Reverting postmitotic cells:** These are radio-resistant.

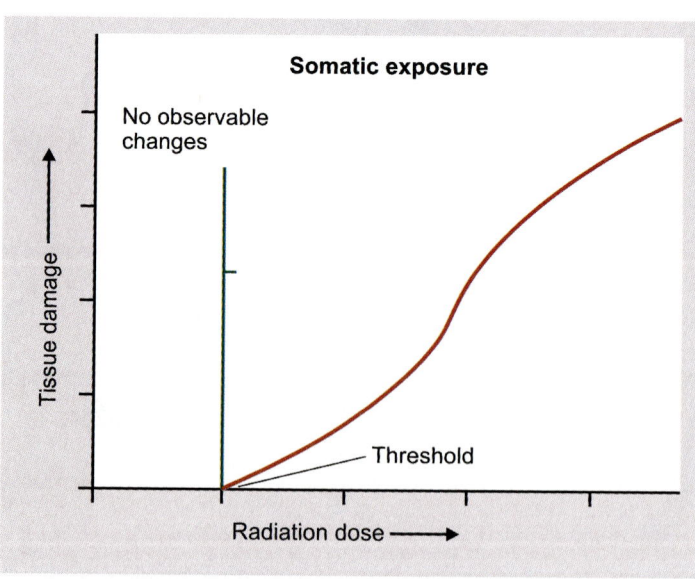

Fig. 26.4: Threshold dose: Dose responsive curve—illustrating curved line type of biological response

TABLE 26.1: Comparison of deterministic and stochastic effects of radiation	
Deterministic effects	*Stochastic effects*
For example: Radiation-induced mucositis resulting from radiation therapy to oral cavity Radiation-induced cataract	For example: Radiation-induced cancer Heritable effects: Gene mutations
Caused by killing of many cells	Sublethal damage to DNA
Threshold plays a key role for sufficient cell killing and clinical response	Threshold does not play role—even one photon could cause a change in DNA that leads to a cancer or heritable effect
The severity of clinical effects is proportional to the dose. Greater the dose, greater the effect	The severity of clinical effects is independent of dose. All-or-none response; an individual either has effect or does not
All individuals show effect when dose is above threshold	Frequency of effect is proportional to dose. The greater the dose, the greater the chance of having the effect

TABLE 26.2: Radiosensitivity of various organs in the body		
High	*Intermediate*	*Low*
Lymphoid organs	Fine vasculature	
Bone marrow	Growing cartilage	Optic lens
Testes	Growing bone	Muscle
Intestines	Salivary glands	
Mucous membranes	Lungs Kidney Liver	

- Oxygenation
- Chemical protectors
- Stage of development of the tissue
- Tissue threshold
- Part of the body exposed
- Species and individuals

Long-term effects: The long-term deterministic effects of radiation on tissues and organs depend primarily on the extent of damage to the fine vasculature. The relative radiosensitivity of capillaries and connective tissue is intermediate (Fig. 26.5).

Irradiation of capillaries causes swelling, degeneration and necrosis

Increases capillary permeability and progressive fibrosis

Leading to deposition of fibrous scar tissue and premature narrowing of vascular lumens

Impairs transport of oxygen, nutrients and waste products resulting in cell death

Loss of cell function with reduced resistance of the irradiated tissue causing infection and trauma

- **Fixed postmitotic cells:** These are most radio-resistant.

Factors Effecting the Biological Tissues

- Nature of tissue irradiated
- Area irradiated
- Rate of dose
- Fractionization
- Latent period: Period between the time of irradiation and the appearance of the effect.
- Recovery power of the tissue
- Type of cell
- Type of irradiation

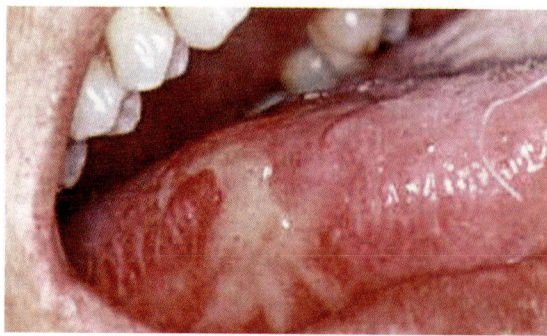

Fig. 26.5: Radiation mucositis representing pseudomembranous slough on lateral border of tongue (right)

Modifying factors: The response of cells, tissues, and organs to irradiation depends on exposure conditions and the cell environment.

1. Nature and area of tissue irradiated
2. Fractionation
3. Type of cell receiving radiation
4. Oxygenation
5. Stage of development of tissue
6. Part of body exposed with radiation

Dose: The severity of deterministic damage seen in irradiated tissues and organs depends on the amount of radiation received. If clinical threshold dose exists below the level, no adverse effects are seen. In all individuals receiving doses above the threshold level, the amount of damage is proportional to the dose. Radiotherapy is frequently used as an adjuvant form of treatment in the management of head and neck cancers.

Dose rate: The term dose rate indicates the rate of exposure. Dose of 5 Gy may be given at a high dose rate (5 Gy/min) or a low dose rate (5 mGy/min). Exposure of biologic systems to a high dose rate causes more damage than exposure to the same total dose given at a lower dose rate.

Oxygen: The radio resistance of many biologic systems increases by a factor of 2 or 3, when the exposure is made with reduced oxygen (hypoxia). Greater cell damage results in the presence of oxygen, which in turn results in increased amounts of hydrogen peroxide and hydroperoxyl free radicals. This is important clinically because hyperbaric oxygen therapy may be used during radiation therapy of tumors having hypoxic cells.

Linear energy transfer: The dose required to produce a certain biologic effect is reduced as the linear energy transfer (LET), higher LET radiations (e.g. α particles) are more efficient in damaging biologic systems because high ionization density is more than X-rays to induce double-strand breakage in DNA. Low LET radiations such as X-rays deposit their energy more sparsely, thus more likely cause single strand breakage and less biologic damage.

Radiotherapy in Oral Cavity

Oral cavity is irradiated during radiation therapy for oral malignant tumors, advanced or deeply invasive usually squamous cell carcinomas

⬇

Fractionation of the total X-ray dose into multiple small doses provides greater tumor destruction than is possible with large single dose

⬇

Fractionation characteristically allows increased cellular repair of normal tissues, thereby inherently greater capacity for recovery than tumor cells. It increases the mean oxygen tension in an irradiated tumor, rendering the tumor cells more radiosensitive

⬇

Thereby, killing rapidly dividing tumor cells and shrinking the tumor mass after the first few fractions, reducing the distance that oxygen must diffuse from the fine vasculature through the tumor to reach the remaining viable tumor cells

Radiocurability: Is defined as the ability of radiations to reduce the number of malignant cells below a critical level such that no further clinical manifestation of their presence will occur during the remaining lifetime of the host.

Radiosensitivity: It is defined as the ability of radiations to biologically change (i.e. cell killing or a destruction of reproduction integrity) cells comprising a tumor or other tissue.

Radioresponsiveness: This refers to the time required for any change to occur and can be measured in terms of the rate at which the clinical manifestations of radiation-induced biologic change occur.

Effects of radiation on oral tissues: The complications of radiotherapy in due course are the best example for deterministic effects. Typically 2 Gy is delivered daily, bilaterally through 8 × 10 cm fields over the oropharynx, for weekly exposure of 10 Gy. This continues typically for 6 to 7 weeks until a total of 64 to 70 Gy is delivered. Cobalt is often the source of radiation; at times small implants containing radon or iodine-125 are placed directly in a tumor mass. Such implants deliver a high dose of radiation to a relatively small volume of tissue in a short time. Recently, a three-dimensional technique called intensity modulated radiotherapy (IMRT) has been used to control the dose distribution with high accuracy.

Oral Mucous Membrane

The basal layer of oral mucosa is composed of rapidly dividing radiosensitive stem cells

In the second week of therapy, as some of these cells die, the mucous membranes begin to show areas of redness and inflammation (mucositis)

As the therapy continues, the irradiated mucous membrane separates from the underlying connective tissue, with the formation of a white to yellow pseudomembrane (the desquamated epithelial layer)

At the end of therapy, the mucositis severe, discomfort is at a maximum, and food intake is difficult. Good oral hygiene minimizes infection

After irradiation is completed, the mucosa begins to heal which completes by 2 months

Later the mucous membrane tends to become atrophic, thin, and relatively avascular

This long-term atrophy results from progressive obliteration of the fine vasculature and fibrosis of the underlying connective tissue. These may cause oral ulcerations of the compromised tissue.

Treatment: Topical anesthetics may be required at mealtimes. Secondary yeast infection by *Candida albicans* is a common complication and may require treatment with antifungals.

Taste Buds

Doses in the therapeutic range cause degeneration of the normal histologic architecture of taste buds, as they are sensitive to radiation

Loss of taste acuity during the second or third week of radiotherapy

Bitter and acid flavors are affected when the posterior two-thirds of the tongue are irradiated and salt and sweet when the anterior one-third of the tongue is irradiated

Taste acuity decreases by factor of 1000 to 10,000 during radiotherapy. Alterations in the saliva partly accounts for reduction, hence proceeding to a state of virtual insensitivity

Taste loss is reversible and recovery takes 60 to120 days

Salivary Glands

Major salivary glands are at times unavoidably exposed to 20 to 30 Gy during radiotherapy for cancer in the oral cavity or oropharynx

Hyposalivation is usually seen in the first few weeks after initiation of radiotherapy

The mouth becomes dry xerostomia and tender, and swallowing is difficult and painful

⬇

The serous cells are more radiosensitive than mucous cells; the residual saliva is more viscous than usual. pH value 5.5

⬇

Dryness of the mouth usually subsides in 6 to 12 months because of compensatory hypertrophy of residual salivary gland tissue

⬇

Few months after irradiation, the inflammatory response becomes more chronic, and the glands demonstrate progressive fibrosis, adiposis, loss of fine vasculature, and concomitant parenchymal degeneration, thus accounting for the xerostomia

Treatment: Various saliva substitutes are available to help restore function.

Teeth: Children receiving radiation therapy to the jaws may show defects in the permanent dentition such as retarded root development, dwarfed teeth, or failure to form one or more teeth.

Adult teeth are resistant to the direct effects of radiation exposure. Pulpal tissue may exhibit fibroatrophy after irradiation. Radiation has no discernible effect on the crystalline structure of enamel, dentin or cementum and radiation does not increase their solubility.

Radiation Caries

Radiation caries is a rampant form of dental decay that occurs in individuals who receive radiotherapy that includes exposure of the salivary glands

⬇

After radiotherapy, the major salivary glands, the microflora undergo a pronounced change, rendering them acidogenic in the saliva and plaque. Patients receiving radiation therapy have increase in *Streptococcus mutans*, *Lactobacillus*, and *Candida*

⬇

Caries results from changes in the salivary glands and saliva, including reduced flow, decreased pH, reduced buffering capacity, increased viscosity, and altered flora

⬇

Finally, because of the reduced or absent cleansing action of normal saliva, debris accumulates quickly. Irradiation of the teeth by itself does not influence the course of radiation caries

⬇

Clinically, three types of radiation caries exist. The most common is widespread superficial lesions attacking buccal, occlusal, incisal, and palatal surfaces. Another type involves primarily the cementum and dentin in the cervical region. These lesions may progress around the teeth circumferentially and result in loss of the crown. A final type appears as a dark pigmentation of the entire crown

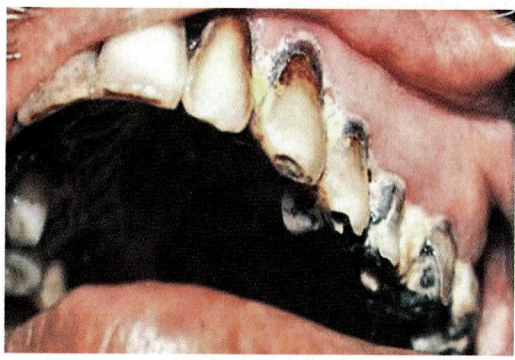

Fig. 26.6: Radiation caries—representing type I and II carious lesions on the cervical, buccal and occlusal aspects of the teeth

Treatment: The best method of reducing radiation caries is daily application of a viscous topical 1% neutral sodium fluoride gel in custom-made applicator trays for 5 min. Use of topical fluoride causes a 6-month delay in the irradiation-induced elevation of *S. mutans*.

Avoidance of dietary sucrose, in addition to the use of a topical fluoride, further reduces the concentrations of *S. mutans* and *Lactobacillus*. The best result is achieved from a combination of restorative dental procedures, excellent oral hygiene, a diet restricted in cariogenic foods, and topical applications of sodium fluoride.

Bone

Treatment of cancers in the oral region includes irradiation of the mandible or maxilla. The primary damage to mature bone results from radiation-induced damage to the vasculature of the periosteum and cortical bone

⬇

Radiation also acts by destroying osteoblasts. Subsequent to irradiation, normal marrow may be replaced with fatty marrow and fibrous connective tissue

⬇

The marrow tissue becomes hypovascular, hypoxic, and hypocellular

⬇

The endosteum becomes atrophic, showing lack of osteoblastic and osteoclastic activity, and some lacunae of the compact bone are empty, indicating necrosis

⬇

The degree of mineralization may be reduced, leading to brittleness, or little altered from normal bone. When these changes are so severe that bone death results and the bone is exposed, the condition is termed osteoradionecrosis

⬇

The decreased vascularity of the mandible is easily infected by microorganisms. This bone infection may result from radiation-induced breakdown of the oral mucous membrane, by mechanical damage to the weakened oral mucous membrane such as denture sore or tooth extraction, through a periodontal lesion, or from radiation caries. This infection may cause a nonhealing wound in irradiated bone that is difficult to treat

Treatment: Initiating preventive techniques of good oral hygiene and daily topical fluoride should be given. The risk for osteoradionecrosis and infection can be minimized by removing all teeth. The dentist

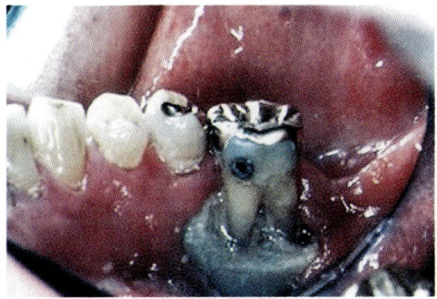

Fig. 26.7: Osteoradionecrosis owing to radiation

should use atraumatic surgical technique to avoid elevating the periosteum and provide antibiotic coverage. Taking radiographs during the first 6 months should be avoided after completion of radiotherapy, to allow time for the mucous membrane to heal.

Musculature: Radiation may cause inflammation and fibrosis resulting in contracture and trismus in the muscles of mastication. Restriction in mouth opening usually starts about 2 months after radiotherapy is completed and progresses thereafter. An exercise program helps in increasing opening distance (Table 26.3).

TABLE 26.3:	Deterministic effects of whole-body irradiation
Dose (Gy)	Effects of radiation on different body systems
1 to 2	Prodromal symptoms
2 to 4	Mild hematopoietic symptoms
4 to 7	Severe hematopoietic symptoms
7 to 15	Gastrointestinal symptoms
50	Cardiovascular and central nervous system symptoms

ACUTE RADIATION SYNDROME

The acute radiation syndrome is a collection of signs and symptoms occur due to whole-body exposure to radiation.

Management of acute radiation syndrome: Antibiotics are indicated when the granulocyte count falls. Fluid and electrolyte replacement is used as necessary. Whole blood transfusions are used to treat anemia, and platelets may be administered to arrest thrombocytopenia.

Prodromal period: Within the first minutes to hours after exposure to whole-body irradiation of about 1.5 Gy, symptoms of anorexia, nausea, vomiting, diarrhea, weakness, and fatigue are noticed. These early symptoms constitute the prodromal period of the acute radiation syndrome. The higher the dose, the more rapid the onset and the greater the severity of symptoms.

Latent period: After the prodromal reaction, a latent period where no signs or symptoms of radiation sickness occur. The extent of the latent period is dose related. It extends from hours or days after supralethal exposures (greater than 5 Gy) to a few weeks after exposure of about 2 Gy.

Hematopoietic syndrome: Whole-body exposures of 2 to 7 Gy cause injury to the hematopoietic stem cells of the bone marrow and spleen. The high mitotic activity of these cells makes bone marrow a highly radiosensitive tissue. A rapid fall in the numbers of circulating granulocytes, platelets, and finally erythrocytes is noticed. The clinical signs of the hematopoietic syndrome include infection from lymphopenia and granulocytopenia, hemorrhage from loss of platelets, and anemia from erythrocyte depletion (Fig. 26.8).

Gastrointestinal syndrome: The gastrointestinal syndrome is caused by whole-body exposures in the range of 7 to 15 Gy. The rapidly proliferating basal epithelial cells of the intestinal villi lead to rapid loss of the epithelial layer of the intestinal mucosa. Because of the denuded mucosal surface, there is loss of plasma and electrolytes, loss of efficient intestinal absorption, and ulceration of the mucosal lining with hemorrhaging into the intestines. These changes are responsible for the diarrhea, dehydration, and loss of weight. The combined effects of damage to these hematopoietic and gastrointestinal stem cell systems cause death within 2 weeks from fluid and electrolyte loss, infection, and nutritional impairment.

Cardiovascular and central nervous system syndrome: Exposures in excess of 50 Gy usually cause death in 1 to 2 days. Collapse of the circulatory system with a precipitous fall in blood pressure in the hours preceding death.

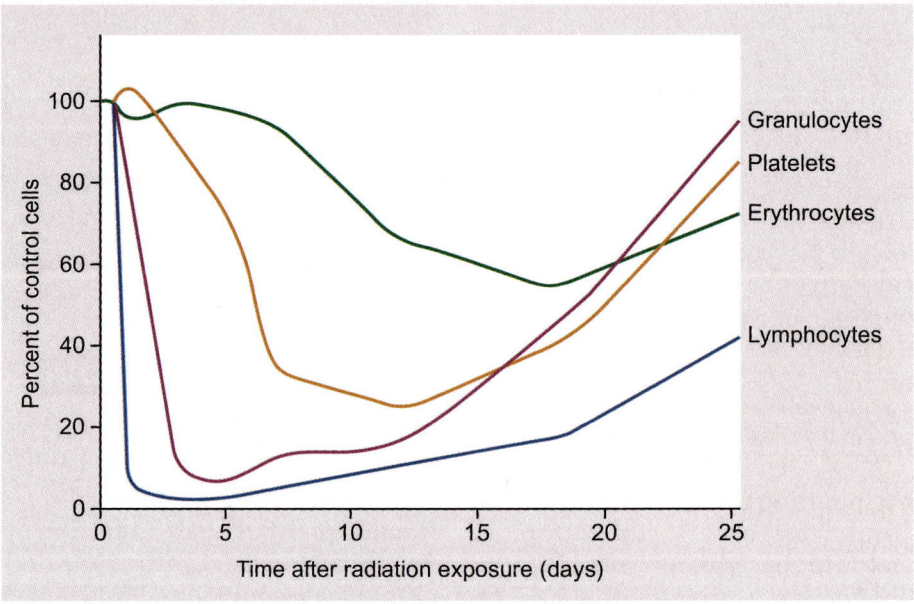

Fig. 26.8: Depletion of granulocytes, platelets, and lymphocytes due to whole body radiation

Chronic exposure: This occurs when small amounts of radiations are absorbed repeatedly over a long period of time.

Somatic damage: These are lifespan injuries. The most important are the radiation-induced cancers. The exact mechanism of induction of cancer by ionizing radiation is not well known but school of thought is radiation causes cancer by modifying the DNA. The most commonly found cancers are thyroid cancer, oesophageal cancer, brain and nervous system cancers, cancer of other organs, like skin, paranasal sinuses and bone marrow also shows excess neoplasia after exposure.

Other late somatic changes:
a. Growth and development
b. Mental retardation
c. Cataract
d. Genetic damage

RADIATION EFFECTS ON EMBRYOS AND FETUSES

The effects of radiation on human embryos and fetuses in women exposed to diagnostic or therapeutic radiation during pregnancy and those exposed to radiation from the atomic bombs dropped at Hiroshima and Nagasaki. Embryos and fetuses are considerably more radiosensitive than adults because most embryonic cells are relatively undifferentiated and rapidly mitotic.

Late Effects

A number of late deterministic effects have been found in the survivors of the atomic bombing of Hiroshima and Nagasaki.

Growth and development: Children exposed in the bombings showed impairment of growth and development. They have reduced height, weight, and skeletal development. The younger the individual at the time of exposure, the more pronounced the effects.

Cataracts: The threshold for induction of cataracts opacities in the lens of the eye ranges from about 0.6 Gy, when the dose is received in a single exposure to more than 5 Gy, when the dose is received in multiple exposures over a period of weeks.

Short lifespan: The survivors of the atomic bombings show a clear decrease in median life expectancy with increasing radiation dose. Survivors demonstrate increased frequency of heart disease, stroke, and diseases of the digestive, respiratory, and hematopoietic systems.

Stochastic effects: Stochastic effects result from sublethal changes in the DNA of individual cells. The most important consequence of such damage is carcinogenesis.

Carcinogenesis

Radiation causes cancer by modifying DNA. The mechanism is radiation-induced gene mutation, where premalignant cells convert into malignant ones, conversion of proto-oncogenes to oncogenes. Gene mutations may also involve a loss of function in the case of tumor suppressor genes.

Leukemia: The incidence of leukemia rises after exposure of the bone marrow to radiation. Atomic bomb survivors and patients irradiated for ankylosing spondylitis show a wave of leukemias after exposure around 7 years. For individuals exposed under age 30 years, the risk for development of leukemia ceases. They appear sooner than solid cancers because of higher rate of cell division and differentiation of hematopoietic stem cells compared with the other tissues.

Thyroid cancer: The incidence of thyroid carcinomas (arising from the follicular epithelium) increases in humans after exposure. Susceptibility to radiation-induced thyroid cancer is greater early in childhood than at any time later in life, and children are more susceptible than adults.

The fallout from the accident at the Chernobyl nuclear power plant, primarily iodine-131, is thought to have caused about 4000 cases of thyroid cancer in children and 15 fatalities.

Esophageal cancer: Data pertaining to esophageal cancer are relatively sparse. Excess cancers are found in the Japanese atomic bomb survivors and in patients treated with X-radiation for ankylosing spondylitis.

Brain and nervous system cancers: Patients exposed to diagnostic X-ray examinations *in utero* and to therapeutic doses in childhood or as adults (average midbrain dose of about 1 Gy) show excess numbers of malignant and benign brain tumors.

Salivary gland cancers: The incidence of salivary gland tumors is increased in patients treated with irradiation for diseases of the head and neck, in Japanese atomic bomb survivors, and in persons exposed to diagnostic radiation. Only individuals who received an estimated cumulative parotid dose of 0.5 Gy or more showed a significant correlation between dental radiography and salivary gland tumors.

HERITABLE EFFECTS

Heritable effects are changes seen in the offspring of irradiated individuals. They are the consequence of damage to the genetic material of reproductive cells leading to heritable changes.

Effects on humans: To date, no such radiation-related genetic damage has been demonstrated. No increase has occurred in adverse pregnancy outcome, leukemia or other cancers, or impairment of growth and development in the children of atomic bomb survivors. Similarly, studies of the children of patients who received radiotherapy show no detectable increase in the frequency of genetic diseases. These findings do not exclude the possibility that such damage occurs but do show that it must be at a very low frequency.

Doubling dose: One way to measure the risk from genetic exposure is by determining the doubling dose, which is the amount of radiation a population requires to produce in the next generation. In humans, the genetic doubling dose is estimated to be approximately 1 sievert (Sv). For comparison, the background dose is about 0.003 Sv per year and the gonadal dose to males from a full-mouth radiographic examination is about 0.001 Sv or less. This exposure is contributed largely by the maxillary views, which are angled caudally. The dose to the ovaries is about 50 times less, in the range of 0.00002 Sv.

FREQUENTLY ASKED QUESTIONS

Write short note on:

1. Direct and indirect effects of radiation
2. Effects on radiotherapy on oral tissues.
3. Radiation caries
4. Radiation mucositis
5. Acute radiation syndrome.

BIBLIOGRAPHY

1. White and Pharoah's Oral Radiology Principles and interpretation South Asia, 2nd ed. Elsevier; 2009, Chapter no. 2, Part II.
2. Freny R Karjodkar, Textbook of Dental and Maxillofacial Radiology 2nd edition, Jaypee Brothers Medical Publishers (P) Ltd.
3. Eric Whaites and Nicholas Drage, Essentials of Dental Radiography and Radiology 5th ed. Churchill Elsevier.
4. Principles of Dental imaging Langland OE, Langlais RP, Preece JW. 2nd ed. Lippincott. Williams and Wilkins, USA.
5. Essentials of Dental Radiology. Pramod John 2nd ed., Jaypee Publishers, India.
6. Aya Fujishiro, Yasuo Miura, Masaki Iwasa, Sumie Fujii Noriko Sugino, Akira Andoh. Effects of acute exposure to low-dose radiation on the characteristics of human bone marrow mesenchymal stromal/stem cells. Inflammation and Regeneration. 2017; 37:19:1–12.
7. Igor Akushevich V, Galina Veremeyeva A, Georgy Dimov P, Svetlana V. Ukraintseva, Konstantin G Arbeev, Alexander Akleyev V. Modeling deterministic effects in hematopoietic system caused by chronic exposure to ionizing radiation in large human cohorts. Health Phys. 2010; 99(3): doi:10.1097/HP.0b013e3181c61dc1.

Radiation Safety and Protection

INTRODUCTION

Ionizing radiation is extensively used in dentistry in the form of IOPA and radiograph, OPG, extraoral radiographs and cone beam computed tomography. All are crucial diagnostic aids which help in diagnosis of disease and other abnormalities, and to monitor the disease progression. Use of ionizing radiation can present a major health risk by causing microscopic damage to living tissue and carries the risk of harm. Radiation protection is defined by the International atomic energy agency (IAEA) as "The protection of people from harmful effects of exposure to ionizing radiation, and the means for achieving this". Basic to radiation safety and protection is the decrease of expected dose and the measurement of dose uptake.

Although radiation doses in dental radiography are low, dentists should reduce patient's exposure to radiation. The low dose received by the patient from dental radiography leads to very small damage, but damage does occur. The risk of radiation in dental radiography is associated to the radiosensitive structures in the head and neck region. Sensitive structures include brain, bone marrow, thyroid glands and salivary glands. The primary aim of dental radiography is to get diagnostic information by keeping the exposure to the patient and dental staff at minimum level and also taking all safety measures necessary to provide reasonably enough protection to the health and safety of persons who are subjected to radiation exposure.

BASIC PRINCIPLE OF RADIATION SAFETY

The aim of radiation safety is to keep all radiation exposures as low as reasonably achievable (ALARA). This means that even if exposures are acceptable, if there is a reasonable way to decrease the exposure even further, those measures should be used. While there are lots of components to an efficient radiation safety program, three basic principles to reduce radiation exposure are:

i. **Justification:** No practice involving exposure to radiation shall be adopted unless its introduction to the exposed persons gives a positive net advantage.

ii. **Optimisation:** All exposures shall be kept as low as reasonably achievable (ALARA), taking economic and social factors into account. The fundamental of optimisation of radiation protection is to adjust the protection measures relating to the application of a radiation source in such a way that the net advantage is maximized.

iii. **Dose limitation:** The dose equivalent to persons shall not go beyond the limits recommended by the International Commission on Radiological Protection

(ICRP). The exposure of persons resulting from the combination of all the pertinent practice should be subject to dose limits.

There are three factors that control the amount, or dose of radiation received from a source. Radiation exposure can be managed by an amalgamation of these factors (Fig. 27.1):

1. **Time:** Reduce time duration working with sources of X-ray. It is the simplest way of protection from ionizing radiations to spend as little time as possible around radiation source. This is valid even when other protection methods are adopted. Reducing the exposure time by one half, reduces the dose received by one half.

2. **Distance:** Increase distance between the source of radiation and yourself. Doubling the distance between the person and the source helps to decrease the exposure to a quarter of its original value. Maintaining a safe distance is important when working near inadequately shielded sources of radiation.

3. **Shielding:** Shielding implies that certain materials (lead, concrete) will attenuate X-rays when they are placed between X-ray source and operator. Shielding includes X-ray tube, room and personnel shielding. The more mass that is placed between a source and a person, the less radiation the person will receive. When decreasing the time or rising the distance may not be possible, one can prefer shielding material to reduce the external radiation exposure.

METHODS OF RADIATION PROTECTION IN DENTISTRY FOR PATIENT

Proper Prescription of the Dental Radiograph (Patient Selection)

The dentist selects the patient who needs radiographs, determines which radiographs are needed, takes or supervises the exposure of the films and interprets the images. An important method for keeping patient exposure as low as reasonably achievable is the appropriate prescription of radiographs.

Collimation

Collimator is a metallic (lead) barrier with an opening in the center and serves to limit the size and shape of the useful X-ray beam reaching the patient. This will not only reduce dose, but may also improve image quality. This is generally done with a lead diaphragm (collimator) within the tube head or at the end of a lead lined cylinder. Decreasing the size of the X-ray beam to the minimum size needed to image the area of interest is an obvious means of reducing the dose to patients. Reducing the beam area on the skin surface also reduces the volume of the patient that is irradiated. Restriction of the X-ray beam size reduces the total area of exposure and helps avoid unnecessary exposure of sensitive areas.

The rectangular and circular collimation is used in dental radiography. The rectangular collimator is preferred over circular collimator, as it is more efficient in reduction of radiation dose to patient (Fig. 27.1A and B). The other advantage of rectangular collimator is that, it improves the diagnostic quality of the resultant image by lessening the amount of image degradation (fog) caused by scatter radiation.

Filtration

The primary X-ray beam is made up of X-rays of different energies. Only the X-rays with higher energies can go through the tissue of the individual's face and react with the image receptor and play an important role in image formation. Low energy X-rays that have no role on image creation and are absorbed by the tissues can lead to tissue damage.

Filtration is the process of absorption of the long wavelength (low energy) X-rays by a sheet of material called a filter. The reason for using filter is to remove the low energy (long wavelength) X-rays. A filter is an absorbing material (generally aluminum) placed in the path of the X-ray beam to

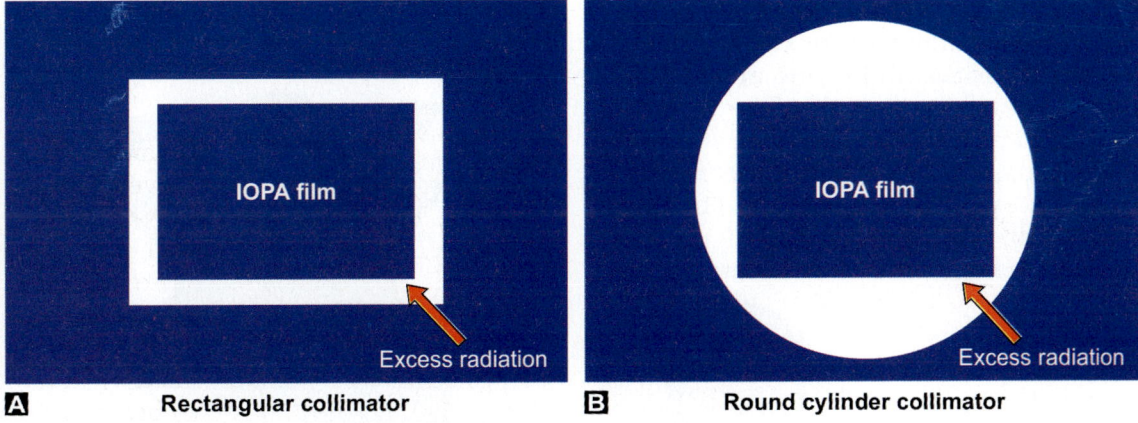

Fig. 27.1A and B: Collimators

remove a low energy (long wavelength) X-rays and decrease patient radiation dose (Fig. 27.2A and B)

A filter functions by absorbing more of the low-energy (long wavelength) X-rays before they reach the individual, while allowing more of the high-energy (short wavelength) X-rays to pass through. The quantity of filtration should be in harmony with the machine's operating range. Below 50 kVp, 0.3 to 0.5 mm thickness of aluminum, 50–70 kVp 1.2–1.5 mm thickness of aluminum and above 70 kVp 2.1–4.1 mm thickness of aluminum is used. The total filtration of an X-ray beam consists of inherent filtration and added filtration. Inherent filtration includes X-ray tube housing, oil and the glass envelope. The quantity of inherent filtration produced by most diagnostic X-ray tubes generally ranges from 0.5 to over 2.0 mm aluminum-equivalent. Added filtration includes sheets of metal (generally aluminum) placed in the path of the X-ray between the port and the patient (Fig. 27.2).

Source to Film Distance

X-ray source to film distance plays a significant role in limiting the radiation doses. Because of the divergence of the X-ray beam, increasing this distance between X-ray source and the film reduces the divergence

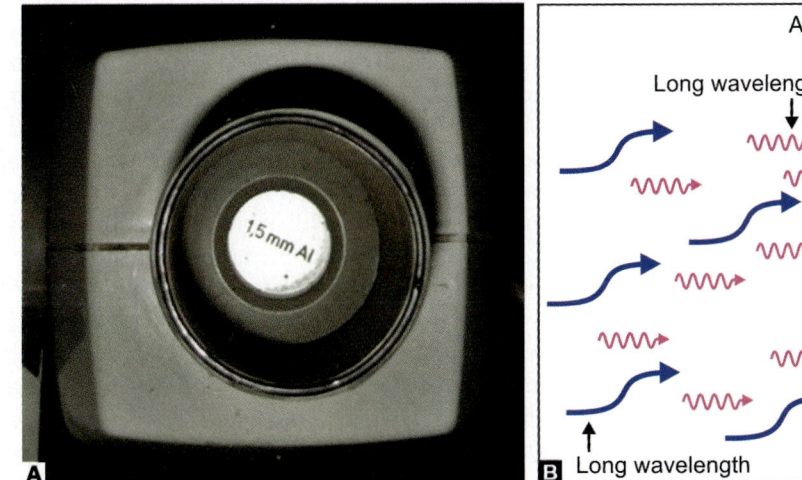

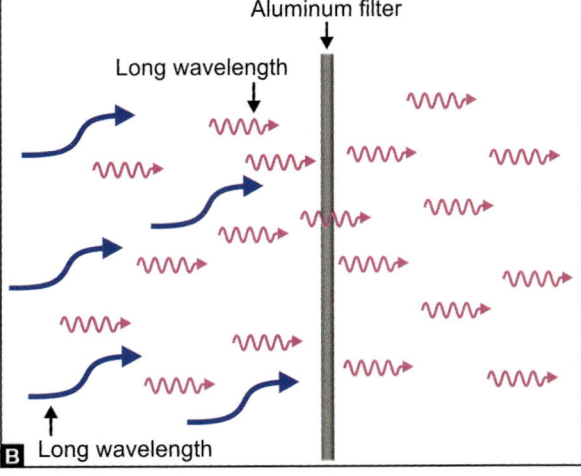

Fig. 27.2A and B: Filter

within the patient and, therefore, reduces the volume irradiated. This can be achieved by using position indicating device (PID). Longer source to film distance results in 32% reduction in exposed tissue volume. As compared to the short PID (8 inch) (Fig. 27.3A). The longer PID (16 inch), (Fig. 27.3B) is preferred because it produces less divergence of the X-ray beam.

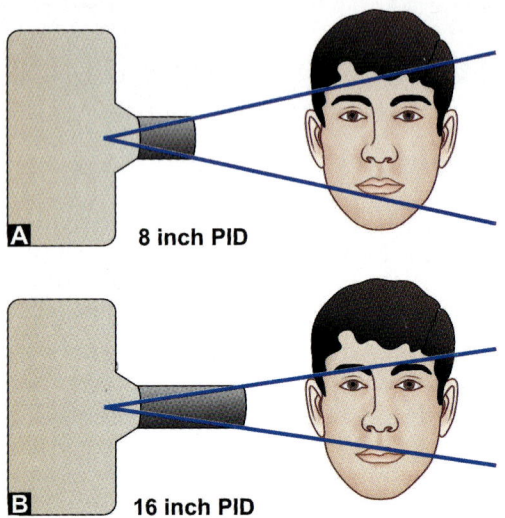

Fig. 27.3: Position indicating devices (PID)

Lead Apron

Lead aprons help to reduce the amount of primary radiation reaching areas of the body that are in the straight path of the primary beam. Lead apron or leaded apron is a type of protective clothing that acts as a radiation shield (Fig. 27.4). It is constructed of a thin rubber exterior and an interior of lead in the shape of a hospital apron. The purpose of the lead apron is to reduce exposure of a hospital patient to X-rays to vital organs that are potentially exposed to ionizing radiation during medical imaging that uses X-rays. A lead apron with at least 0.25 mm thickness of lead has been recommended. When a lead apron is provided, it must be properly stored (over an appropriate hanger) and not folded. Its condition must be routinely checked including a visual inspection at annual intervals. Lead aprons do not protect

against radiation scattered internally within the body.

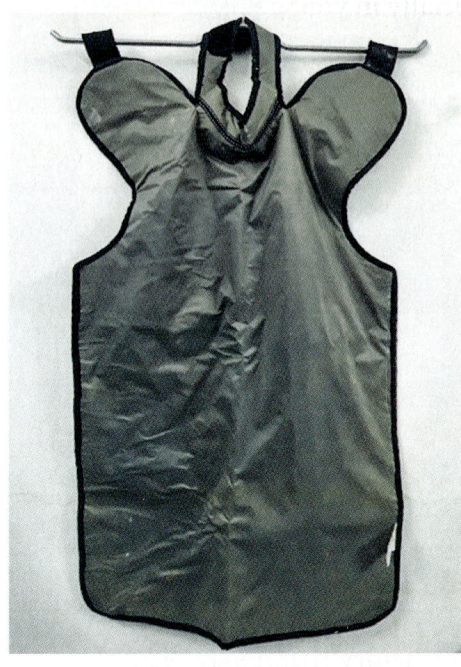

Fig. 27.4: Lead apron

Thyroid Collar

The thyroid gland is one of the more radiosensitive organs in the head and neck region. It is frequently exposed to scattered radiation and occasionally to primary beam during dental radiography. Because people under age 30 are at greater risk of radiation-induced thyroid cancer than older individuals, some have argued that thyroid collars should be used when intraoral radiographic examinations are made on this population (Fig. 27.5). However, it is probable that rectangular collimation for intraoral radiography offers similar level of thyroid protection to lead shielding, in addition to its other dose reducing effects. Thyroid shielding is inappropriate for panoramic radiography, as it may interfere with the primary beam. In cephalometric radiography lead thyroid protection is necessary, if the beam collimation does not exclude the thyroid gland. Thyroid shielding was found to reduce radiation doses of 45% during CT of the head and is strongly recommended, especially in younger age groups.

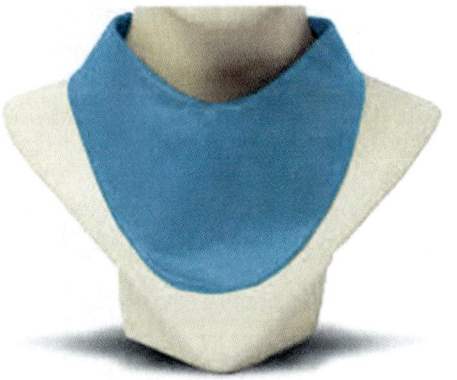

Fig. 27.5: Thyroid collar

Choice of Image Receptor

* **Use of fast film:** For intraoral radiography, the fastest available films consistent with satisfactory diagnostic results should be used. Changing film speed has a significant effect on the exposure required to produce an image. Just switching from D-speed to F-speed, film can reduce patient exposure by 60%. Intraoral films of speed groups E or F are recommended because they reduce the radiation dose to patient as compared with group D-speed films.
* **Digital receptor:** Using digital sensors can further decrease the exposure by approximately 25%, but this is subject to variances, e.g. the type and manufacturer of the sensor, and the make of X-ray machine being used. The digital images are supposed to achieve images of high diagnostic quality, at least equal to that of conventional radiographic film. Furthermore, the images are displayed immediately on the computer monitor and no processing chemicals or equipment is needed.
* **Use of intensifying screen:** Intensifying screens are used in the extraoral X-ray cassette to intensify the effect of the X-ray by producing light. It reduces the

mAs required to produce the image of a particular density and hence reduces the patient dose significantly.

Proper Handling and Proper Film Processing and Interpretation

Improper handling and film processing has impact on patient radiation exposure. It leads to repetition of dental radiograph subsequently causes further unnecessary radiation exposure to patient. One can avoid repetition of radiograph by proper handling and processing of the film and appropriate interpretation of radiograph.

METHODS OF RADIATION PROTECTION IN DENTISTRY FOR OPERATOR

Lead Partition

When decreasing the time or increasing the distance may not be possible, one can use shielding material to reduce the external radiation risk. Lead shielding refers to the use of lead as a form of radiation protection to shield people or objects from radiation so as to reduce the effective dose (Fig. 27.6).

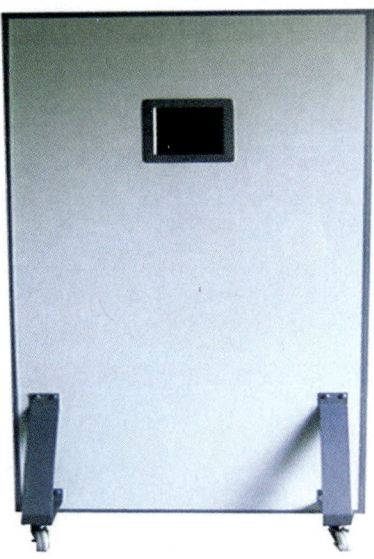

Fig. 27.6: Lead partition

Always operate the equipment from behind the protective barrier. Lead is a common shielding material for X-rays because it has a high density, is inexpensive, and is comparatively simple to work with it.

Position and Distance Rule

The best radiological practice is that operators should always stand behind a lead barrier having 0.5 mm lead equivalent, and barriers should contain a leaded glass window which allows the operator to observe the patient during X-ray exposure.

Position and distance rules rate that if protective barrier is not available then operator should stand at least six feet away from the source of radiation at an angle of 90° to 135°, with respect to the direction of the central ray during the period of X-ray exposure. This area is called the zone of greatest safety which ranges from 90° to 135° with respect to the primary central X-ray beam (Fig. 27.7). This rule not only takes the advantage of inverse square law as the distance increases the intensity of X-ray decreases but also takes the benefit of the fact that in this position the patient's head absorbs most scatter radiation.

- The film should not be hold by the operator in the patient's mouth during exposure.
- During exposure, the operator should not stabilize the X-ray machine.
- The operator should not stand directly in the path of the primary central beam.
- Radiation exposure to the operator should be monitored periodically by using film badges or personnel monitoring devices.
- Rotation of duties of the operator is necessary so that continuous accidental exposure to one operator can be avoided.

Quality Assurance Programme

Quality assurance may be defined as any planned activity to ensure that a dental office will consistently produces high quality images with minimum exposure to patient and the personnel.

Continuing Dental Education

Operator should gain knowledge regarding new information about radiation safety, advancement in equipment, recent material and technique used through continuing dental education programs to reduce the radiation exposure to both patient and operator.

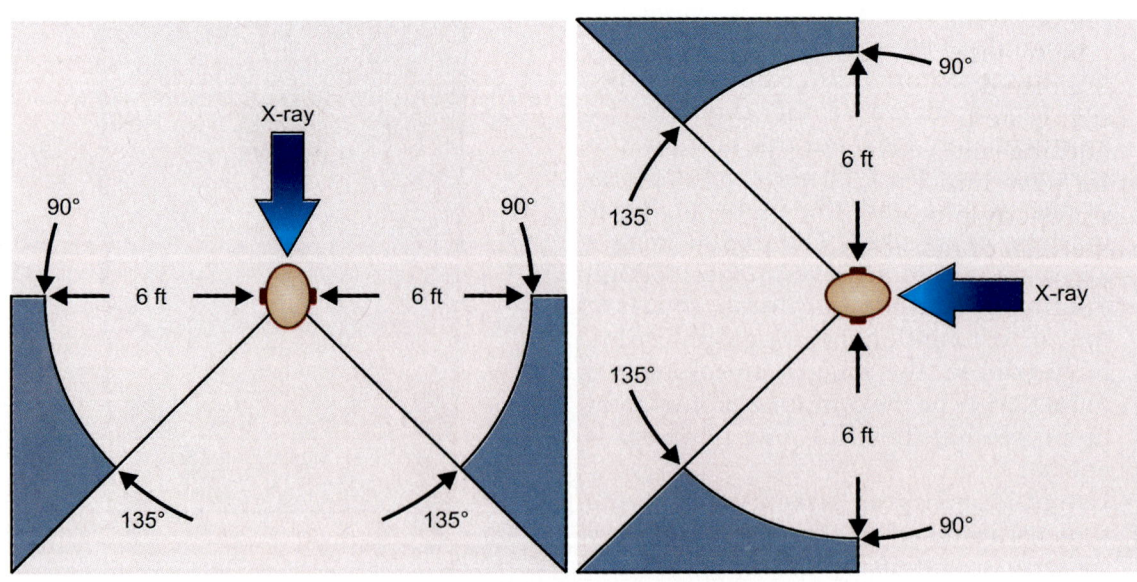

Fig. 27.7: Position and distance rule

Radiation protection methods
Before exposure
• Proper prescribing the dental radiograph
• Patient's instruction (explain the procedure)
During exposure
• Collimation
• Filtration
• Long PID
• Leaded aprons
• Thyroid collar
• Fast film
• Use of intensifying screen
After exposure
• Proper handling
• Proper film processing
• Appropriate interpretation of radiograph

Summary

Diagnostic information from dental X-rays can be obtained by minimizing patient exposure with appropriate use of modern film, equipment and technology. Radiation protection can be achieved at different level before, during and after X-ray exposure (Box 27.1) starting from the selection of the patient. Before X-ray exposure one can properly prescribe the appropriate dental radiograph according to need. Proper collimation, filtration and use of extended source to film distance (PID) are the useful radiation protection measures. Use of leaded aprons, thyroid collars, and fast film or uses of digital receptors are the excellent tools to minimize the radiation dose to individuals during actual X-ray exposure. Proper handling and processing of the exposed film have impact on radiation protection. Improperly processed radiograph result in repetition of radiograph and causes further radiation exposure. Though dental exposure is low as compared to medical exposure, every effort is to be made to reduce the radiation exposure for patient, healthcare worker and operator.

FREQUENTLY ASKED QUESTIONS

Write a short note on:

1. Radiation protection for patient
2. Radiation protection for operator
3. Position and distance rule

BIBLIOGRAPHY

1. Whaites E. Essentials of Dental radiography and Radiology. 4th edition. Spain: Churchill Livingstone Elsevier; 2007.
2. White S., Pharoah Medicine Oral Radiology. Principles and Interpretation. 6th edition. Elsevier Inc; 2011.
3. White S., Pharoah Medicine Oral Radiology. Principles and Interpretation. 5th edition. Mushy; 2004.
4. Goaz P, White. Oral Radiology Principles and Interpretation. 2nd edition: BI Publishers; 1998.
5. Whaites E. Essentials of Dental Radiography and Radiology. 2nd edition. Churchill Livingstone; 1997.
6. Langland O, Langlais R., Preece J. Principles of Dental Imaging, 2nd edition. Lippincott: Williams and Wilkins; 2002.
7. Langland O, Langlais R., Principles of Dental Imaging 1st edition: Lippincott. Williams & Wilkins; 1997.
8. Wood N, Goaz P. Differential Diagnosis of Oral and Maxillofacial Lesions. 5th edition. Elsevier; 2007.
9. Karjodkar F. Textbook of Dental and Maxillofacial Radiology. 2nd edition. Jaypee Brothers Medical Publishers; 2009.

X-Ray Film, Intensifying Screen and Grid

There is a changing trend from conventional film-based radiography to digital radiography, even then the use of X-ray films is common.

The X-ray film is the conventional image receptor system. It receives or records the image after the radiation exposure. The X-ray film is the term that may be used before it is processed, once exposed and processed, it is referred to as radiograph.

FILM PACKET

The film is placed in the packet made of plastic vinyl, moisture proof cover. On one corner of the film packet, there is a small raised dot or convexity known as the identification dot (Fig. 28.1).

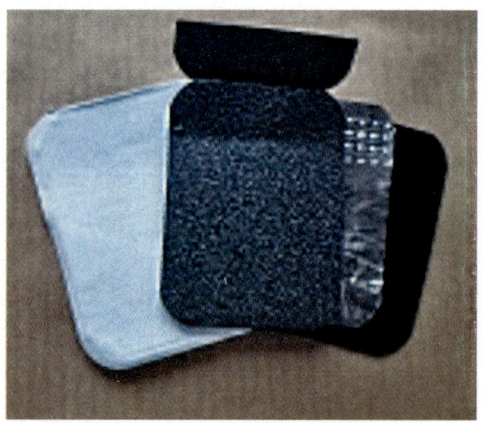

Fig. 28.1: Contents of film packet

Film packet has the following contents along with X-ray film.

- *Outer cover:* Outermost packet wrapping made up of soft plastic vinyl.
- *Black paper:* Placed on both the sides of film.
- *Thin lead foil:* Placed on one side that is tube side of X-ray film.
- *X-ray film:* Innermost component in the packet, placed between two black papers.

Film packet content	Function
Outer cover	Covers the film and other components to protect it from moisture
Black paper	Shields the film from light and protects film inside packet
Lead foil	Shields the film from back-scatter that may fog the film
X-ray film	Image receptor to record the image

Positioning of Film and Side Determination

The outer cover of the film packet has two sides—a colored side and a white side. The white side is the tube side and it has the raised embossed dot or convexity on one corner (Fig. 28.2).

When placed in the mouth, the white side (tube side) of the film must face the teeth and tube head with raised dot placed toward the incisal or occlusal surface of the teeth.

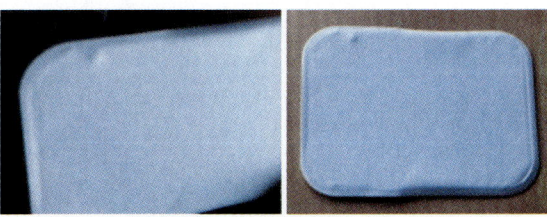

Fig. 28.2: Embossed dot

Types of X-ray Films

The X-ray films are classified as follows:

I. **According to region of exposure:**
   × *Intraoral:* It is placed inside the mouth during X-ray exposure.
   × *Extraoral:* Placed outside the mouth during X-ray exposure and used to examine large areas of the head or jaws. The films are placed in the cassette which is a rigid metal or plastic case available in various sizes as 5/6 × 12 inches, 5 × 7 inches, and 8 × 10 inches. The intraoral film records smaller intraoral areas while extraoral films are used to examine large areas of the skull or jaws. The films are placed in the rigid case which can be of metal or plastic. Extraoral film can be used in combination with or without intensifying screen (screen and non-screen films). The rigid cassette holds the film and protects it from exposure to light. Usually, the film is sandwiched between the intensifying screens. Intensifying screen intensifies the effect of the radiation and thus decreases the amount of exposure needed.

II. **According to exposure:**
   × *Direct exposure:* Exposed directly to radiation.
   × *Indirect exposure/Screen film:* Extraoral film is used with intensifying screen.

Intraoral Films

Intraoral films are classified as follows.

I. **According to use** (Fig. 28.3)
   × Periapical films
   × Bitewing film
   × Occlusal film

1. **Periapical films:** The periapical films should record full length of the tooth, that is, crown and root with at least 2 mm of periapical bone surrounding the root of one arch, either maxillary or mandibular arch. It clearly shows the alveolar crest, lamina dura, periodontal ligament and the supporting bone.

2. **A bitewing film** records the crowns, only adjacent root portion and alveolar crest of both the arches, that is, maxillary and mandibular arches in single image.

   The bitewing packet has a bite tab that resembles like a wing on the side on which the patient bites. The films can be placed with their long axis vertical or horizontal. Routinely, the intraoral films are used to take bitewing radiograph.

   It is used to record the coronal portions of the maxillary and mandibular teeth in one image used for detection of the interproximal caries and evaluate the height of the alveolar bone. While X-ray exposure, patient bites on a paper tab projecting from the middle of the film which helps to hold the film in place.

3. **The occlusal film** shows the occlusal view which is taken at right angle to the periapical or bitewing film. This film is considerably larger than the periapical film; 5 × 7.5 cm/57 × 76 mm (about 2 × 3 inches). The objective of the occlusal view is to show larger segments of the maxillary or mandibular arches or the floor of the mouth. The image field consists of occlusal view of maxillary and mandibular arches, adjacent palatal areas, floor of the mouth, partial or complete dentition as per the type of view and projection.

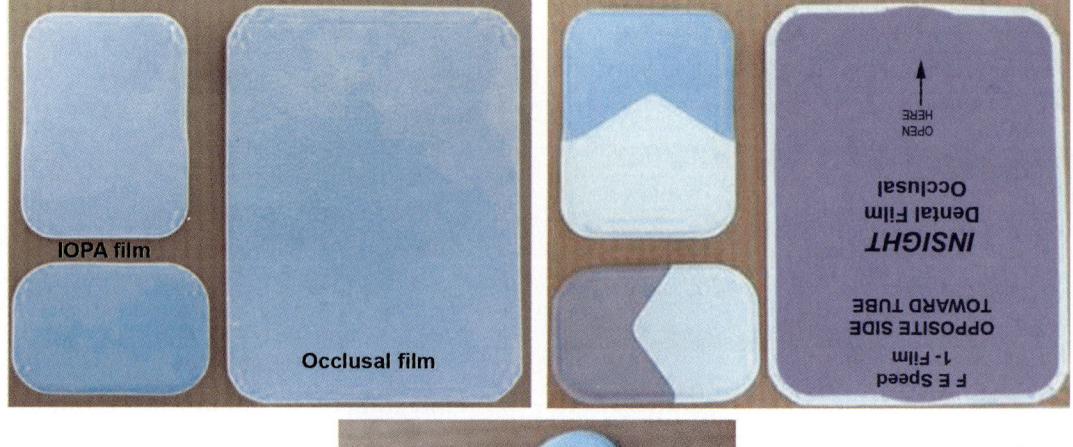

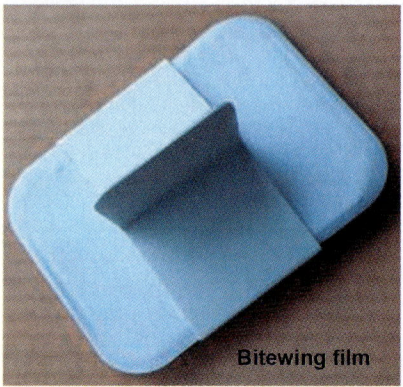

Fig. 28.3: Various intraoral films

II. **According to size** (Fig. 28.3): Intraoral film packets come in sizes as follows:
- For child (size 0)—22 × 35 mm
- For anterior teeth (size 1)—24 × 40 mm
- For adult (size 2)—30.5 × 40.5 mm
- For occlusal radiograph—57 × 76 mm

The type of dentition and teeth sizes vary according to the age of the patient, accordingly the film sizes also vary. The child may have deciduous or mixed dentition with the smaller jaw size, and hence needs the smaller size film (size 0), which will cover the dentition and will be compatible with oral tissues so that image will be recorded without film impinging on the oral tissues of the child patient. In case of an adult dentition, jaw sizes will be larger; however, the anterior teeth are narrower than posterior teeth, so the size 1 film will be appropriate for them.

For posterior teeth, the larger adult film (size 2) should be used which will cover the desired area of the dentition. The occlusal film is the largest of all intraoral films and has larger image field than intraoral films to cover portion of palatal bone and floor of the mouth along with the dentition.

III. **According to speed:** Speed refers to the amount of radiation required to produce a radiograph of standard density, thus determines how much exposure is required to produce the image.

Speed is denoted by alphabetical letters D, E, F speed films.
- Slow film
- Fast film (requires less radiation compared to slow film)

The F-speed film, the newest and fastest film available today. It reduces radiation exposure to the patient by 20% to 60% as compared to the E and D speed films.

IV. **Single Pack/Double Pack Films:** Intraoral film packet can be single-film packet or double-film packet; it may contain either one or two X-ray films respectively inside the packet. In that case, the second film serves as a duplicate record which can be used to send for storage purpose for future reference for second opinion or to the insurance companies.

Composition Intraoral Film

The dental X-ray film is made up of two basic components: Base and emulsion.

i. **Base:** It is the innermost layer of X-ray film. It is flexible in nature and made up of polyester polyethylene terepthalate. It supports the emulsion and provides the uniform base. It should be able to withstand the exposure to processing solutions and roller in the automatic processor. The thickness of base is approximately 0.007 inch.

ii. **Emulsion:** It is coated on both sides of base. It is made up of radiosensitive crystals distributed in vehicle matrix. The radiosensitive crystals are the silver halide crystals mainly including silver bromide and silver iodide along with free ions and gold or sulfur impurities. The thickness of base is approximately 0.0005 inch.

The dental intraoral X-ray film has emulsion on both sides of the film, as it requires less radiation to produce an image.

iii. **Vehicle matrix:** It contains gelatin and non-gelatinous material. It allows the uniform distribution of silver halide crystals. It absorbs the processing solution and allows the processing chemicals to react with them. An additional layer of vehicle matrix is added on the emulsion as an overcoat to protect it from the chemical, thermal and mechanical damage from processing or improper handling.

Composition of Cassette

It usually contains extraoral film in combination with or without intensifying screen (screen and non-screen films). The rigid cassette holds the film and protects it from exposure to light. In all conventional dental applications, intensifying screens are used in pairs, one on each side of the film, and the film is sandwiched between the intensifying screens. The rigid cassettes are used with a purpose to hold each intensifying screen in contact with the X-ray film to maximize the sharpness of the image.

Intensifying screen intensifies the effect of the radiation and thus decreases the amount of exposure needed.

Composition of Intensifying Screen

The intensifying screen (Fig. 28.5) consists of base, phosphors, reflector (titanium dioxide) and a protective coat.

The screen base is made up of polyester plastic that provides the mechanical support to the screen, is about 0.25 mm thick. The base provides mechanical support for the other layers. In some intensifying screens, the reflector layer is added to the base, in that case, it also acts as a reflector where it reflects light emitted from the phosphor layer back toward the X-ray film. This has the effect of increasing the light emission of the intensifying screen. However, it may add to 'unsharpness' of the film. The omission of reflecting layer in some screens is to improve image sharpness.

Phosphor Layer

The intensifying screen base is coated with phosphorescent crystals suspended in a polymeric binder. When the crystals absorb X-ray photons, they fluoresce that give off light when exposed to X-radiation. The phosphor crystals are made of rare earth elements such as lanthanum and gadolinium and small amount of terbium, thulium and niobium to increase the fluorescence.

The rare earth elements in the screen convert each absorbed X-ray photon into around 4000 visible light photons which in turn expose the adjacent film. In dental radiography, the intensifying screens absorb about 60% of the photons that reach the cassette after passing through a patient. These phosphors are about 18% efficient in converting this X-ray photon to visible light. The phosphor grain size in the screen, thickness of phosphor layer and coating weight affect this conversion efficiency of intensifying screens.

The overcoat protects phosphor layer and makes it easy to clean. It is essential to clean the intensifying screen surface of the debris as dirt and scratches may cause spots on resultant image.

Thus, the extraoral film is affected by both the X-radiation and visible light produced by the phosphor in the intensifying screen.

Digital Film/Image Receptor

The image receptor is a thin flexible plate of size of the conventional X-ray film that has been coated with phosphor crystals. The phosphor layer is able to store the energy of the X-ray photons for some time. A scanner is required to "read" the information stored on the plate by using a laser beam to release the energy from the plate and convert it into a digital image.

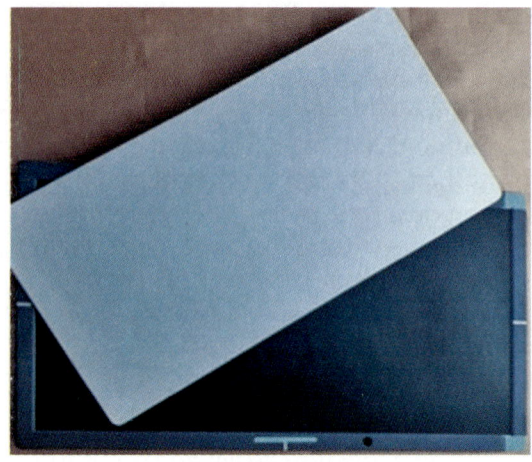

Fig. 28.5: Intensifying screen

Proper Storage

The proper storage of the film is essential as the X-ray film is sensitive to X-rays visible light, pressure, fumes, heat and moisture; even the aging causes a gradual fogging of the film.

Grid

Image quality can be improved by grid. The function of grid is to reduce scattered radiation which in turn reduces the fog; however more exposure is needed. For image acquisition as compared to the film alone. Therefore, grids should be used only when the improvement in diagnostic image quality is sufficient to justify the added exposure.

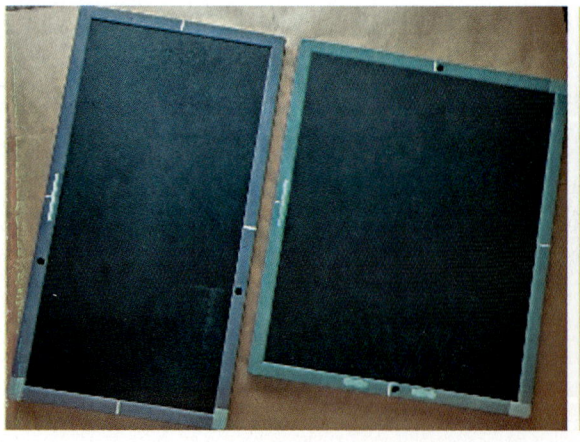

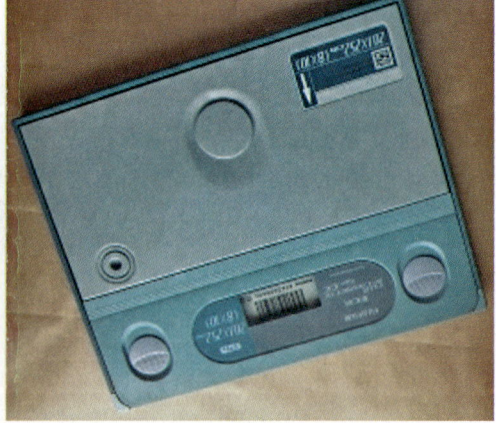

Fig. 28.4: Extraoral films

When an X-ray photon strikes a patient, many photons undergo Compton interactions and produce scattered photons, these may reach and strike the film many times to fog the film and reduce the subject contrast.

Composition of the grid: The grid is made up of alternating strips of radiopaque (lead) and radiolucent material (plastic). While taking radiograph, the grid is placed between object and the film. The X-rays pass through the grid first, where scattered radiation is removed before it reaches the film sparing the primary photons. This happens because the direction of the scattered photons deviates from that of the primary beam, and hence they cannot pass through the parallel plates of the grid. The generated scattered photons are absorbed by the radiopaque material in the grid, thus reducing the secondary or non-imaging exposure.

The grids are broadly classified into:
A. Linear grids
B. Crossed grids

Also, there are other types of grids, as:
C. Focused grids
D. Pseudofocused grids
E. Bucky grids

However, in dentistry, the focused grids are commonly used in which the strips of radiopaque material are directed towards a common point.

Grids are manufactured with a varying number of line pairs of absorbers and radiolucent spaces per inch. Grids with 80 or more line pairs per inch do not show objectionable grid lines on the image.

Grid ratio is the ratio of thickness of the grid to the width of the radiolucent spacer. Higher ratio removes scattered radiations more effectively. The ratio of '8 or 10' is preferred.

FREQUENTLY ASKED QUESTIONS

Write a short note on:

1. Composition of film packet/cassette/intensifying screen

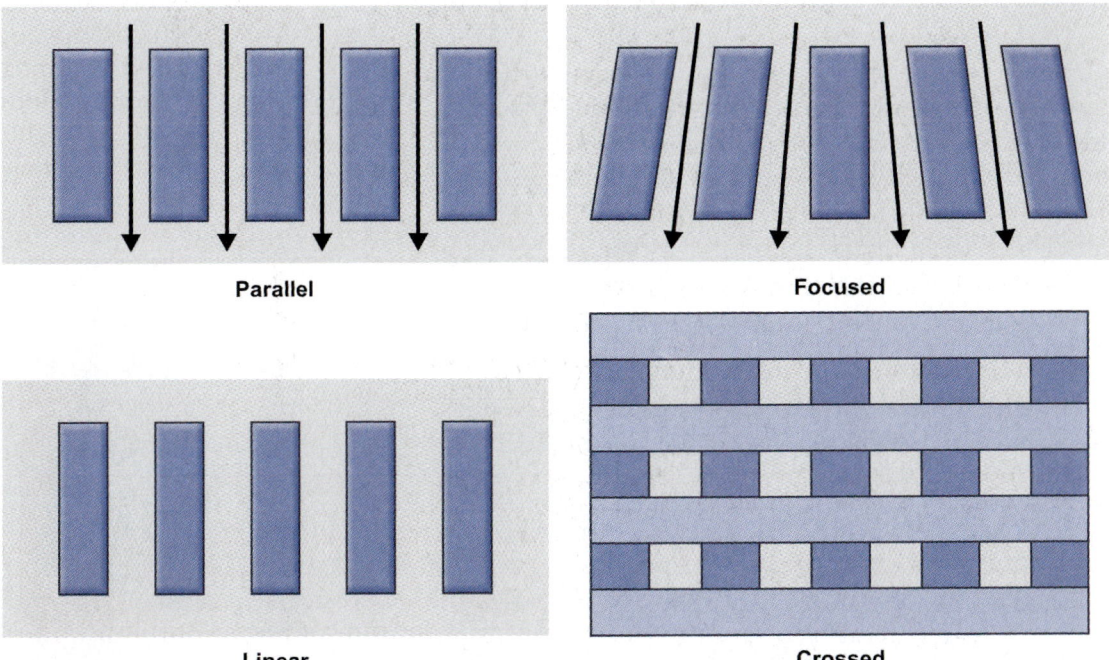

Parallel

Focused

Linear

Crossed

Fig. 28.6: Linear crossed

2. Types of films
3. Advanatges and disadvantages of intensifying screen
4. Grids used in dentistry

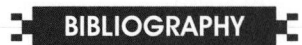

BIBLIOGRAPHY

1. White and Pharoah, Textbook of Oral Radiology, Principles and Interpretation. 5th ed.
2. Haring and Howerton. Dental Radiography—Principles and Techniques, 3rd edition.
3. Eric Whaites: Essentials of Dental Radiography and Radiology, 3rd edition.
4. Tani T. Photographic Sensitivity, Oxford University Press, 1995, 31–32, 84–85, 89–91.
5. Mitchell, JW Evolution of the concepts of photographic sensitivity. J Imag Sci Tech, 1999; 43: 38–48.

Film Processing

Processing the radiograph transforms the latent image into a visible image, thus the invisible image is made visible by processing. The operator must thoroughly understand the procedures and techniques necessary to process films into diagnostic quality images.

FORMATION

When dental X-ray film is exposed to radiation, the image is produced. Once emitted from X-ray tube, rays passed through teeth and the adjacent tissues and form the image on the film. The image formed after exposure of the film is invisible, that invisible image before processing is known as the latent image.

Wherever photon strikes the film, that areas together form the latent image sites. X-ray photons when exit the object and strike the X-ray film, they interact with the silver halide crystals in the film emulsion to produce chemically altered neutral silver halide grains, this together constitutes the invisible latent image.

Mechanism of Formation

The photons primarily react at the sensitivity sites in the emulsion. The crystals are chemically sensitized by the addition of trace amounts of sulfur compounds, which bind to the surface of the crystals. The sulfur compounds play a crucial role in image formation. Along with physical irregularities in the crystal produced by gold and iodide ions, sulfur compounds create sensitivity sites. These sites in the crystals are sensitive to radiation. Each crystal has many sensitivity sites, where the process of image formation begins by trapping the generated electrons.

Steps in Latent Image Formation (Fig. 29.1)

Sensitivity sites: Areas of emulsion with impurities (free Ag ions, iodine, gold, sulphur)
1. X-ray photon interacts with bromide ion
2. Bromide ion $\rightarrow e^- =$ Bromine atom $+ e^-$
3. $e^- +$ Sensitivity site = Negatively charged sensitivity site
4. Negative sensitivity site + Free silver = Latent image

The incoming photon liberates an electron, called a photoelectron, from a silver halide crystal. Photoelectrons migrate to an electron trap site (a sensitivity site), where the electrons reduce silver ions to form a metallic silver speck. One very important way to increase photographic sensitivity is to manipulate the electron traps in each crystal. The shallow electron traps are created by sulfur sensitization, introduction of a crystalline defect, and incorporating a trace amount of non-silver salt. The location, kind and number of shallow traps have a huge influence on the efficiency by which the photoelectrons create latent image centers, and consequently, on photographic sensitivity. The presence of gold is known to reduce the number of metallic silver atoms necessary to render the crystal developable. This can be another mean to increase photographic sensitivity.

Exposure to radiation chemically alters the photosensitive silver halide crystals to produce the latent image.
The X-ray photons interact primarily with the bromide ions in emulsion by photoelectric and Compton interactions, this results in the removal of an electron from the bromide ions. This loss of an electron converts bromide ion into a neutral bromine atom. The free electrons move through the crystal until they reach a sensitivity site, where they become trapped and impart a negative charge to the site.

The sensitivity sites that are negatively charged attract positively charged free interstitial silver ions to reduce them to a neutral atom of metallic silver. The sites containing these neutral silver atoms are now called latent image sites. This process occurs several times within a crystal, the overall distribution of latent image sites in a film after exposure constitutes the latent image.

Once the film is exposed and the latent image is formed, the exposed films are processed in the darkroom. Film processing is carried out in well-equipped darkroom.

Darkroom Requirements

- A conventional darkroom in dental radiology should be at least 4 feet × 5 feet.
- Light-tight or lightproof—no light leaks in the room
- Processing tanks for the developer and fixer solution (master tank and insert tanks)
- A circulating water bath with running water (Fig. 29.2)
- Stirring rods to mix the chemicals
- Source of safelight and white light
- Thermometer and timer
- Film hangers
- Film dryer
- Separate disposal containers for lead foil, film packets or barriers/infection-control items (e.g. gloves, disinfectant spray, paper towels) labeled with a biohazard label
- Safe storage space for chemicals/films
- No source of stray lights should be there, to ensure this the door should be tightly closed.
- For heat and moisture to escape, the dark-room should be well ventilated.
- Room temperature is attained to maintain optimal condition for solutions.

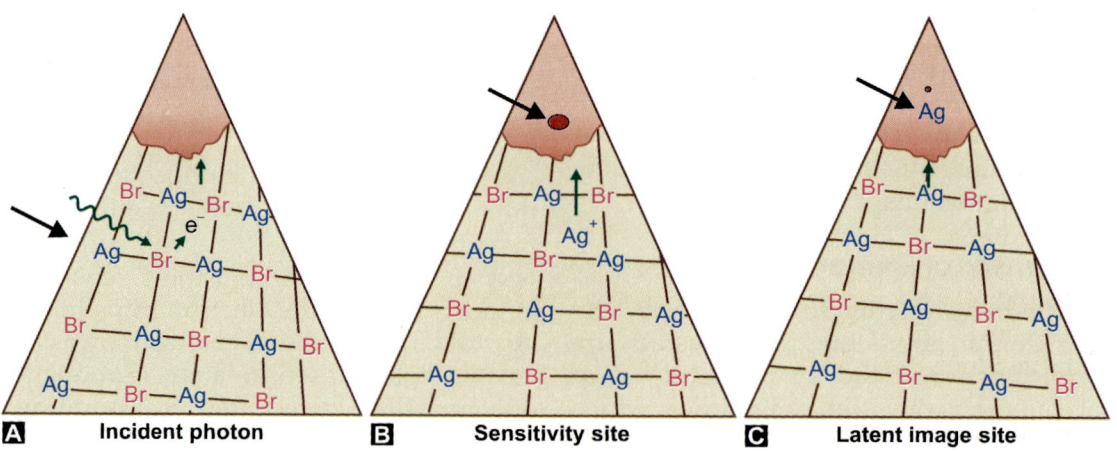

| A | Incident photon | B | Sensitivity site | C | Latent image site |

Fig. 29.1: Latent image formation

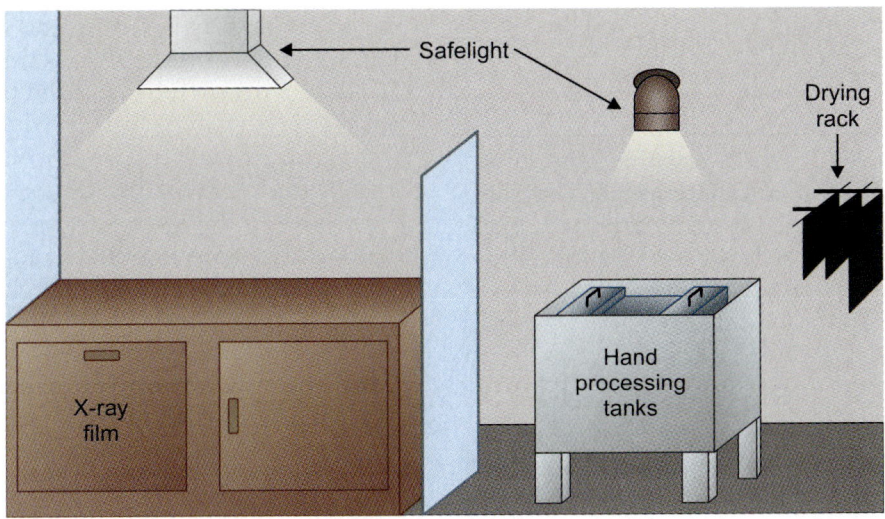

Fig. 29.2: Darkroom

- A 15 watt safelight which is of low intensity and long wavelength is used. It is mounted 4 feet above the surface where open films are handled.
- Film handling is preferably limited to 5 minutes under safe lighting.

Coin test or penny test: Used to evaluate darkroom safe lighting.

Under the monthly checks of quality assurance, the darkroom should be inspected regularly and the integrity of the safelights (preferably GBX-2 filters with 15-watt bulbs) should also be assessed on the monthly basis.

Light leaks or inefficient safelight filters can lead to film fog (low contrast and dark films).

The coin test or penny test can be used to evaluate the inappropriate safe lighting conditions in the darkroom.

1. The coin test is to be performed in the darkroom.
2. Open the packet of an exposed film and place the test film in the area where the films are usually unwrapped and clipped on the film hanger.
3. Place a penny on the film and leave it in this position for the approximate time required to unwrap and mount a full-mouth set of films, usually about 5 minutes.
4. Process the test film by routine method.
5. If the image of the coin is visible on the resultant film, the room is not light-safe for the particular film tested.

Laws by government should be followed to manage radiographic wastes in dental operatory. Dissolved silver in processing solution and lead foil in the film packet are primary ingredients of concern for waste disposal. Licensed companies pick up these waste material to prevent environmental damage.

DEFINITION OF PROCESSING

Processing is a series of steps that changes the latent image on the exposed film into a radiograph by producing a visible image on the film. It refers to several procedures collectively done to produce the visible image.

Types or Methods of Processing

- Visual method/manual method
- Time-temperature method
- Automatic processing

- Rapid processing
- Daylight processing
- Digitized processing
- **Visual/manual method:** It is the manual method in which the X-ray film is immersed in developing solution for about 10 sec and then removed and observed in the safe light. If required image has been obtained, then it is put for rinsing, otherwise reinserted in the developing solution till adequate image is obtained. However, the drawback with this method is that it is highly subjective in nature.
- **Time-temperature method:** It is the manual processing in which a thermometer, a timer and the time-temperature chart are essential. The ideal time to process radiographs in the developer is 68°F for 5 minutes. A time-temperature chart is used to determine the time, temperature of the solution.
- **Automatic processing:** In this method, the processing is done in the automatic processor.
  - *Mechanism:* The automatic processor consists of an in-line transport mechanism that picks up the unwrapped film and passes it through the various small insert tanks contained in the processor device. The tanks are meant for developing, fixing, and washing solutions encased in the chamber. The series of rollers enclosed in the processor propels the film from one tank to another. The top rollers squeeze the film and remove developing solution minimizing carryover of developer into fixing solution. The dried film is recovered from the slots provided in the automatic processor. The chemical compositions of processing solutions are altered to operate at higher temperatures than those used for manual processing. Also, the fixer has higher amount of hardener as compared to the conventional solutions.
- **Rapid processing:** It is used for emergencies as well as in endodontics. The film is developed for 15–20 seconds and may be ready within 1–2 minutes to deliver. The films do not have the same amount of contrast and will discolor over time period.
- **Daylight processing method:** It is the processing method that doesn't require a darkroom. It involves stripping the film inside a lightproof pouch/chamber; the processing steps are carried out manually in daylight-loading chamber. Hence, it eliminates the need of a darkroom.
- **Digitized processing:** The image receptor has been coated with phosphor crystals that record the image. A scanner is required to 'read' the information stored on the plate by using a laser beam to release the energy from the plate and convert it into a digital image.

Manual Processing Methods

- Visual method
- Time-temperature method

Processing Armamentarium

- Well-equipped darkroom, processing tanks and processing solutions
- Intraoral films are being processed by manual, automatic or digitized processing. In the darkroom, it is customary to place the developer tank on the left side and fixer tank on right side in the water bath.

Series of Events in Film Processing Producing Radiograph

Exposure creates invisible/latent image
1. **Development:** Converts latent image to black metallic silver
2. **Rinsing:** Removes excess developer
3. **Fixing:** Dissolves out unexposed silver halide crystals.
4. **Washing:** Removes products of processing
5. **Drying:** Removes water
   Five steps in manual processing are:
   - Development
   - Rinsing
   - Fixation

- Washing
- Drying

The film packets are opened only in the darkroom under safe light conditions. The film is attached to the film hanger at the corner or edge of the film firmly.

At the beginning, check the levels of developer and fixer solution and replenish them, if needed.

1. Development

Firstly the film hanger is placed in the developer solution. The basic reaction is reduction (addition of an electron) of the silver ion, which changes it into black metallic silver.

The films must not contact one another or the sides of the processing tanks during development. The film must be completely immersed in the developer. Once in the developer, gently agitate the film hanger to prevent air bubbles from clinging to the film.

The negative charge attracts positively charged free silver ions and is reduced to black metallic atoms. This precipitation corresponds to the black (radiolucent) areas on the radiograph.

The reducing agents used as developers are catalyzed by the neutral silver atoms at the latent image sites. The silver atoms act as a bridge by which electrons from the reducing agents reach silver ions in the crystal and convert them to solid grains of metallic silver. Individual crystals are developed completely or not at all during the recommended developing times. Variations in density on the processed radiographs are the result of different ratios of developed (exposed) and undeveloped (unexposed) crystals. Areas with many exposed crystals are denser because of their higher concentration of black metallic silver grains after development.

The developing solution contains four components, all dissolved in water:
1. Developer
2. Activator
3. Preservative
4. Restrainers.

▶ Developer

Developing solution acts on the exposed silver halide crystals. The primary function of the developing solution is to convert the exposed silver halide crystals into metallic silver grains. This process begins at the latent image sites, where electrons from the developing agents are conducted into the silver halide crystal and reduce the constituent silver ions (approximately 1 billion to 10 billions) to solid grains of metallic silver.

Two developing agents are used in dental radiology:
- Phenidone (1-phenyl-3-pyrazolidone)
- Hydroquinone (paradihydroxy benzene)

Functions
- Phenidone is a pyrazolidone-type compound; it serves as the first electron donor that converts silver ions to metallic silver at the latent image site. This electron transfer generates the oxidized form of phenidone.
- Hydroquinone provides an electron to reduce the oxidized phenidone back to its original active state so that it can continue to reduce silver halide grains to metallic

TABLE 29.1: Contents of developer	
Chemical	*Action*
Phenidone/elon or metol	Acts faster, as a first electron donor
Hydroquinone	Brings out sharp contrast
Sodium or potassium hydroxide Sodium bicarbonate	Alkalizer provides alkaline medium to accelerate the reaction
Sodium sulphite, preservative	Slows oxidation
Potassium bromide and benzotriazole	Acts as an antifogging agent, restrains the development of unexposed crystal
Water, vehicle	Provides a means for the chemicals in the developer to react, water helps to soften gelatin

silver. Unexposed crystals, those without latent images, are unaffected during the time required for reduction of the exposed crystals.

× This reaction can only occur in an alkaline medium

When an exposed film is developed, the developer initially has no visible effect. After this initial phase, the density increases, very initially. Eventually all the exposed crystals develop (become reduced to black metallic silver), and the developing agent starts to reduce the unexposed crystals. The development of unexposed crystals results in chemical fog on the film. The interval between maximal density and fogging explains why a properly exposed film does not become overdeveloped, although it may be in contact with the developer longer than the recommended interval. Thus, dark films usually are the result of overexposure rather than overdevelopment.

▶ **Activator**

The developers are active only at alkaline pH values, usually around 10.

Hence, some alkalizer or alkali compounds added to the developing solution accelerate or activate this developing effect. The compounds such as sodium or potassium hydroxide are added as an activator and sodium bicarbonate added as a buffer.

Functions

× It accelerates or activates the developing reaction

× The buffers added help to maintain alkaline condition.

× The activators also cause the gelatin to swell so that the developing agents can diffuse more rapidly into the emulsion and reach the suspended silver bromide crystals.

▶ **Preservative**

Sodium sulfite is added as a preservative to the developing solution. In addition to preservation, it has the antioxidant effect.

Functions

× The preservative protects the developers from oxidation by atmospheric oxygen thus preserves the strength of the developer solution

× It extends the shelf life.

× The preservative also combines with the brown oxidized developer to produce a colorless soluble compound.

× Solution without antioxidant/preservative would rapidly weaken, with darkening of the solution.

▶ **Restrainer**

Potassium bromide and benzotriazole are added to the developing solutions which act as a restrainer.

Functions

× It restrains development of unexposed reduction of both exposed and unexposed crystals; it is much more effective in depressing the reduction of unexposed crystals.

× Acts as antifog agents

× Serves to increase contrast.

If the restrainer is not added, developing agent will deposit silver in the unexposed crystals causing silver deposits on the film leading to its fogging.

Considerations in relation to film developing solution

i. Replenishing of the developing solution is needed.

ii. The concentration of the developer slowly weakens due to the number of films processed and with time by oxidation of the developer by exposure to air.

iii. Traditionally, the developer tank is placed on the left side of the other chemicals solutions.

iv. Developing solution acts on the exposed silver halide.

v. To produce a diagnostic image, this reduction process must be restricted to crystals containing latent image sites.

vi. If the developer remains too long in contact with silver bromide halide crystals that do not contain a latent image, it slowly reduces these crystals also, thereby overdeveloping the image.

vii. The reaction does not occur unless alkalizer is present. The alkali 'opens the doors' and permits the developing agents to enter the pores of the emulsion.

viii. If the lid is left off the developing tank, the preservative will be rapidly become exhausted by oxidation.

1. Developer–Replenisher

The developing solution of both manual and automatic developers should be replenished with fresh solution each morning to prolong the life of the seasoned developer.

In the normal course of film processing, phenidone and hydroquinone are consumed, and bromide ions and other byproducts are released into solution. Developer also becomes inactivated by exposure to oxygen. These actions produce a 'seasoned' solution, and the film speed and contrast may get compromised.

The recommended amount to be added daily is 8 ounces of fresh developer (replenisher) per gallon of developing solution. This assumes the development of an average of 30 periapical or 5 panoramic films per day. Some of the used solution may need to be removed to make room for the replenisher.

2. Rinsing Process

After development, the chemicals that are carried along with the film are removed by rinsing the film by placing the film in a water bath. The film should be rinsed for 10–15 seconds in a bath of fresh running water.

By rinsing the film in the water, the chemicals are removed, the development reaction is stopped and the alkalinity of the residual developer is reduced.

3. Fixing

After rinsing, immerse the film hangers in fixer solution and gently agitate it for 5 seconds every 30 seconds to eliminate air bubbles. This will bring the fresh fixer in contact with emulsion to have the action of fixer solution on film. The fixing solution dissolves and removes the unexposed silver halide crystals to render clear areas of the film. If film kept longer time in fixer it will start affecting the exposed crystals thus affecting the image formed.

The acidic fixing solution removes the unexposed and undeveloped silver bromide crystals from the film emulsion and re-hardens the emulsion that has softened during the development process.

Fixing solution also contains four components, all dissolved in water:

× Clearing agent
× Acidifier
× Preservative
× Hardener

TABLE 29.2: Contents of fixer	
Chemicals	Action
Ammonium thiosulfate	Removes unexposed crystals
Acetic acid	Provides acid medium. Alum reacts better in acid medium Stops developing process
Sodium sulfite	Prevents deterioration of solution
Aluminum sulfate	Shrinks and hardens the gelatin
Water, vehicle	Provides a means for the chemicals in the fixer to react, water helps to soften gelatin

Fixing solution: The primary function of fixing solution is to dissolve and remove the undeveloped silver halide crystals from the emulsion. The presence of unexposed crystals causes film to be opaque. If these crystals are not removed, the image on the resultant radiographs is dark and non-diagnostic. A second function of fixing solution is to harden and shrink the film emulsion. As with developer, fixer should be replenished daily at the rate of 8 ounces per gallon.

▶ Clearing Agent

Ammonium thiosulfate is added as clearing agent in the fixing solution. An aqueous solution of ammonium thiosulfate dissolves the silver halide grains. It forms stable, water-soluble complexes with silver ions, which then diffuse from the emulsion.

Functions

- It acts on unexposed silver halide crystals
- After development the film emulsion must be cleared by dissolving and removing the unexposed silver halide.

The clearing agent does not have a rapid effect on the metallic silver grains in the film emulsion, but excessive fixation results in a gradual loss of film density because the grains of silver slowly dissolve in the acetic acid of the fixing solution.

▶ Acidifier

Acetic acid is added to the fixing solution, which has specific functions as clearing agent. The fixing solution contains an acetic acid buffer system (pH 4 to 4.5) to keep the fixer pH constant. The acidic pH is required to promote good diffusion of thiosulfate into the emulsion and of silver thiosulfate complex out of the emulsion.

Functions

- It provides acid medium.
- Stops developing process of unexposed crystals.

The acid-fixing solution also inactivates any carryover developing agents in the film emulsion, blocking continued development of any unexposed crystals while the film is in the fixing tank.

▶ Preservative

Ammonium sulfite is the preservative in the fixing solution. It preserves the fixing solution by preventing it from deterioration, which is unstable in the acid environment.

Functions

- It prevents oxidation of clearing agent.
- It also binds with any colored oxidized developer carried over into the fixing.

It effectively removes the carried over developer from the solution; which prevents the staining of the film.

▶ Hardener

The aluminum sulfate is used as the hardening agent. Aluminum complexes with the gelatin during fixing and prevents damage to the gelatin during subsequent handling.

Functions

- Shrinks the gelatin.
- Hardens the gelatin.

Both of these actions of hardener are very crucial, first of all, it hardens the gelatin which lessens mechanical damage to the emulsion. Secondly, it reduces swelling of the emulsion by shrinking it during the final wash that limits water absorption, thus shortening drying time.

Considerations in relation to fixing

- Replenishing fixing solution is required.
- Proper washing of the film after fixing.
- Fixing is the slower effect than developing hence film needed to be kept for longer than developing.
- The acidic pH required for good diffusion of thiosulfate into the emulsion and for silver thiosulfate complex out of the emulsion.
- Any silver compound or thiosulfate that remains because of improper washing discolors and causes stains, which are most apparent in the radiopaque (light) areas.
- The thiosulfate reacting with silver to form brown silver sulfide, which can obscure diagnostic information.
- Exhaustion of the fixing solution causes poor clearing of the film, insufficient hardening of the emulsion, and unreliable transport from the fixer assembly through the drying operation.

Replenishing fixer solution: It is important to maintain the constituents of the fixer carefully to preserve the optimal physical properties of the film emulsion within the narrow limits imposed by the speed and temperature of automatic processing. As the activity of the fixing solutions lessens, its effect on the film diminishes.

To compensate for this loss of activity, some automatic processors include an automatic replenishment system that adds fresh developer to the developer tank and fresh fixer to the fixer tank. As with manual processing, 8 ounces of fresh developer and fixer should be added per gallon of solution per day. This assumes an average workload of 30 intraoral or 5 extraoral films per day.

4. Washing the Film

After fixing, the films are then placed in running water for at least 10 minutes. The purpose of the final wash is to remove residual fixer chemicals from the film which may stain and contaminate the image if not washed.

5. Drying

Before putting in the dryer, the surface moisture of film is removed by gently shaking off the excess water from the film and the hanger.

The processed wet film emulsion is soft and gets easily damage by improper handling. It is better, if the processed films are dried in cabinet dryers in moderately warm air to protect it from scratching, dust and excessive air flow. The cabinet dryers are available which are equipped with a fan and heating elements for uniform and complete drying of the film.

The film must be completely dried before they can be handled for mounting and viewing.

TIME-TEMPERATURE METHOD

This method of processing is dependent on time of developing of film and temperature of the solution. The temperature of the processing solution affects the developing of the film; rise in the temperature of processing solution speed up the processing, thus lessens the processing time.

Time-temperature method is the manual processing in which a thermometer, a timer and the time-temperature chart are essential. The steps in the processing are similar to the visual manual method except for the use of the time-temperature chart. The ideal time to process radiographs in the developer is 68°F for 5 minutes.

Time-temperature Chart

Temperature (°F)	Time of development of film (minutes)
68	5
70	4½
72	4
76	3
80	2½

Steps in Time-temperature Manual Processing

- Check the temperature of the developing solution before the film is immersed in developer solution. The hot water in the master tank and thermometer will help to monitor the temperature of the solution.
- Development: After unwrapping of the film in the darkroom, the film is inserted in the developing solution as in manual processing. The time for which developing is performed is dependent on the temperature of the solution, time-temperature chart is to be followed.
- Rinsing
- Fixation with the increase in the temperature reduces the processing time.
- Washing
- Drying

Automatic Processing

In this method, the processing is done in the automatic processor which has solution tanks encased in the chamber and the series of roller that propels the film from one tank to another. The film is inserted and recovered from the slots provided in the automatic processor. Although, it is time-saving and may process the film in 4–6 minutes, the rollers may produce marks on the film (Fig. 29.3).

Automatic film processing is a fast and simple method used to process dental X-ray films. Other than opening the film packet, all steps of film processing are handled by the automatic processor. Automatic film processing requires only 4 to 6 minutes for processing, whereas manual processing techniques require approximately 1 hour.

The automatic processor maintains the correct temperature of the solutions and adjusts the processing time. Proper maintenance of the automatic processor reduces the chance of errors during film processing.

Components of the Automatic Processor

- The processor housing covers all of the component parts.
- The film feed slot is for the unwrapped films to be inserted into the automatic processor.
- The roller film transporter is a system of rollers that rapidly moves the film through the compartments.
- The developer and fixer compartments hold the solutions.
- The film is transported directly from the developer into the fixer without a rinsing step.
- The water compartment holds circulating water.
- The drying chamber holds heated air and dries the wet film.

Advantages of Automatic Film Processing

- Less processing time is required.
- Time and temperature are automatically controlled.
- Less equipment are used.
- Less space is required.

Disadvantages of Automatic Processing

- Expensive
- The rollers may produce marks on the film.
- Higher temperature of processing solutions leads to errors.
- Needs frequent cleaning of equipment.

ERRORS

These are visible on processed radiographs due to various causes like insufficient processing and film placement or projection errors.

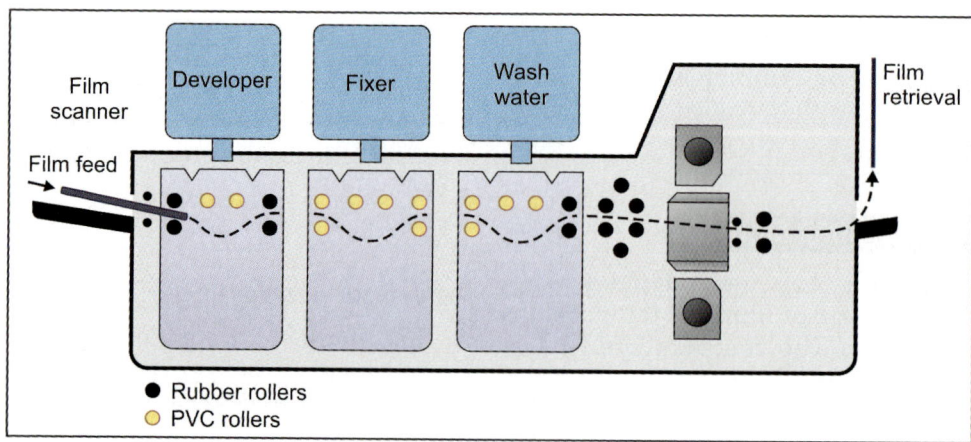

Fig. 29.3: Automatic processor

Errors during Processing (Manual)

× High contrast image

Causes: High developing time and temperature, strong developing solution.

It is necessary to monitor the developing time especially when processing solutions are freshly prepared, it will lead to over-development of the film.

× Black and white spots on film

Causes: Film contaminated with either developer/fixer before processing, dirty rollers/excessive roller pressure, film in contact with another film while in fixer/developer in the tank.

× Stains on film

Causes: Brown/yellow—insufficient washing, contaminated processing solutions

While shifting the film from developer to fixer and from fixer for drying, it is necessary to wash the film properly for carried processing solution. The insufficiently washed film will stain in due course of time.

If the lid is left off the developing tank, the preservative will be rapidly become exhausted by oxidation. If not removed, oxidation products interfere with the developing reaction and stain the film.

× Film fogging (dark radiograph)

Causes: Improper safe light, light leaks in darkroom, contaminated processing solutions.

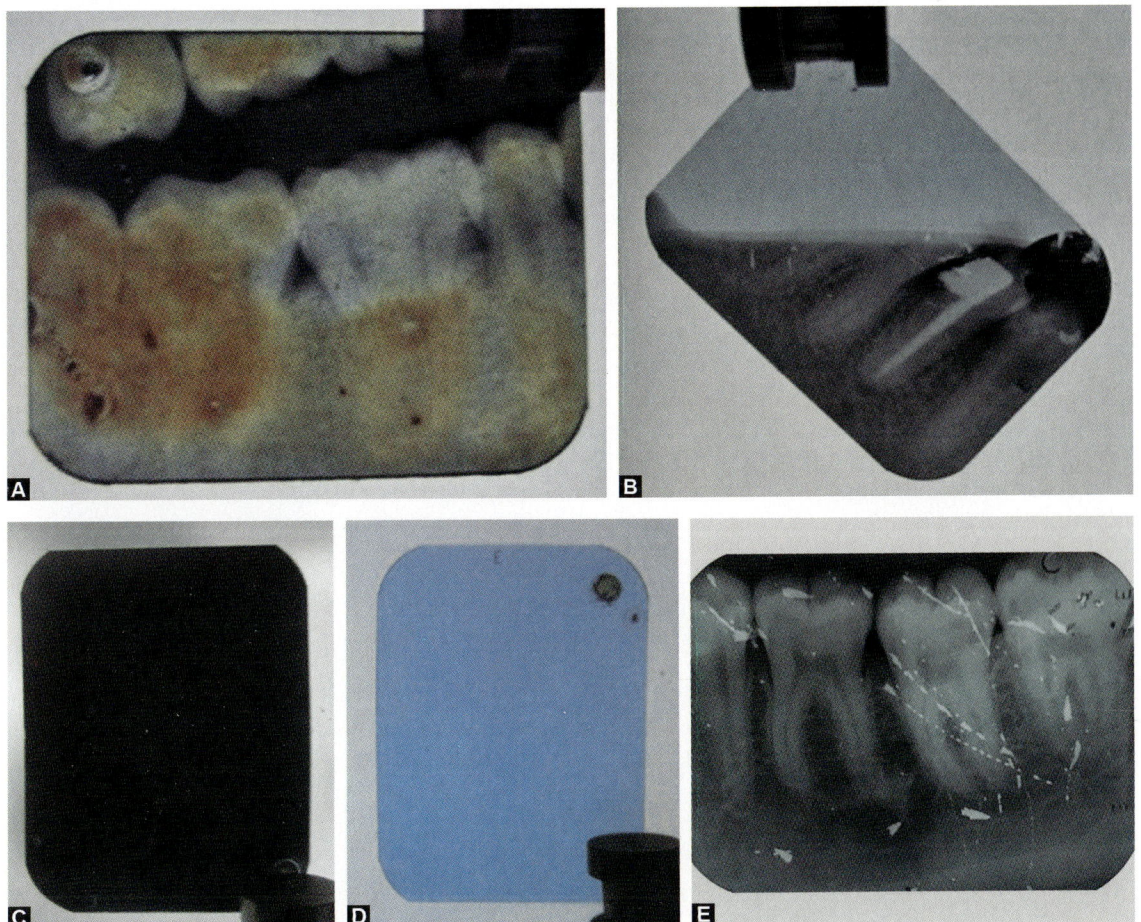

Fig. 29.4A to E: A. Yellow/brown stains on film; **B.** Incompletely developed film; **C.** Dark film; **D.** Clear film; **E.** Emulsion peel

TABLE 29.2: Errors in film processing

Error—patient preparation	Causes	Radiographic image
1. Radio-opaque artefacts	✖ Presence of dental appliances, body piercings, jewellery and eyeglasses during exposure leads to appearance of radio-opaque artefacts superimposed over the dental image	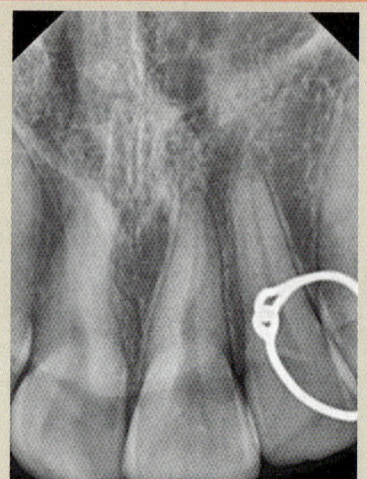
2. Blurred image	✖ Movement of the film/patient/tube head during exposure ✖ Motion blurring: Image sharpness is also lost due to movement of the film, subject or X-ray source	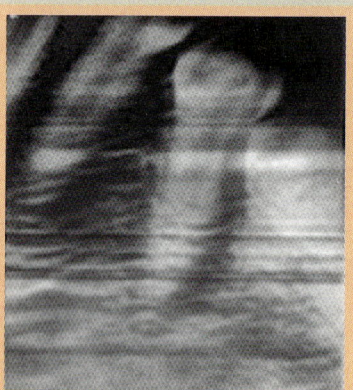
3. Incomplete exposure/ partial image: Apical ends of teeth are not visible on the radiograph Partial image/coronal ends not visible on the radiograph	✖ The film is not positioned apically enough to record the entire tooth	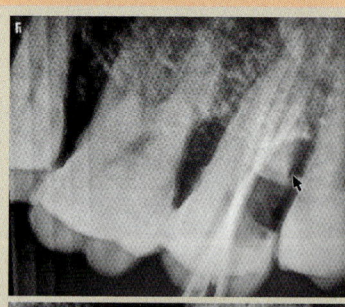 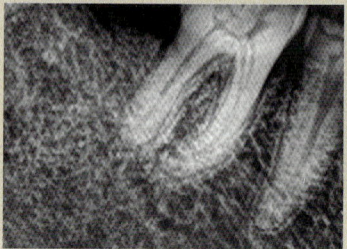

Contd.

TABLE 29.2: Errors in film processing (*Contd.*)

Error—patient preparation	Causes	Radiographic image
4. Cone cut	✗ Cone of X-ray source/cylinder not covering area of interest	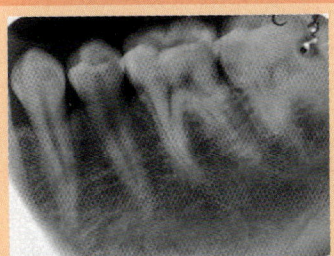
5. Overlapping of teeth	✗ Incorrect horizontal angulation	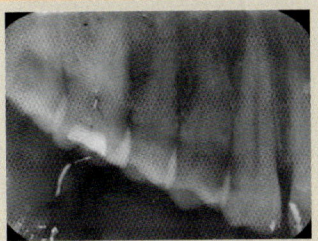
6. Foreshortening	1. In the bisecting angle technique when vertical angulation is increased. 2. The film is not placed parallel to the long axis of the teeth	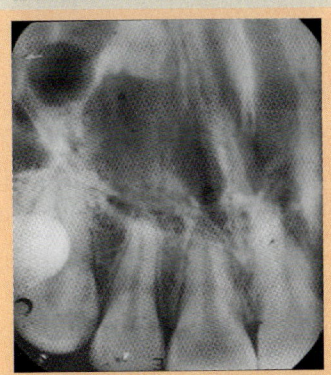
7. Elongation	✗ In the bisecting angle technique when vertical angulation is decreased ✗ The film is not placed parallel to the long axis of the teeth	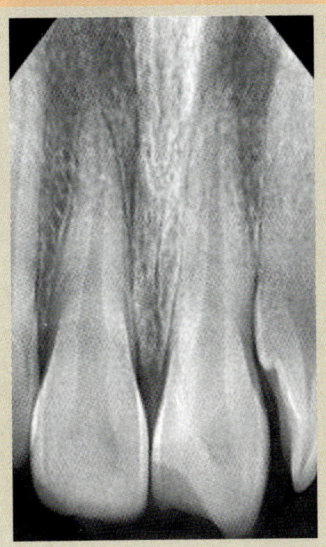

Contd.

TABLE 29.2: Errors in film processing (*Contd.*)

Error—patient preparation	*Causes*	*Radiographic image*
8. Magnification	✗ Decreased focal spot to object distance ✗ Increased object to film distance	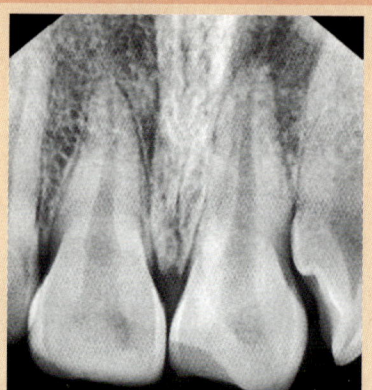
9. Tire track appearance	✗ Back side of the film with the lead foil placed facing towards the cone	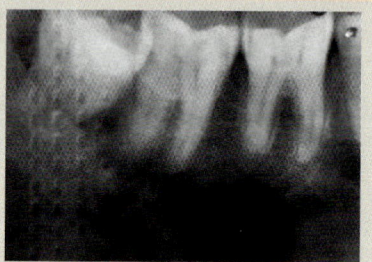
10. Black lines on the radiograph (bending marks)	✗ Excessive bending of the film (to reduce patient discomfort)	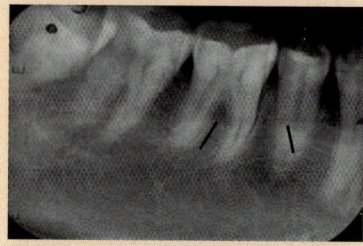
11. Dark radiographs	a. Prolonged exposure time b. Increased mA c. Increased kVp d. Decreased source to film distance	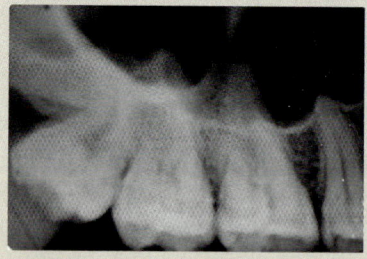
12. Light radiographs	a. Reduced exposure time b. Decreased mA c. Decreased kVp d. Increased source to film distance	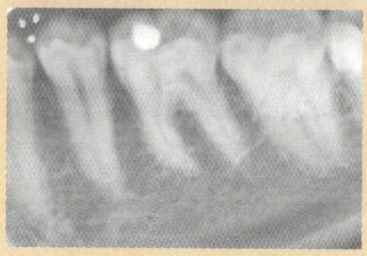

The darkroom, where the processing of film is carried out should be light-tight or light-safe. Any kind of light leakage either from the darkroom or from safelight will lead to the fogging of the film. The periodic checks for the light leaks should be done under quality assurance.

× Partial image

Causes: Inadequate level of developer

The level of the processing solution should be adequate, so that the film hangers and the film should be immersed completely in the solution. The insufficient levels will leave the portion above the solution undeveloped leading to partial image.

× Emulsion peel

Causes: Depleted fixer, too high temperature of developing solution, film in contact with tank, film for long time in wash water will soften the emulsion and render it vulnerable for peeling.

× Dark or clear film

Causes: Overdevelopment/film exposed in darkroom, unexposed film subjected to processing.

If the unexposed film get processed, it will appear clear on processing.

× Blisters/reticulation on film

Causes: Drying film at too high temperature, high processing temperature

The drying of the film should be done in the dryer that is moderately and uniformly hot. The drying or processing at excessively high temperature will lead to cracking of emulsion and reticulation on the resultant radiograph.

× Finger/nail mark on film

Causes: Finger/nail in contact with film while processing.

The finger or finger nail if in contact with the film while developing may cast mark on the soften emulsion to appear on the resultant radiograph, this may interfere with the minute details of diagnostic value (Fig. 29.4).

Film Placement and Projection Errors

Technique errors or projection errors include; elongation, shortening and blurring due to patient movement (motion blurring). Other causes of blurring are:

1. **Geometric blurring:** Image sharpness is influenced by several geometric factors. Larger the focal spot, lesser the image sharpness. Sharpness is improved by:
   i. Increasing the distance between focal spot and distance.
   ii. Decreasing the distance between object and image receptor.
2. **Image receptor blurring:** The size and number of silver grains in the film emulsion determine image sharpness. Fine image is produced by fine grains.

Mounting Radiographs

In case of multiple or full mouth radiographs of the same patients, the radiographs should be mounted and preserved in the film mount to avoid the confusion and related errors. In the film mount, the films can be mounted as per the anatomical relationship or sequence in the oral cavity and have the same relationship to the viewer as when the viewer faces the patient. Mounts are made of plastic or cardboard and may have a clear plastic window that covers the film. This way radiographs can be handled with greater ease reducing the damage while handling. To ensure optimum exposure and radiographs of diagnostic quality, it is necessary to follow quality control program laid by health regulatory bodies. This program includes tasks to be done in dental radiography section periodically. Yearly calibration of dental X-ray machines and verification of digital sensors; monthly evaluation of darkroom safelight, intensifying screens, thyroid collar and lead aprons is recommended. Few significant measures are more frequently practiced which includes; replacing processing solutions and cleaning of processing equipment and view boxes weekly while checking, temperature and replenishing processing solutions and comparing processed film with standard radiograph are advised daily.

Infection control in dental radiography is highly recommended. Maintaining pathogens free environment must be practiced strictly like, wear and change gloves during all radiographic procedures, disinfect dental chair, X-ray machines and lead apron, sterilize equipment.

BIBLIOGRAPHY

1. White SC, Pharoah MC. Oral Radiology, Principles and Interpretation; 2011:6th ed.
2. Haring J, Lannucci M, Howerton LJ. Dental Radiography—Principles and Techniques; 2006: 3rd edition.
3. Langland OE, Langlais RP, Preece JW. Principles of Dental Imaging; 2002:2nd ed. Lamba M. published on August 31, 2013.
4. Serman N. Processing the radiograph. The stages in the production of the radiograph, Sept. 2000, Chapter 6.
5. FrenyR.Karjodkar 2nd Edition. Textbook of Dental and Maxillofacial Radiology.

Projection Geometry

INTRODUCTION

Conventional radiographic technique provides us with a two-dimensional image of 3-dimensional structure of teeth and associated structures. There are numerous elements that affect the formation of this image which include visual characteristics (density and contrast) and geometric characteristics (sharpness, magnification, and distortion). Thus, an image so obtained should have proper degree of density and contrast, detailed sharpness, and minimal magnification and distortion (ideal radiograph). These factors should be able to delineate most of the diagnostic information from the image for the amount of radiation used. Thus a diagnostic dental radiograph should not be too light or too dark and provide complete information of the object radiographed.

The purpose of this chapter is to describe in detail the visual and geometric image characteristics and to discuss how these image characteristics are influenced by different imaging and processing factors.

A dental radiograph when viewed on a source of light (view box) reveals various shades of gray in a black-and-white image, with the darkest area appearing black, and the lightest area appearing white. There are two terms, viz. radiolucent and radiopaque, to describe the black and the white areas on a radiograph, respectively.

A radiolucent structure lacks density and permits the passage of the X-ray beam without any resistance. For example, air space freely transmits X-rays, casts a dark area and appears radiolucent on the radiograph. On contrary, radiopaque structures are dense and absorb X-ray photons. For example, enamel, dentin, and bone cast a light area and appear radiopaque on the film.

PRINCIPLES OF IMAGE PROJECTION

The purpose of the receptor is to capture the image of the exposed area of interest. Certain principles of image projection are required to follow, whether the operator is using a digital receptor or conventional film. The purpose of these principles is to obtain the best possible image of the area of interest and called principles of projection geometry. These principles are related to use and direction of the source of X-rays (focal spot), film placement and object orientation. These principles can be summarized as follows:

Principle 1: It states that the X-rays should be emitted from the smallest area of focal spot as possible. The smaller the focal spot, the greater is the resolution of the resultant image. However, the size of focal spot is fixed for the machines and it cannot be changed by the operator. Periodic quality check is required to evaluate the focal spot. Resolution test devices can identify the focal spot size and indicate the need to replace the tube head.

Principle 2: It states that the focal spot-to-object distance should be as long as possible. The focal spot-to-object distance refers to the distance between the focal spot and the object to be imaged. The use of a long cone or position indicating device allows X-ray photons to travel in a straight line generating an accurate image. The more the X-ray photons travelling in straight line, the less divergent the X-ray beam will be and more sharper the resultant image will be.

Principle 3: This principle states that the object-to-receptor distance should be as minimal as possible. Here the object refers to area of interest or the tooth and its surrounding structures that are being exposed. The closer the area of interest to the image receptor/film, the lesser will be the magnification and greater will be the image sharpness.

Principle 4: In this principle, the film and long axis of the object (tooth) should be parallel to each other. This minimizes the shape distortion of the radiographic image as in the paralleling technique.

Principle 5: This principle suggests that the X-ray beam should be directed perpendicular to the long axis of the tooth and receptor.

Principle 6: There should be no movement of the tube, film or patient during exposure.

Inference

In bisecting angle or short cone technique the film is placed in close proximity with the tooth. However, it does not follow to the fourth principle and the resultant image is more prone to shape distortion (deviation from the actual shape or dimension of the object). The bisecting angle technique is considered a secondary method but may be a necessary compromise in certain clinical situations. Further, in this technique fifth principle is not followed as vertical angulation is operator sensitive. Therefore, resultant image will appear either foreshortened (shorter than the actual object) or elongated (longer than the actual object) when increase or decrease in vertical angulation respectively.

In paralleling technique, the object to film distance is increased as parallel orientation of the film is difficult due to anatomic shape or palate and mandible. However the amount of magnification in resultant image is acceptable.

VISUAL CHARACTERISTICS

As discussed earlier, density and contrast are visual characteristics of the radiographic image and directly influence the diagnostic quality of a radiographic image. Let us understand about their role in image interpretation.

Density

Density can be defined as the overall blackness or darkness of a dental radiograph. When a dental radiograph is mounted on the viewbox, the light is transmitted through the transparent areas on the film. These transparent areas on the radiographic image are formed due to distribution of black silver particles in the emulsion. Darker areas represent heavier deposits of black silver particles and this degree of silver blackening is termed as density.

Adequate density is required to visualize images of teeth and surrounding structures. If the image appears too dark or too light, it is difficult to separate the objects in the film visually. A radiograph with the optimal density enables to view the black areas formed due to air spaces, the white areas resulted from enamel, dentin, and bone; and the gray areas produced by soft tissue (Fig. 30.1).

Factors directly affecting the density of a dental radiograph include the exposure factors and the thickness of the subject. Any increase or decrease in exposure factors individually or in combination influences the density of radiograph (Table 30.1).

Exposure Factors

Milliamperage (mA): Although modern dental X-ray machines do not permit adjustment of mA certain machines may allow for adjustment. As mA is directly proportional to quantity of X-ray photons, increasing mA will result in more number of photons reaching the film and will increase density. On contrary, if mA is decreased, the radiograph will appear lighter.

Kilovoltage Peak (kVp): The quality or the energy (penetration power) of X-ray beam is governed by kVp. An increase in kVp will increase density by producing photons of higher energy. On the other hand, if kilovoltage is decreased, the radiograph will appear lighter.

Exposure time: Density is directly proportional to exposure time. An increase in exposure time will increase density as the number of photons that reach the film are increased. The longer the exposure time, the more will be the film exposure and darker the image.

Although in the above discussion the mA and the exposure time are discussed separately the amount of radiation reaching the film and hence the film density is controlled by product milliamperage and second (mAs) rather than by their individual values.

Subject thickness: Increase in the thickness of soft tissue (buccal fat) or density of bone will increase the attenuation of X-ray beam and fewer photons will reach the film producing lighter image. If the exposure parameters set for children are used in adult patient, the radiograph will have less density as thickness of the adult tissue is more.

Adjustments in setting of kVp, mA, or exposure time should be made to compensate for variations in subject thickness.

Subject density: Distinctions in the density of the structures in subject influence the resultant radiographic image. The greater the density of a structure, the greater the attenuation of the X-ray photons will occur. The relative densities of various dental structures, in order of decreasing density are enamel, dentin and cementum. Metallic restorations have higher density than enamel and therefore completely attenuate the X-ray photons (Fig. 30.1).

Contrast

The difference in the degrees of darkness (densities) between adjacent areas on a dental radiograph is termed contrast. It is the difference in densities between adjacent

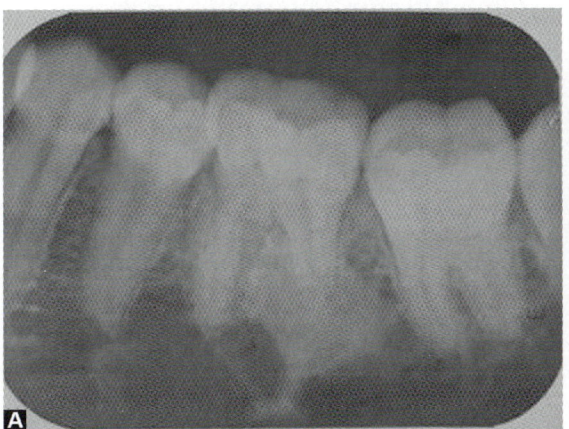 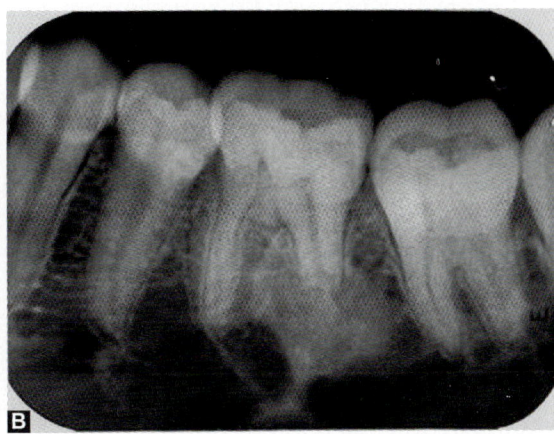

Figs. 30.1A and B: Image A is having lower density than image B

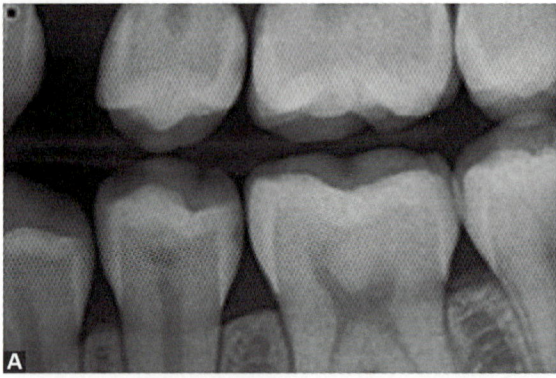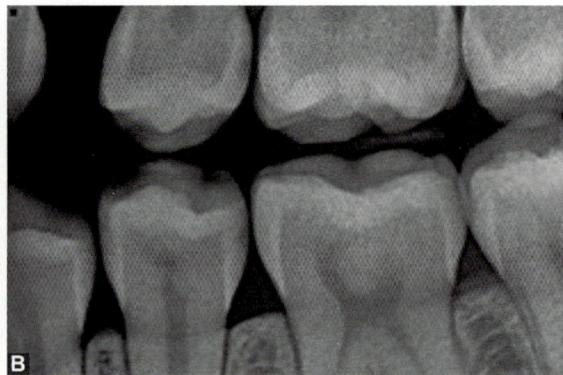

Fig. 30.2A and B: (A) Bitewing radiograph revealing low contrast and (B) high contrast

areas. In other words, it tells us how well can we differentiate between the light and dark areas from each other. For instance, when considering two areas like pulp chamber and dentin, if there is just a small difference in density, then they do not really stand out from each other (low contrast). On the other hand, if the difference in densities is more, they are clearly defined from each other (high contrast).

Contrast can also be described as the differences in the amount of light transmitted through neighboring areas of radiographic image. On a viewbox, an image with very dark areas and very light areas is said to have high contrast wherein the dark and light areas are remarkably different. On contrary, image with many shades of gray is said to have low contrast.

One should attempt to obtain an image between low contrast and high contrast. The general contrast of a dental radiograph is governed by film contrast, and by the subject contrast (area of subject radiographed).

Film contrast: Film contrast is affected by the inherent qualities of the film which are directly controlled by the manufacturer. Further the conditions for processing the film also govern the film contrast; however, it can be very well controlled by the operator. The developing time, the temperature and strength of the developing solution can affect the film contrast. Increase in time and/or temperature of developing will increase the contrast of the film (Fig. 30.2).

Subject contrast: The characteristics of the subject do influence radiographic contrast and include thickness, density, and composition (atomic number) of the subject. Subject contrast can be changed by increasing or decreasing the kilovoltage. Subject contrast is inversely related to kilovoltage. When a high kVp is selected, subject contrast decreases, and many shades of gray are visible on the image. Equally, with low kVp, high subject contrast is obtained and black and white areas are seen on the image. Increasing or decreasing the exposure time with keeping constant kVp, can influence the subject contrast (Table 30.1).

GEOMETRIC CHARACTERISTICS

Geometric characteristics of the radiographic image influence the diagnostic quality of a dental radiograph and they need to be minimized to obtain an accurate image. These geometric characteristics include image sharpness, magnification and distortion.

Umbra is defined as that part of the shadow when all light is absorbed, or area of total darkness.

Penumbra is that part of the shadow of an object which is larger than a point and yet represents a single point of the object. It is thus the unsharpness of the image.

TABLE 30.1: Factors affecting density and contrast

Parameter	Influencing factor	Effect of influencing factor	
Density	Miliampere (mA) Kilovoltage (kVp) Exposure time (S) Subject thickness	$\uparrow$ mA = $\uparrow$ D $\uparrow$ kVp = $\uparrow$ D $\uparrow$ S = $\uparrow$ D $\uparrow$ Thickness = $\downarrow$ D	$\downarrow$ mA = $\downarrow$ D $\downarrow$ kVp = $\downarrow$ D $\downarrow$ S = $\downarrow$ D $\downarrow$ Thickness = $\downarrow$ D
Contrast	Kilovoltage (kVp)	$\uparrow$ kVp = Low contrast	$\downarrow$ kVp = High contrast

Legends: D—density, $\downarrow$ — decrease, $\uparrow$ — increase

Sharpness

Image sharpness can be defined as the characteristic of the film to reproduce the distinct outlines between adjacent objects. It is also referred to as resolution or definition of the image and contributes to image clarity. However, a certain amount of unsharpness does occur in every dental image. The indistinct, unclear area generally occurs at the edges of a radiographic image. For radiographic diagnosis, it is desired to get images with high sharpness and resolution.

The sharpness of an image is influenced by the factors like focal spot size, film composition and movement.

Focal spot size: Focal spot, target of the anode, produces X-ray photons when high speed electrons are bombarded from the cathode of X-ray tube. As photons originate from all points over the surface of focal spot and travel in straight line, their projection of any portion of the object do not register at the same location on the image receptor. This results in blurring of the edge of the object radiographed and contributes to unsharpness of the image. This suggests that image sharpness is related to the size of the focal spot. As the size of the focal spot reduces, the sharpness will increase.

Ideally, it can be expected that if the target of the anode is a single point source, no unsharpness will be present in the image. But as the limitations in capacity of X-ray machine, a single point source cannot be created.

Figure 30.3 shows the direction of X-ray beam originating at the margins of the focal spot and provides an image of the edges of an object. The resulting blurred zone of unsharpness on an image causes a loss in image clarity by reducing sharpness and resolution. The larger the focal spot area, the greater the loss of clarity.

Film composition: The size of the silver halide crystals in the film emulsion impacts sharpness of radiographic image. As the crystal size increases, the speed of the film increases relatively. So, the slower films produce sharper image than the faster films. However, the radiation exposure to patient is relatively higher in slower films, thus the amount of unsharpness in faster films can be acceptable.

Motion blur: Movement in X-ray tube head, the film, or the patient during exposure affects image sharpness. Patient movement can be minimized by stabilizing the patient's head with the chair head rest during exposure. Use of a higher mA and kVp and correspondingly shorter exposure times also help to minimize motion blur.

MAGNIFICATION (SIZE DISTORTION)

When a radiographic image appears larger in dimensions than the actual size of the object, it is termed as magnification. Magnification results from the divergent paths of the X-ray beams, as they radiate from the focal spot. Because of these diverging paths, some degree of image magnification is present in every dental radiograph. Factors influencing image magnification include focal spot–film distance and object–film distance (Fig. 30.4).

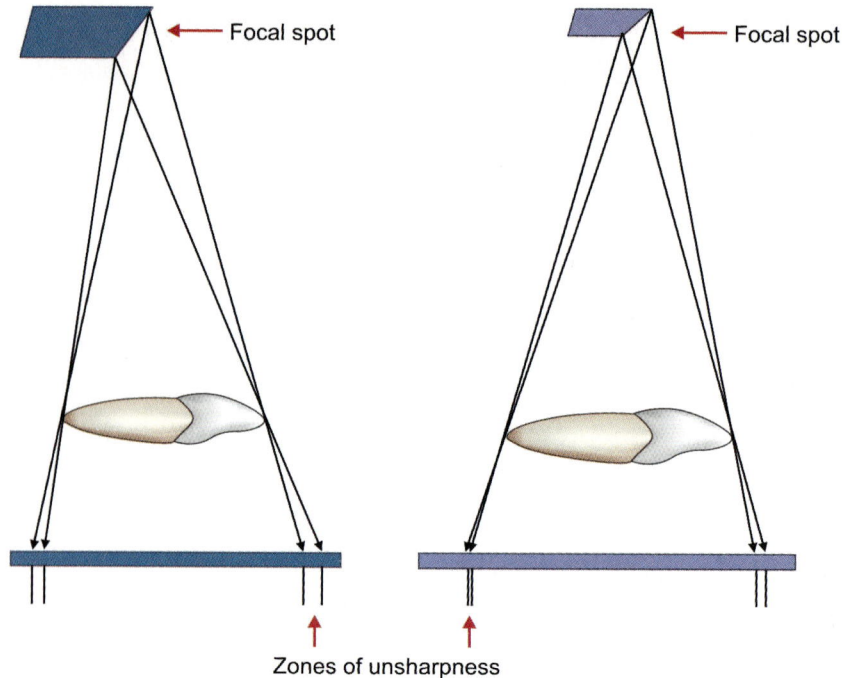

Zones of unsharpness

Fig. 30.3: Photons originating at different places on the focal spot result in a zone of unsharpness on the radiograph. On the left a large focal spot size results in a wide zone of unsharpness compared with a small focal spot size on the left that results in a narrow zone of unsharpness.

Focal spot–film distance: The focal spot–film distance (FSFD) is the distance between the source of X-rays and the film. This distance is determined by the length of the position-indicating device (PID). Use of long PID enables the central beam to strike the object while eliminating divergent X-rays from the periphery of the beam. This results in less image magnification. Use of shorter PID will result in more image magnification.

Object–film distance: The object–film distance is the distance between the object to be imaged (the tooth) and the film. The object to film distance should always be as close as possible. As the distance will increase, there will be more magnification.

SHAPE DISTORTION

Shape distortion is an unequal magnification of the object and will have variation in size and shape. Incorrect alignment of film and beam angulation are the influencing factors.

Object–film alignment: As stated in the principles of shadow casting, the object and film must be parallel to each other. If there is an angular relationship, the resultant image will have shape distortion due to unequal distance between parts of the object and the film.

X-ray beam angulation: The X-ray beam must be directed perpendicular to the object and film. This helps in record the images of adjacent structures in their actual three-dimensional relationships.

Paralleling versus Bisecting Angle Technique

The primary objective of dental radiography is to acquire a near accurate image of teeth and their adjacent structures. In bisecting angle technique, the film is placed as

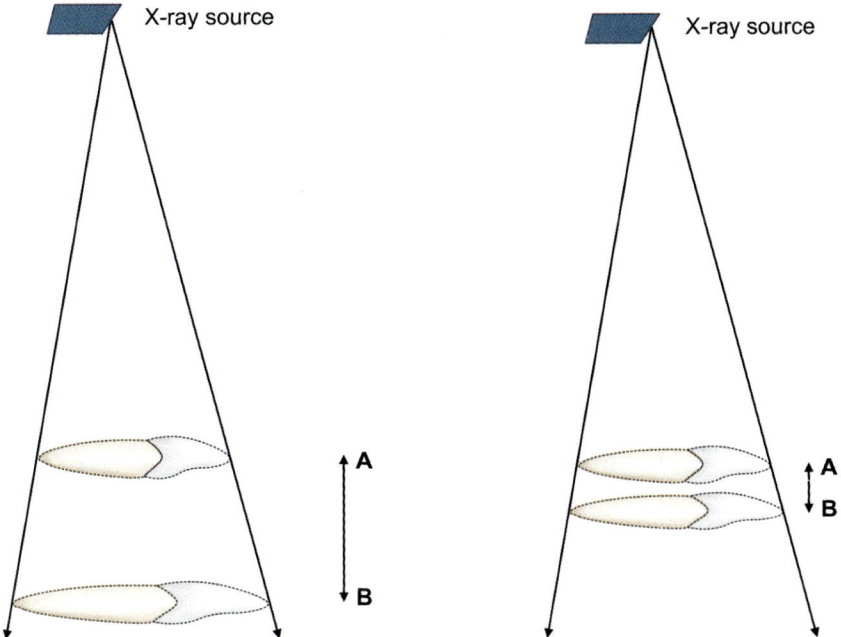

Fig. 30.4: Increase in the film to object distance (A–B) causes image magnification (image on the left)

closed to the tooth as possible without any film deformation and the central rays are perpendicular to the bisector of long axis of tooth and the film. The image so obtained can exhibit shape distortion although the size of the image may be near accurate. As discussed earlier, the distance between apex of the tooth and the film will be more than the crown and the film that will add to shape distortion. Further, use of more positive angle for central beam will result in shorter length of the image and is termed as foreshortening and using less positive angle will result in image elongation (Fig. 30.5).

In paralleling technique, the object and the film are placed parallel to each other, while the central rays are perpendicular to both. This orientation helps to minimize the shape distortion of the image. However, the operator has to place the film in the middle of the oral cavity to obtain parallel position with the tooth and causes increase in the distance between them. This leads to the image magnification and loss of image sharpness. Nonetheless, this technique

uses long cone or long PID, it helps to overcome these shortcomings by directing more parallel and central rays of the beam perpendicular to the film and the tooth. Availability of sophisticated film holding and beam aligning devices have made this technique very simplified. Thus paralleling technique is recommended over bisecting angle technique.

LOCALIZATION TECHNIQUES

Radiographs are two-dimensional images of three-dimensional structures; they only provide antero-posterior and supero-inferior aspect. Therefore, missing buccal-lingual dimensions or depth of the object, sometimes necessitate localizing impacted teeth or foreign materials in the jaws. Change in angulation of X-ray tube head for making another projection at right angle can help to delineate these structures. Such a technique used is known as object localization technique to provide a three-dimensional view. These projections can be

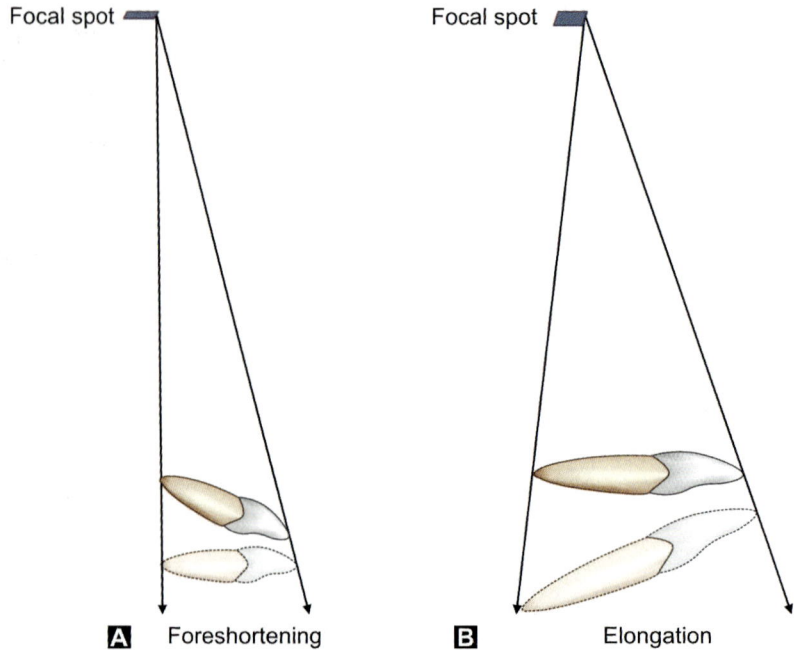

A Foreshortening   **B**   Elongation

Fig. 30.5A and B: Image A shows foreshortening (central rays perpendicular to film and object is not parallel to film), image B shows elongation (central rays perpendicular to object but not to the film)

Parameter	Affecting factor	Consequences of affecting factor	
TABLE 30.2: Factors affecting sharpness, magnification and distortion			
Sharpness	✗ Focal spot size ✗ Film composition ✗ Motion	✗ ↑ Size = ↓ Sharpness ✗ ↑ Size = ↓ Sharpness ✗ ↑ Motion = ↓ Sharpness	✗ ↓ Size = ↑ Sharpness ✗ ↓ Size = ↑ Sharpness ✗ ↓ Motion = ↑ Sharpness
Magnification	✗ Target–film distance ✗ Object–film distance	✗ ↑ Distance = ↓ Magnification ✗ ↑ Distance = ↑ Magnification	✗ ↓ Distance = ↑ Magnification ✗ ↓ Distance = ↓ Magnification
Distortion	✗ Object–film alignment ✗ X-ray beam angulation	✗ Object-film parallel = ↓ distortion ✗ Beam perpendicular to object and receptor = ↓ distortion	✗ Object-film not parallel = ↑ distortion ✗ Beam not perpendicular to object and receptor = ✗ ↑ distortion
Legends: ↓ — decrease, ↑ — increase			

helpful in treatment planning for removal of impacted teeth, during endodotic procedures to localize root canal and trauma. There are two basic techniques used to localize objects and are as follows:

- Tube shift technique
- Right angle technique

Tube Shift Technique

The tube shift technique or Clark's rule is used for object localization, when there is need to ensure the location of the object either buccal or lingual (buccal-object rule). This is an easy to use method for dental practitioner and can be carried out by using standard periapical radiography. To establish the apparent buccal to lingual relationship between two structures which are superimposed on standard periapical radiograph, a second radiograph should be taken with a different horizontal angulation. One should keep all parameters (like point of entry, film position, and vertical angulation) same for the second exposure, except that the X-ray tube is shifted about 20° either mesially or distally (Fig. 30.6).

On comparison between two radiographs, we can observe that the object has moved in the opposite direction from initial place due to tube shift in second film. If the tube is shifted mesially in horizontal plane, the object will appear to have moved mesially. On contrary, a distal shift will result in mesial movement of the object. Therefore, this method is termed buccal-object rule and the key phrase is "same lingual, opposite buccal" which is short formed as SLOB.

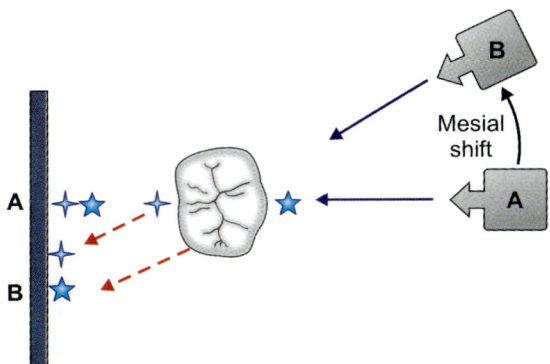

Fig. 30.6: Buccal-object rule. Position A is a standard radiograph showing overlap. As the tube position is shifted to mesial (position B), the buccal object (star) is moved relatively in the opposite direction, distally.

Right-angle Technique

This technique uses two radiographic projections taken at right angles to each other, for example, first a periapical view and then an occlusal view of the same area.

This technique is used to locate an object in the third dimension. For instance, in a radiograph showing impacted tooth, one can visualize mesial or distal location of impaction and its vertical position from the alveolar crest, but the depth in the bone in a buccal-lingual dimension is difficult to differentiate. In right-angle technique, the central ray is directed at an angle of 90° to the primary film. Thus, an occlusal radiograph at 90° angulation will provide buccal-lingual dimensions of impacted tooth that was found on periapical radiograph.

EGG SHELL EFFECT

It is an appearance of corticated structures of the jaws on the radiographs, as the image projected is a three-dimensional volume on a two-dimensional receptor. The top photon has a tangential and a much longer path through the shell of the egg than the lower photon. The lower photon strikes the surface of the egg at right angles and travels through two thicknesses of the shell. So, photons travelling at periphery are more attenuated than photons travelling at right angles to the surface. This eggshell effect demonstrates why normal structures such as lamina dura, border of maxillary sinuses and nasal fossa as well as abnormal structures such as corticated walls of cysts and benign tumors are well demonstrated. Soft tissue structures (such as nose) do not show eggshell effect, as they are not composed of a dense layer surrounding soft tissue core.

FREQUENTLY ASKED QUESTIONS

Write a short note on:

1. Principle of projection geometry
2. Image characteristics
3. Object localization

BIBLIOGRAPHY

1. White SC, Pharoah MJ. Oral Radiology: Principles and Interpretation. 6th edition. St. Louis, Mo: Mosby/Elsevier, 2009

2. Iannucci JM, Howerton LJ. Dental Radiography: Principles and Techniques, 4th edition. St. Louis, Mo: Elsevier Saunders, 2012.

3. Whaites E. Essentials of Dental Radiography and Radiology. 5th edition. Edinburgh: Churchill Livingstone, 2007.

4. Meredith WJ, Massey JB. Fundamental Physics of Radiology. 3rd edition. John Wright and Sons Ltd. 1977.

5. Frommer HH, Stabulas-Savage JJ. Radiology for the Dental Professional. 9th Edition. St. Louis, Elsevier Mosby 2011.

6. Reynolds T. Basic Guide to Dental Radiography 1st edition. John Wiley and Sons, 2016.

7. Watanabe PCA, Camargo AJ, Pardini LC. Radiographic Density and Contrast of Images of Individual Films from Double Film Packets. Cosmetol and Oro Facial Surg 2016; 2: 110.

8. Barnes GT. Contrast and Scatter in X-ray Imaging. RadioGraphics 1991; 11:307–23

9. Campos GM, Tamburus JR. A Method to Evaluate and Compare Roentenograms. Braz Dent J, 1991; 2: 95–102.

10. American Dental Association Council on Scientific Affairs: An Update on Radiographic Practices: Information and Recommendations, J Am Dent Assoc. 132:234–38.

11. Nikneshan S, Hosseinzadeh M, Dehghanpourbarooj M, Kheirkhahi M. Localization of Impacted Maxillary Canine Teeth: A Comparison between Panoramic and Buccal Object Rule in Intraoral Radiography. J Dent Sch. 2017; 35(1): 31–40.

Intraoral Radiographic Techniques

INTRODUCTION

Radiographs are two-dimensional image of three dimensional objects. Intra oral radiographic technique is mainly to show all the teeth and surrounding structures apical to the teeth. In these techniques a radiographic film is placed near the area to be radiographed and exposed to X-rays, in a radiographic film almost 3–4 teeth can be seen.

Types of intraoral radiographic techniques
1. **Periapical radiographs:** It shows teeth and the periapical area of the teeth to be radiographed.
2. **Bitewing radiographs:** It shows crowns of the maxillary and mandibular teeth to be radiographed and the adjacent alveolar crests.
3. **Occlusal radiographs:** Where occlusal films are placed between the occlusal surfaces of the teeth with the central beam directed at 90° or at 50–60° to the plane of the film depending on the area of maxilla or mandible is to be visualized.

Periapical radiographs should show all of a tooth and surrounding bone. To ensure diagnostic quality radiographs one must properly align the X-ray film, the area to be radiographed, and the position indicating device of the X-ray machine. Alignment can be accomplished by using either the parallel film placement (paralleling technique/long cone technique), or the bisecting angle technique (short cone technique).

Indications for Periapical Radiographs

- To detect dental caries
- Assessment of periodontal status/diseases
- Evaluation of periapical infection
- Evaluation of cysts and tumor
- Post trauma to the teeth and associated alveolar bone
- Assessment of unerupted teeth
- Evaluation of root morphology before extraction
- During endodontic procedures
- Preoperative and postoperative implant surgery

There are two techniques used to take periapical radiographs
a. The bisecting angle technique or short cone technique
b. The paralleling or long cone technique

THE BISECTING ANGLE TECHNIQUE OR SHORT CONE TECHNIQUE

Bisecting angle technique is based on the geometric principle that states that two triangles are equal, if they have two equal angles and a common side. This is called Dr. Cieszynski's rule of isometry **(Fig. 31.1)**. When rule of isometry is used in dental radiography, it is used to determine the correct vertical angulation of the cone (PID).

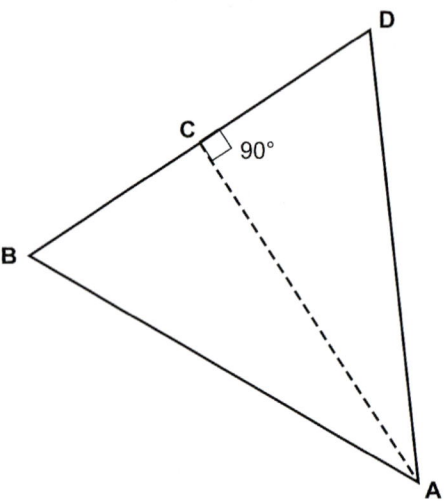

Fig. 31.1: Cieszynski's rule of isometry

Basic Concepts

* The film is placed as close as possible to the tooth of interest to be radiographed.
* Film should not be bent.
* The angle formed between the long axis of the tooth and the long axis of the film packet should be assessed and bisected.
* The X-ray tube head is positioned at right angle to this bisecting line with the central ray of the X-ray beam aimed through the tooth apex **(Fig. 31.2)** .

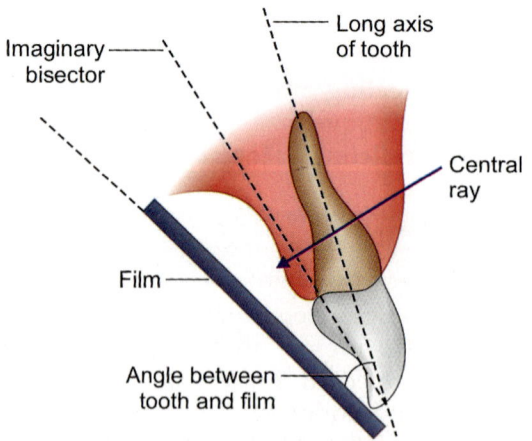

Fig. 31.2: Angle formed between the long axis of the tooth and the long axis of the film packet

* Using the geometrical principle, actual tooth length will be equal to the length of image of the tooth on the film.

Vertical Angulation of X-ray Tube Head

Refers to the positioning of the PID in vertical direction or in up and down plane. It differs according to the technique used in short cone technique; the vertical angulation is determined by the imaginary bisector. The central ray is directed perpendicular to imaginary bisector.

The angle formed by the continuing line of the central ray until it meets the occlusal plane determines the vertical angulation of the X-ray beam to the occlusal plane.

If the central ray is directed perpendicular to tooth (decreased vertical angulation), an elongation is seen **(Fig. 31.9)**.

If the central ray is directed perpendicular to the imaginary bisector → ideal image is seen **(Fig. 31.11)**

If the central ray is directed perpendicular to the film (increased vertical angulation), a foreshortening is seen **(Fig. 31.10)**.

Horizontal Angulation of X-ray Tube Head

In the horizontal plane, the central ray should be aimed through the interproximal area to avoid overlapping of the teeth. Horizontal angulation is determined by the shape of the arch and size of the teeth **(Fig. 31.3)**.

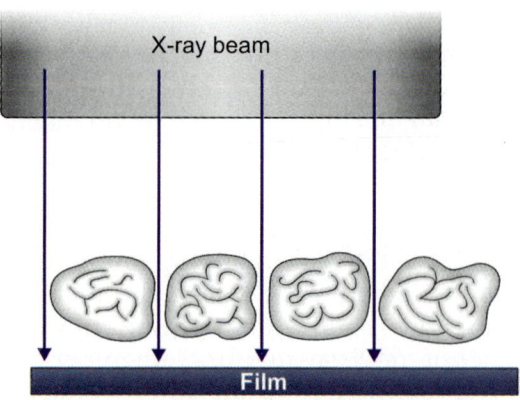

Fig. 31.3: Proper horizontal angulation

Incorrect horizontal angulation → Overlapping of the teeth will be seen (Fig. 31.4).

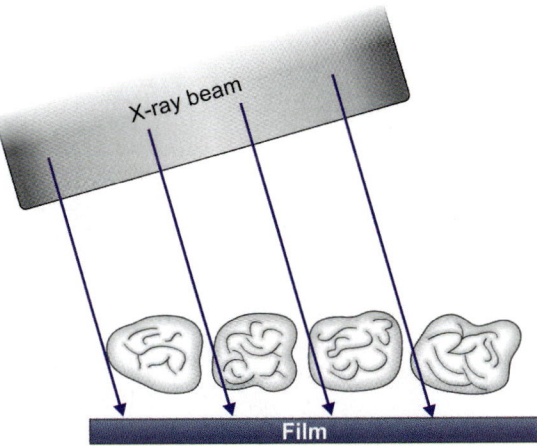

Fig. 31.4: Incorrect horizontal angulation

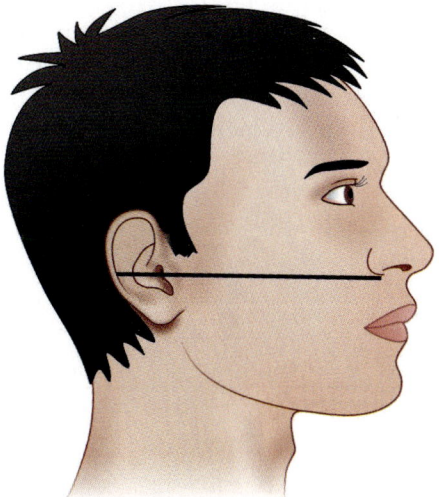

Fig. 31.5: Patient head position during maxillary arch projection

Radiographic film used
Size 2 is the size of intraoral film used.

Film holders used for bisecting angle technique
1. Rinn XCP instruments
2. Snap-A-Ray
3. Rinn greene stable disposable film holder
4. Rinn greene bite block

PROCEDURE OF BISECTING ANGLE TECHNIQUE

Patient Positioning

- Procedure to be explained to the patient.
- Patient should be seated in upright position.
- Patient head should be positioned in such a way that the arch to be radiographed should be parallel to the floor and the mid-sagittal plane should be perpendicular to the floor (Figs 31.5 and 31.6)
- Lead apron and thyroid collar should to placed.
- Metal objects should be removed in and around the jaws.

Film Placement

Radiographic film should be placed to cover the tooth of interest to be radiographed.

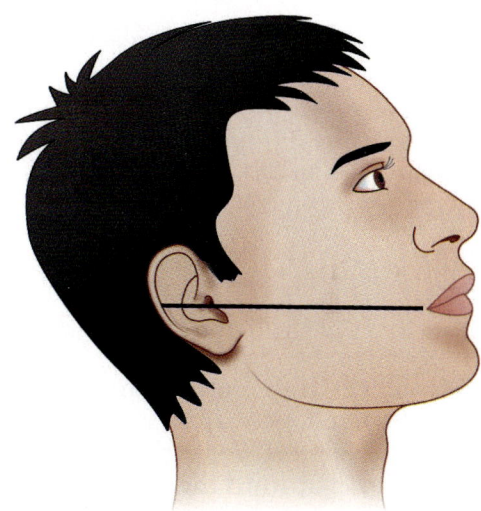

Fig. 31.6: Patient head position during mandibular arch projection

Film Position

- Film should be placed against the lingual surface of the tooth. The occlusal/incisal end of the film must extend approximately 1/8th inch above the incisal/occlusal surface of the tooth.
- If the film holder is not used, patient is asked to hold the film gently against the cervical portion of the tooth.

Positioning the PID

- **Vertical angulations** (Fig. 31.7) should be proper in the bisecting angle technique. Angulations are mentioned in **Table 31.1**.

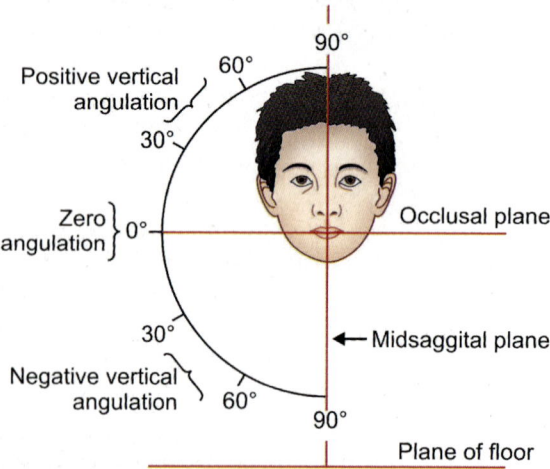

Fig. 31.7: Positive and negative vertical angulations

Table 31.1: Vertical angulation

Projection	Maxilla	Mandible
Incisors	+40	−15
Canines	+45	−20
Premolars	+30	−10
Molars	+20	−5

- **Positive vertical angulation:** It is the angulation in downward direction.
- **Negative vertical angulation:** It is the angulation in upward direction.
- Horizontal angulations should be 0°.

Point of Entry (Figs 31.12 and 31.13)

- The X-ray beam should be directed through the center of the area of interest. Point of entry is different for different teeth in the upper and lower jaws.
- Maxillary central incisors and lateral incisors: Tip of the nose.
- *Maxillary canines:* Ala of the nose.
- *Maxillary premolars:* Point of intersection of ala-tragus line and a perpendicular line from the pupil of the eye.

- *Maxillary molars:* Point of intersection of ala-tragus line and perpendicular line from outer canthus of the eye.

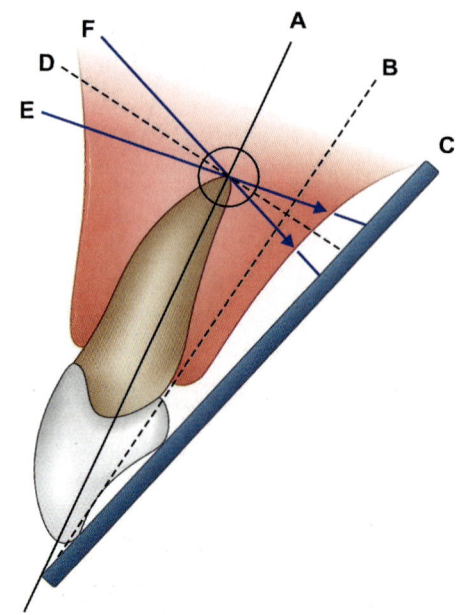

Fig. 31.8: Depicting ideal positioning of tooth and film. **A.** Long axis of the tooth **B.** Imaginary bisector. **C.** Long axis of the tooth. **D.** Central ray is perpendicular to the long axis of imaginary bisector. **E.** Central ray is perpendicular to the long axis of tooth causing elongation of the resultant image. **F.** Central ray is perpendicular to the long axis of the film causing foreshortening of the resultant image

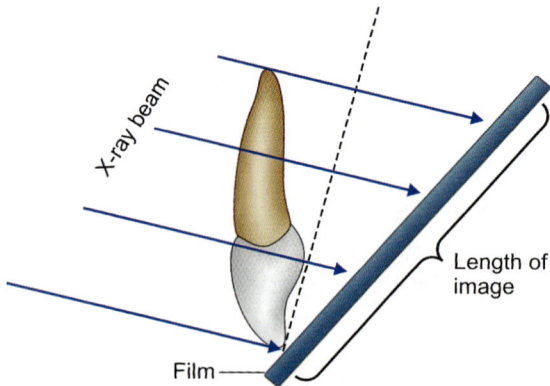

Fig. 31.9: Central ray perpendicular to the long axis of tooth causing elongation of the resultant image

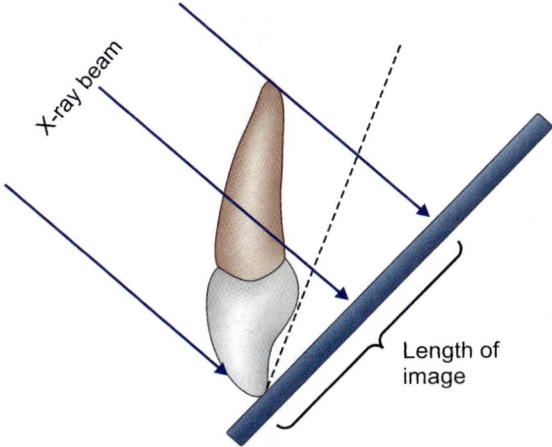

Fig. 31.10: Central ray perpendicular to the long axis of the film causing foreshortening of the resultant image

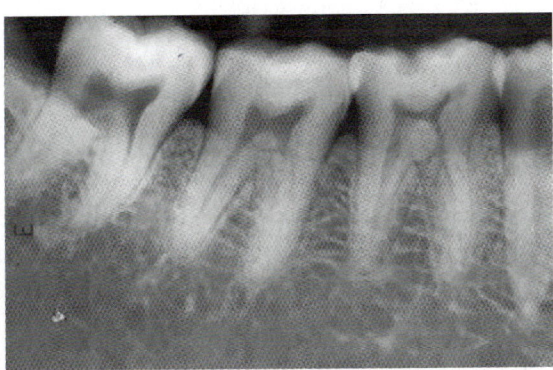

Fig. 31.11: IOPA radiograph in bisecting angle technique

* *Maxillary third molars:* Point of intersection of ala-tragus line and perpendicular line from distal to the outer canthus of the eye.
* *Mandibular central incisors and lateral incisors:* Tip of the chin.
* *Maxillary canines:* Point of intersection of 0.5 mm above the lower border of the mandible to a perpendicular line from the pupil of the eye.
* *Maxillary premolars:* Point of intersection of 0.5 mm above the lower border of the mandible to perpendicular line from distal to the outer canthus of the eye.

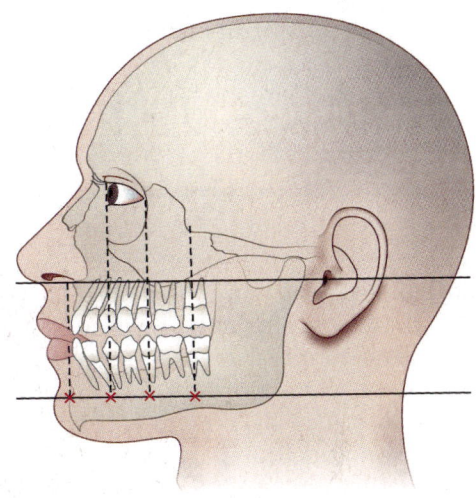

Fig. 31.13: Point of entry for mandibular teeth projection

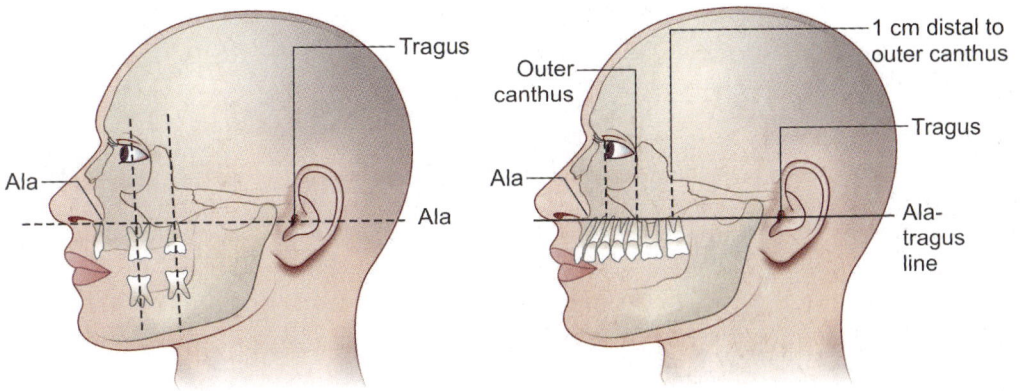

Fig. 31.12: Point of entry for maxillary teeth projection

× *Maxillary molars:* Point of intersection of 0.5 mm above the lower border of the mandible to perpendicular line from the outer canthus of the eye.

× *Maxillary third molars:* Point of intersection of 0.5 mm above the lower border of the mandible perpendicular line from distal to the outer canthus of the eye.

Advantages

× Positioning of the film is comfortable.
× Method is simple and quick.
× If angulations are correct, ideal image will be formed.

Disadvantages

× Incorrect angulation—image will be distorted.
× Cone cut and foreshortening of buccal roots are common.

THE PARALLELING OR LONG CONE TECHNIQUE

The paralleling technique is a standard for intraoral radiographic technique. It has many diagnostic advantages. The paralleling technique requires holders that align the radiographic film at a right angle to the central beam and thus parallel to the tooth axis.

Basic Concepts

× Radiographic film packet is placed in the film holder and positioned in the mouth parallel to the long axis of the tooth which is the area of interest.
× The central ray of the X-ray beam should be directed perpendicular or at right angle to both log axis of the tooth and the radiographic film.
× To achieve parallelism between the film and the long axis of the tooth object to film distance should be increased.
× To avoid unsharpness and magnification source to film distance should be increased, so long cone (16 inches PID) is used.

Film holders used for paralleling technique

1. Rinn XCP instruments
2. Snap-A-Ray
3. Eezee grip film holder
4. Stable disposable film holder
5. Rectangular collimating instrument

Procedure for Paralleling Cone Technique

× Selection of correct film holder should be done for the appropriate size of the radiographic film according to the tooth of interest to be radiographed.

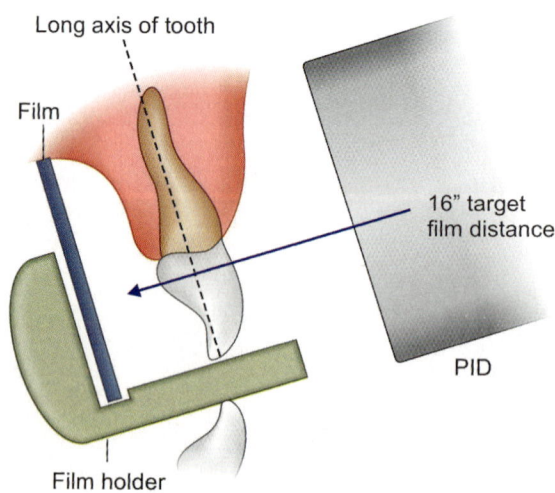

Long axis of tooth

Film

16" target film distance

PID

Film holder

Fig. 31.14: Technique for paralleling or long cone method

× White surface of the film packet should always face the X-ray tube head.
× Patient should be positioned with the head supported and occlusal plane horizontal to the floor.
× Film holder and film packet are placed in oral cavity as follows:
   a. **Maxillary incisors and canines:** Film should be placed sufficiently posterior to enable its height to be accommodated in the palatal vault.
   b. **Maxillary premolars and molars:** Film packet should be placed in the midline of the palate to accommodate its height in the palatal vault.
   c. **Mandibular incisors and canines:** Film packet should be placed on the floor of the mouth, approximately covering incisors and canine teeth.

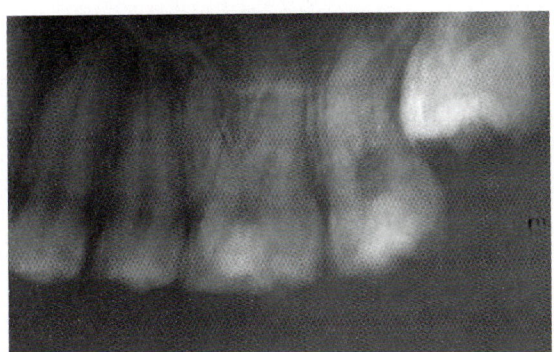

Fig. 31.15: IOPA radiograph in paralleling cone technique

   d. **Mandibular premolars and molars:** Film packet should be placed in the lingual sulcus next to the appropriate tooth to be radiographed.
× Patient should be asked to bite gently to stabilize the film holder in position.
× The aiming rings moved down the indicator rod until it contacts the patient's face.
× Next the position indicating the device is aligned with the aiming ring this will automatically set the vertical angulation as well as horizontal angulation and centers the X-ray beam on the film packet.
× Later exposure should be made.

TABLE 31.2: Comparison between bisecting angle technique and paralleling cone technique

Bisecting angle technique	Paralleling cone technique
× Also known as short cone technique	× Also known as long cone technique and right angle technique
× Central ray is perpendicular to an imaginary bisector plane between the long axis of the tooth and image receptor	× Central ray is perpendicular to the long axis of the tooth
× Film is placed as close to the tooth as possible	× Film is placed parallel to the long axis of the tooth
× Vertical angulation is different for different teeth	× Vertical angulation is zero
× Patient's finger is used to hold the film, unnecessary radiation exposure	× Difficult for distal molar as film holders are used
× Elongation and foreshortening of the images is possible with variation in the vertical angulation.	× Less chances of elongation and foreshortening, as it is guided by aiming ring (geometrically accurate images)
× Bending of the film is common	× Bending of the film is uncommon
× Shadow of the alveolar bone fills the interproximal spaces	× Alveolar crest is seen in the true relationship with the teeth
× Superimposition of zygomatic arch on the molar teeth	× Superimposition of zygomatic arch on the molar teeth will not be seen
× Cone cut is common	× Uncommon
× Distortion of the film occurs due to bending of the film	× Bending of the film is not possible as film holders are used.
× Images are not reproducible	× Images formed are reproducible

Advantages
* Geometrically accurate images are formed
* Periodontal bone level is well appreciated.
* Periapical area is well appreciated.
* Angulation is automatically determined by the PID.

Disadvantages
* Positioning of the film holders are technique sensitive.
* Positioning the film holders for lower 3rd molars are very difficult.

BITEWING RADIOGRAPHY

It is also called interproximal imaging. The image of bitewing radiograph includes the crown of maxillary and mandibular teeth and the alveolar crest. In this technique, the patient bites on a small wing attached to an intraoral film packet. Modern film holders have eliminated the need for the wing but terminology remains the same.

There are two types of bitewing radiographs—premolar bitewing and molar bitewing

Indications for bitewing radiography
1. Detection of interproximal caries
2. Monitoring the progression of dental caries
3. Detection of secondary caries
4. Evaluation of existing restoration
5. Assessment of periodontal status/crestal alveolar bone.

Advantages of bitewing radiography
1. Very simple
2. Not expensive
3. Tabs can be disposable/autoclavable
4. Can be used easily in pediatric patient.
5. Not much discomfort to the patient.

Disadvantages of bitewing radiography
1. Technique is operator dependent.
2. Radiographs are not accurately reproducible.
3. Cone cut is the most common.
4. Film packet can be displaced by the tongue

Basic principle of bitewing radiography
a. The film should be placed parallel to the crowns of both the upper and lower teeth in the area of interest (premolar region or molar region).
b. Patient should bite on bitewing tab or bitewing film holder to stabilize the film.
c. Central ray should be directed through the occlusal plane, using a vertical angulation of +10°.

Film Holder and Bitewing Tab

Film holders: Rinn XCP bitewing instruments include plastic bite blocks, plastic aiming rings and metal indicator arms.

Bitewing tab: It is a heavy paper board tab or loop fitted around a periapical film and used to stabilize the film during exposure (Fig. 31.16)

Films used: Size 0, size 1, size 2, size 3 films can be used for bitewing radiography.

Point of entry: The central ray should be directed through the occlusal plane of the teeth towards the center of the film packet.

Angulation of PID
* Horizontal angulation—central ray is directed perpendicular to the contact area of the teeth
* A vertical angulation of +10° is used.

Procedure
1. *Patient positioning*
   * Explain the procedure.
   * Seated upright
   * Head position to be adjusted in such a way that upper arch is parallel to the floor and midsagittal plane is perpendicular to the floor.
   * Lead apron and thyroid collar to be placed
2. *Film placement:* Film should cover the area of interest and stabilized by biting on the bitewing film holder or bitewing tab
3. *Film position:* Parallel to the crowns of both the upper and lower teeth.
4. *PID angulation:* + 10° vertical angulation (Fig. 31.17).

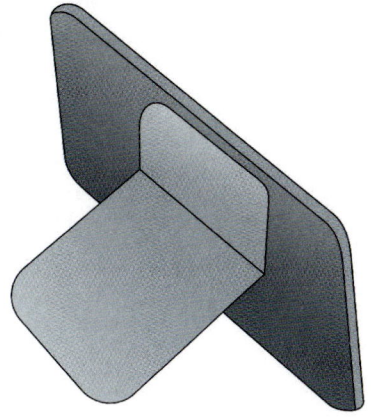

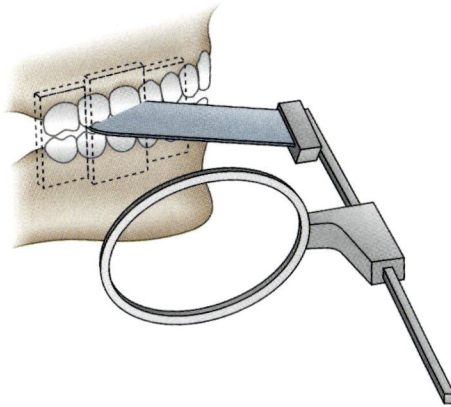

Fig. 31.16: Bitewing tab

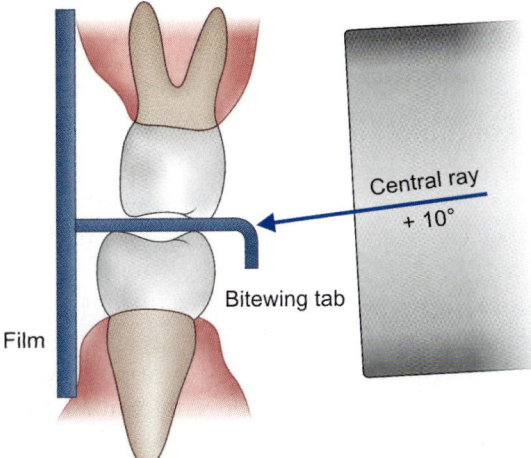

Fig. 31.17: Bitewing radiography with +10° vertical angulation

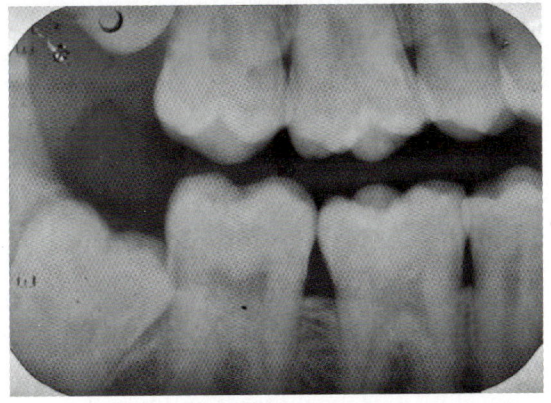

Fig. 31.18: Bitewing radiograph

5. *Exposure:* X-ray pointed towards the middle of the X-ray film.

OCCLUSAL RADIOGRAPHY

Occlusal radiography is an intraoral radiographic technique that shows a larger occlusal area of maxillary and mandibular arch. Used in patients who are unable to open mouth wide. Steep angulation used to determine the location of an object in all three dimensions. This technique is also called sandwich technique. This is an additional radiographic technique usually used along with periapical or bitewing radiograph.

Types of Occlusal Radiographs

Maxillary Arch

- Anterior maxillary occlusal projection (topographic anterior)
- Cross-sectional maxillary occlusal projection
- Lateral maxillary occlusal projection (oblique occlusal)

Mandibular Arch

- Anterior mandibular occlusal projection (topographic anterior)
- Cross-sectional mandibular occlusal projection (true occlusal)
- Lateral mandibular occlusal projection (oblique occlusal)

Indication for Occlusal Radiography

- To evaluate the patient with limited mouth opening
- Detecting the presence of unerupted teeth
- To localize the unerupted teeth—bucco-lingual position
- Evaluation of size and extent of cysts and tumors
- Evaluation of fractures of teeth and alveolar bone
- Evaluate the condition of maxillary sinus/antral floor
- Assessment of presence and position of sialolith
- To assess the buccolingual expansion of the body of the mandible.
- To evaluate cleft lip and cleft palate.

Basic Principles of Occlusal Radiography

- Radiographic film should be placed with the white side facing the arch to be radiographed.
- Radiographic film should be placed between the upper and the lower arch.
- Radiographic film should be stabilized by biting gently on the surface of the film.

Radiographic Films Used

Large receptors of size 57 × 76 mm are used, placed in the plane of occlusion and tube is positioned towards the jaw to be examined with steep angulations.

Procedure

Maxillary Occlusal Radiograph

Anterior maxillary occlusal projection (Figs 31.19 and 31.20)

- *Patient position:* Midsagittal plane should be perpendicular to the floor and occlusal plane should be parallel to the floor.
- *Film placement:* Radiographic film should be placed with the white surface of the film towards the maxilla.

- *Film positioning:* Radiographic film should be stabilized by gently closing the mouth and biting the film.
- *PID angulation:* +45° vertical angulation and 0° horizontal angulation
- *Point of entry:* Central ray should pass though the tip of the nose.
- *Exposure:* Exposed towards the middle of the X-ray film.

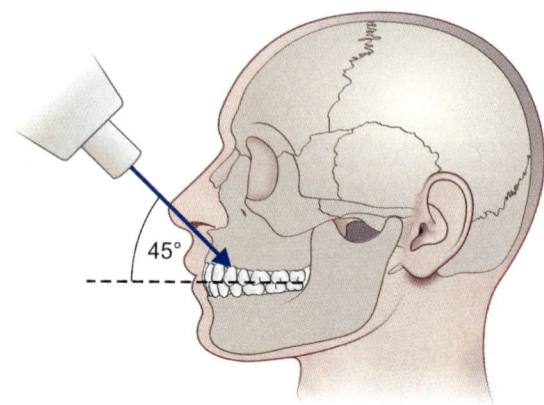

Fig. 31.19: Anterior maxillary occlusal projection

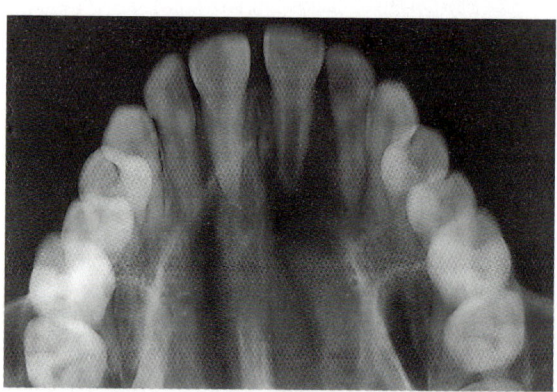

Fig. 31.20: Anterior maxillary occlusal radiograph

Cross-sectional occlusal projection view (Figs 31.21 and 31.22)

- *Patient position:* Midsagittal plane should be perpendicular to the floor and occlusal plane should be parallel to the floor.
- *Film placement:* Film should be placed with the white surface towards the maxilla with posterior border touching the ramus.

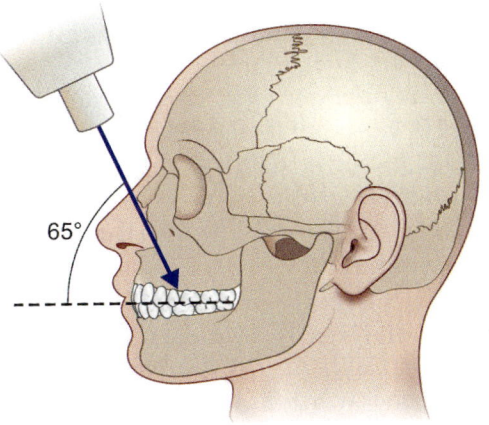

Fig. 31.21: Cross-sectional occlusal projection view

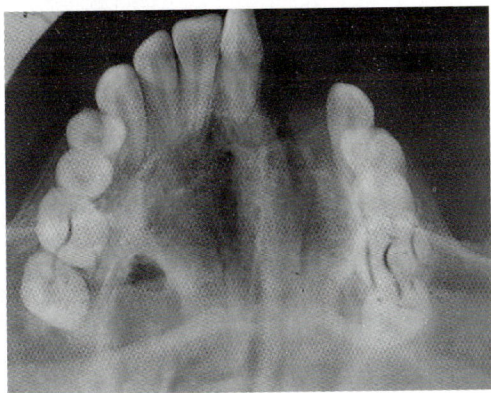

Fig. 31.22: Cross-sectional occlusal radiograph

the maxilla and lateral border of the film should be parallel with the buccal surface of the posterior teeth with extending 1 cm past the buccal cusp.

× *Film positioning:* Film should be stabilized by gently closing the mouth and biting the film.
× *PID angulation:* +60° vertical angulation and 0° horizontal angulation
× *Point of entry:* Central ray should pass approximately 2 cm below the lateral canthus of the eye directed towards the center of the film.

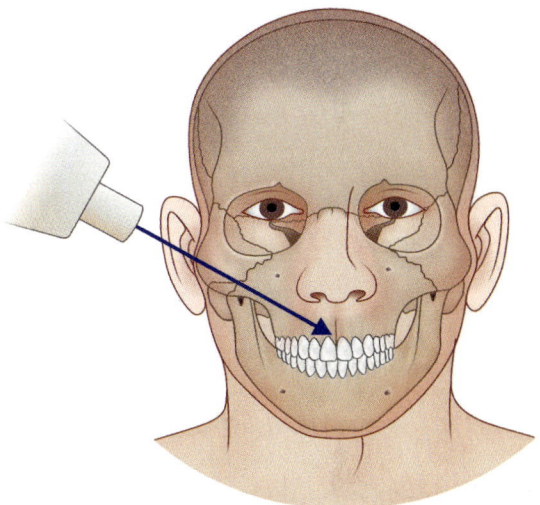

Fig. 31.23: Lateral occlusal projection view

× *Film positioning:* Film should be stabilized by gently closing the mouth and biting the film.
× *PID angulation:* +65° vertical angulation and 0° horizontal angulation
× *Point of entry:* Central ray should pass though the bridge of the nose.
× *Exposure:* Exposed towards the middle of the X-ray film.

Lateral occlusal projection view (Figs 31.23 and 31.24)
× *Patient position:* Midsagittal plane should be perpendicular to the floor and occlusal plane should be parallel to the floor.
× *Film placement:* Film should be placed with the white surface of the film towards

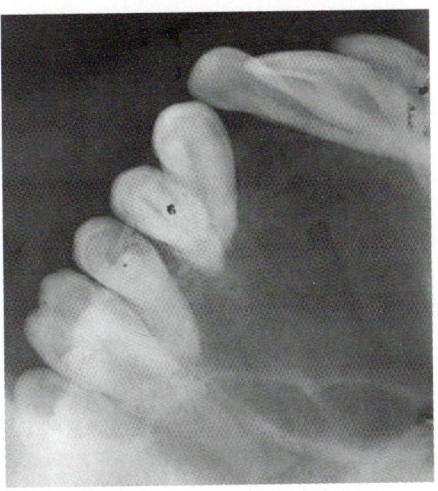

Fig. 31.24: Lateral occlusal radiograph

* *Exposure:* Exposed towards the middle of the X-ray film.

Mandibular Occlusal Radiograph

Anterior mandibular occlusal projection (Figs 31.25 and 31.26)

* *Patient position:* Patient seated with head supported with occlusal plane parallel to the floor.
* *Film placement:* Film should be placed with the white surface of the film facing downwards on the occlusal surfaces of the mandibular teeth.

* *Film positioning:* Film should be stabilized by gently closing the mouth and biting the film.
* *PID angulation:* +45° vertical angulation and 0° horizontal angulation
* *Point of entry:* Central ray should pass through the chin.
* *Exposure:* Exposed towards the middle of the X-ray film.

Cross-sectional mandibular occlusal projection (Figs 31.27 and 31.28)

* *Patient position:* Patient head should be tilted backwards as far as it is comfortable, where it is supported.
  * The mandibular arch should be perpendicular to the floor.

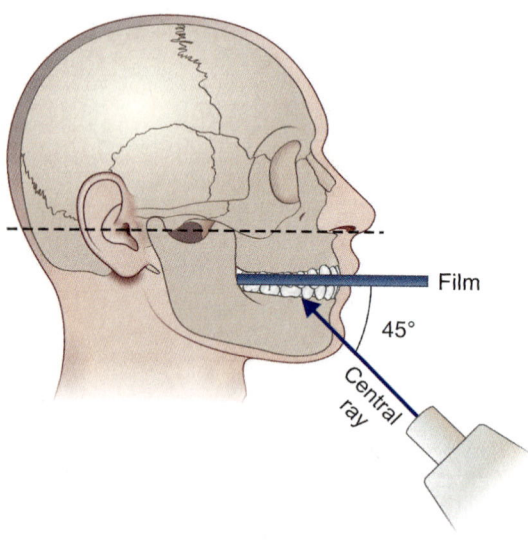

Fig. 31.25: Anterior mandibular occlusal projection

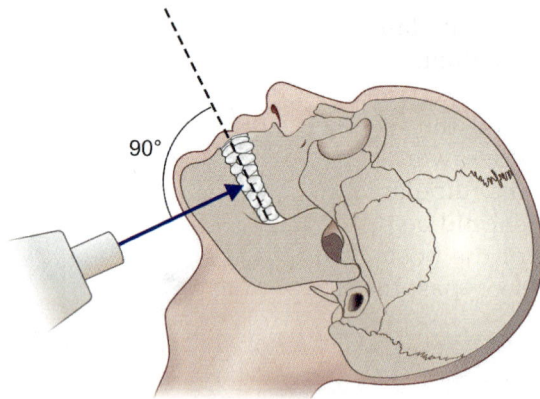

Fig. 31.27: Cross-sectional mandibular occlusal projection

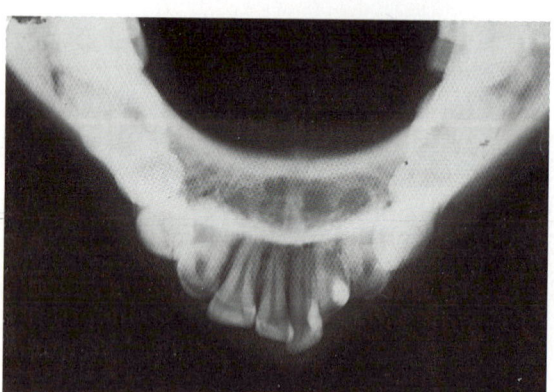

Fig. 31.26: Anterior mandibular topographic occlusal radiograph

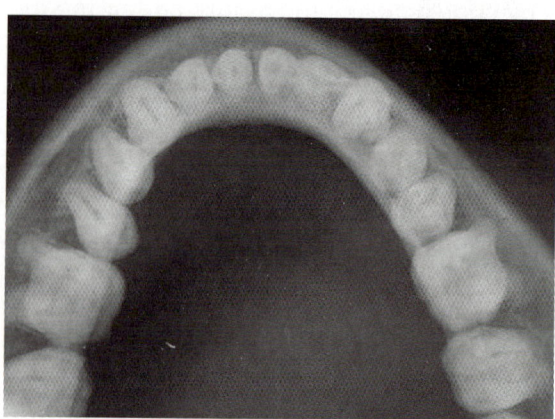

Fig. 31.28: Cross-sectional mandibular occlusal radiograph

* *Film placement:* Film should be placed with the white surface of the film facing downwards on the occlusal surfaces of the mandibular teeth.
* *Film positioning:* Film should be stabilized by gently closing the mouth and biting the film.
* *PID angulation:* 90° to the occlusal radiographic film and 0° horizontal angulation
* *Point of entry:* Central ray should pass through the floor of the mouth approximately 3 cm below the chin.
* *Exposure* is directed at right angles to the center of the X-ray film.

Lateral mandibular occlusal projection

* *Patient position:* Patient head should be tilted backwards in semi-reclining position, so that ala-tragus line is perpendicular to the floor.
* *Film placement:* Film should be placed with the white surface of the film facing downwards on the occlusal surfaces of the mandibular teeth. Lateral border of the film should be parallel with the buccal surface of the posterior teeth extending laterally 1 cm past the buccal cusps.

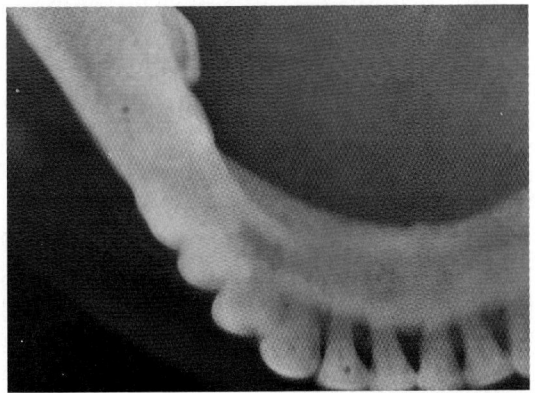

Fig. 31.29: Lateral mandibular occlusal radiograph

* *Film positioning:* Film should be stabilized by gently closing the mouth and biting the film.
* *PID angulation:* 90° to the occlusal radiographic film and 0° horizontal angulation.
* *Point of entry:* Central ray should pass through the 3 cm posterior to the chin and 3 cm lateral to the midline.
* *Exposure* is directed at right angles to the center of the X-ray film.

FREQUENTLY ASKED QUESTIONS

1. What are the different types of intraoral radiographic techniques?
2. What is Dr. Cieszynski's rule of isometry?
3. What are the various types of film holders used in intraoral radiographic techniques?
4. What are the indications of the bisecting angle technique?
5. Comparison between the bisecting angle technique and paralleling technique.
6. Name different types of occlusal views and write indications of occlusal radiography.
7. Write indications of bitewing radiography.

BIBLIOGRAPHY

1. Whaites E. Essentials of Dental Radiography and Radiology. 4th edition. Spain: Churchill Livingstone Elsevier; 2007
2. White S., Pharaoh Medicine Oral Radiology. Principles and Interpretation. 6th edition:. Elsevier Inc; 2011.
3. Langland O, Langlais R, Preece J. Principles of Dental imaging. 2nd edition. Lippincott Williams and Wilkins; 2002.
4. Karjodkar F. Textbook of Dental and Maxillofacial Radiology. 2nd edition. Jaypee Brothers Medical Publishers; 2009.

Digital Imaging

Digital radiography has been available since the late 1980s and has recently been refined with better hardware and more user-friendly software. It has grown in popularity to become the mainstay of radiography given the current 'filmless' digital age in radiology departments. It has the ability to capture, view, magnify, enhance, and store radiographic images in an easily reproducible format that does not degrade over time. Digital radiography uses no X-ray film and requires no chemical processing. Instead, a sensor is used to capture the image created by the radiation source. This sensor is either directly or wirelessly attached to a local computer, which interprets the signal and using specialized software, translates this signal into a two-dimensional digital image that can be displayed, enhanced, and analyzed. The image is stored in the patient's file, typically in a dedicated network server and can be recalled as needed.

A variety of different terms are used to describe the characteristics of digital imaging and varies somewhat from the film-based imaging. Definitions are listed in Table 32.1.

TERMINOLOGIES IN DIGITAL RADIOGRAPHY

Sensor

A sensor is an electronic device that is constantly measures a physical variable and transforms the physical variable into an electric signal.

There are two kinds of *sensors*: Digital and Analog.

1. **Digital sensors:** The signal produced or reflected by the sensor is binary. A digital sensor only detects two possible status: If it is working at 100% or at 0%.
2. **Analog sensors:** The signal produced by the sensor is continuous and proportional to the measurement. An analog sensor measures continuously the variable and detects any proportional value between 100% and 0%. For this reason, the measure provided by the analog sensor is more precise than the one provided by the digital sensor.

The terms 'sensors', 'detectors' and 'receptors' are used synonymously in this chapter.

Digital Radiography: A filmless imaging system; method of capturing a radiographic image using a sensor, breaking it into electronic pieces and presenting and storing the image using a computer.

Digital Image: A numerical representation of an image via a set of picture elements known as pixels. There are three parameters of a digital image that moderate resolution.

  i. *Image matrix:* The image matrix is comprised of columns (M) and rows (N) that define the elements or pixels within an image. The size of an image is:

TABLE 32.1: Comparison of film-based imaging and digital imaging	
Film-based imaging	Digital imaging
Density: The overall degree of darkness of an exposed film	**Brightness:** Digital equivalent to density or overall degree of image darkening
Latitude: Measure of range of exposures that will produce usefully distinguishable densities on the film	**Dynamic range:** The numerical range of each pixel; in visual terms, it can be referred to as the number of shades of gray that can be represented
Film speed: Amount of radiation required to produce an image of a standard density; refers to the sensitivity of the film to produce radiation. Faster the film, lesser the radiation required	**Linearity:** Linear or direct relationship between exposure and image density. Contrast can be altered but density cannot be affected after image exposure
Contrast: The difference in the densities between light and dark regions on the radiographs. High contrast images will have a few shades of gray between the black and white while low contrast areas will demonstrate a wider range of gray	**Contrast resolution:** Ability to differentiate the small varies in density as displayed on the image
Resolution: Ability to distinguish between small objects that are close together, measured in line pairs per millimeter.	**Spatial frequency:** Measure of resolution in line pairs per millimeter
Radiographic mottle (noise): Appearance of uneven density in a uniformly exposed film	**Background electronic noise:** Small electrical current that conveys no information but serves to obscure the electronic signal
Sharpness: Ability of a radiograph to define and edge or display density boundaries	**Signal to noise ratio:** Ratio between the fraction of the output signal (voltage or current or charge) that is directly related to the diagnostic information (signal) and the fraction that does not contain diagnostic information (noise)

Contd.

$$Matrix = M \times N \times k \text{ bits}$$

The field of view (FOV) is the size of the displayed image. However, if you maintain the same FOV and increase the matrix size, the pixels will be smaller and hence spatial resolution is improved.

ii. *Pixel:* The pixel is the element that makes up the image matrix, each pixel is a respective value that will represent a brightness level. The size is determined via: Pixel size = FOV/matrix

A decreased FOV means the pixel is smaller and hence an improvement in spatial resolution.

iii. *Voxel:* The voxel is a pixel that represents information that is contained in a volume.

$$Bit \text{ depth (k bit)}$$

The k bit is the number of bits per pixel, the gray scale of an image is equal to 2k bit, for example:

× k bit of 2 = 4 shades of gray
× k bit of 8 = 256 shades of gray

The higher the bit depth, the more gray scale and therefore, higher the contrast resolution.

DIGITAL DETECTORS

Digital radiography can be divided into solid state detectors and photostimulable phosphor plate (PSP) systems.

Solid State Detectors

Solid state detectors have the ability to generate a digital image in the computer without any other external device. The use of solid state detectors in medicine is referred as digital radiography and intraoral solid state detectors in dentistry are called sensors.

The key clinical feature of these detectors is the rapid availability of the image after exposure. The matrix and its associated read-out and amplifying electronics of intraoral detectors are enclosed within a plastic housing to protect them from oral environment. These elements of the detector consume a part of the real estate of the sensor, so that the active area of the sensor is smaller than the total surface area. Detectors also incorporate an electronic cable to transfer data to the computer. The wireless detector consists of a radiofrequency transmitter which frees the detector from a direct tether to the computer but adds to the sensor bulk.

Different solid state detectors described are the charged coupled device, charged metal oxide conductor and flat panel detectors.

Charged Coupled Device

The charged coupled device (CCD) (Fig. 32.1) was introduced to dentistry in 1987 and was the first digital image receptor to be adapted for intraoral imaging.

Principle: The CCD is a solid-state detector composed of an array of X-ray or light sensitive pixels on a pure silicon chip for image recording (Fig. 32.2 and 32.3). The

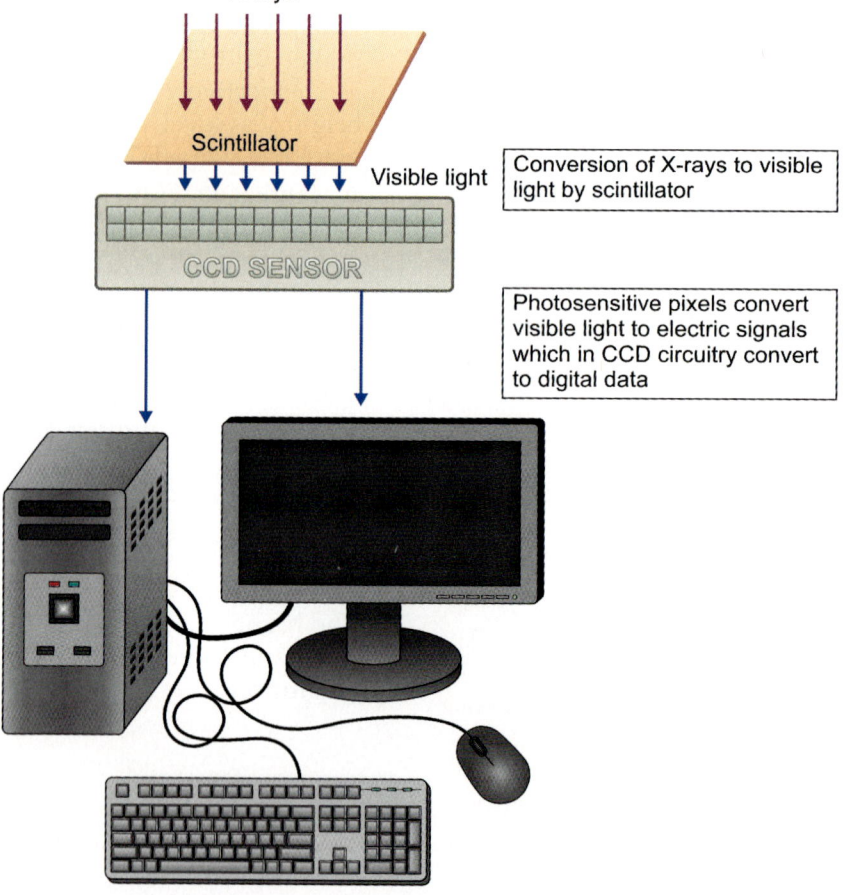

X-rays

Scintillator

Visible light — Conversion of X-rays to visible light by scintillator

CCD SENSOR

Photosensitive pixels convert visible light to electric signals which in CCD circuitry convert to digital data

Fig. 32.1: CCD with computer system

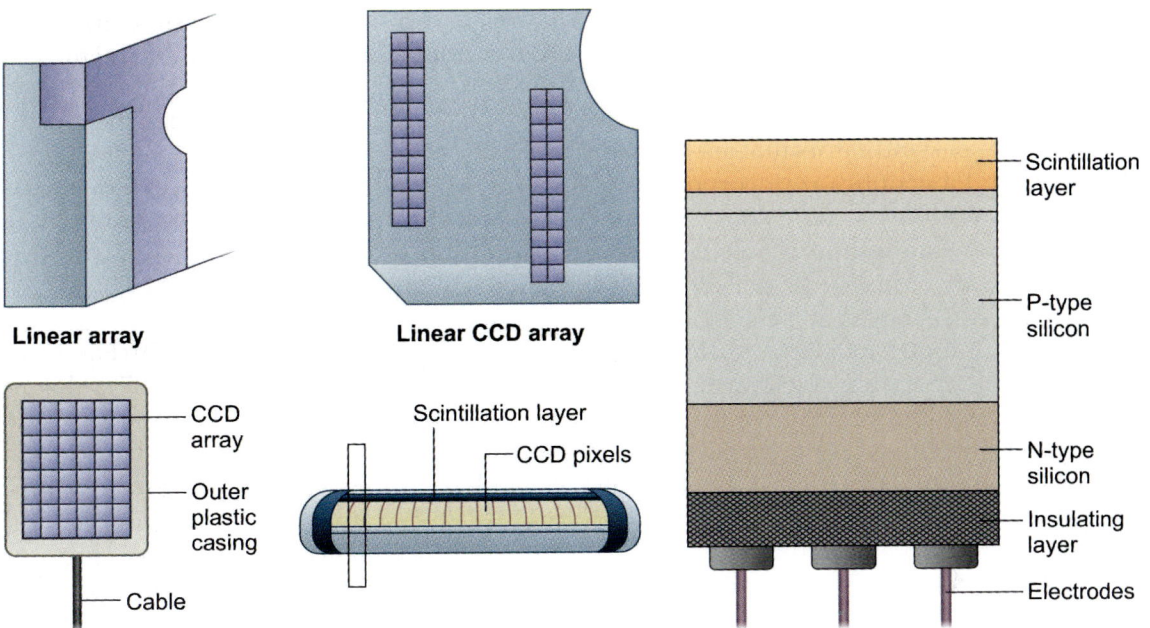

Linear array **Linear CCD array**

CCD array

Outer plastic casing

Cable

Scintillation layer

CCD pixels

Scintillation layer

P-type silicon

N-type silicon

Insulating layer

Electrodes

Fig. 32.2: A slot-scan CCD-based system. The patient is scanned with a fan-shaped beam of X-rays. A simultaneously moving CCD detector of the same size collects the emitted light and converts the light energy into electrical charges

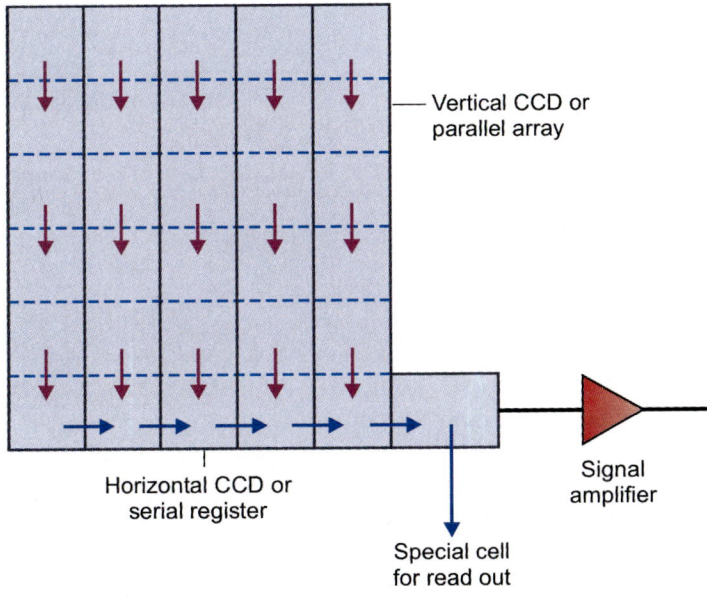

Vertical CCD or parallel array

Signal amplifier

Horizontal CCD or serial register

Special cell for read out

Fig. 32.3: Read out of CCD in a 'bucket-brigade fashion'

surface of the silicon may incorporate a scintillating material to minimize scatter and improve X-ray efficiency. Gadolinium oxybromide compounds or cesium iodide are examples of scintillators that are used for this purpose. Fiber optics are incorporated to improve resolution.

A pixel consists of a small electron well into which the X-ray or light energy is deposited upon exposure. Charge coupling is a process whereby the number of electrons deposited in each pixel are transferred from one well to the next in a 'bucket brigade fashion' to a read-out amplifier and transmitted as a voltage to the analog to digital converter (ADC) located within the computer for image display on the monitor.

The individual CCD pixel size is approximately 40 μ with the latest versions in the 20 μ range. The rows of pixels are arranged in a matrix of 512 × 512 pixels.

There are two types of digital sensor array designs: Area and linear.

Area arrays are used for intraoral radiography, while linear arrays are used in extraoral imaging. Area arrays are available in sizes comparable to size 0, size 1, and size 2 film, but the sensors are rigid and thicker than radiographic film and have a smaller sensitive area for image capture. The sensor communicates with the computer through an electrical cable. Area array CCDs have two primary formats: Fiberoptically-coupled sensors and direct sensors. Fiberoptically-coupled sensors utilize a scintillation screen coupled to a CCD. When X-rays interact with the screen material, light photons are generated, detected, and stored by CCD. Direct sensor CCD arrays capture the image directly.

Unfortunately, some CCD sensors are still bulky, inflexible and, in use, have a cable extension out of the oral cavity. The recent development of a semiconductor chip allows high speed wireless communication. Care must be exercised as CCD sensors are fragile and expensive to replace.

Complementary Metal Oxide Semiconductors *(CMOS, Fig. 32.4)*

The complementary metal oxide semiconductors appear identical to CCD detectors, but they use an active pixel technology (APS) that reduces the system power by a factor of 100 to process the image as compared to the CCD. CMOS-APS is the latest development in direct digital sensor technology.

Principle

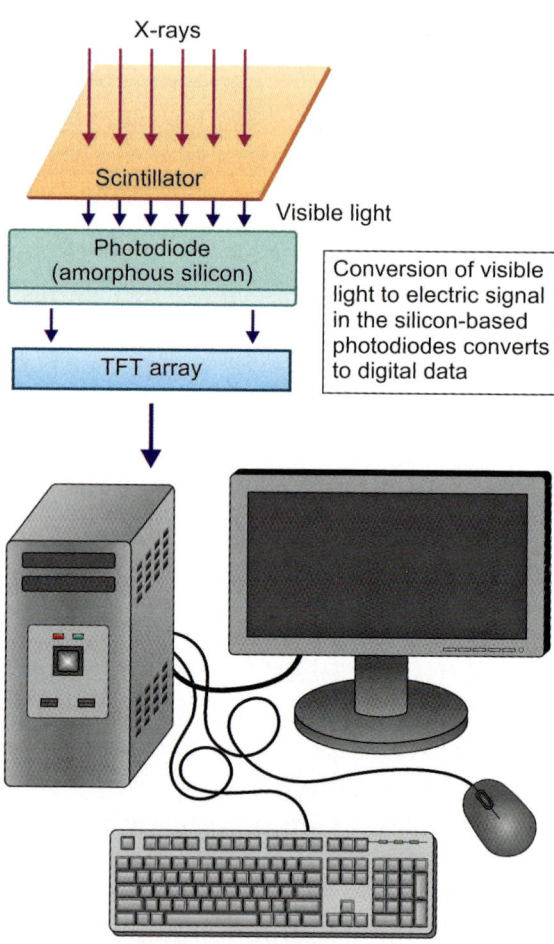

Fig. 32.4: An amorphous silicon-based CMOS system. X-ray energy is converted into visible light in a scintillator layer. The emitted light is then converted into electrical charges by an array of silicon-based photodiodes and read out by a TFT array

CMOS detectors are also silicon-based conductors, but they fundamentally differ from the CCDs in the way the pixel charges are read. Each pixel is isolated from its neighboring pixels and is directly connected to the transistor. The electron hole pairs are generated in proportion to the amount of X-ray energy that is absorbed. The charge is transferred to a thin film transistor (TFT) as a small voltage. The voltage in each transistor can be addressed separately, read by a frame grabber and then stored and displayed as a digital gray value.

Uses

1. Intraoral imaging
2. Construction of computer central processing unit chips and video cameras.

Advantages

1. Offers greater durability than CCD
2. Low power requirements
3. Lower cost than CCD
4. Design integration

Disadvantages

1. More fixed pattern noise
2. Smaller active area for image acquisition

Flat Panel Detectors

Flat panel detectors (FPD) are used in medical imaging and several extraoral imaging devices. The detectors can provide relatively large matrix areas with pixel sizes less than 100 μm. FPDs are of two types:

1. Direct conversion FPDs
2. Indirect conversion FPDs

Direct conversion FPDs

Principle: The flat panel detectors make use of a layer of selenium with a corresponding underlying array of thin-film transistors (TFTs). During exposure, a charge pattern proportional to that of the incident X-rays is generated on the surface of the amorphous selenium and recorded by the TFT array, which accumulates and stores the energy of the electrons. The energy is released and read out by applying appropriate row and column voltages to the particular pixel's transistor. Direct detectors using selenium provide

a higher resolution but lower efficiency in comparison to indirect detectors using gadolinium or cesium.

Figs 32.5 and 32.6 show a selenium-based flat-panel detector system. Incident X-ray energy is directly converted into electrical

Flat panel detectors

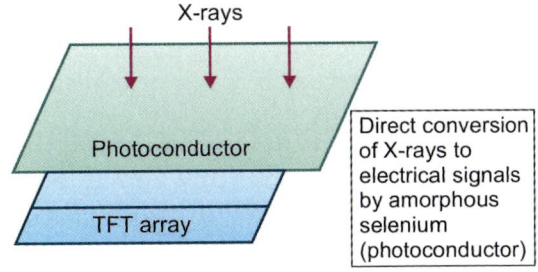

Fig. 32.5: Direct conversion FPDs

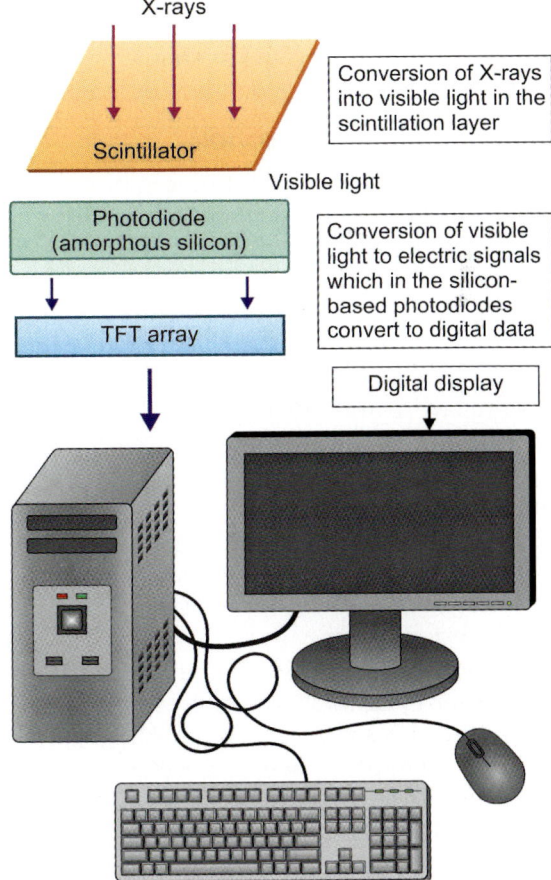

Fig. 32.6: Indirect conversion FPDs

charges within the fixed photoconductor layer and readout by a linked TFT array beneath the detective layer.

Indirect conversion FPDs

Principle: Indirect conversion FPDs are "sandwich" constructions consisting of a scintillator layer, an amorphous silicon photodiode circuitry layer, and a TFT array. When X-ray photons reach the scintillator, visible light proportional to the incident energy is emitted and then recorded by an array of photodiodes and converted to electrical charges. The performance of these devices is determined by the thickness of the intensifying screens. Thicker screens are more efficient but allow greater diffusion of X-ray photons leading to image unsharpness. These charges are then read out by a TFT array similar to that of direct conversion digital radiography (DR) systems.

Photostimulable Phosphor

Imaging using a photostimulable phosphor (PSP) can also be described as an indirect digital imaging technique. The image is captured on a phosphor plate as analog information and is converted into a digital format when the plate is processed. Photostimulable phosphor radiographic systems were first introduced in 1981 by the Fuji Corporation (Tokyo, Japan).

X-ray luminescence is the physical mechanism by which X-ray energy is converted into light in a phosphor screen. It involves two mechanisms that both occur to some degree when a phosphor screen is irradiated:

* **X-ray fluorescence:** The immediate emission of light. This is the mechanism that predominates in screen film radiography.
* **X-ray phosphorescence:** This is when the emission of light is delayed over a timescale of many minutes, hours or days and can be accelerated by shining specific colored light onto the phosphor. This is the mechanism exploited in PSP. It allows

X-ray energy to be temporarily stored in a phosphor screen to be read-out later.

Principle (Fig. 32.7)

Image Processing (Fig. 32.8)

1. **Latent image formation:** PSP is a layer of phosphor crystals (made of barium fluorohalide activated with divalent europium ions) embedded in a polymer binder with the top surface protected by a layer of toughened plastic. It is typically 0.3 mm thick.

   During exposure, X-ray photons are absorbed into a phosphor crystal giving rise to a high energy photoelectron. The electrons become temporarily trapped at higher energy levels at specific sites throughout the layer of phosphor crystals producing the latent image. In this way, X-ray energy can be stored for several hours, depending on the specific physical properties of the phosphor crystal used.

2. **Laser simulated emission:** If left long enough, the electrons spontaneously relax back to their ground state and the image decays over time. During read-out the image plate is scanned with a red laser beam stimulating the trapped electrons to immediately relax back to their ground state and release their stored energy as light photons in the blue part of the spectrum. The light photons are then collected by optical fibers to a photomultiplier (PM) tube. The PM tube produces an electrical current.

3. **Resetting cassette:** Read out is 'destructive', as it eliminates the latent image. The film is then exposed to bright light to erase any residual signal before re-using the cassette. The read-out process should start immediately after exposure because the amount of stored energy decreases over time.

4. **Post-processing of image:** After exposure and read out, the raw imaging data must be processed for display on the computer. Image processing is one of the key features

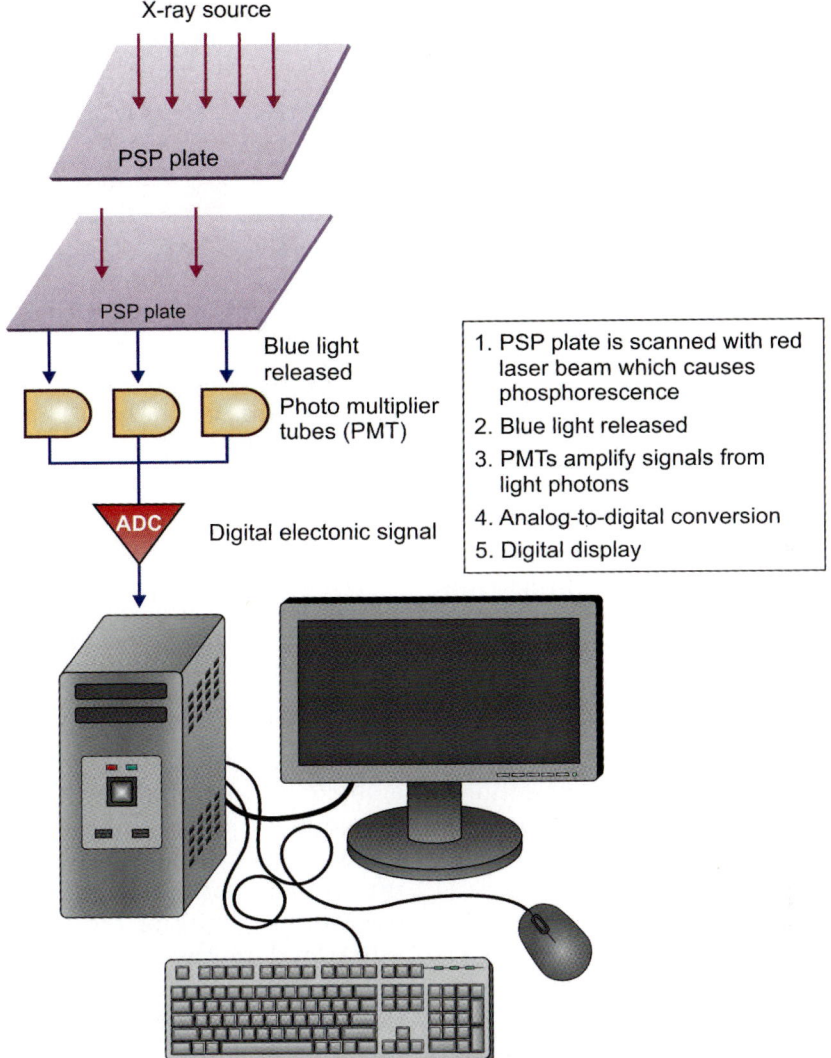

X-ray source

PSP plate

PSP plate

Blue light released

Photo multiplier tubes (PMT)

ADC   Digital electonic signal

1. PSP plate is scanned with red laser beam which causes phosphorescence
2. Blue light released
3. PMTs amplify signals from light photons
4. Analog-to-digital conversion
5. Digital display

Fig. 32.7: Indirect system using photostimulable storage—phosphor. Image generation is separated into two steps. First, the image plate (IP) is exposed to X-ray energy, part of which is stored within the detective layer of the plate. Second, the image plate is scanned with a laser beam, so that the stored energy is set free and light is emitted. An array of photomultipliers collects the light, which is converted into electrical charges by an analog-to-digital (A/D) converter

of digital radiography, greatly influencing the way the image appears to the radiologist. Although software products from several manufacturers use similar algorithms such as edge enhancement, noise reduction, and contrast enhancement to alter the appearance of the image, the resulting impressions may differ considerably. Image processing is used to improve image quality by reducing noise, removing technical artifacts, and optimizing contrast for viewing. Spatial resolution (the capacity to define the extent or shape of features within an image sharply and clearly) cannot be influenced by the processing software because it is dependent on the technical variables of the detector (e.g. pixel size). However,

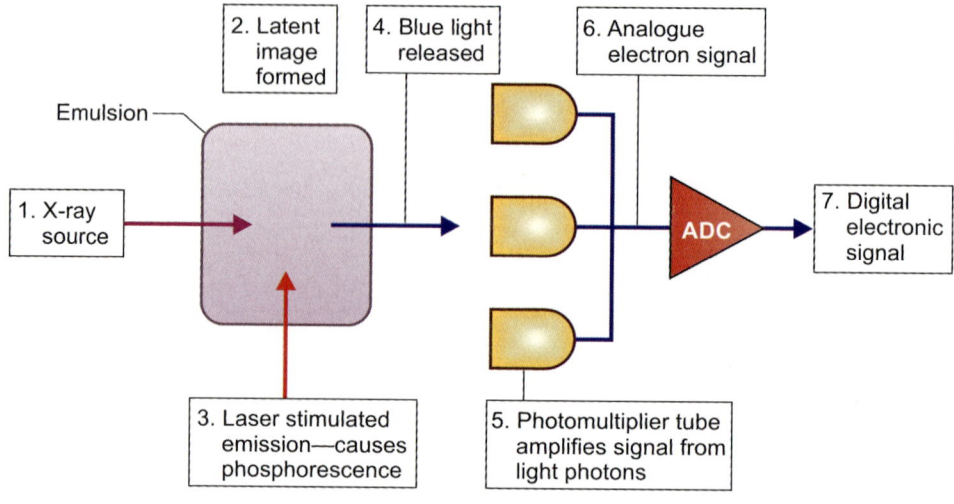

Fig. 32.8: Image processing

with optimization of other processing variables, lack of spatial resolution can be partially counteracted.

Digital Image Viewing

The principal viewing means of a digital image is a computer monitor. Conventional computer monitors use a cathode ray tube (CRT) whereas, the thin film transistor (TFT) technology used in flat panel detectors is also used in laptop and flat panel computer displays. The liquid crystal display (LCD) and modern CRT monitors are sufficient in quality for display of digital radiographs. They all display a maximum of 256 shades of gray. The radiographs contain many more shades of gray than the human eye is able to perceive. The process of adjusting the gray scale and brightness on a digital radiograph is known as windowing and leveling.

The LCD or CRT monitors are most appropriate for viewing digital radiographs.

The output of laptop displays is limited in intensity and does not have a dynamic range or contrast found in conventional CRT or LCD. The viewing angle of laptop display is also limited and the observer needs to be positioned squarely in front of the display for optimum viewing quality.

The digital radiographs should be viewed in a darkened or dimly lit room and not in bright sunlight.

Image Processing

Any operation that acts to improve restore analyze or in some way change a digital image is a form of image processing. The use of digital imaging in dental radiography involves a variety of image processing operations. Some of these operations are integrated in the image acquisition and image management software and are hidden from the user. Others are controlled by the user with the intention to improve the quality of the image or to analyze its contents.

Image Restoration

The raw data needs a number of preprocessing steps to correct the image before display on the computer screen. For example, some of the pixels in a CCD sensor are always defective. The image is restored by substituting the gray values of the defective pixels with some weighted average of the gray values from the surrounding pixels. Similarly, a wide range of operations are performed rapidly before it comes to display and are unnoticed by the user. Most of these operations are set by the manufacturer and cannot be changed.

Image Enhancement

The term 'image enhancement' implies that the adjusted image is an improved version of the original one. This can be accomplished by increasing the contrast, optimizing the brightness and reducing unsharpness and noise which makes the image visually more appealing. Subjective image enhancement does not necessarily improve the accuracy of the image interpretation and they are usually task specific. For example, increasing the contrast between enamel and dentin for caries detection may make it more difficult to identify the contour of the alveolar crest. Image enhancement operations are viewer specific.

Image Analysis

Image analysis operations are designed to extract diagnostically relevant information from the image. The analysis can range from simple linear measurements to fully automated diagnosis. The use of image analysis tools is useful but has its limitations. The accuracy and precision of the measurements are limited by the extent to which the image is a truthful and reproducible representation of the patient and by the operator's ability to make an exact measurement.

Image Storage

Digital images are stored in the hard drive of the computer interfaced with the radiographic equipment. Primary storing of the original file is done by the software.

In order to preserve the data for posterity, a regular backup is mandatory. The backup should be performed on an external drive and not the hard drive of the computer as a crash of the drive may lead to complete loss of data. The data may also be stored on CD-ROM, DVDs or zip drive depending on the required durability and practical considerations.

In order to save the storage space, files can be compressed. These compression algorithms are termed "lossless". Lossless methods do not discard any image data and

an exact copy of the image is produced after decompression. However, their potential for size reduction is limited to a factor of 2:1 or 4:1. "Lossy" compression, on the other hand, achieves a higher compression rate at the cost of a loss of image information. A compression of 80:1 or more can be achieved in the Joint Photographic experts group (JPEG) format.

For medicolegal reasons, the original image must be stored and protected separately. If the image is processed for additional diagnostic or treatment purposes, it must be stored as an additional file. Many countries have set-up regulations dealing with these issues (Table 32.2).

Infection Control

Sensors are categorized as semi-critical items and they should be cleaned and ideally be heat-sterilized or high-level disinfected in between the patients. However, these items vary by manufacturer or type of device in their ability to be sterilized or high-level disinfected. The following apply for digital radiography sensors:

a. Barriers like disposable plastic envelope covering the sensor and the wire is mandatory.

b. To minimize the potential for device-associated infections, after removing the barrier, clean and disinfect using a disinfectant with an intermediate-level activity after each patient.

As the sensors and associated components vary by manufacturer and are expensive, manufacturers should be consulted regarding specific disinfection products and procedures. Some manufacturers recommend against using certain chemicals on their sensors. Also, some manufacturers allow immersion of their sensors while others do not.

Uses of Digital Radiography

1. **Caries detection:** Contrast resolution is an important parameter in the diagnostic accuracy of caries detection. Software

TABLE 32.2: Clinical comparison of intraoral imaging alternatives

Imaging procedure	Film	CCD/CMOS	PSP
Receptor preparation	✗ None	✗ Placement of a protective plastic sleeve over the receptor ✗ Receptor must be connected to the computer and patient details to be entered for acquisition/archiving software	✗ Erase plate ✗ Package plates in protective plastic cover
Receptor placement	✗ Use film holders ✗ Films may be bent according to patient's anatomy	✗ Specialized film holders are used. However, due to the different specifications of the manufacturer, options are limited. ✗ Patient discomfort due to inflexible and bulky receptor ✗ Receptor cable needs to be directed out of the mouth. Due to the increased bulk, cordless receptors add to the patient discomfort	✗ Film holders used for film may be used for PSP. ✗ Bending of PSP can irreversibly damage the plates
Exposure	✗ Simple	✗ Computer activation required	✗ Simple
Processing	✗ Light safe, darkroom environment or light safe loader required ✗ Chemicals must be prepared and replenished as per requirement ✗ Chemical temperature has to be monitored ✗ Film must be removed from wrapper; lead foil must be separated for recycling	✗ Immediate image acquisition and display.	✗ Dim light ✗ Prior programming with patient information, so that images can be stored and retrieved when required ✗ Protective plastic cover must be removed before use
Display	✗ The films after drying and processing need to be mounted and labeled	✗ The software in the computer aids in viewing of the image. Image manipulation is possible to achieve maximum diagnostic information	
Image duplication	✗ Resultant image quality is inferior with loss of diagnostic information	✗ Multiple copies of the original image may be made without loss of image quality and diagnostic information	

TABLE 32.3: Intraoral receptor comparison

Feature	Film	CCD	PSP
Spatial resolution	Intraoral systems: Film>CCD = CMOS>PSP Panoramic systems: Film = CCD = PSP Cephalometric systems: Film> CCD = PSP		
Exposure latitude	PSP>>CCD = CMOS ≥ Film		

Contd.

TABLE 32.3: Intraoral Receptor Comparison (Contd.)

Feature	Film	CCD	PSP
Receptor dimensions	For equivalent imaged area, Film = PSP<CCD = CMOS		
Time for image acquisition	CCD = CMOS<<PSP = Film		
Image quality	Subjective quality is best when carefully exposed and well processed		
Image adjustment/ processing	Improves appearance of digital images		
Cost	Initial costs of digital systems are greater than film. Subsequent costs vary greatly depending on receptor wear and tear or abuse		
Reliability	Mechanical problems affect digital PSP and film systems. Software reliability varies greatly among manufacturers. Changes in unrelated computer components and software can cause digital systems to malfunction		
Image storage and retrieval	Data backup is critical for digital systems		
Image transmission	Achieved rapidly in digital systems		

allows image manipulation by applying specific filters to detect carious lesions.

2. **Diagnosis of periodontal lesions:** The high resolution of intraoral radiography helps the visualization of the bony supporting tissues, including small details such as periodontal ligament space, lamina dura, and bony trabecularization.

3. **Measuring the extent of bone loss** using image analysis tools.

4. High-resolution technology and/or dedicated endodontic filtering improves the visibility of small file tips as small as 0.06 mm.

5. Serial radiographs with identical geometric projection and exposure settings can be subtracted using digital subtraction radiography. This allows for qualitative evaluation by underscoring small changes such as caries progression, periapical lesions, or even quantitative evaluation of periodontal bone loss.

6. **Forensic dentistry:** Determination of the age of an individual by assessing the stage of eruption of teeth as well as for evidence in the identification of the suspect, to determine the cause of death, to find faulty charting of teeth, legal matters, body identification, postmortem examination, and for non-accidental injuries of children and forensic anthropology.

7. **Evaluation of cysts or benign tumors:** Multiplanar sections (axial, coronal, and sagittal planes) are helpful to locate deeper tissues.

8. It is also helpful in **postsurgical follow-ups** of lesions with high recurrences.

Advantages

1. Digital radiography requires 90% lesser dose compared to E-speed film.

2. In digital imaging, image quality may be interactively manipulated after image acquisition, i.e. contrast, blur and noise may be altered digitally. Filtering of the digital image may result in a reduction of blur of structure boundaries.

3. Diagnostic accuracy of the detection of carious lesions is increased by digital contrast enhancement and filtering.

4. Measurements of length, angle, and area can be made on a digital image. Three-dimensional reconstruction of radiographic images is of importance for the diagnosis and treatment planning in malformations, trauma, tumor investigation, and surgery planning.

5. Low-pass spatial filtering (smoothing) reduces the image noise. However, it decreases image resolution. High-pass spatial filtering (hardening) enhances edges to create a crisper image, but with

more noise. It facilitates the detection of boundaries of low-contrast regions.

6. In digital radiography, the same image can be used for various diagnostic purposes. For example, marginal bone loss which requires lighter images and caries detection requiring darker images. With the CCD system, the image is displayed immediately postexposure. Although, there is a lag time between scanning and the appearance of an image, it is faster than the conventional method.

7. DICOM standard facilitates a common method of transmission for medical radiographic images. DICOM compliant system utilizes common file formats that are universally recognized. For example, when one is contemplating digital image submission to insurance companies.

Disadvantages

1. **Cost of devices:** Initial costs of digital systems are greater than film. Subsequent costs vary greatly depending on receptor wear and tear or abuse.

2. **Learning to use the concept:** After receiving initial education to begin using digital radiography, staff members still will require significant time to master the use of the software.

3. **Thickness of the sensor:** CCD sensors vary in thickness, from more than 3 mm to more than 5 mm. Although this seems to be a major disadvantage, it is surprising to note the relative ease of use of CCD sensors inspite of their thickness.

4. **Rigidity of the sensors:** CCD sensors are rigid and can irritate the oral soft tissues and can cause pain.

5. **Lack of standardization:** A CDROM can hold over 30,000 images. This means that images can be stored cheaply and indefinitely.

6. **Infection control:** The CMOS and CCD sensors are used on multiple patients and must be covered by barriers. Sensors that become contaminated are incapable of being sterilized.

Other considerations

1. Company service/support, system cost, length of warranty, and ease of use/capability of imaging software.

2. Compatibility with open platform imaging software will be a consideration for those clinics utilizing these software packages.

3. Adequate cable length and sensor size/shape is another consideration. Sensors with rounded edges may be more comfortable. Sensor wires exiting from the back of the sensor may make for easier placement in some situations compared to configurations where the wire exits from the end of the sensor.

4. Sensor thickness disadvantages may be minimized when sensors are positioned properly (more towards the center of the mouth).

Multiple considerations come into play when selecting a digital radiography package and there are advantages and disadvantages to all systems.

FREQUENTLY ASKED QUESTIONS

Write short note on:

1. CCD
2. CMOS
3. Advantages and disadvantages of digital imaging
4. Uses of digital radiography

BIBLIOGRAPHY

1. Markus Körner, Christof H Weber, Stefan Wirth, Klaus-Jürgen Pfeifer, Maximilian F Reiser, Marcus Treitl. Advances in Digital Radiography. Physical Principles and System Overview. 2007;27:3:675–86

2. Ludlow JB, Andre Mol (2009). Digital Imaging. In: White, SC and Pharoah MJ (Eds.) Oral Radiology: Principles and interpretation. (pp 78–100) St. Louis, Mo: Mosby/Elsevier.

3. Parks ET, Williamson GF. Digital Radiography: An Overview. J Contemp Dent Pract. 2002; November; (3)4:23–39.

4. Karjodkar Freny R. Digital Radiography. Textbook of Dental and Maxillofacial Radiology, 2006 (Pp 336–46) Jaypee Brothers Medical Publishers.
5. Rowlands JA. The physics of computed radiography. Phys Med Biol. 2002; 47:R123–R166.
6. Iannucci, J. M., and Howerton, L. J. Digital Radiography. Dental radiography: Principles and techniques 2012. (pp 343–56) St. Louis, Mo: Elsevier Saunders.
7. Jayachandran S. Digital Imaging in Dentistry: A Review. Contemp Clin Dent. 2017;8(2):193–4.
8. Bansal GJ. Digital radiography. A comparison with modern conventional imaging. Postgrad Med J. 2006; 82:425–8.
9. Stamatakis HC, Welander U, McDavid WD. Physical properties of a photostimulable phosphor system for intra-oral radiography. Dentomaxillofac Radiol. 2000; 29:28–34.
10. Schaefer-Prokop CM, Prokop M. Storage phosphor radiography. Eur Radiol. 1997; 7:58–65.
11. Yaffe MJ, Rowlands JA. X-ray detectors for digital radiography. Phys Med Biol. 1997; 42:1–39.
12. Van der Stelt PF. Principles of Digital Imaging. In: Miles DA, editor. Applications of Digital Imaging Modalities for Dentistry. Dent Clin North Am. 2000 Apr; 44(2):237–48, v.
13. Sanderink GC, Miles DA. Intraoral Detectors. In: Miles DA, editor. Applications of Digital Imaging Modalities for Dentistry. Dent Clin North Am. 2000 Apr; 44(2):249–55, v.
14. Paurazas SB, Geist JR, Pink FE, et. al. Comparison of diagnostic accuracy of digital imaging using CCD and CMOS-APS sensors with E-speed film in the detection of periapical bony lesions. Oral Surg Oral Med Oral Pathol Oral Radiol Endod. 2000 Mar; 89(3):356–62.

Normal Anatomical Landmarks

INTRODUCTION

Radiographs play an important role in diagnosis and treatment of a disease. Since a wide range of variation in the appearance of normal anatomic structures may mimic the pathologies, a sound knowledge of radiographic appearance of normal structures is necessary.

On radiograph the structures appear as radiopaque or radiolucent. The calcified structures absorb the X-ray and hence appear radiopaque while the soft tissues allow the X-rays to pass through them and hence appear radiolucent.

Anatomical landmarks are broadly categorized into:
- Landmarks common to both maxilla and mandible
- Landmarks seen in maxilla
- Landmarks seen in mandible

Landmarks common to both maxilla and mandible

- **Teeth**
  - Enamel
  - Dentin
  - Pulp chamber and root canal
  - Cementum

- **Supporting structures**
  - Alveolar process
  - Periodontal ligament space
  - Cortical bone

Teeth

Enamel: Enamel is the dense homogenous radiopaque cap of greater whiteness than dentin and hardest calcified tissue in the human body. It consists mainly of inorganic material of approximately 96%, hence causes the greatest attenuation of the X-ray photons. Hence enamel characteristically appears more radiopaque than any other tissue.

Dentin: A large portion of the tooth is made up of dentin. Dentin consists of comparatively lesser amount of inorganic material than enamel (i.e. approx. 65%), hence appears less dense than the latter. The dentinoenamel junction appears as a distinct interface that separates these two structures. Physical and chemical qualities of dentin closely resemble bone, hence its radiographic appearance can be roughly comparable to bone. Caries involving dentin or operative procedures induce changes in the dentin.

Cementum: It is the mineralized dental tissue covering the anatomic roots of human teeth. It has a mineral content of around 50%, comparable to that of dentin. Also its physical properties are similar to that of dentin. Hence, cannot be differentiated from dentin on radiographs.

Pulp chambers and root canals
- Pulp is broadly divided into
  - Coronal pulp
  - Radicular pulp (root canal)

- It is composed of soft tissue and absorbs fewer X-rays than surrounding dentin and appears radiolucent on radiographs. The protrusions that extends into the cusps of each tooth, called *pulp horns* are seen commonly in young pulp. With aging, the pulpal walls in the apical region begin to constrict and finally come into close apposition.
- In some, the root canal can be traced till the extreme apex. In others, the foramen may be visible for only few millimeters. With aging, the shape of the pulp chambers and canals may change. Diffuse calcifications appear as irregular calcific deposits in the pulp tissue. Diffuse calcifications usually are seen in root canals whereas pulp stones (denticles) are common in the coronal pulp.

Supporting Structures

Alveolar Process

Alveolar process may be defined as the part of the maxilla or mandible that forms and supports the sockets of the teeth. Depending upon the adaptation and function, two parts of the alveolar process are distinguished:
- Alveolar bone proper (lamina dura)
- Supporting alveolar bone
  - Cortical plates
  - Medullary bone

Anatomically, no distinct boundary exists between the body of the maxilla or the mandible and their respective alveolar processes. An alveolar process forms with the development and eruption of teeth, and conversely, it gradually diminishes in height after the loss of teeth.

Alveolar processes are subdivided into various parts depending on their anatomic relation with the teeth they surround, as
- *Interproximal bone or interdental septum:* Bone located between adjacent teeth.
- *Inter-radicular bone:* Bone between the roots of multirooted teeth.
- *Radicular bone:* Alveolar process located on the facial or lingual surfaces of roots.

- *Alveolar crest:* The coronal margin of the alveolar process.

▶ Lamina Dura

Radiographically, lamina dura appears as a thin radiopaque line surrounding the roots of the teeth. It appears more radiopaque than the adjacent cancellous bone, as it is not more mineralized than cancellous bone.

Thickness and density of lamina dura:
- It varies with the amount of occlusal stress to which the tooth is subjected. It is wider and dense around the roots of teeth in heavy occlusion and thinner and less dense around teeth subjected to week occlusal forces. Sometimes, when the mesial or distal surfaces of roots present two elevations in the path of X-ray beam, it results in the appearance of double lamina dura.
- Appearance of lamina dura on radiograph varies in thickness, density, shape, and number which depends on
  - Position of tooth in the arch
  - Angulation of the beam
  - Numerous foramina that carry blood vessels through lamina dura
- These differences have no clinical significance as long as the lamina dura is continuous around the root.

▶ Alveolar Crest

The coronal margin of the alveolar bone processes are called alveolar crests. They are covered with a thin layer of dense cortical bone, seen as a thin radiopaque line. Its level is considered normal when it is not more than 1.5 mm from CEJ of the adjacent tooth. Its appearance is influenced by the interproximal cementoenamel junction of the teeth. It appears radiopaque when CEJ is straight and wide buccolingually and less radiopaque when CEJ is peaked and thin buccolingually.

Shape of the alveolar crest

Anteriorly between the incisors, the crest is reduced to only a point of bone while posteriorly it is flat, aligned parallel with and slightly below a line connecting the CEJ of the adjacent teeth.

Cancellous or Spongy Bone

The bone surrounding the tooth socket and lamina dura is the cancellous bone. It is made of thin strands of bone called trabeculae which appear radiopaque. Between these trabeculae are the medullary spaces, which appear radiolucent. The radiographic pattern shows considerable intrapatient and interpatient variations.

Maxillary Trabecular Pattern

* Trabecular pattern is almost always finer than that in the mandible, and lacks the distinct trajectory pattern seen in the latter. It is made of numerous delicate inter-dental and inter-radicular trabeculae. The size of the marrow spaces vary between 1 to 4 mm.
* Anterior maxilla shows numerous fine, granular, and dense trabecular pattern with relatively small and numerous marrow spaces.
* Posterior maxilla shows trabecular pattern may be quite similar, but marrow spaces are slightly larger.

Mandibular Trabecular Pattern

Trabecular pattern varies between different parts of the same bone and in different persons as well. Greater part of the mandible shows linear trabeculation with the strands running in a relatively horizontal pattern, with a distinct trajectory pattern. The trabecular network between the roots of mandibular molar and sometimes between the central incisors, shows stepladder pattern.

Trabecular Pattern in Senile Bone

Bone of the elderly is often more radiolucent with thinner trabeculae and wider medullary spaces. The bone loses some of its calcific contents due to various reasons such as nutritional deficiencies, disease atrophy, hormonal changes, and osteoporosis. Following the tooth extraction, bone experiences less stress, hence trabeculae are less organized leading to the radiolucent appearance of the bone.

Periodontal Ligament Space

The space between the tooth and lamina dura is called the periodontal ligament space. It appears as a thin uniform radiolucent structure surrounding the root of the tooth (Fig. 33.1).

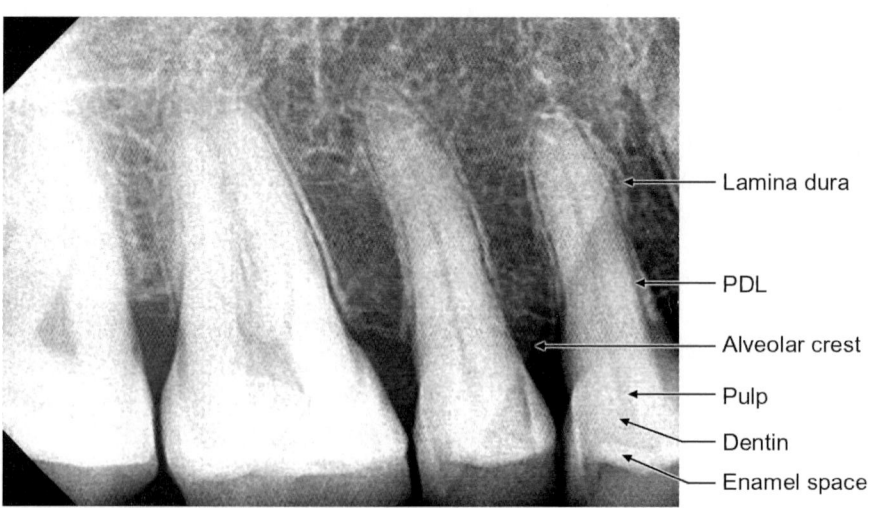

Fig. 33.1: Teeth and its supporting structures

TABLE 33.1: Maxillary anatomic landmarks

Maxillary landmark	*Radiographic appearance*
1. **Intermaxillary suture (median maxillary suture):** It appears as thin radiolucent line in the midline from the alveolar crest between the central incisors. It has uniform width. The appearance, however, depends on both anatomic variability and the angulation of the X-ray beam through the suture	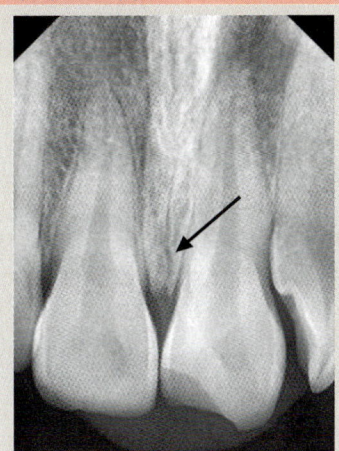
2. **Anterior nasal spine:** It is seen on the periapical views of the maxillary central incisors. It is located in the midline. It lies approximately 1.5 to 2 cm above the alveolar crest between the central incisors, below the junction of the inferior end of the nasal septum and the inferior outline of the nasal fossa.	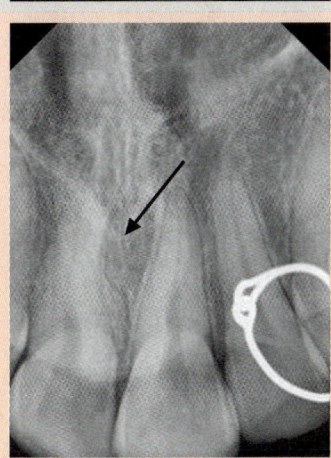
3. **Nasal fossa:** It appears as radiolucent image on the periapical projections in the region of central incisors. The anterior floor of the nasal fossa is radiopaque and extends laterally from anterior nasal spine. The nasal septum appears as a radiopaque structure within the nasal fossa.	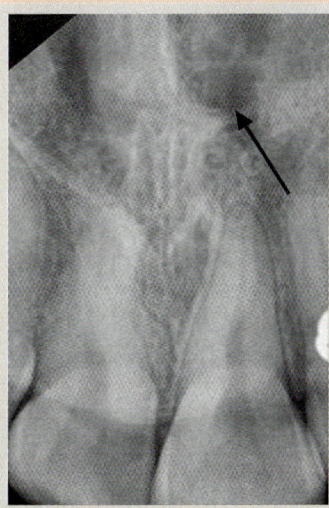

Contd.

TABLE 33.1: Maxillary anatomic landmarks *(Contd.)*

Maxillary landmark	*Radiographic appearance*

4. **Nasal septum:** Nasal septum appears as a radiopaque structure directly above the anterior nasal spine. It divides the nasal cavity into two halves. The mucosal covering of the inferior concha may occasionally be seen in the nasal fossa extending from right and left lateral wall towards the septum.

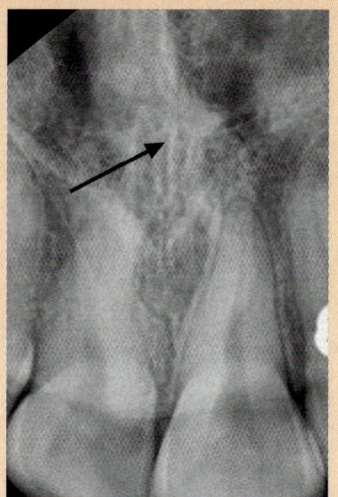

5. **Incisive foramen (nasopalatine foramen):** It is the opening of the nasopalatine canal. It appears as radiolucent image between central incisors. It doesn't have any cortical outline. It is usually round, oval, heart or diamond shaped in appearance. It is present almost always in the midline and mostly seen in between the roots of two central incisors. Sometimes, it is seen very near to alveolar crest.

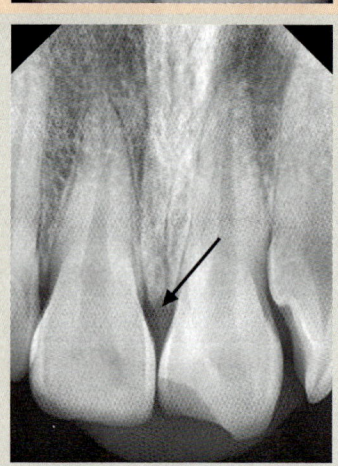

6. **Lateral fossa (incisive fossa):** It is a gentle depression in the maxilla, near the apex of the lateral incisor medial to canine eminence. It appears as a diffusely radiolucent zone in the region of lateral incisor.

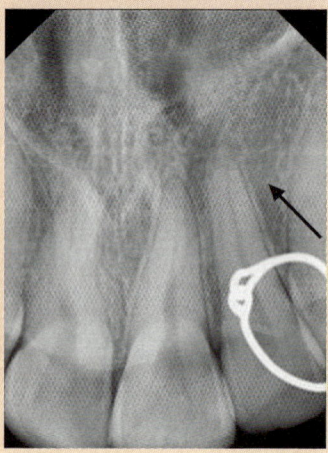

Contd.

TABLE 33.1: Maxillary anatomic landmarks (*Contd.*)

Maxillary landmark	Radiographic appearance
7. **Nose:** It is a soft tissue shadow of the tip of the nose. It is sometimes seen in the maxillary central-lateral incisor projections. It is seen as a uniform, slightly radiopaque shadow with uniform outline.	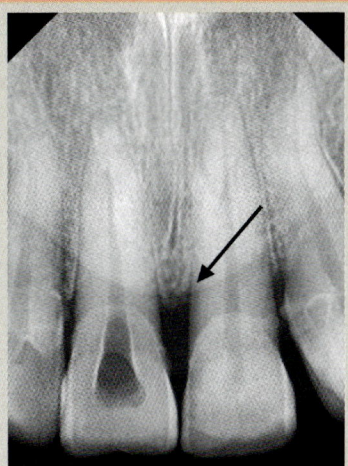
8. **Nasolabial fold:** It is a soft tissue shadow of the nasolabial fold seen in the maxillary lateral incisor and canine projections. It is seen as a uniform, slightly radiopaque extending across canine-premolar region. 9. **Nasolacrimal canal:** It is seen in maxillary occlusal radiograph and sometimes in maxillary molar X-ray. It is seen as a round radiolucent shadow on palatal aspect of second molar.	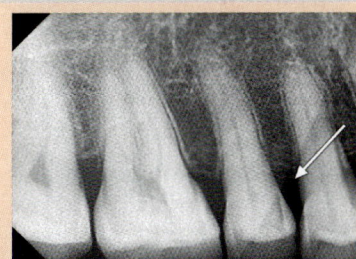
10. **Maxillary sinus** ✗ Maxillary sinuses are pyramid-shaped cavity in maxillary bone that contains air and hence, they appear as dark radiolucent image. Its borders appear as a thin, delicate, tenuous radiopaque line (actually, a thin layer of cortical bone). In posterior periapical radiographs, the maxillary sinus is usually seen extending from the premolar area to the maxillary tuberosity. ✗ The anterior wall of maxillary sinus meets the nasal fossa in canine and premolar region and forms an inverted 'y' shaped appearance on radiograph. One wing of 'y' is made up of nasal fossa and another is of anterior wall of maxillary sinus and leg is made by lateral cortex of nasal fossa . This is known as 'inverted y line of ENNIS'.	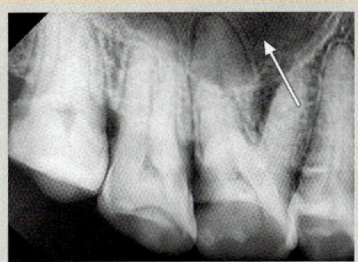 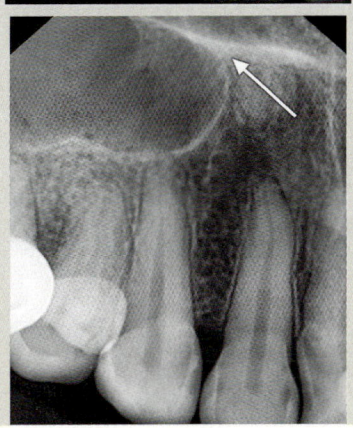

Contd.

TABLE 33.1: Maxillary anatomic landmarks *(Contd.)*

Maxillary landmark	*Radiographic appearance*

* Many times septae are present in the maxillary sinus. These septae vary in number, thickness and length. Septae usually divide the sinus either partially or completely.
* Premature removal of maxillary molar may cause the pneumatization of antrum into the alveolar bone. Maxillary sinus floor extends towards the crest of the alveolar ridge in response to edentulousness.

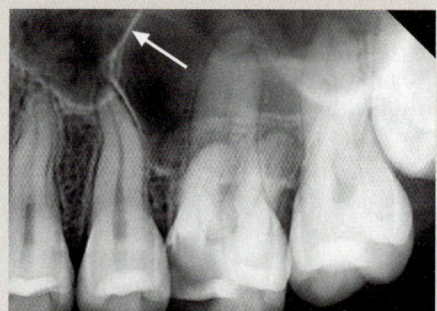

11. **Maxillary tuberosity:** This a bony prominence distal to last molar in maxillary arch. It appears as a radiopaque dense structure.

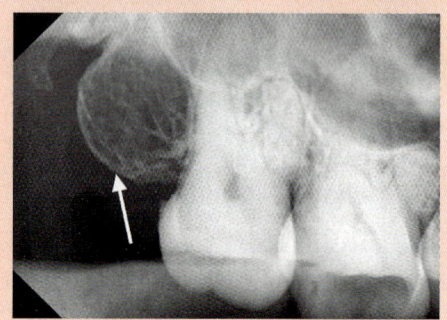

12. **Zygomatic process and zygomatic bone:** It is a dense corticated bone. It appears as a U-, J- or V-shaped radiopaque thick line with its open end directed superiorly. Usually, we see superimposition of the zygomatic arch over the roots of the maxillary molars due to vertical angulation of X-ray beam.

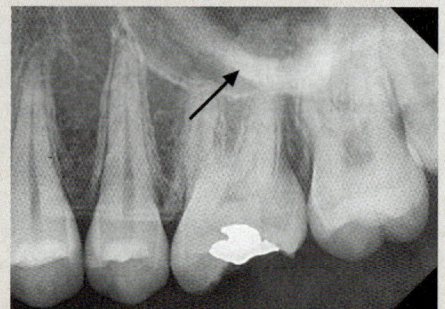

13. **Pterygoid plates:** Medial and lateral pterygoid plates lie immediately posterior to the maxillary tuberosity. They are thin bone projections which provide attachment to the pterygoid muscles. On radiograph, they appear as two tiny radiopaque projections of corticated bone in distal direction.

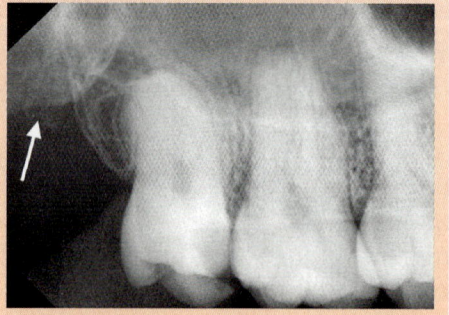

Contd.

TABLE 33.1: Maxillary anatomic landmarks (Contd.)	
Maxillary landmark	**Radiographic appearance**
14. **Hamular process:** It is a bony depression behind the maxillary tuberosity. It is present between the pterygoid plates and maxillary tuberosity.	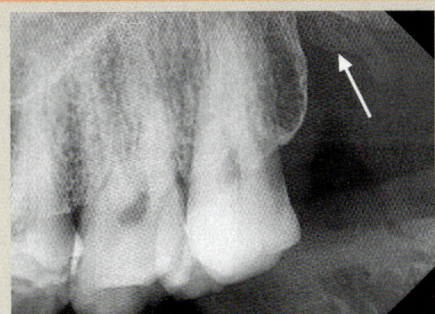
15. **Coronoid process:** The coronoid process of mandible appears as a thick dense radiopaque structure either superimposed or lies inferior to maxillary tuberosity. It usually occurs in maxillary molar X-rays. It is a part of the mandible which is visualized in maxillary molar X-rays. This occurs when the patient opens his mouth, the coronoid process of the mandible moves forward and lies in the line of X-rays.	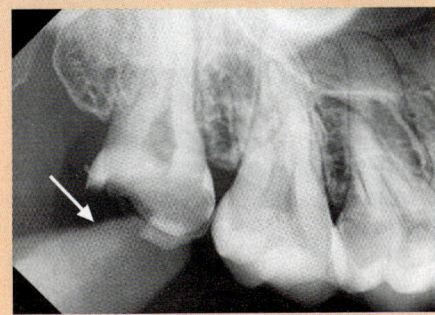

Mandibular Anatomical Landmarks

Symphysis: Symphysis is a radiolucent landmark which appears in anterior region of mandible in infants. It is seen as a broad radiolucent area in mandibular anterior region between forming deciduous central incisors. It is a suture in midline of mandible which fuses by 18 months of age (Fig. 33.2).

Restorative Materials

The restorative materials used cast their shadow on the X-ray. They may occur as radioapaque or radiolucent shadow depending on their composition. Most of the restorative materials are radioapaque in nature. Commonly used restorative materials like amalgam, gold, stainless steel crown and other orthodontic brackets, silver points used in root filling, Gutta percha points used in root canal filling, and cements

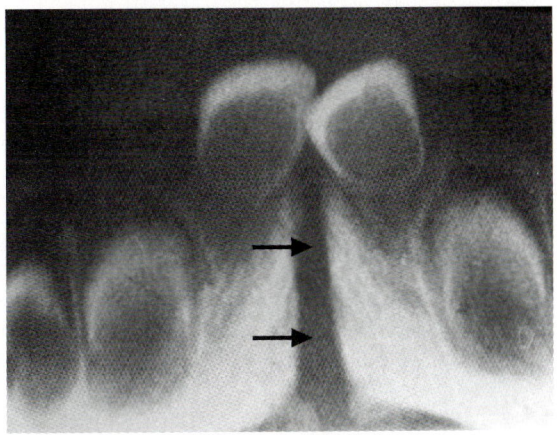

Fig. 33.2: Radiograph of infant's symphysis

like silicates appear radiopaque. Composites and porcelain are radiolucent, but nowadays radioapaque additives are added to these and hence they appear radiopaque. The density of radiopacity is more compared to the teeth for all these restorative materials.

TABLE 33.2: Mandibular anatomic landmarks

Mandibular landmark	Radiographic appearance
1. **Genial tubercles:** These are radiopaque shadows appear on lingual surface of mandibular anterior region. They can be either one or two in number. Mostly seen in midline. These are present slightly above the lower border of mandible. They have a small conical or sharp spine shaped appearance. These cast dense shadow on teeth in IOPA while in occlusal radiograph appear on lingual side of the X-ray.	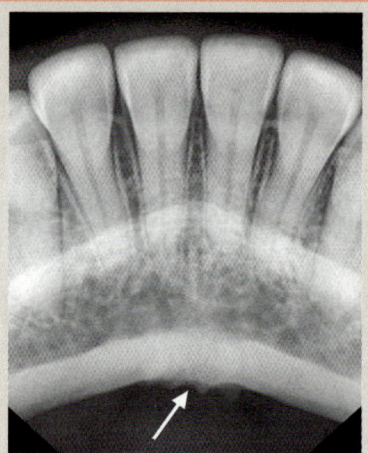
2. **Mental ridge:** Mental ridge is a thick band of radioapaque shadow present in mandibular anterior region. They are superimposed over the mandibular incisor teeth. They extend laterally from midline towards lower border of mandible in oblique direction. Their density and width often varies.	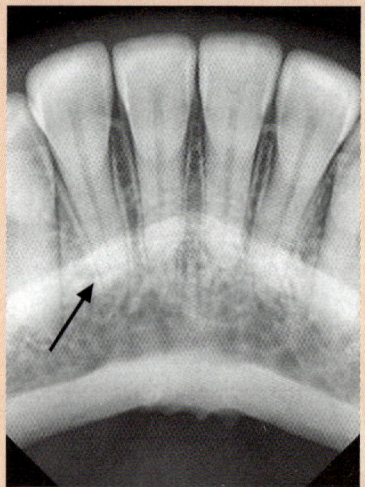
3. **Mental fossa:** Mental fossa is a radiolucent landmark seen in mandibular anterior region above mental ridge. It causes a depression on labial aspect of mandible. This casts a faint radiolucent shadow on the mandibular incisors.	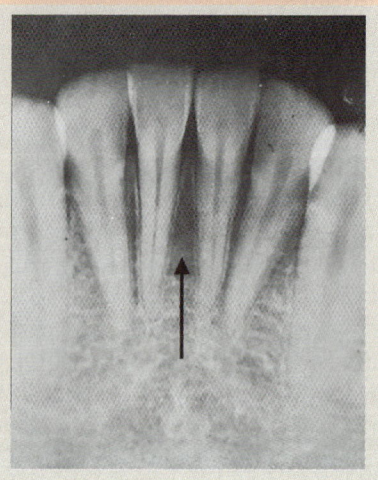

Contd.

TABLE 33.2: Mandibular anatomic landmark *(Contd.)*

Mandibular landmark	*Radiographic appearance*
4. **Mental foramen:** Mental foramen is a small round radiolucent shadow present below the roots of 1st premolar or between the 1st and 2nd premolars. The inferior alveolar nerve divides into mental nerve and exits from it along with blood vessels. The image of mental foramen is often variable in its location. It is mostly identified because of continuity with inferior alveolar nerve canal. Rarely multiple mental foramina are seen on an X-ray. When it is projected on the roots of the tooth, it may mimic as a periapical pathology.	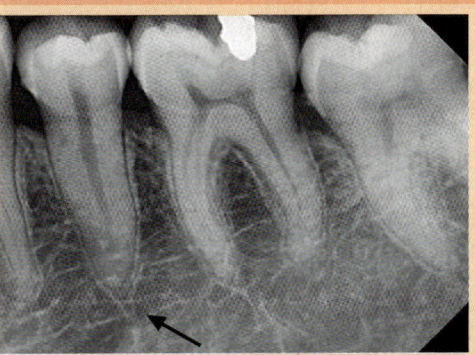
5. **Mandibular canal:** Mandibular canal is a radiolucent landmark present in posterior region of mandible. It appears as a radiolucent linear band present below the roots of molars and premolar. It extends from mandibular foramen to mental foramen and contains inferior alveolar nerve and blood vessels. It forms a most prominent structure in mandible. Relationship of third molar tooth to mandibular canal: Depending upon the angulation of the X-rays projection, the roots of mandibular molar teeth vary in their relation to mandibular canal.	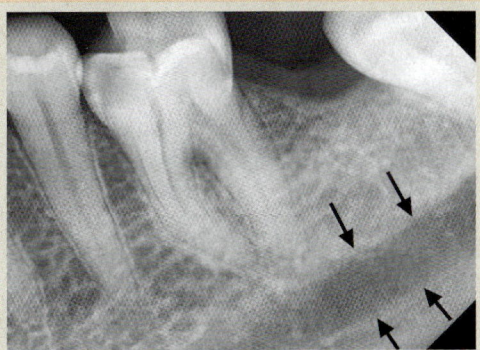
6. **Mylohyoid ridge:** Mylohyoid ridge is a radioapaque landmark present in posterior region of mandible. It is a thick band of radiopaque shadow seen over the apices of mandibular posterior teeth. It usually runs downwards and forwards from third molar region to premolar region. This ridge serves as an attachment for mylohyoid muscle.	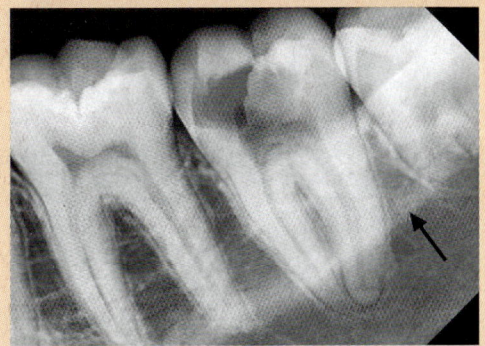
7. **Nutrient canals:** Nutrient canals are radiolucent landmark present just superior to the root apex. These are thin radiolucent lines extending vertically below the root apices. They contain blood vessels and nerves. These are seen more predominantly in mandibular anterior region.	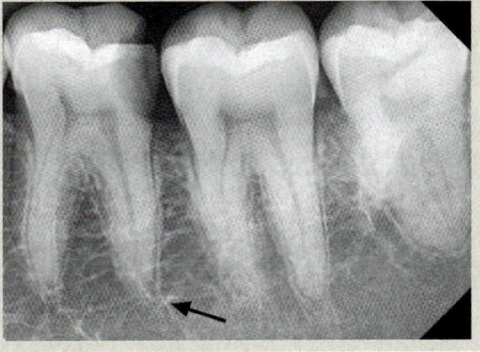

Contd.

TABLE 33.2: Mandibular anatomic landmark *(Contd.)*

Mandibular landmark	Radiographic appearance
8. **Submandibular gland fossa:** Submandibular gland fossa is radiolucent landmark present in posterior region of mandible. It appears as a thin radiolucent shadow with sparse trabecular pattern between the mylohyoid ridge and lower border of mandible. It is seen below the second and third molar region. In some patients the submandibular gland fossa is more prominent and forms a large depression in the mandible.	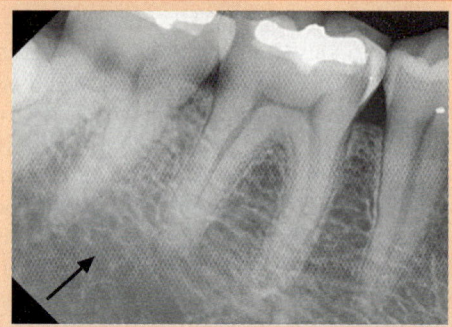
9. **External oblique ridge:** External oblique ridge is a radioapaque landmark present in posterior region of mandible. It is a continuation of anterior border of ramus of mandible running downwards and forwards from third molar region to premolar region.	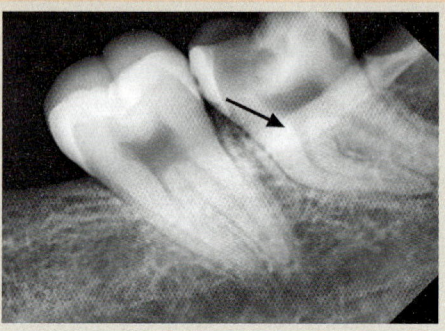

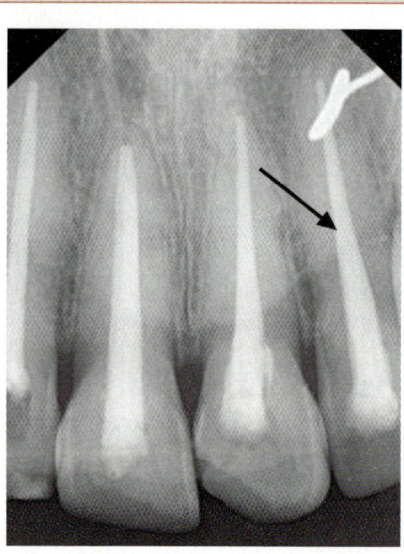

Fig. 33.3: Incisors with radiopaque restorations

FREQUENTLY ASKED QUESTIONS

1. Enumerate RO/RL landmarks of maxilla/mandible.
2. Enumerate landmarks in mandibular posterior/anterior region.
3. Enumerate landmarks in maxillary posterior/anterior region.

BIBLIOGRAPHY

1. Karjodkar F. Textbook of Dental and Maxillofacial Radiology, 2nd edition. Jaypee Brothers Medical Publishers; 2009.
2. Whaites E. Essentials of Dental Radiography and Radiology, 4th edition. Spain: Churchill Livingstone Elsevier; 2007.
3. White S, Pharoah Medicine Oral Radiology. Principles and Interpretation. 6th edition. Elsevier Inc; 2011.
4. White S, Pharoah Medicine Oral Radiology. Principles and Interpretation. 5th edition. Mushy; 2004.
5. Goaz P. wwtes. Oral Radiology Principles and Interpretation. 2nd edition: BI Publishers; 1998.
6. Whaites E. Essentials of Dental Radiography and Radiology. 2nd edition. Churchill Livingstone; 1997.
7. Karjodkar F. Textbook of Dental and Maxillofacial Radiology. 1st edition : Jaypee Brothers Medical Publishers; 2006.

Extraoral Radiography

Extraoral radiography or imaging techniques are practiced using X-ray image receptor placed outside the oral structure/cavity.

Anatomic 'baselines' are used for accurate positioning of the cassette/film which helps in acquisition of the required image.

* **Radiographic baseline** or the orbitomeatal line extends from outer canthus of eye to external auditory meatus.
* **Midsagittal plane:** The median plane of the head passing through the sagittal suture and dividing the head into right and left halves.
* **Frankfort horizontal plane (FH plane):** Extends from the superior border of the external auditory meatus to the infraorbital rim.
* **Canthomeatal line/orbitomeatal line:** The line extending from the outer canthus of the eye to the center of the external auditory meatus. It is also called the radiographic baseline/Reid's baseline.
* **Infraorbital line:** The line running from one infraorbital margin to the other.
* **Camper's line/Ala-tragus line:** Line running from the ala of the nose to the center of the tragus of the ear.

Equipment used for extraoral radiography are:
1. Intraoral X-ray machine
2. Extraoral X-ray machine
3. Cephalometric X-ray unit
4. Digital sensors equipped with computer assembly

FILMS

* Screen films are routinely used in extraoral radiography which use the film cassettes and grid. Screen films sensitive to blue or green light are commonly used.
* Digital setups need dry-fix films.
* Screen films sensitive to blue or green light are commonly used.
* Conventional methods use the film cassettes and grid.

General Indications

1. Evaluation of facial and jaw bones (trauma/pathology)
2. Evaluation of eruption pattern of teeth including skeletal growth and development.
3. Temporomandibular evaluation.
4. In patients with trismus, where intraoral radiographs are not possible.
5. For larger lesions involving jaws.
6. Investigation of paranasal sinuses
7. Diseases affecting the skull base and vault.

Exposure Parameters

* kVp
  * 70 to 80 for intraoral units.
  * 60 to 100 for extraoral units.
* mA
  * Up to 8 mA for intraoral unit
  * Up to 100 mA for extraoral unit with grids.

TABLE 34.1: Imaging techniques for skull

Sr. No.	Maxillofacial imaging view	Patient's position	Film position	Central ray	Indication/structure seen
1.	Lateral cephalogram	☓ Upright with area of interest towards film/sensor	☓ Parallel to patient's midsagittal plane (left side towards film)	☓ Perpendicular to midsagittal plane, centered over external auditory meatus	☓ Evaluation of facial growth and developmental trauma, diseases or anomalies ☓ To evaluate treatment prognosis 1. Evaluation of the skull and facial bones 2. Evaluation of the soft tissue profile of the face
2.	True lateral	☓ Mid-sagittal plane parallel to film	☓ Film is placed close to cheek covering entire skull	☓ Perpendicular to midsagittal plane and film	☓ Evaluation of skull and facial bones.
3.	PA skull	☓ Mid-sagittal plane perpendicular to film, forehead and nose	☓ In front of patient ☓ Canthomeatal line perpendicular to film	☓ Perpendicular to midsagittal plane/cassette (ray directed PA)	☓ Skull vault, frontal sinuses cranium and intracranial calcifications
4.	PA cephalogram	☓ Midsagittal plane perpendicular to film, forehead and nose touch the film lips in the center of film	☓ Canthomeatal line is 10° to horizontal plane and FH plane is perpendicular to film ☓ In front of the patient	☓ Perpendicular to film centered at bridge of the nose	☓ To access instead of assess facial asymmetry ☓ To analyse effect of orthognatic surgeries
5.	Towne's projection (antero-posterior view)	☓ Back of patient head touches film ☓ CM line is perpendicular to film	☓ Perpendicular to the floor	☓ 30° to CM line and passes from midpoint of line joining two external auditory meatus	☓ To visualize occipital region of skull

Commonly Practiced Views in Dental Radiography:

Maxillofacial Imaging Views

1. **Skull:** Lateral cephalogram
   ☓ True lateral view
   ☓ PA (posteroanterior) cephalogram
   ☓ Towne's projection
2. **Paranasal sinuses**
   ▪ PA (posteroanterior)-occipitofrontal view
   ▪ Occipitomental projection (0° and 30°)
   ▪ PA Water's view

TABLE 34.2: Imaging techniques for paranasal sinuses

Sr. No.	Maxillofacial imaging view	Patient's position	Film position	Central ray	Indication/structure seen
1.	PA projection/ occipito-frontal view—0°	✗ Patient faces the image receptor ✗ FH plane at 45° to film	✗ Cassette in front of the patient	✗ Central ray passes from occipital region (posterior to anterior).	✗ Facial skeleton and maxillary antra ✗ Le Fort-I Le Fort-II Le Fort-III ✗ Coronoid process and its pathologies
2.	Occipito-mental projection (0° and 30°)	✗ Patient faces the image receptor ✗ FH plane at 45° to film	✗ Cassette in front of the patient	✗ Central ray is directed by shifting tube head upward and passing beam through lower border of orbit making 30° angle to the horizontal plane.	✗ Shows facial skeleton but from different angle than 0° view. (Two views, 0° and 30°, can be taken at a time to diagnose facial pathologies)
3.	PA Water's view	✗ Patient's head is tilted upward ✗ CM line is 37° with film (in open mouth position, sphenoid sinuses can also be visualized)	✗ Film is placed in front of patient with rays perpendicular to image receptor	✗ Beam centered at the level of maxillary sinuses	✗ Primarily for maxillary sinuses ✗ Frontal and ethmoidal sinuses ✗ Orbit and coronoid process can also be seen

TABLE 34.3: Imaging techniques for mandible

Sr. No.	Maxillofacial imaging view	Patient's position	Film position	Central ray	Indication/ structure seen
1.	Lateral oblique projection—body of mandible	✗ Head is tilted to the side of interest with protruded mandible (sufficient tilt should be given to avoid superimposition)	✗ Cassette is placed against patient's cheek on the side of interest. ✗ The center of film should be at PM and M region ✗ Lower border of cassette is 2 cm below lower border of mandible and parallel to it	✗ PM-M region of opposite side ✗ The beam passes 2 cm below the angle of mandible (opposite side)	✗ To evaluate pathologies or developmental disorders in PM-M region or body of mandible

Contd.

TABLE 34.3: Imaging techniques for mandible *(Contd.)*

Sr. No.	Maxillofacial Imaging view	Patient's position	Film position	Central ray	Indication/ Structure seen
2.	Lateral oblique projection— body of ramus	˟ Head is tilted towards the side of interest with protruded mandible	˟ Cassette is placed in a way to cover the ramus region including posterior aspect as much as possible to include condyle	˟ Centered over ramus from opposite side, i.e. 2 cm below inferior border of mandible in the first molar region	˟ For ramus region. Pathologies like developmental anomalies, impacted teeth, etc.
3.	PA-mandible	˟ Midsagittal plane is perpendicular to the film ˟ Head is tilted to touch the cassette with forehead and nosetip ˟ FH plane is perpendicular to the film	˟ Film is perpendicular to the floor	˟ X-ray beam passes through vertebrae at the level of midpoint of angle of mandible	˟ To evaluate body and ramus for various pathologies as well as mediolateral expansion of posterior one-third of the body of ramus

TABLE 34.4: Imaging techniques for zygomatic arches

Sr. No.	Maxillofacial imaging view	Patient's position	Film position	Central ray	Indication/structure seen
1.	Submento-vertex (SMV) projection	Head is extended behind the maximum limit possible by keeping CM line 10° with respect to image receptor	Cassette is placed parallel to patients axial those and perpendicular to midsagittal plane.	Beam is perpendicular to film directed from an imaginary line joining mandibular molars, i.e. 3 cm below chin approx.	˟ To evaluate the base of the skull and anatomic structures ˟ Axial inclination (of condyles (palate, pterygoid plates, sphenoidal sinuses)
2.	Jug handle or modified SMV	–	–	–	˟ To evaluate zygomatic arch fracture

(Underexposed SMV or low exposure parameters are required for jug handle view)

TABLE 34.5: Reverse Towne's projection

Maxillofacial Imaging view	Patient's position	Film position	Central ray	Indication/structure seen
Reverse Towne's (PA) view	✗ Head tipped forward with mouth opened ✗ FH plane is perpendicular to receptor ✗ Opening the mouth positions the condyles out of glenoid fossa which helps in their visualization	✗ In front of the patient	✗ Beam aims upwards 30° to FH plane through line joining the condyles in center	✗ Condylar heads and neck (bilaterally)

TABLE 34.6: Various radiographic technique

Maxillofacial imaging view	Beam and patient position	Images	Radiographs
Lateral cephalogram	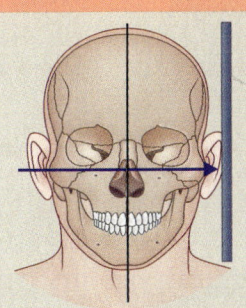	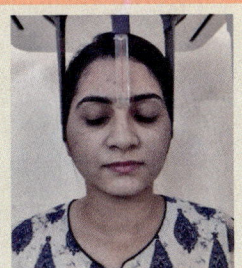	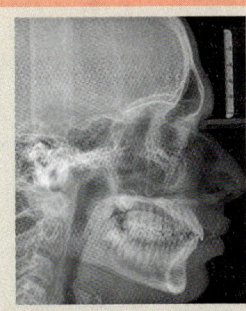
PA skull	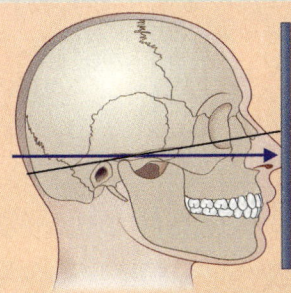	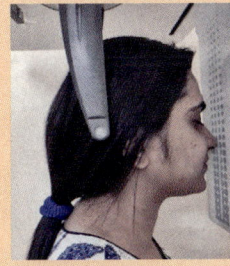	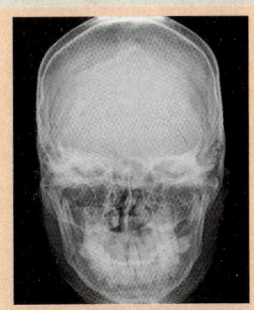
Water's view	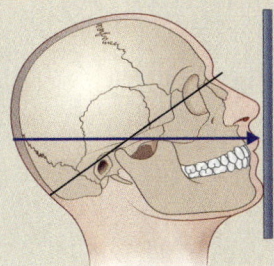	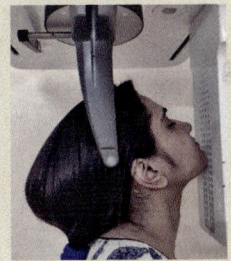	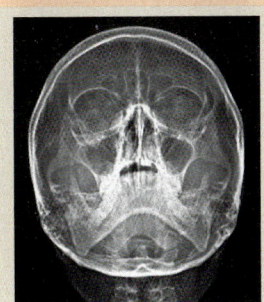

Contd.

TABLE 34.6: Various radiographic techniques *(Contd.)*

Maxillofacial imaging view	Beam and patient position	Images	Radiographs
SMV			
Reverse Towne's view			
Lateral oblique projection—body of mandible			
Lateral oblique projection—ramus			

3. **Mandible**
   - Lateral oblique projection—body and ramus
   - PA mandible
4. **Base of the skull:** Submentovertex projection (SMV)
5. **Zygomatic arches:** Jug handle view on modified SMV
6. **Temporomandibular joint**
   - Transcranial ⎫
   - Transorbital ⎬ TMJ views are discussed in Section I
   - Transpharyngeal ⎭
   - Reverse Towne's

FREQUENTLY ASKED QUESTIONS

Write short note on

1. Indications of lateral cephalogram
2. Indications of Water's view
3. Indications of submentovertex
4. Indications of reverse Towne
   or
   Indications and patient positioning of extraoral views can be asked as SAQ, MCQ, LAQ or viva voce questions.

BIBLIOGRAPHY

1. Karjodkar F. Essentials of Oral and Maxillofacial Radiology. 1st edition New Delhi: Jaypee Brothers Medical Publishers; 2014.
2. Karjodkar F. Textbook of Dental and Maxillofacial Radiology 2nd edition: Jaypee Brothers Medical Publishers; 2009.
3. Whaites E. Essentials of Dental Radiography and Radiology, 4th edition, Spain: Churchill Livingstone Elsevier; 2007.
4. White S., Pharoah Medicine Oral Radiology. Principles and Interpretation. 6th edition: Elsevier Inc; 2011.
5. White S., Pharoah Medicine Oral Radiology. Principles and Interpretation. 5th edition: Mushy; 2004.
6. Goaz P. White. Oral Radiology Principles and Interpretation. 2nd edition: BI Publishers; 1998.
7. Whaites E. Essentials of Dental Radiography and Radiology 2nd edition Churchill Livingstone; 1997.
8. Langland O, Langlais R, Preece J. Principles of Dental imaging 2nd edition : Lippincott Williams and Wilkins; 2002.
9. Langland O, Langlais R, Principles of Dental imaging 1st edition : Lippincott Williams and Wilkins; 1997.
10. Wood N, Goaz P. Differential diagnosis of Oral and Maxillofacial Lesions. 5th edition, Elsevier; 2007.

Orthopantomography

INTRODUCTION

* Panoramic radiography, as the name suggests, is "an unobstructed view of a region in every direction" that is displaying of entire maxillomandibular region on a single film.
* The use of extraoral source of radiation, i.e. rotational panoramic radiography was first proposed by Dr. Hisatsugu Numata of Japan in1933 and experimented in 1934.

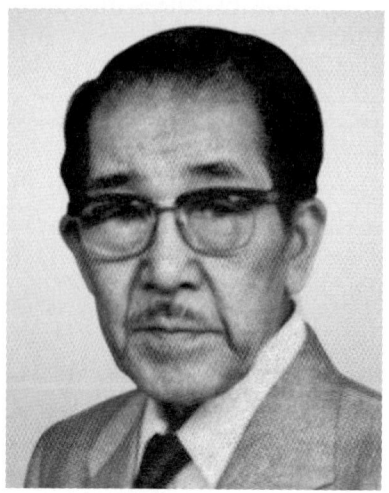

Hisatsugu Numata

* He placed a curved film in the mouth lingual to the teeth and used a slit or narrow X-ray beam that rotated around the patient's jaws to expose the film.

* Another method for panoramic radiography (PR) was intraoral which employed an intraoral source of radiation. The radiation is directed from inside the mouth through the jaws and exposes a film molded to the outside of the face of the patient.
* The X-ray source, patient, and film are stationary during the exposure. Maxilla and mandible are exposed separately.
* Horst Berger of Germany was the inventor of this machine who received patent to his firm producing such machines in 1943.
* In 1946, Dr. Y Paatero from Finland proposed, experimented (1948) and demonstrated a slit beam method of PR for the dental arches (1949).
* Tomography—X-ray tech, for making radiographs of tissues in depth, without the interference of tissue above and below that level.
* In 1950, Dr. Robert Nelsen and machinist technician John W. Kumpula developed technique of PR similar to Paatero'sparabolographic intraoral film method and called it panographic radiography.

PRINCIPLE OF ORTHOPANTOMOGRAPHY

Orthopantomography (OPG) is a single tomographic image of maxillomandibular structures including teeth and supporting hard tissue. OPG principle involves synchronized movement of X-ray tube head and the sensor/film with common center/s of rotation, rotating in a horizontal plane in a circular path around patients' head.

This reciprocal movement of an X-ray source and an image receptor around one point at a time which is called image layer (focal trough). OPG obtains given image in sections (tomosections). Drawback of tomography is, only structures within the sections will be evident on the resultant radiograph. The section of focal trough is horseshoe shaped (as per dental arches in OPG).

Slit Beam Technique

OPG machines have slit shaped lead collimators at X-ray source and image receptor. This restricts the shape of the beam or makes it narrow. The narrow beam traverses the film exposing sections of film during movement of machine. Entire film shows the image after completing rotation or at the end of one exposure cycle.

Process of Image Acquisition in Pantomograph

X-ray source and image receptor are moving in orthopantomograph while patient is stationary. X-ray tube head orbits around the back of patients' head while image receptor orbits in front of the face. When X-ray source is at left side of patient's jaw, receptor is at right side and vice versa. In new generation machines, there are multiple center of rotations. Rate of speed of receptor rotation is same as speed of X-ray beam passing through the anatomic structures on the side of the patient, nearest to the receptor. Structures on the opposite side of the patient, which are near X-ray source appear blurred as X-ray beam sweeps through them in opposite direction to image receptor motion. Structures near the X-ray source are magnified and cannot be appreciated separately on the image. These are called phantom on ghost images.

Image receptors for OPG
- Cassette with intensifying screen (fast film with high speed rare earth material)
- Digital sensors
  - Charged couple device (CCD)
  - Phosphor storage plates (PSP)

Patient's Position

Patient is prepared for X-ray exposure by removing dental prosthesis, earrings, necklaces, hairpins and other metallic objects in head region.
- New generator machines have FH plane and midline aligners. They help to position midsagittal plane (midline) and horizontal plane of patient. Biteblock (with a small

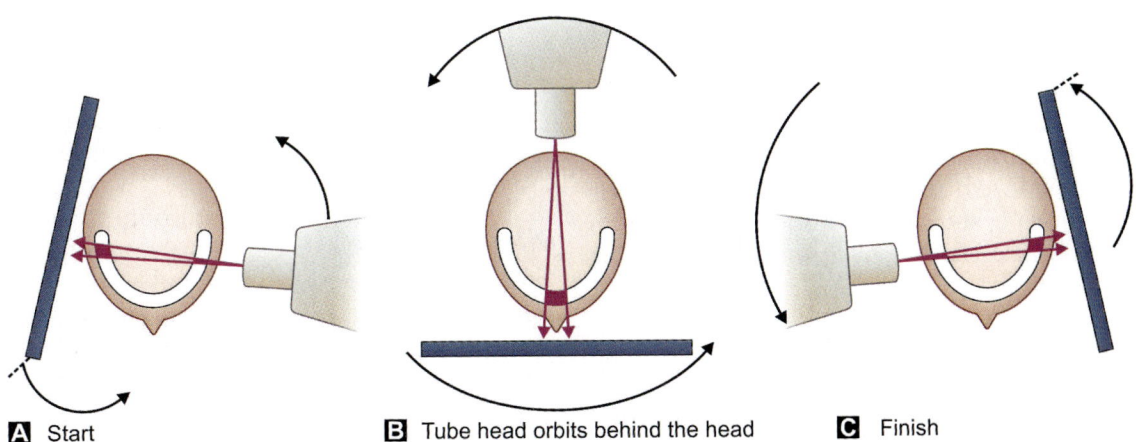

A Start   **B** Tube head orbits behind the head   **C** Finish

Fig. 35.1(A to C): Diagrammatic representation of image acquisition in pantomography

notch) guides to position incisal edge of anterior teeth into notch.

- Patient is placed upright either in standing or sitting position with slightly extended neck.
- After positioning patient in machine, they are instructed to swallow and hold the tongue to the roof of the mouth. This aids in visualization of a portion of maxillary teeth due to rising of dorsum of tongue to the hard palate.

Focal Trough

The focal trough or image layer or 3D curve zone where anatomic structures are reasonable when appreciated on final radiograph. The simple circular rotatory movement with a single center of rotation produces a curved circular focal trough.

Object or structures outside the image layer or focal trough appear magnified, reduced or distorted. So, it is important to position the patient accurately while scanning which allows the visualization of required structure in focal trough.

Different brands of machine may have different focal trough and positioning device as well. But failure to place anatomic structure in focal trough results in various errors in resultant radiograph.

Indications

- As a substitute for full mouth intraoral periapical radiographs.
- For evaluation of tooth development for children, the mixed dentition and also the age.
- To assist and assess the patient for and during orthodontic treatment.
- To establish the site and size of lesions such as cysts, tumors and developmental anomalies in the body and rami of the mandible.
- Prior to surgical procedures such as extraction of impacted teeth, enucleation of cyst, etc.
- For detection of fractures of the middle third face and the mandible after facial trauma.

- For follow-up of treatment, progress of pathology or postoperative bony healing.
- Investigation of TM joint dysfunction.
- To study the antrum, especially to study the floor, posterior and anterior walls of the antrum.
- Periodontal disease, as an overall view of the alveolar bone levels.
- Assessment for underlying bone disease before constructing complete or partial dentures.
- Evaluation of developmental anomalies.

Contraindications

- Panoramic films are not as defined or sharp as the images seen on intraoral films.
- They cannot be used to assess:
  - Finer details of anatomic landmarks.
  - Small carious lesions
  - Fine structures of the marginal periodontium
  - Periapical diseases

Advantages of OPG

- Simple procedure requiring very little patient compliance.
- Convenient for the patient.
  - Useful in patients with trismus and gagging problems.
  - Time required is minimal compared to full mouth intraoral periapical radiographs.
  - Portions of the maxilla and the mandible lying within the focal trough can be visualized on a single film.
  - The patient dose is relatively low. Panoramic radiographs taken for diagnostic purpose are valuable visual aids in patient education.

Disadvantages of OPG

- Areas of diagnostic interest outside the focal trough may be poorly visualized, e.g. swelling on the palate, floor of the mouth.
- Comparatively this radiograph is of a poor diagnostic quality, in terms of magnification, geometric distortion, poor definition and loss of detail.

- There is an overlapping of the teeth in the bicuspid area of the maxilla and the mandible.
- Number of radiopaque and radiolucent areas may be present due to the superimposition of real/double or ghost images and because of soft tissue shadows and airspaces.

Errors

Common patient positioning errors are discussed in Table 35.1

Errors	Reason	Radiographic appearance
a. Ghost image	Produced when a radiodense object is penetrated twice by the X-ray beam	 Failure to remove earrings
b. Reverse smile appearance	Chin is positioned too high or tipped up	
c. Exaggerated—smile appearance shortening of lower incisors	Chin is positioned too low	
d. Patient positioned too forward on bite block	Anterior teeth appear narrow	

TABLE 35.1: Common patient positioning errors

Contd.

TABLE 35.1: Common patient positioning errors (Contd.)

Errors	Reason	Radiographic appearance
e. Patient is positioned too far back on the bite block	Anterior teeth appear widened and blurred	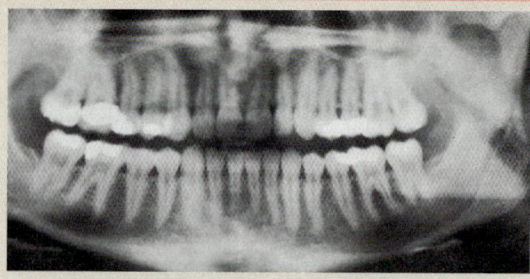
f. Patient head tilted to one side	The side tilted towards the X-ray tube is enlarged	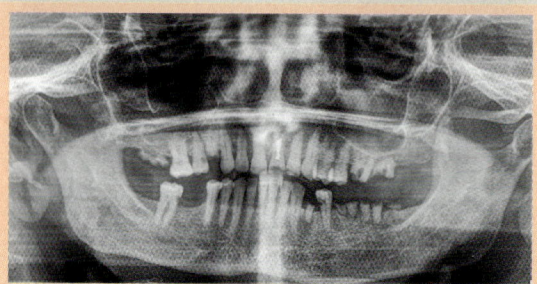
g. Positioning of the spine	If the patient is not sitting or standing with a straight spine, the cervical spine appears as a pyramid-shaped radiopacity in the center of the film and obscures diagnostic information	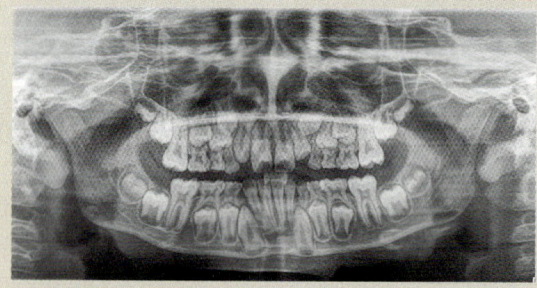
h. Continuous shaking movement throughout the cycle	Due to movement of patient during exposure, image appears blurred	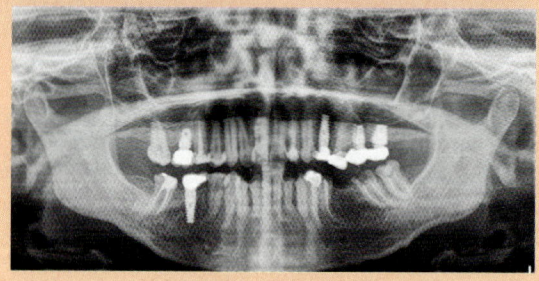

FREQUENTLY ASKED QUESTIONS

1. Define focal trough.
2. Explain principle of OPG.
3. Enumerate advantages and disadvantages of OPG.
4. Give 5 indications of OPG.

BIBLIOGRAPHY

1. Whaites E. Essentials of Dental Radiography and Radiology, 4th edition. Spain: Churchill Livingstone, Elsevier; 2007.
2. White S., Pharoah Medicine Oral Radiology. Principles and Interpretation. 6th edition: Elsevier Inc; 2011.

3. White S., Pharoah Medicine Oral Radiology. Principles and Interpretation. 5th edition: Mushy; 2004.

4. Goaz P White. Oral Radiology Principles and Interpretation.2nd edition: B.I Publishers; 1998.

5. Whaites E. Essentials of Dental Radiography and Radiology, 2nd edition, Churchill Livingstone; 1997.

6. Langland O, Langlais R, Preece J. Principles of Dental Imaging, 2nd edition : Lippincott Williams and Wilkins; 2002.

7. Langland O, Langlais R. Principles of Dental Imaging. 1st edition. Lippincott Williams and Wilkins; 1997.

8. Wood N, Goaz P. Differential Diagnosis of Oral and Maxillofacial Lesions. 5th edition, Elsevier; 2007.

9. Karjodkar F. Textbook of Dental and Maxillofacial Radiology. 2nd edition. Jaypee Brothers Medical Publishers; 2009.

Advance Imaging

INTRODUCTION

Imaging has evolved from conventional radiography to recently developed more sophisticated imaging techniques like magnetic resonance imaging. Imaging will always remain a mainstay in the diagnosis of any disease, particularly in preoperative assessment. With the advent of continuous research going on in the field of radiology, newer techniques, computer assisted programs, newer sequences, better contrast agents are being introduced, thus increasing accuracies in diagnosing specific pathology.

In this chapter, we will discuss the basics of advance imaging techniques and their utility with special reference to dental imaging.

Imaging techniques like sialography, arthrography will be discussed in other chapters.

ULTRASONOGRAPHY (USG)

Use of ultrasound in medical practice was made since 1940. It is continuously going through modifications and new additions so as to increase its efficacy in the diagnosis of different medical conditions.

Ultrasound uses sound waves of higher frequency, i.e. above 20 kHz and it needs medium to transmit. Interaction of ultrasound waves within the body is the basis of image formation and it depends on scattering of sound waves by the different tissues.

Basic Concept of Ultrasound

In simple language, sound waves are transmitted to the body through ultrasound transducer (probe), they get reflected or refracted depending upon the tissue through which they travel and then return to the probe. While returning to the probe, they carry information about the tissue travelled which is converted by the image software into an image.

Sound Frequencies

Whenever sound travels through a medium, it undergoes compression and relaxation depending upon the medium and it produces a sound wave (Fig. 36.1).

The distance between two points on the time-pressure curve is a wavelength (λ), and the time (T) to complete a single cycle is called period. The number of complete cycles in a unit time is the frequency which is termed hertz (Hz).

Audible frequencies range from 20 to 20,000 Hz. Acoustic frequencies used for diagnostic purposes range from 2 to 15 MHz, i.e. much higher than the audible one.

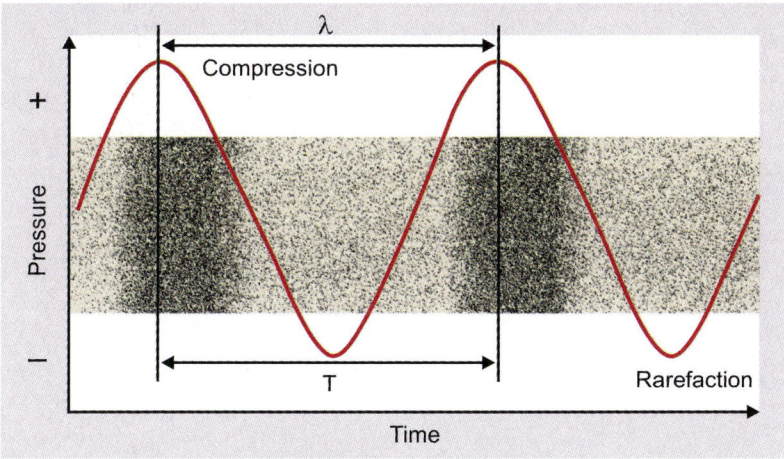

Fig. 36.1: Sound waves

Instrument

Ultrasound scanners (**Fig. 36.2**) consist of:
- Transmitter to energize the transducer
- Ultrasound transducer
- Receiver
- Display
- Image storage.

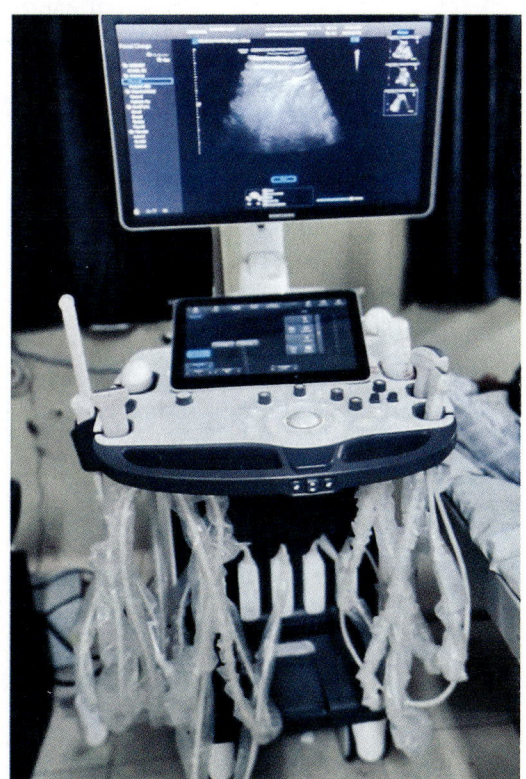

Fig. 36.2: USG machine

Transmitter: The ultrasound transducer is energized by application of high-amplitude voltage.

Transducer: In diagnostic ultrasound, transducer converts electric energy provided by the transmitter to the acoustic pulses directed into the patient and receives reflected echoes, converting them into electric signals.

Ultrasound transducer uses piezoelectric crystals (**Fig. 36.3**).

Piezoelectric materials, under the influence of electricity change the shape.

When stimulated by the application of a voltage difference, the transducer vibrates. The ultrasound pulse generated by a transducer will propagate in tissue to get clinical information. Special transducer coatings and ultrasound coupling gels are necessary to allow efficient transfer of energy from the transducer to the body.

Receiver: The returning echoes strike the transducer and weak currents are produced. These weak signals are detected and amplified by the receiver. Another important function of the receiver is the compression of the wide range of amplitudes returning to the transducer into a range that can be displayed to the user.

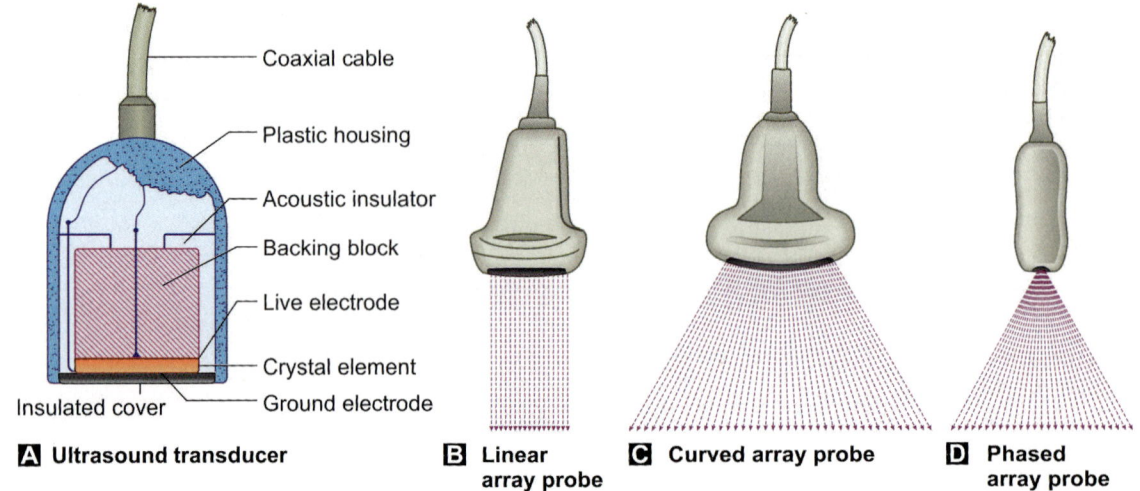

Coaxial cable
Plastic housing
Acoustic insulator
Backing block
Live electrode
Crystal element
Insulated cover — Ground electrode

A Ultrasound transducer   **B** Linear array probe   **C** Curved array probe   **D** Phased array probe

Fig. 36.3(A to D): USG transducers

Image display: Images can be displayed in various forms ranging from spectrum in A and M mode to high resolution, real time gray scale images in B mode.

Transducer selection: For superficial vessels and organs, such as the thyroid, breast, or testicle, lying within 1 to 3 cm of the surface, imaging frequencies of 7.5 to 15 MHz are typically used. For evaluation of deeper structures in the abdomen or pelvis more than 12 to 15 cm from the surface, frequency as low as 2.25 to 3.5 MHz may be required.

For head and neck region frequencies ranging from 2.9 MHz are used.

Terminologies Used in USG

Anechoic: Any structure which is dark (black) image, e.g. cyst.

Hypo-echoic: Any structure that appears dark as compared to the surrounding tissue.

Hyper-echoic: Any structure that appears bright as compared to the surrounding tissue.

Advantages of Ultrasound

* As the frequency of ultrasound is above the audible human hearing, it is comfortable for patients.

* It is easily available and can be used as primary screening modality in most of the medical conditions.
* Less expensive.
* Less time consuming.
* Readily reproducible.
* Ultrasound uses non-ionizing radiations.
* It provides clear image of soft tissues which are not seen in X-ray images.
* It noticeably differentiates between solid and cystic structures.
* Ultrasound guided diagnostic/therapeutic procedures can be done under real time.

Disadvantages of Ultrasound

* USG is an operator-dependent modality. Image quality totally depends on the skills of the operator and machine.
* Ultrasound poorly penetrates through the air and bone and hence pathologies related to the lung and bone could not be evaluated with the USG.
* Image quality is less as compared to CT and MRI.
* Artifacts in USG can hamper the detailing of the pathology.
* Tissue heating is one of the adverse effects of long time use, prolonged, repeated use of ultrasound.

Color Doppler Imaging

It is the imaging of blood vessels and their abnormalities by using real time ultrasound.

The Doppler effect in diagnostic imaging is used to study blood flow in vessels, i.e.

× Presence or absence of flow
× Direction of blood flow
× Velocity of blood flow.

Uses of Ultrasound in Dental Practice

× Evaluation of salivary glands and their pathologies.
× Identification of the salivary gland ducts and calculi, so it can obviate the need for sialography, hence avoiding radiation.
× Lymph nodal status in infective and malignant conditions.
× Status of the vessels in the neck.

COMPUTED TOMOGRAPHY

Computed tomography (CT) scanning, also known as computerized axial tomography (CAT) scanning, is the diagnostic imaging modality which uses X-rays to construct a cross-sectional image of a particular portion of the body. CT scanners were first introduced in 1971 by Sir Godfray Hounsfield, an electrical engineer at Electric and Musical Industries Ltd.

CT image is produced by the process of reconstruction—X-rays which will pass through the patient at different angles and attenuated in different tissue depending upon their attenuation coefficient. This image is digital and consist of many pixels which is viewed as gray scale image.

CT Acquisition

In CT, as the X-rays pass through the tissue in different directions and information is collected by many detectors which moves in synchronization with the X-ray tube. The finale data acquired carries more information which helps in reconstruction of images in three dimensions (Fig. 36.4).

The detectors of the CT scanner measure the transmission of a thin beam of X-rays through full scan. The image of that section is taken from different angles and this allows to retrieve the information in the depth, i.e. the third dimension (as oppose to radiograph only two dimensions are measured).

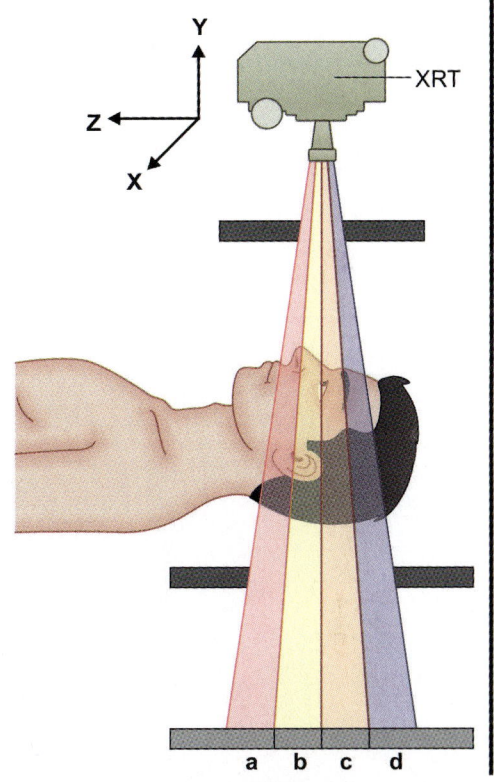

Fig. 36.4: Image acquisition in CT

In modern CT scanners, there is continuous movement of the detectors which are arranged in multiple rows to create image of multiple sections.

In order to obtain CT images of the patient from the data in 'raw' scan, the computer uses complex mathematical algorithms for image reconstruction. All these methods use computerized mathematical operation to get 2D image.

The CT image is a map of tissue attenuation and these maps are quantified by using **CT number** scale named after Sir Hounsfield as

Hounsfield unit scale. Each tissue in a body has specific CT number depending on linear attenuation of X-rays.

There are four basic densities,

* Air = –1000 HU
* Fat = –60 to –120 HU
* Water = 0 HU
* Compact bone = +1000 HU

Window level and window width are adjusted according to the study to identify the smaller difference in the adjacent structures.

Instrumentation

Gantry: Modern CT scanner uses slip ring technology to get continuous rotation (Fig. 36.5). Due to evolution through years, data acquisition time has been reduced from hours to less than a second.

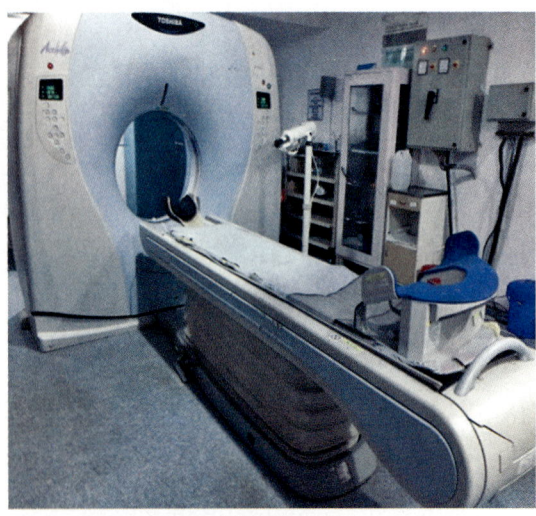

Fig. 36.5: CT gantry

X-ray generators and tube: High frequency X-ray generators, i.e. power rating of 80 to 120 kilowatts are used to generate high frequency beam used in CT scans.

X-ray tubes of modern CT scanner have rotating anodes and uses innovative cooling methods to continuous high X-ray output.

Filters: They are used to modify the shape and spectrum of the X-ray beam. The filters used in CT are combination of Teflon or copper with aluminum. They are thicker than the filters used in the conventional radiography. The filters are arranged such that the radiation dose to the patient is less without compromising on image quality.

Detectors: CT scanners are scintillation crystals to convert X-rays into light which is then converted to the digital image by the proper electronic circuit. CT detectors are crystals of fast scintillator ceramics, i.e. cadmium telluride and gadolinium oxysulphide. These detectors moves in synchronized fashion with the X-ray tubes and can cover approx. 80 to 160 mm in single tube rotation. This system needs to be stable, uniform and should be capable of tracking wide dynamic range. Slight error in this will result in an artifact.

The typical number of detectors in the array ranges from about 600 to more than 900.

Data acquisition systems: Data acquisition systems (DAS) are the mainstay of CT scanners. In DAS,

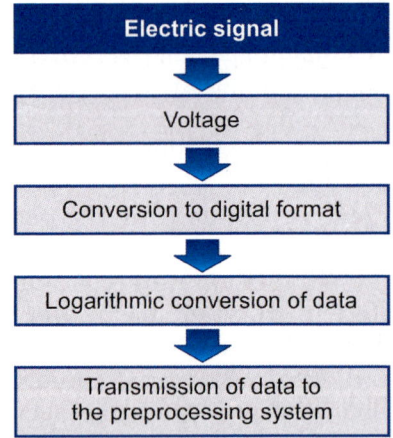

Reconstruction: Reconstruction produces an image from the digital data provided by the data acquisition system.

The typical CT image is composed of 512 rows, each of 512 pixels, i.e. a square matrix of $512 \times 512 = 262144$ pixels (one for each voxel). In the process of the image, the value of the attenuated coefficient for each voxel is calculated.

The simplest and most common method of producing a cross-sectional image from CT data is called filtered back projection.

Before the data are presented on the screen, the conventional rescaling is done into CT numbers.

Data display: Image display includes components necessary to convert the digital data provided by the reconstruction system to electrical signals. It consists of display monitor, graphic display of individual CT numbers representing attenuation values of individual sections of anatomy. The display system also provides patient information, scan protocol, and reconstruction parameters.

Terminologies used in CT Physics

Slice: CT image formed by individual rotation of the gantry are called **slice** because the tissue displayed appears as thin slice of the particular portion of the body.

Scanner geometry: It is the combination of the X-ray tube and detector movement. Best combination is rotate–rotate type, i.e. both tube and detector rotate during the scan. It is best for high-speed scanning in multidetector CT.

Spiral CT: In spiral/helical CT, the patient table moves through the gantry while the scan frame rotates continuously around the patient, sampling data as a volume. Spiral CT has many advantages over conventional or axial CT, viz. reduced scan time, decreased motion artifacts, reduced radiation dose, improved image quality and enhanced multiplanar or 3D reconstruction.

Acquisition is the entire volume of data collected during a continuous spiral scan.

Revolutions refer to the number of 360° rotations of the X-ray tube during a single acquisition.

Pitch is the distance the table travels during one 360° revolution of the X-ray tube divided by a length.

Interpolation is a reconstruction method for the realignment of spiral/helical scan data for reconstruction of an axial image.

Multidetector CT. Multidetector-row scanners are design to cover large regions of anatomy in short times without affecting image quality. This is achieved by arranging multiple narrow detector rows side-by-side along the z-axis and connecting them to a data acquisition system with multiple input channels.

Terminologies used while Describing CT Scans

Hypo-dense: Any structure that appears dark as compared to the surrounding tissue.

Hyper-dense: Any structure that appears bright as compared to the surrounding tissue.

Iso-dense: The structure that appears in same density as that of surrounding tissue.

Contrast used in CT is iodinated contrast agent which are excreted through kidney and cannot be given in patient with renal insufficiency.

Advantages of CT
* Accessibility is more as compared to MRI.
* Less expensive (compared to MRI).
* Less time consuming (compared to MRI), so can be done in unstable patients.
* Accuracy in diagnosing pathologies helps in proper management of the patient.
* Multiplanar reconstruction of the volume data can be done.
* Three-dimension surface shaded rendering is also possible for bones and soft tissues.
* Volume rendering is an advanced rendering technique that displays an entire volume.
* Maximum intensity projection (MIP) helps for easy viewing of vascular structures or air-filled cavities.
* Diagnostic as well as therapeutic procedure can be done in CT.

Disadvantages of CT
* It uses ionizing radiation, hence repeated use is not recommended.

- Not used in pregnant female and lactating mothers.
- The contrast agents given in CT can lead to anaphylactic reactions, so should be avoided in elderly patient with compromised renal function, asthma and multiple myeloma.
- Artifacts are known in CT scans, so radiologist should be aware of them.

Uses of CT in dental practice

- **Cone beam CT:** It is particularly used in dental imaging. It differs from routine CT in that it uses cone-shaped X-ray beam rather than fan-shaped beam. The advantage of cone beam CT is its low cost and less radiation dose.
- **Staging of head and neck malignancies.**
- **In case of facial trauma,** three-dimensional CT views are important to get an idea of exact nature of fracture.

MAGNETIC RESONANCE IMAGING (MRI)

The basic concept of magnetic resonance imaging (MRI) or previously called nuclear magnetic resonance (NMR), was first introduced by C J Gorter in 1934. Bloch and Purcell got Nobel prize for their work on NMR in solids and liquids in 1946. In 1974, Paul Lauterbur used MRI for the first time in animal imaging. It took almost 50 years for MRI to be introduced in medical practice.

Basic Concept of Image Formation in MRI

MRI does not use X-rays for image formation as in CT. The image formation in MRI is due to interaction of body tissue with radiofrequency waves in the presence of strong magnetic field and this forms the basis for MR image generation.

The present MR imaging is based on imaging of proton. Proton is a positively charged ion in human body. Hydrogen is only ion made of only protons (H^+) and it is abundant in human body. These protons are in constant rotator motion in the body called **spin**. Whenever they come under the influence of any external magnetic field, sudden change in the movement of the proton is seen. This change in the movement will depend on the strength of the magnetic field. In the body, we have both high and low energy protons. When external magnetic field is applied to the body, the low energy proton will give their energy to the external magnetic field and align parallel to it while protons with higher energy level align antiparallel to the external magnetic field. This movement is called **precession**.

We have three axes, i.e. X, Y and Z and external magnetic field is applied along the Z axis. The protons in parallel and antiparallel direction will cancel each other and there will be always more protons in the parallel direction which is called *longitudinal magnetization*. However, for generation of a measurable signal, we need *transverse magnetization*, i.e. magnetization in opposite direction. To get this, a radiofrequency pulse (RF pulse) is sent and weak energy proton will gain energy and go to the higher level so that the magnetization in transverse plane will be more (i.e. protons in antiparallel direction are more). This energy transfer occurs only if the frequency of RF pulse and processional frequency of proton is same. This is called *resonance*.

Transverse magnetization forms vector along X-Y axis and it produces electric signal which can be received by the **receiver coils.**

When the RF pulse is switched off, the protons will give energy to the surrounding and there will be gain in longitudinal magnetization. With this there will be reduction in transverse magnetization. **T1** is time taken for longitudinal magnetization to recover to its original after RF pulse is switched off. **T2** is time taken for transverse magnetization to reduce to its original after RF pulse is switched off. And this T1 and T2 time will decide the type of sequence (image).

K space: The raw data is stored in this space and then it is used to construct images by **Fourier transformation.**

Summarizing, how image is produced in MRI:

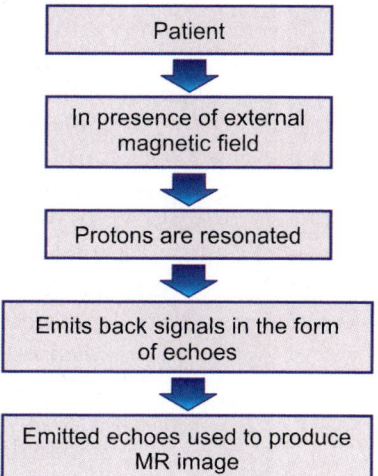

```
┌──────────────────────────────┐
│           Patient            │
└──────────────────────────────┘
              ↓
┌──────────────────────────────┐
│   In presence of external    │
│      magnetic field          │
└──────────────────────────────┘
              ↓
┌──────────────────────────────┐
│   Protons are resonated      │
└──────────────────────────────┘
              ↓
┌──────────────────────────────┐
│  Emits back signals in the   │
│      form of echoes          │
└──────────────────────────────┘
              ↓
┌──────────────────────────────┐
│  Emitted echoes used to      │
│      produce MR image        │
└──────────────────────────────┘
```

Instrumentation

Basic components of the MR systems are:
- External magnetic field
- Gradient coil
- Coils
- Image display system

External magnetic field: Magnetic field strength is expressed in terms of Gauss or Tesla. In medical practice, strength ranges from 0.2 to 0.7 Tesla. It is expressed as B0. Three types of magnet are used in clinical MRI, viz. permanent magnet, electromagnet and super conducting magnet.

Depending upon the strength of magnetic field used, MRI system is labeled as 1 T, 1.5 T or 3 T (Fig. 36.6).

Faraday cage: Entire MRI unit embedded in copper wire, which blocks radiofrequency signal from outside interfering with the MR signal.

Gradient coil: These are used to change the magnetic field strength superimposed on superconducting magnet. They are applied in X, Y & Z axes perpendicular to each other.

Coils: RF coils are antennae that serve to transmit energy to and receive energy from the patient. Coils are circular or cylindrical in shape to localize the transmission and reception. Larger coils are better for

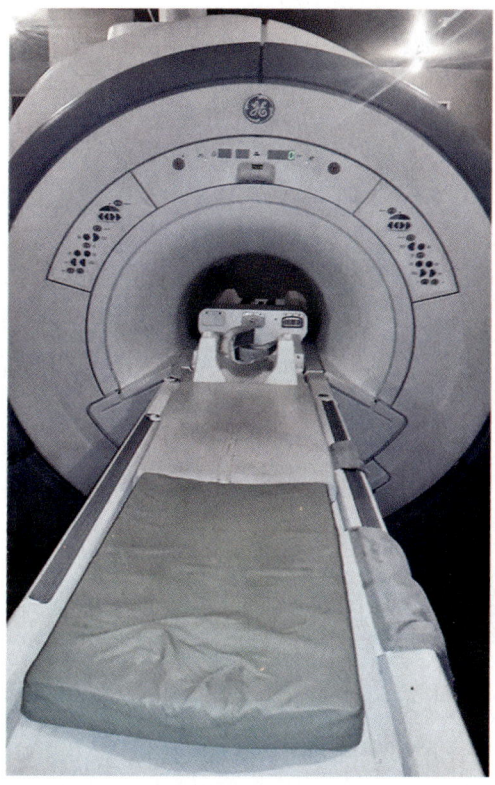

Fig. 36.6: MRI gantry

transmission, smaller coils are better for reception. Different coils are used according to the body part under study, viz. head coil, surface coil, body coil, knee coil, endorectal coil, breast coil (Fig. 36.7).

Image display system: It is computer-assisted data collection, modification and display of the images.

Terminologies to Understand Image Formation in MRI

Matrix: Number of rows and columns of pixels in a given area.

SNR: Signal to noise ratio.

Flip angle: Angle by which longitudinal magnetization vector is rotated from Z axis.

FOV: Area from which signal is produced.

Bandwidth: Range of frequencies.

Shimming: Removing magnetic field inhomogenity.

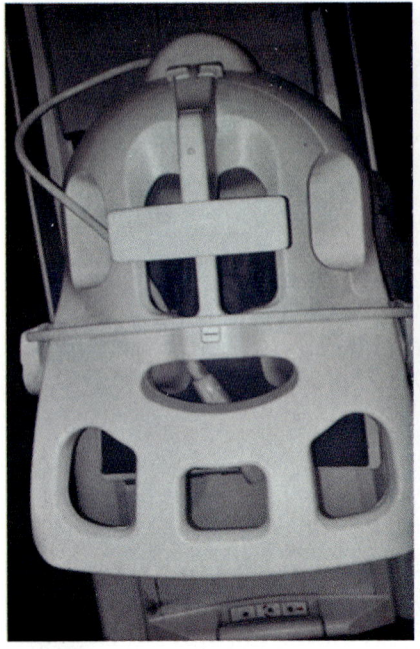
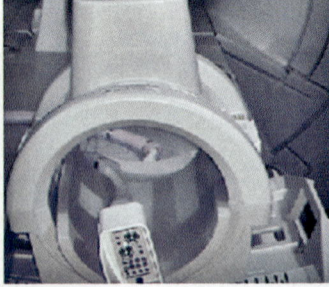
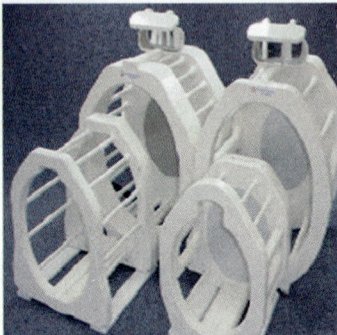
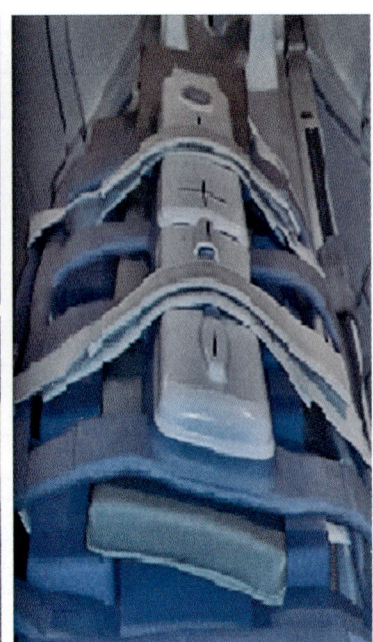

Fig. 36.7: Different coils

Time to repeat (TR): Time interval between start of one RF pulse and start of next RF pulse.

Time to echo (TE): Time interval between one RF pulse and maximum echo (signal).

The following combinations of TR and TE will give images accordingly.
- Short TR and short TE = T1-weighed images (Fig. 36.8).
- Long TR and long TE = T2-weighed images (Fig. 36.9).
- Long TR and short TE = Proton density images

Pulse sequences: A pulse sequence is mainstay of MR image formation which takes into account different parameters, interaction with RF pulse and gradients.

Terminologies used while describing MRI scans

Hypo-intense: Any structure that appears dark as compared to the surrounding tissue.

Hyper-intense: Any structure that appears bright as compared to the surrounding tissue.

Iso-intense structure that appears in same density as that of surrounding tissue.

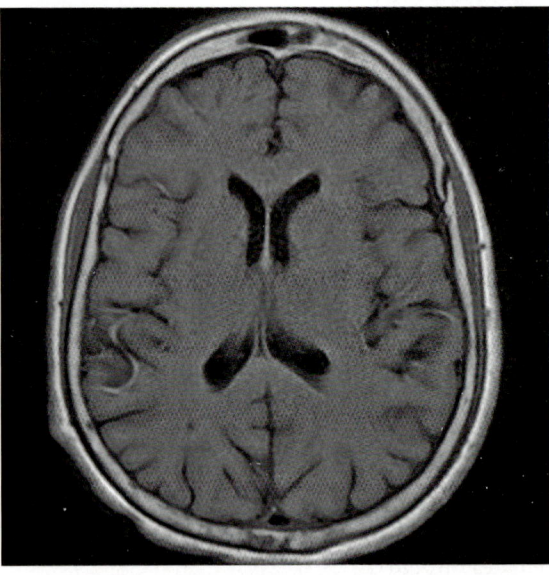

Fig. 36.8: T1 weighted brain image

MRI Contrast Agent

Gadolinium chelates are used.

Advantages of MRI
- It uses non-ionic radiation, so it is relatively safe.

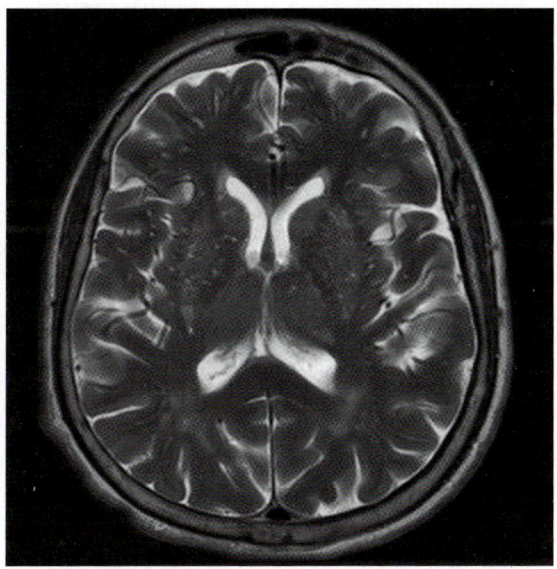

Fig. 36.9: T2-weighted brain image

- It is excellent for soft tissue evaluation.
- It gives multiplanar imaging, hence exact morphology and site of the lesion can be assessed.
- MRI has replaced CT in most of the cases of neuroimaging.
- It is the modality of choice in bone marrow pathologies, internal derangement of various joints.
- Non-contrast angiography is possible with MRI.

Limitations of MRI
- It is costly as compared to CT.
- Time consuming
- It has low sensitivity to pick calcification.
- Inferior in diagnosing fractures.
- Cannot be done in claustrophobic patients.

Absolute Contraindications to MRI
- Internal cardiac pacemakers
- Implantable cardiac defibrillators
- Cochlear implants
- Neurostimulators
- Bone growth stimulators
- Electrically programmed drug infusion pumps
- Intraocular metallic foreign body
- Aneurysmal clips

Uses of MRI in Dental Practice
- Because of excellent soft tissue resolution MRI has become the modality of choice in **evaluating and staging of head and neck malignancies.**
- It helps in study of **internal derangement of temporomandibular joint.**
- **Neural spread of the malignancy** is well evaluated with MRI.

POSITRON EMISSION TOMOGRAPHY (PET)

Positron emission tomography (PET) was developed in the early 1970s. PET is a non-invasive imaging technique to quantify radioactivity in the human body. In PET, positron-emitting radiopharmaceutical agent is injected in the body and after specific time period the distribution and quantification of patterns of radiopharmaceutical accumulation in the different parts of the body are imaged.

During PET Scanning

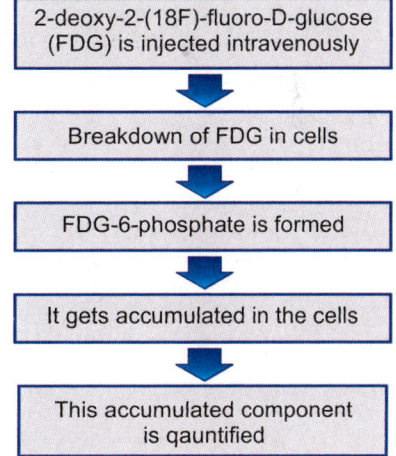

- A positron emission tomography (PET) scan is done to detect the metabolic activity in the cancer cells and accordingly helps in deciding the management.

Advantages of PET
- PET imaging is unique in that it shows the metabolic activity of the cells in organs *in vivo*.
- Increased sensitivity and precise diagnosis.

Disadvantages of PET

- Diagnosis of perticular pathology.
  - Uses ionizing radiation.
  - Needs due care as it deals with radio-nuclides
- PET images are degraded by number of factors like attenuation, scatter, random coincidences, dead time, limited resolution and noise.
- It is expensive.

PET-CT

It is the combination of PET with CT scan to enhance the diagnostic accuracy. PET-CT has totally replaced dedicated PET. The major role of PET-CT is in cancer patient and their follow-up to look for the exact location of the metabolically active cancer cell.

FREQUENTLY ASKED QUESTIONS

1. Write indications of: CT/MRI/USG/PET
2. Write about advantages of: CT/MRI/USG.

BIBLIOGRAPHY

1. Chivers RC, Parry RJ. Ultrasonic velocity and attenuation in mammalian tissues. J Acoust Soc Am. 1978;63(3):940–53.
2. Merritt CR, Kremkau FW, Hobbins JC. Diagnostic ultrasound: Bioeffects and safety. Ultrasound Obstet Gynecol. 1992;2(5):366–74.
3. Merritt CR. Technology update. Radiol Clin North Am. 2001;39(3):385–97.
4. Carol M Rumack, Stephanie R. Wilson, J. Willian Charboneau and Dedorah Levine. Diagnostic ultrasound, Vol 1, 5th edition.
5. Merritt CR. Doppler US: The basics. Radiographics. 1991;11(1):109–19.
6. Merritt CR. Doppler color flow imaging. J Clin Ultrasound. 1987;15(9):591–97.
7. CT and MRI of the Whole Body, John R Haaga, Daniel T Boll, Volume 1. Chapter 1, Pp 3–27. 6th edition,
8. Cody DD. AAPM/RSNA physics tutorial for residents: Topics in CT. Image processing in CT. Radiographics 2002: 22:1255–68.
9. Peter M Som, Hugh D Curtin. Head and Neck Imaging, Section V, Chapter 23, Volume 1, 5th edition. Pp 1443–59.
10. John R Haaga, Daniel T Boll. CT and MRI of the Whole Body, Chapter 3, Volume 1, 6th edition, Pp 46–114.
11. Dr. Govind Chavan. MR Made Easy (for beginners). Section 1, Chapters 1, 2, 3. Pp 3–140.
12. Dr. Govind Chavan. MR Made Easy (for beginners). Section 1, Chapter 7. Pp 105–114.
13. Votaw JR. The AAPM/RSNA physics tutorial for residents. Physics of PET. Radiographics. 1995;15 (5): 1179–90.
14. Grainger and Allison's Diagnostic Radiology Essentials. Churchill Livingstone. ISBN:0702034487.
15. Pooley RA, McKinney JM, Miller DA. The AAPM/RSNA physics tutorial for residents: digital fluoroscopy. Radiographics. 2001 Mar-Apr;21(2):521–34.
16. Allisy-Roberts PJ, Williams J. Farr's Physics for Medical Imaging. 2nd edition. 2008 Pp 98–102.

CBCT: Principles and Applications in Dentistry

INTRODUCTION

Traditionally, the computed tomography used in hospitals have fan-shaped X-ray beam. Cone beam computed tomography (CBCT) is a medical imaging technique where the X-rays are divergent in a 'cone' shape.

Different nomenclatures have been used to describe CBCT by different researchers. To name a few, C-arm CT, cone beam volume CT, cone beam volumetric tomography and digital volume tomography.

Pioneers, who invented the CBCT technology, were Attilio Tacconi, Piero Mozzo, Daniele Godi and Giordano Ronca. On July 1st, 1994, two NewTom engineers, Giordano Ronca and Daniele Godi, performed the first complete CBCT scan on a skull. It was only in the last decade, CBCT gained wide acceptance in the field of dentistry and changed the world's dental radiology scenario.

Four research advances have converged to make CBCT possible.
* Computers capable of computational complexity
* X-ray tubes capable of continuous exposure
* Compact high-quality two-dimensional detector arrays
* Advances in 3D reconstruction

PRINCIPLES OF IMAGE FORMATION

In medical CT, slices are acquired to reconstruct the volume. In CBCT, volume is acquired to reconstruct the slices. The 'cone'-shaped beam helps this volume acquisition. To give an analogy, medical CT gets the data in the form of 'slices of bread' and then reconstructs these slices into a 'loaf of bread' (Fig. 37.1A). Contrast to this, CBCT captures the data as a 'bread loaf' and then reconstructs the images by slicing (Fig. 37.1B).

CBCT image production can be explained under three steps:
a. Image acquisition
b. Image reconstruction
c. Image display

a. **Image acquisition:** X-rays penetrate the patient from different angles and reach the image receptor (usually flat-panel detector). These receptors measure the amount of X-rays penetrating the patient from various angles and this process is known as image acquisition.

b. **Image reconstruction:** Once these attenuated X-rays reach the image receptor, they are transferred to the computer. Here the software, mathematically calculates the attenuated X-ray information and produces a CT image volume. This process is known as image reconstruction.

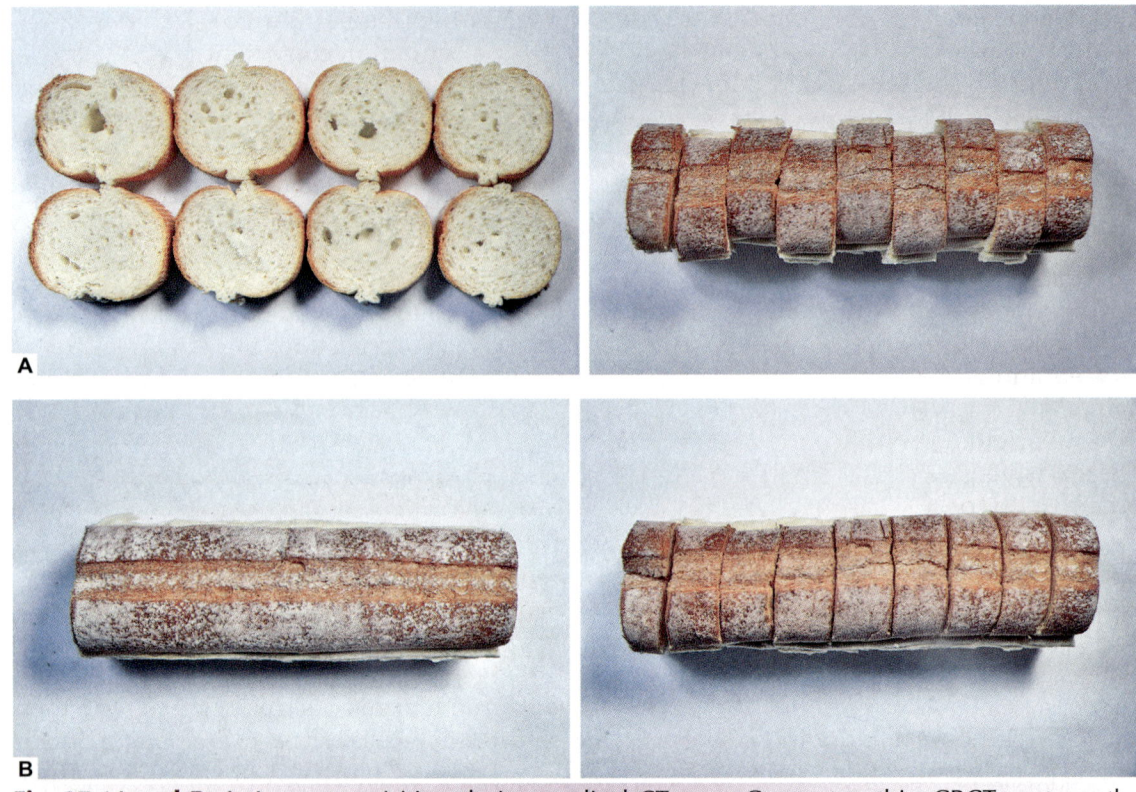

Fig. 37.1A and B: A. Image acquisition during medical CT scan. Contrast to this, CBCT captures the data as a 'bread loaf' and then reconstructs the images by slicing. **B.** Image acquisition during CBCT scan.

c. **Image display:** After the image reconstruction, the computer will enable the display of the image in axial, sagittal, coronal sections and 3D format using any image viewing software. These images are displayed in DICOM format (digital imaging and communications in medicine).

Unlike CT machines, CBCT uses a conical beam which can capture limited anatomical area depending on the 'field of view' of the machine. In other words, 'field of view' or FOV is the area of the patient irradiated. Currently the smallest FOV available in the market is 5 × 3.8 cm and largest FOV is 23 × 26 cm. FOV is selected based on the clinical requirement or size of the lesion. Smaller the FOV, lesser is the radiation dose.

CBCT machine captures the cylindrical images in the form of three-dimensional data blocks known as 'voxels' (volume element)

which is isotropic (equal x, y and z planes). This gives a high resolution image compared to conventional CT units. The resolution of various available CBCT machines ranges from 0.09 to 0.4 mm.

CBCT software usually displays the images in 'multiplanar reformation' (MPR), which means that in three different sections, 2D images are viewed. They are axial, sagittal and coronal sections. These data can be manipulated and customized based on the direction or based on the section thickness. The ability to give thinner sections varies between manufacturers.

Almost all CBCT machines come with 3D rendering facilities. 3D rendering is the 3D computer graphics process of automatically converting 3D models into 2D images with 3D photorealistic effects or non-photorealistic rendering on a computer. These images play a greater role in patient education rather than diagnosis. Depending on the software used by the machine, different models of 3D rendering are made available. There are two basic types of rendering, namely direct and indirect volume rendering. Direct volume rendering or otherwise known as maximum intensity projection (MIP) is the most preferred form of rendering due to its diagnostic accuracy (Fig. 37.1C and D)

The radiodensity of the structures seen in a CBCT scan explains the nature of the tissue imaged and is measured using Hounsfield units.

Hounsfield unit or CT number is the quantitative scale used to measure the radiodensity of the tissue, named after Sir Godfrey Newbold Hounsfield. A Hounsfield unit (HU) is "the numeric information contained in each pixel of a CT image. It is related to the composition and nature of the tissue imaged and is used to represent the density of tissue". In a voxel, the average linear attenuation coefficient of this value is taken into consideration before calculating the HU. Hounsfield units used in CBCT imaging are actually gray values used with linear attenuation coefficients. Studies have shown strong correlation between gray levels and HU. Accuracy of these Hounsfield units has varied showing differences due to patient positioning, patient size, and image artifacts. When used for implant placement, *the Hounsfield units should be used as a general idea of bone density and not exact units.*

HU can range from –1000 to +3000, where –1000 represents the radiodensity of the air, zero for water and +700 to +3000 for bone.

Region growing (crowing) is another application given by some of the CBCT manufacturers (Romexis). This function helps in identifying the volume of a given lesion/region and its content.

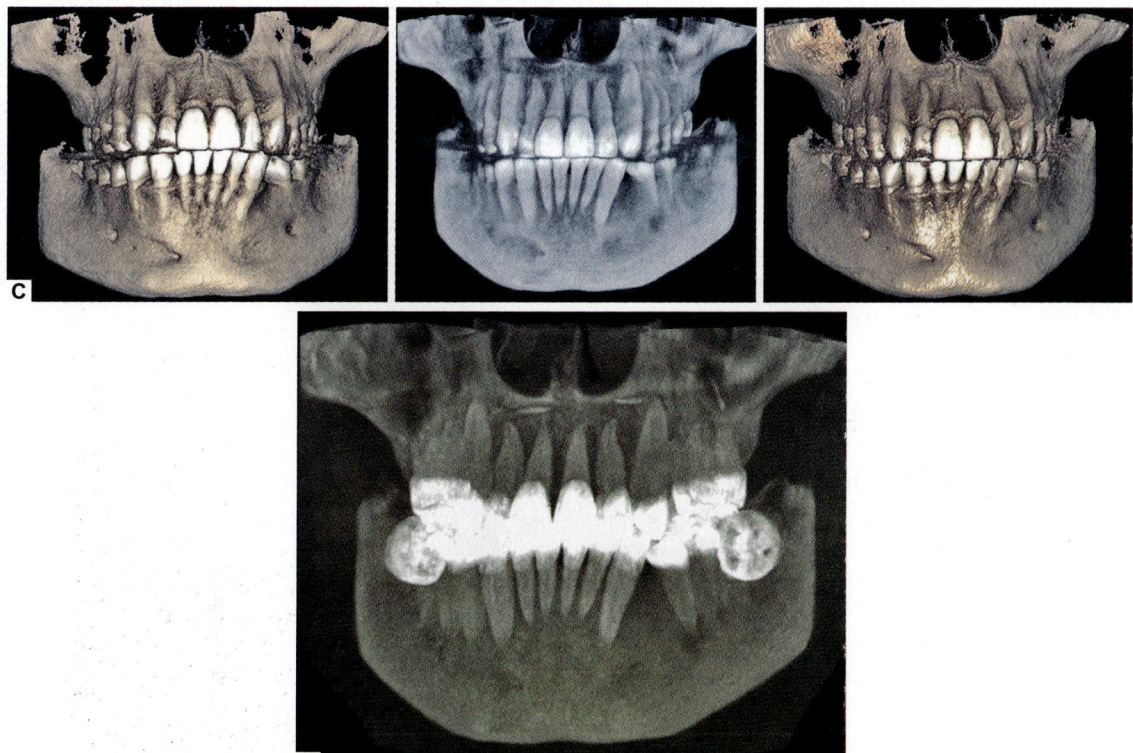

Fig. 37.1C and D: C. Different types of volume rendering and **D.** MIP rendering

Image Receptors

Image receptors in CBCT are of four types:
a. Image intensifier coupled to charge-coupled device (CCD)
b. Complementary metal oxide semiconductor (CMOS)
c. Thin-film transistor (TFT)
d. Flat-panel detectors (FPD)

Most of the presently marketed CBCT machines either use TFT or FPD type of image receptors. Image intensifiers are used only by two manufacturers, namely Biolase (Scanner name DaVinci D3D) and Sirona (Scanner name Scanora 3Dx).

Image intensifier is a vacuum tube device used for increasing the intensity of available light in an optical system to allow use under low-light conditions, such as at night, to facilitate visual imaging of low-light processes. The disadvantage of using such image receptor is the distortion of the images at the periphery. Hence, most of the manufacturers go for either TFT or FPD.

Radiation Dose Concerns

Definitely CBCT gives a higher radiation dose compared to traditional two-dimensional imaging. To make it more understandable and simple, the following comparisons are given:
* Radiation dose received due to smoking per annum is around 320 µSv.
* A return flight journey from Helsinki (Finland) to Tokyo (Japan) gives a cosmic radiation dose equivalent to 61 µSv.
* A one year stay in Denmark can give a background radiation of 4000 µSv.
* Medical CT gives a radiation equivalent to 1200 to 3300 µSv (White S) and a typical panoramic radiograph gives radiation equivalent to 24.5 µSv (ICRP 2007).
* CBCT gives a radiation dose of 20 to 250 µSv which is equivalent to 8 to 10 panoramic radiographs or full mouth radiographs using films.

Artifacts

Like any other imaging modality, CBCT images have artifacts which can limit the diagnostic usage.

The common artifacts seen in CBCT images are:
* Beam hardening
* Metal artifacts
* Radiographic noise
* Motion artifact
* Exomass

Beam hardening: It is caused by the diverse absorption of the (polychromatic) X-ray beam, while it crosses the object being radiographed, whereas the lower energy portion of the spectrum is absorbed more than that at high energy. Consequently, the beam at the exit of the object is 'harder' than at the entrance. In volumetric reconstructions from CBCT, this result in the central part of dense objects being effectively subject to harder X-rays than the periphery, hence the object behaves as if it was less radiodense at the center. This typically manifests as a 'cupping artifact', i.e. the center of a uniformly dense object appears more radiolucent (lower CT numbers) than its outer parts (Figs 37.2 and 37.3).

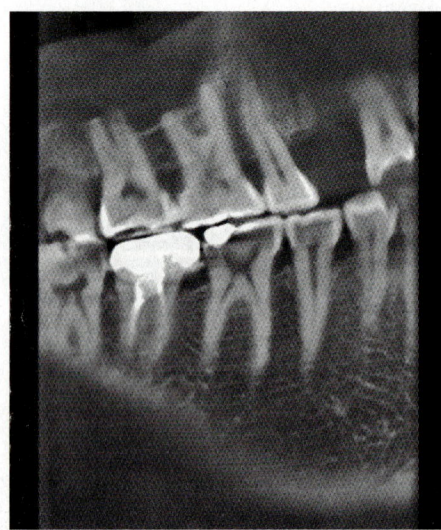

Fig. 37.2: Beam hardening effect seen as 'secondary caries' in #46

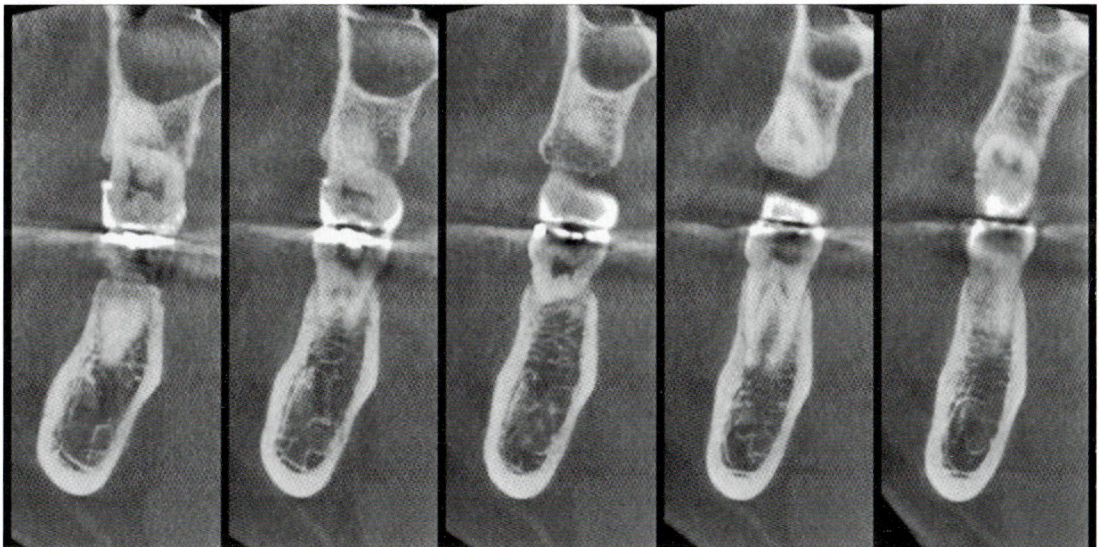

Fig. 37.3: Coronal sections in molar region showing occlusal metallic restoration and radiolucency beneath the restoration giving an impression of 'secondary caries' which is due to beam-hardening effect

Metal artifacts: These occur in the immediate proximity of a (dense) metal object, or in the region in between two such objects, where effectively the X-ray beam may get totally blocked (starbursts or streaking artifact). However, a very dense object may also cause extreme beam hardening manifesting as a dark halo around it (Fig. 37.4).

Radiographic noise: It is usually seen as a result of improper calibration or improper head positioning of the patients (Fig. 37.5).

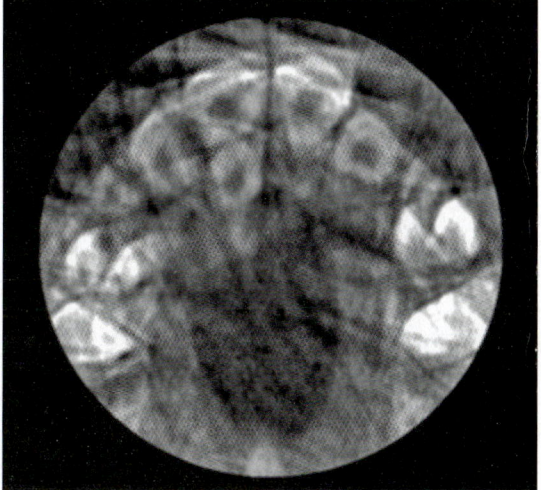

Fig. 37.5: Radiographic noise due to calibration problems or positioning of the head

Motion artifact: If the patient head is not stabilized, this can result in motion artifact characterised by blurring of the edges. Due to the faster image acquisition technology, it is quite rare to see this artifact in the recent models of CBCT.

Exomass: Exomass is the mass present outside the FOV during image acquisition, which is

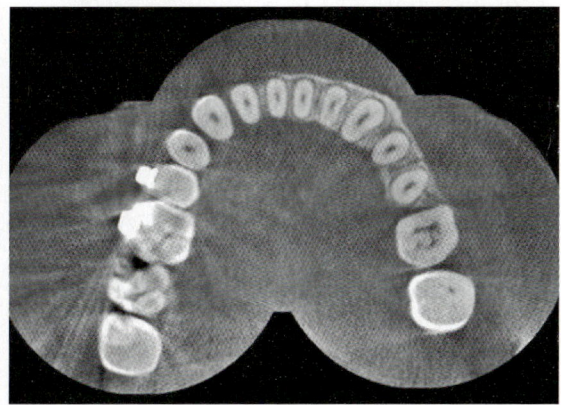

Fig. 37.4: Streaking artifact seen as criss-crossing white lines adjacent to the metallic restorations in third quadrant

associated with the variability of the gray values in CBCT examinations. For example, if any object with a known gray value is subjected to CBCT imaging using different FOV machines, greater the FOV machines, lesser the variability in the gray value. The variability of the gray values associated with the exomass may be explained by the projection data discontinuity caused by the variation of the superimpositions of the non-homogeneous and non-symmetrical tissues outside the FOV along the rotation of the X-ray beam during image acquisition.

Uses in the Field of Dentistry

The current applications of CBCT appear to have impacted all the specialties of dentistry. To name a few:

- Assessment of impacted teeth position
- Inferior alveolar nerve and sinus floor location
- Paranasal sinus evaluation
- Pre-surgical implant site assessment
- Odontogenic lesion visualization
- Trauma evaluation
- Endodontic diagnoses
- Diagnosis of temporomandibular joint disorders (TMD)
- Surgical guide fabrication
- Other CAD/CAM devices (3D models)

Assessment of impacted teeth: It is a common practice to advise either an OPG or a periapical view for impacted third molars or canines. These projections can only give the superioinferior and mesiodistal relation between the impacted tooth and the nearest anatomical structure like mandibular canal or floor of the maxillary sinus. Bucco-lingual relation is always left to the clinical expertise of the dentist. CBCT overcomes this limitation of traditional imaging, thus aiding the dentist to be ready for the proximity of the vital anatomical structure **(Figs 37.6 to 37.8).**

Paranasal sinus evaluation: Due to the proximity of paranasal sinuses to the dental apparatus, it is very common to see different aspects of sinuses routinely and

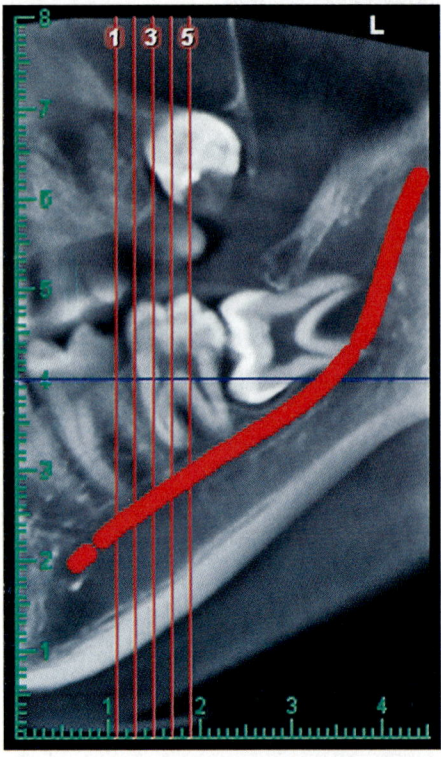

Fig. 37.6: Sagittal section showing the horizontally impacted tooth and its relation to the inferior alveolar canal (marked in red)

hence the dentist should be in a position to identify the anatomical variations and the pathologies affecting the sinuses. Common sinus pathologies like mucosal thickening, polyps and cysts, oroantral fistulae can be well appreciated in CBCT sections **(Figs 37.9 and 37.10)**

Few machines come with additional ENT software enabling the ENT applications.

Implant assessment: Imaging is an integral part of implantology. With increasing demand for accurate implant placement, CBCT imaging for implant site assessment has gained wide popularity. According to the recommendations by AAOMR – 2012, CBCT is the method of choice for 3D imaging in implant assessment. CBCT can aid in implant placement for:

a. Implant site assessment to estimate of available bone height and width **(Figs 37.11 and 37.12).**

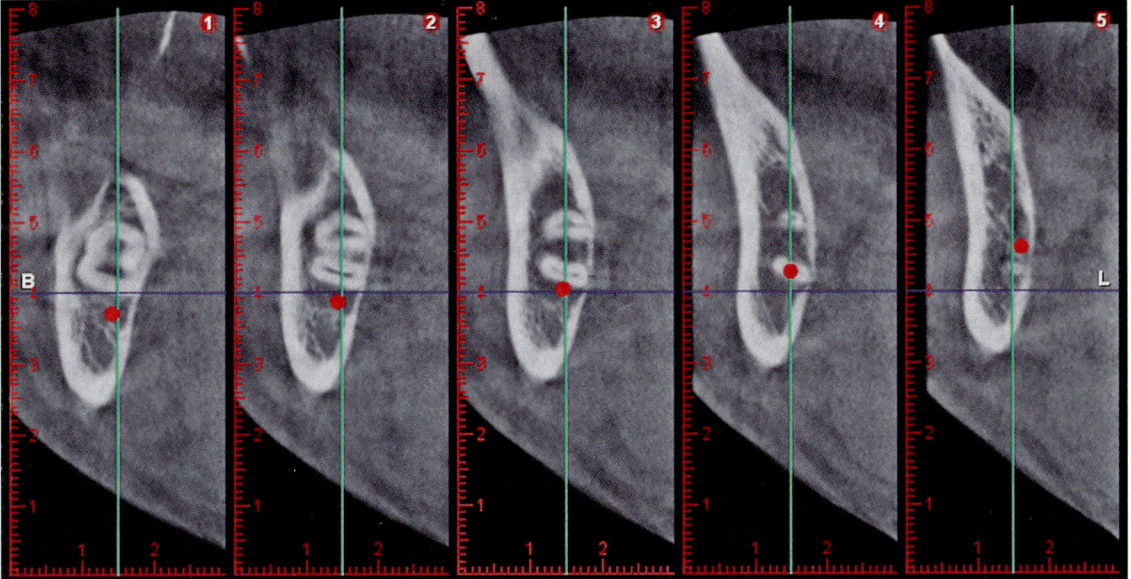

Fig. 37.7: Coronal sections of the impacted #38 roots and its relation to the inferior alveolar canal (marked in red)

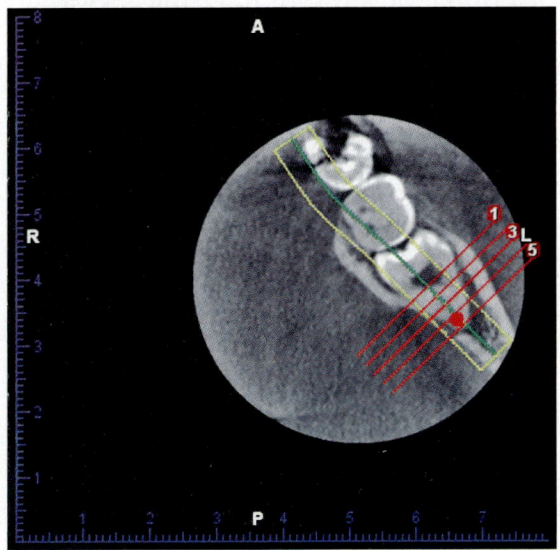

Fig. 37.8: Axial section of impacted #38 and its relation to the inferior alveolar canal (marked as red dot)

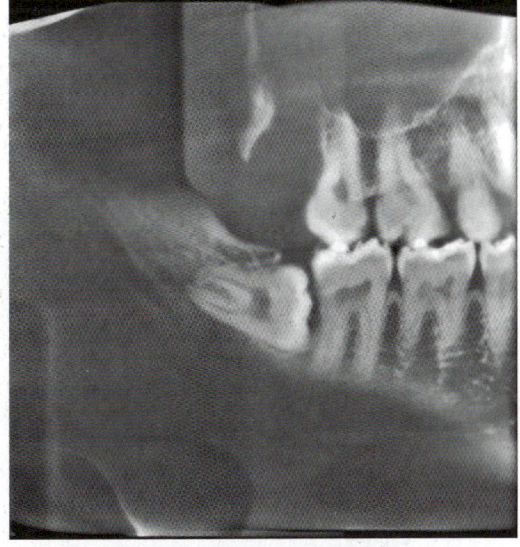

Fig. 37.9: Sagittal section in #28 region showing oroantral communication

b. Assessment of proximity to anatomical structures (inferior alveolar canal, lower border of maxillary sinus)

c. Simulated implant placement (Fig. 37.13)

d. Detection of anatomical variations like bone concavities (Figs 37.14 and 37.15)

e. Quality of bone assessment (Fig. 37.16)

f. Patient education

Odontogenic lesions: CBCT aids in the accurate diagnosis of odontogenic lesions like inflammatory diseases, tumors and

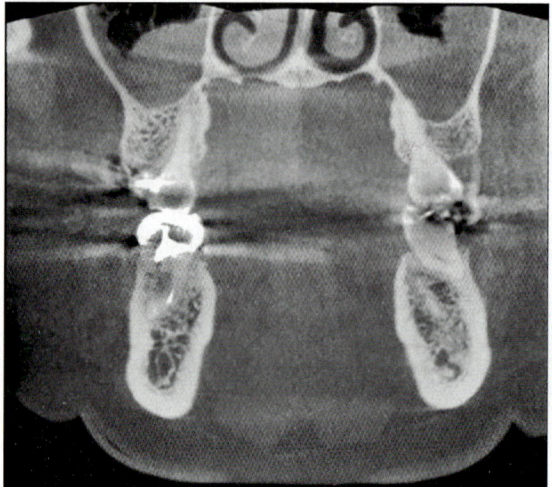

Fig. 37.10: Coronal section showing mucosal thickening in the maxillary sinus bilaterally

developmental anomalies. Region growing (crowing) application helps in the total volume calculation of soft tissue or bone, thereby giving a rough idea about the content (Figs 37.17 to 37.19).

Trauma evaluation: Midfacial and naso-ethmoidal complex fractures are best diagnosed using CBCT due to the regional anatomical complexity and overlapping of bones. Dentoalveolar fractures, especially, if the fracture lines are not perpendicular to the routine X-ray angulations used in periapical views, can be easily detected in CBCT. One of the highly used applications of CBCT is to diagnose vertical/horizontal root fractures (Figs 37.20 and 37.21).

Endodontic diagnoses: Shift cone technique may not be always helpful in detecting the additional root canals. In such cases, CBCT images offer a ready solution. This can be of great advantage for patients who are visiting dental clinics due to endodontic failure. The resolution of CBCT provides additional data like 'C' shape of the canal, additional roots, bifurcation/trifurcation of the canals, any perforations and lateral canals (Figs 37.22 and 37.23).

Diagnosis of temporomandibular joint disorders: Majority of the clinical cases of TMD are related to muscle or disc problems where CBCT is of limited use. Developmental disorders of condyle and condylar surface changes secondary to degenerative disorders and fracture lines are best visualized in CBCT.

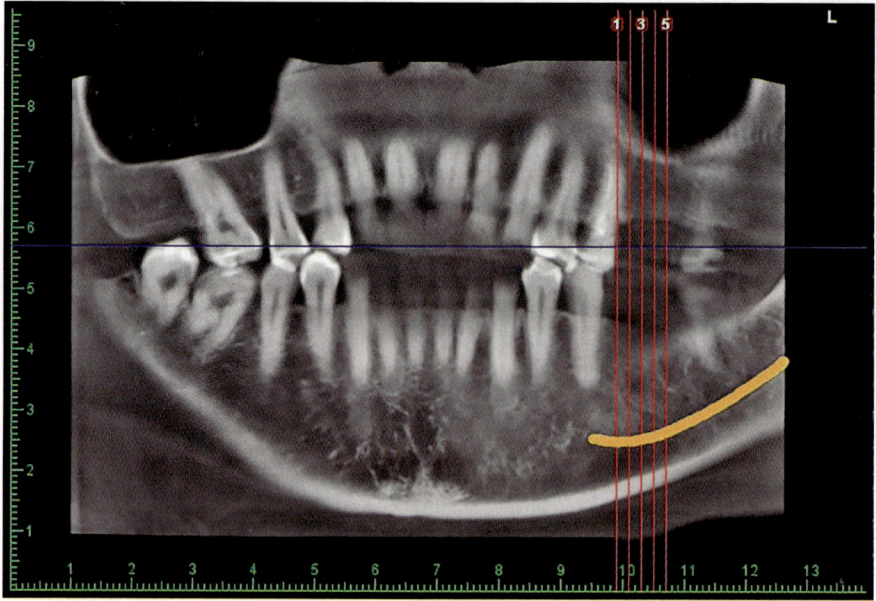

Fig. 37.11: Sagittal section showing the nerve tracing (yellow marking) done prior to implant planning

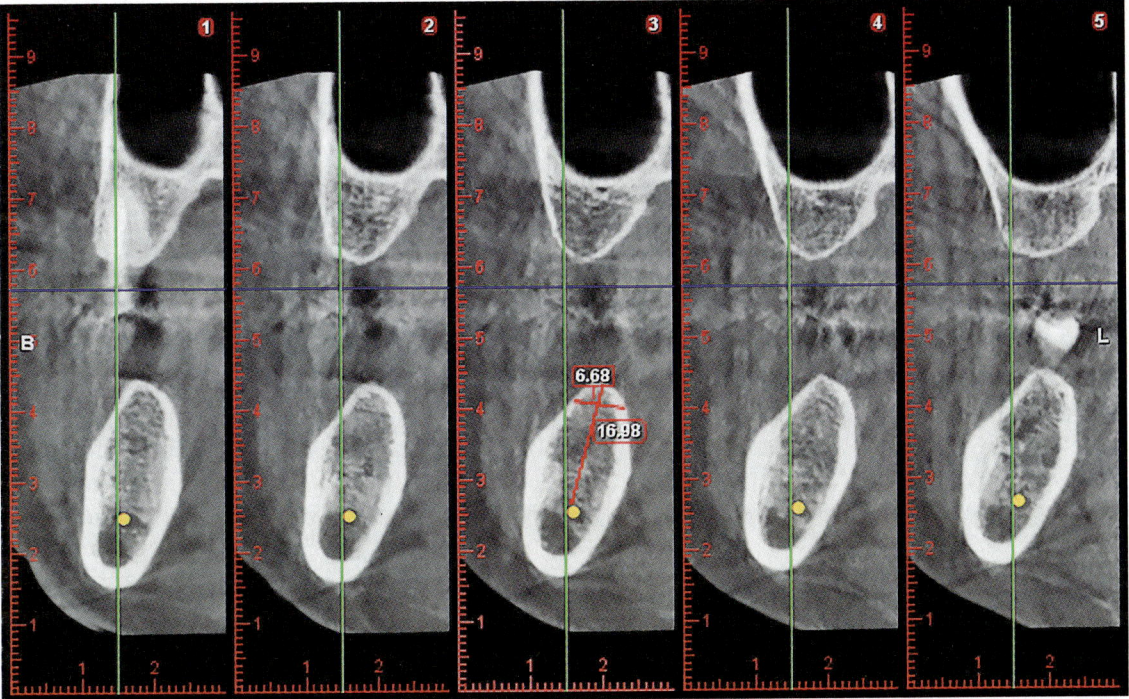

Fig. 37.12: Coronal sections in #36 region showing the available bone height and width (note the red markings representing the measurements). Yellow dots represent the inferior alveolar canal

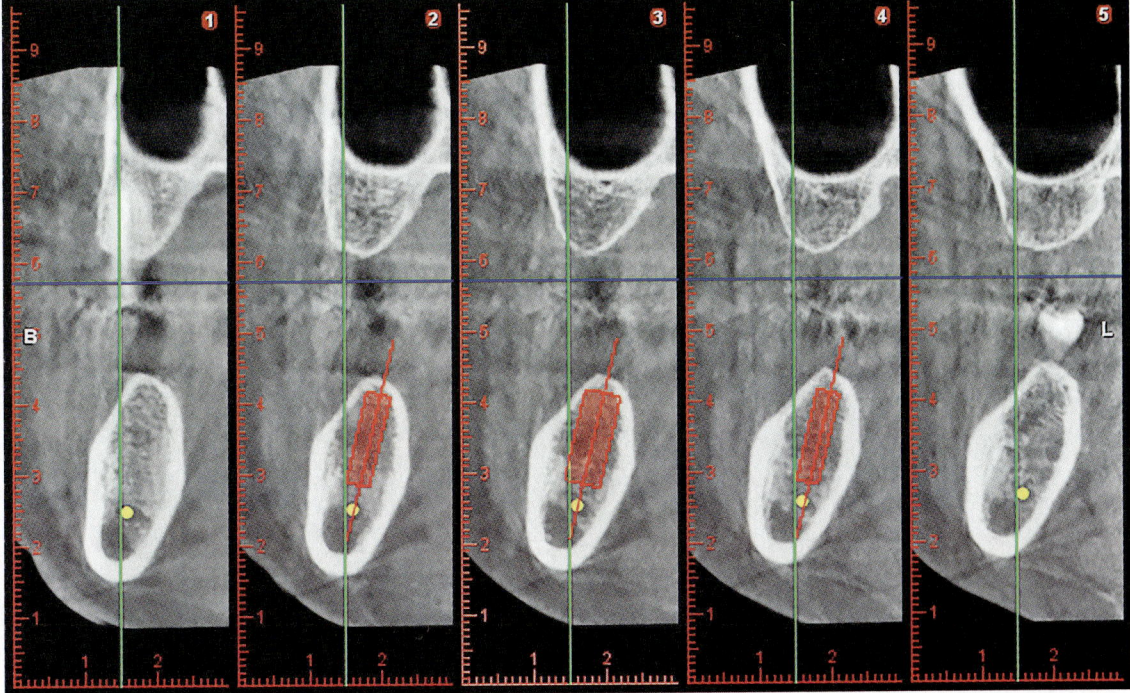

Fig. 37.13: Coronal sections in #36 region showing placement of simulated implant in the planned site

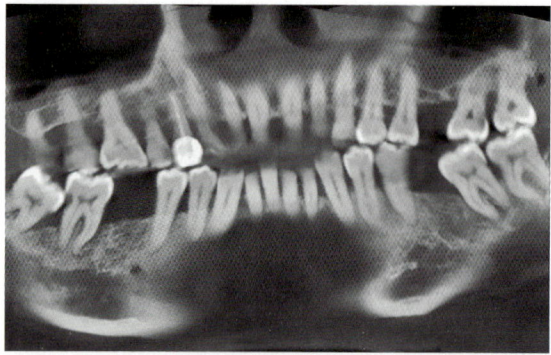

Fig. 37.14: Sagittal section of maxilla and mandible showing good bone height in #46 region

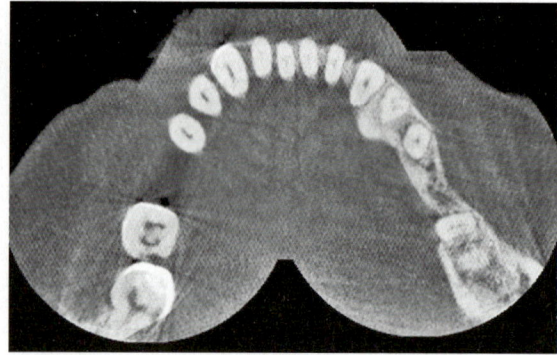

Fig. 37.15: Axial section of mandible showing buccal concavity in #46 region which cannot be appreciated neither in periapical view nor in OPG

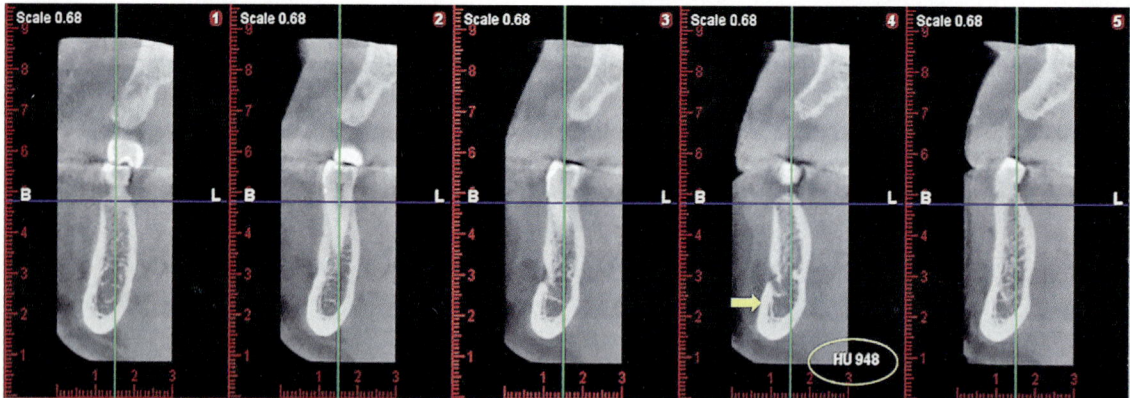

Fig. 37.16: Circled number seen below the second coronal section (from right) denotes the Hounsfield Unit of the bone which denotes the quality of bone

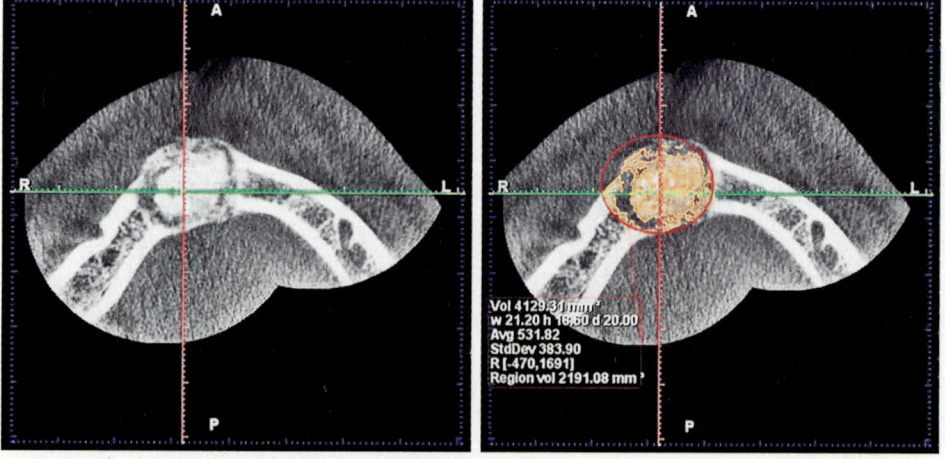

Fig. 37.17: Axial sections showing a mixed radiopaque and radiolucent lesion in the anterior mandible with and without region crowing. Region crowing (colored) shows the volume of the lesion

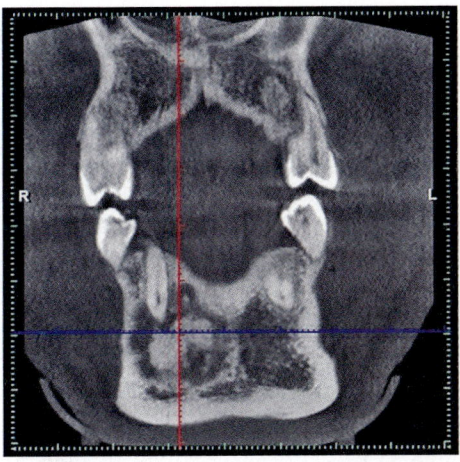
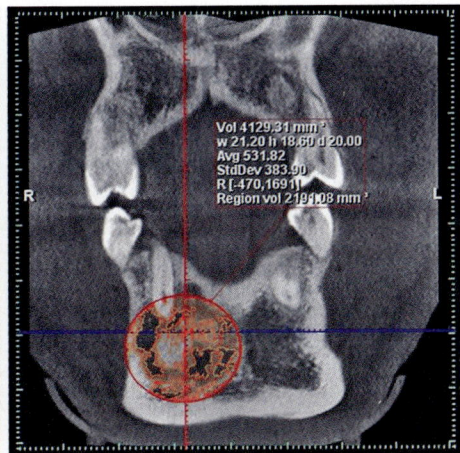

Fig. 37.18: Sagittal sections of the same lesion with and without region crowing

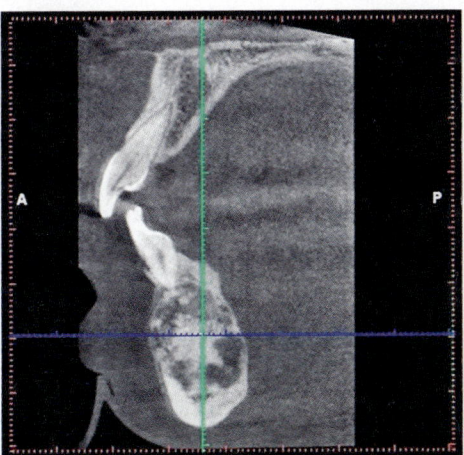
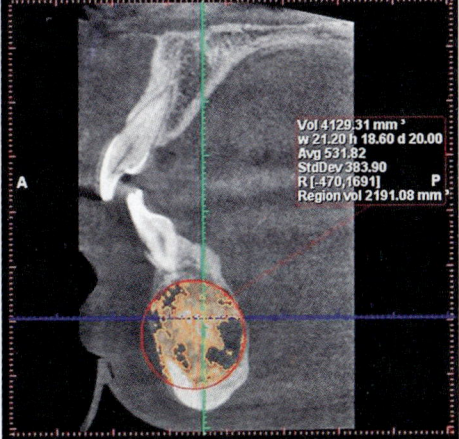

Fig. 37.19: Coronal sections of the same lesion with and without region crowing

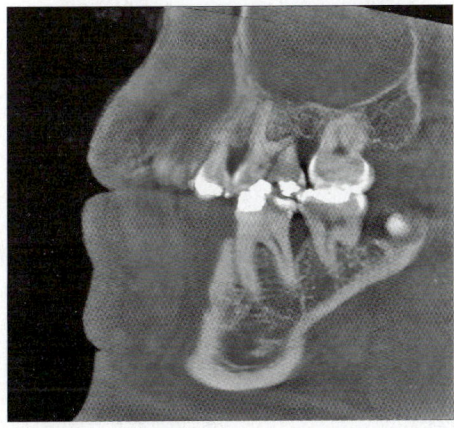
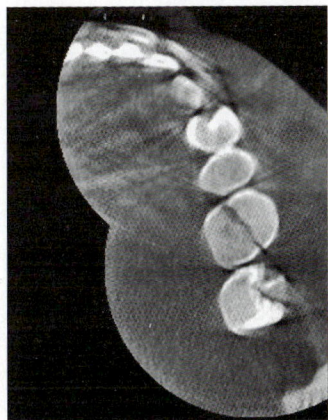

Fig. 37.20: Sagittal section in #26 region showing oblique fracture line

Fig. 37.21: Axial section of #26 showing oblique fracture line

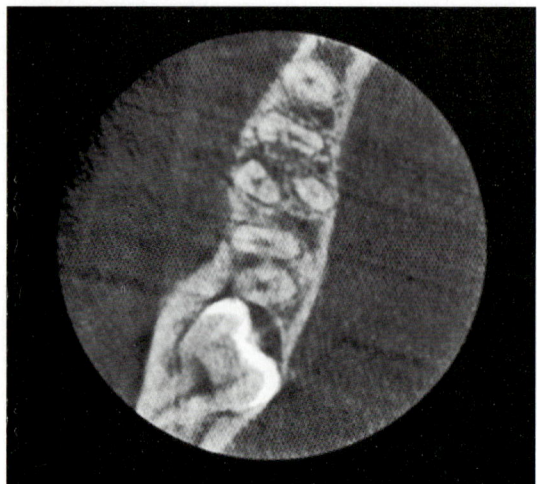

Fig. 37.22: Axial section in #46 region showing three roots. Note the horizontally impacted #48 region

Surgical guide fabrication: Surgical guides are used during dental implant surgery to assist in accurate placement. These guides can be fabricated using traditional free hand method or CAD-CAM technology using milling or stereolithographic principles. Newer CAD-CAM machines can be directly fed with the CBCT images to fabricate surgical stents/guides.

Limitations of CBCT

One of the most important limitations of CBCT is its inability to give details of soft tissues. CBCT machine produces more scatter radiation than the medical CT machines. Majority of the machines provide antiscatter software algorithms. Some of the CBCT machines need to be calibrated more often and this can reduce the productivity of the busy radiology department.

Hounsfield units measured in a CBCT unit are yet to be proven as reliable data for the determination of the bone quality.

Image Retrieval and Storage

CBCT images are default stored in DICOM format in the hard drives. This type of set-up is good enough to cater the needs of a single radiologist/user. In a hospital set-up, where multiple stations need to display the images in DICOM format and store the same safely, PACS (picture archiving and communication system) technology is been used. This system eliminates the need for manual retrieval of images or purchase of multiple viewer licenses. Recently, mini-PACS is developed to cut down the cost and using it in dental hospitals.

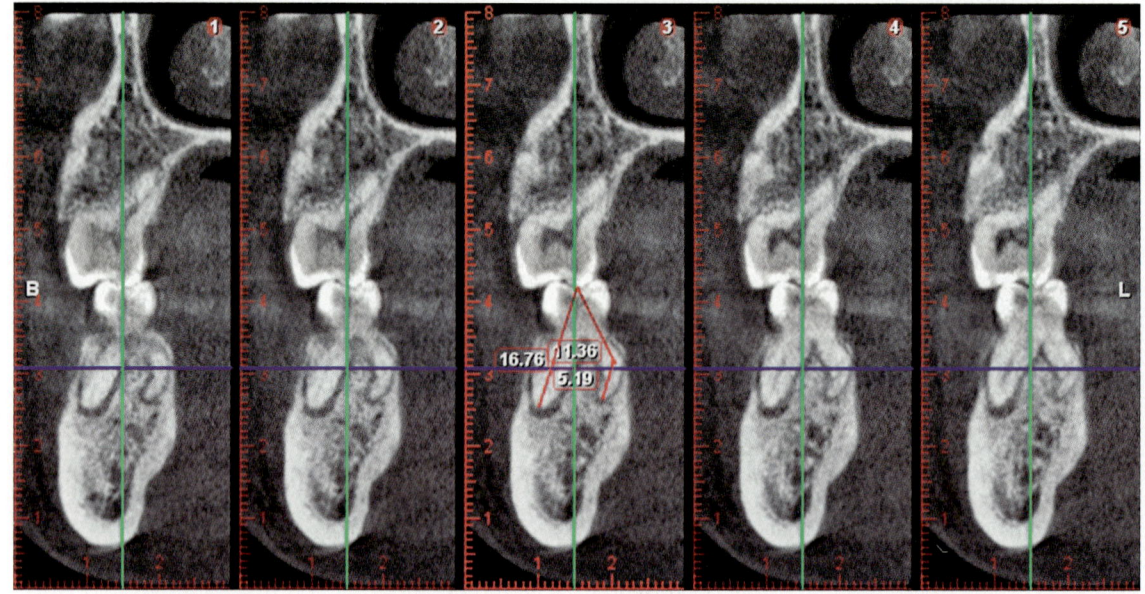

Fig. 37.23: Coronal sections in #46 region showing Radix Entomolaris on the lingual side

Alternatively, single patient images can be stored along with viewer software and the link can be shared through Google drive or DropBox.

CBCT images should be transferred either in STL, OBJ, AMF, and 3MF formats for 3D printing. The file format decides what information goes to the 3D printer. Hence, it is best to decide the format based on the needs.

CBCT Guidelines

The European Academy of Dento-MaxilloFacial Radiology came out with 20 recommendations about CBCT use in dentistry.

1. The referring practitioner must review the patient's history and perform a thorough clinical exam. Documentation of these procedures and justification that the excess radiation will result in a benefit outweighing the radiation risk must be included in the patient's chart prior to prescribing a scan.
2. The referring practitioner should have basic knowledge of CBCT and be aware that a CBCT scan will potentially add new information and aid in the management of the patient.
3. The referring practitioner must use CBCT only when lower-dose traditional 2D radiography does not provide the information necessary to manage a patient.
4. A referring practitioner should not 'routinely' prescribe CBCT scans without determining a risk/benefit for each specific scan.
5. If soft tissues are in question, a conventional CT or MRI should be requested instead of a CBCT.

Use of Cone Beam Computed Tomography Scan

1. When a new CBCT unit is being installed in an office, it should be tested to ensure radiation protection is optimal.

2. A quality assurance program must be created for offices with a CBCT unit. The unit must be routinely tested to ensure proper radiation protection for patients and office members.
3. The guidelines in Section 6 of Radiation Protection 136, European Guidelines on Radiation Protection in Dental Radiology (European Academy DentoMaxilloFacial Radiology) should be followed.
4. All who will be operating the CBCT unit must have theoretical and practical training in radiation protection. Continued education on CBCT and radiation protection is required. Those offices that have not received adequate training should undergo additional training involving a dentomaxillofacial radiologist.
5. The CBCT unit should have a variety of fields of view and resolution options. The smallest field of view should be used with the lowest amount of radiation necessary to capture the area in question.
6. When positioning a patient, positioning lights must be used.
7. If other dentists refer to your office for a CBCT, they must provide you with adequate clinical information regarding the patient's history and examination.

Interpretation of a Cone Beam Computed Tomography Scan

1. All CBCT scans must have a thorough clinical evaluation (radiological report) made of the entire dataset.
2. When a CBCT scan involves the mandible and maxilla up to the floor of the nose, a radiological report should be made by a trained dentomaxillofacial radiologist or, when this is not possible, an adequately trained general dentist.
3. When a CBCT scan involving large fields of view and/or anatomy beyond the teeth and jaws, a radiological report should be made by a trained dentomaxillofacial radiologist or medical radiologist.

FREQUENTLY ASKED QUESTIONS

1. Describe three advantages and disadvantages of cone beam computed tomography.
2. Discuss the various uses of CBCT in dentistry in detail.
3. Differentiate image acquisition principles between medical CT and CBCT.

BIBLIOGRAPHY

1. http://www.newtom.it/it/news-ed-eventi/eventi/2014/20deg-anniversary-of-the-1deg-dental-cbct-complete-scan(accessed on 24th December 2017)
2. Scarfe WC, Farman AG. What is cone beam CT and how does it work? Chapter in Contemporary Dental and Maxillofacial imaging. The Dental Clinics of North America. Edited by Thomas SL and Angelopoulos C. Elsevier Saunders Publications. Pp. 707–30.
3. Jacobson MW. Technology and principles of cone beam computed tomography. Chapter in Cone Beam Computed Tomography – Oral and Maxillofacial Diagnosis and Applications. Sarment D (Editor). Wiley Blackwell publications, Iowa, 2014.
4. Gonzalez SM (Editor). Interpretation Basics of Cone Beam Computed Tomography. Wiley-Blackwell Publications, Iowa, 2014.
5. Miles DA (Editor). Atlas of Cone Beam Imaging for Dental Applications. 2nd edition. Quintessence Publishing Co, Inc, Chicago, 2013.
6. http://www.planmeca.com: CBVT principles 0910 accessed on 26/12/2017.
7. Molteni R. From CT numbers to Hounsefield units in cone beam volumetric imaging: The effect of artifacrts. Presented a 62nd AAOMR, Chicago, 9th December 2011.
8. Katsumata A, Hirukawa A, Okumura S, Naitoh M, Fujishita M, Ariji E, Langlais RP. Effects of image artifacts on gray-value density in limited-volume cone-beam computerized tomography. Oral Surg Oral Med Oral Pathol Oral Radiol Endod. 2007;104:829–836.
9. Tyndall DA, Price JB, Tetradis S, Ganz SD, Hildebolt C, Scarfe WC. Position statement of the American Academy of Oral and Maxillofacial Radiology on selection criteria for the use of radiology in dental implantology with emphasis on cone beam computed tomography. Oral Surg Oral Med Oral Pathol Oral Radiol 2012;113: 817–26.
10. European Academy Dentomaxillofacial Radiology guidelines (2011). http://eadmfr.info/sedentexct (accessed on 4th January 2018).

Dental Caries

Dental caries is an infectious microbial disease of the calcified tissues of the teeth characterized by demineralization of the inorganic portion and destruction of the organic substance of the tooth.

INTRODUCTION

Dental caries represents one of the most widely spread and prevalent conditions affecting around 35% of individuals across all the age group divisions, globally. For the effective prevention and early management of dental caries proper diagnostic approach is essential. Since carious process leads to demineralization and destruction of mineralized components of the tooth, it can be easily located on the radiograph as dark or black area due to inability of demineralized areas to absorb X-rays. But a radiograph fails to determine whether lesion is active or arrested in nature. Also, it needs 30–40% of demineralization of hard tissue for appearance on the radiograph, i.e. lesions cannot be seen until substantial tissue loss has occurred.

Principles of Caries Diagnosis by Radiography

Radiographic investigations provide a superior diagnostic aid in exact carious lesion location and evaluating its extent when compared to clinical detection alone. Essentially, radiographic diagnosis of dental caries is based on the fact that as the carious lesion progresses, the net mineral content of enamel and dentin decreases which leads to a relative decrease in the absorption of the X-ray beam passing through the tooth making the carious area to appear more radiolucent. But the radiographic detection is only possible after 30–40% of demineralization process has occurred.

Various Radiographic Techniques Available for Detection and Diagnosis of Dental Caries

1. **Bitewing radiography:** Ideal method for proximal caries detection for the posterior teeth. Method requires a parallel placement of radiographic film or detector using a holder or stick on tab, on which the patient bites and then image is recorded.
2. **Periapical radiography:** This view provides with a radiographic image containing tooth and its related structures. Carious lesions, and periapical changes can be detected by this technique. The film is placed parallel to the long axis of the tooth but a few number of teeth can be seen per film.
3. **Panoramic radiograph (OPG):** These radiographs are based on extraoral

approach, i.e. recorded outside the oral cavity. Although OPG has low sensitivity in detection of dental caries and not a recommended method for caries detection, it can be an appropriate method for patients with multiple carious lesions.

Radiography and Challenges in Carious Lesion Detection

Accurate diagnosis of caries by using radiographs is a well researched and reliable method, but the radiograph presents a two-dimensional image of a three-dimensional object, thus leading to misdiagnosis. Also carious lesions are larger in size clinically when compared to their appearance on radiographs. Various other parameters related to film detector placement or processing affect the caries detection procedure on radiographs.

Proper placement of the receptor film and horizontal/vertical alignment of the X-ray beam is crucial, as it may lead to over or underestimation of the carious lesion or sometimes the lesions in enamel are projected to be progressed to dentin. Overlapping of teeth on the radiographic image may lead to masking the proximal lesions whereas changes in the exposure factor directly affect the contrast of radiographs and appearance of lesion size.

Superimposition of various anatomic structures like alveolar bone at the neck of the teeth and existing radio opaque restorative material may lead to improper caries estimation, i.e. exact caries site, size, distance from pulp cavity, recurrent caries, and undermined carious lesions. Radiolucent restorations and linings may be mistaken for caries, but these usually have clearly demarcated outlines and can be confirmed clinically. Developmental defects in enamel like hypoplasia may appear as radiolucent dots.

Radiolucent wedge shaped defect called *cervical burnout*, is an artifact seen at the alveolar bone height in cervical region. It is observed on radiographs due to the anatomy of tooth in cervical region and amount of radiation passing for i.e. more amount of exposure leads to burnout appearance. These defects on radiographs may mimic interproximal, cervical or recurrent carious lesions. Whereas an optical illusion which produces fictitious radiolucent areas in dentinal peaks bounded by occlusal and proximal enamel, seen especially in premolar, are known as *Mach Band Effect* on radiograph.

Prerequisites for Radiographic Caries Detection

1. **Proper film or detector placement:** Film or detector should be placed appropriately, so that area of interest can be focused and overlap of buccal or lingual cusps and interproximal areas can be avoided.
2. **Correct positioning of X-ray tube, i.e. horizontal and vertical angulation:** Improper angulations can lead to over and underestimation of size of carious lesion.
3. **Amount and time of exposure:** Over and underexposure can lead to dark or light images on radiographs, respectively. Exposure should be sufficient enough to capture enamel and dentin images properly and avoid cervical burnouts.
4. **Processing of films (manual and digital):** In case of X-ray films, improper use of developer and fixer can lead to over or underdeveloped radiographs. Whereas digital images should be evaluated for contrasts, brightness, enhancement and magnifications.
5. Proper film mounting and viewing conditions can also affect the accuracy of caries diagnosis.
6. Expertise of the evaluator.

Radiographic Appearance of Dental Caries

Occlusal Caries

A carious lesion begins either at base or side walls of pit and fissures on the occlusal surface of posterior tooth. Lesion then spread perpendicularly along the dentino-enamel junction. Sometimes, lesions can go undetected radiographically, until crossing the dentinoenamel junction. Lesions on the occlusal surfaces are best detected on clinical examination rather than using radiographic methods.

Lesions usually begin as dot shaped within the enamel rods, just beneath the pits and fissures and then spread along the dentinoenamel junction. Visualization on the radiographs appears as thin line spreading at dentinoenamel junction. After carious penetration into the dentin surface conical or rounded radiolucency can be seen where apex is towards the pulp chamber and base at the periphery. Occlusal caries can be classified as incipient, moderate and severe on the bases of depth of penetration into enamel and dentin.

a. **Incipient lesions:** Usually not recorded on the radiographic imaging, only clinical detection is possible. If recorded it appears as grayish shadow just beneath the dentinoenamel junction.

b. **Moderate lesions:** Lesion is located under enamel with little or no change seen in the appearance of enamel surface. Thin radiolucent line can be observed at the level of dentinoenamel junction (Fig. 38.1).

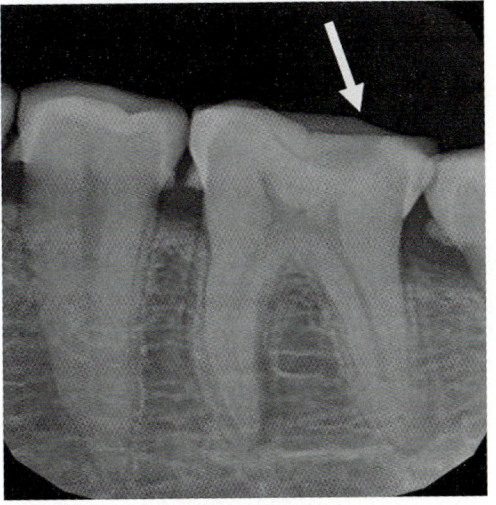

Fig. 38.1

c. **Severe lesions:** Lesion appears as cavitations on clinical examination, radiographically large conical or round-shaped radiolucent area can be seen (Fig. 38.2).

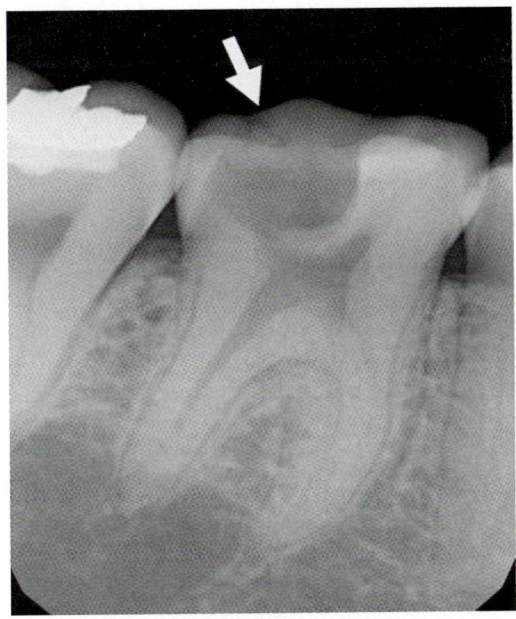

Fig. 38.2: Severe occlusal caries

Differential diagnosis: Buccal caries may mimic as occlusal caries, but latter presents with more extensive and ill-defined radiolucent borders on radiographic imaging, whereas buccal caries presents with well-defined boundaries and uniform non-carious region of enamel tissue around affected region.

Interproximal Carious Lesions

Interproximal carious lesions appear below the contact area and free gingival margin. They are difficult to locate and diagnosed during the routine clinical examination.

Interproximal caries starts as notch on the radiograph which later appears as cone-shaped lesion or hourglass-shaped in appearance. On the basis of extent of the lesions appearing on the radiographs they are classified as incipient, moderate, advanced and severe (Fig. 38.3).

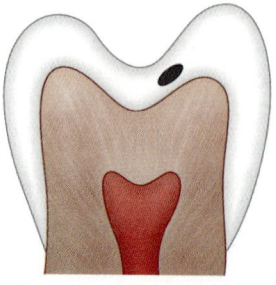 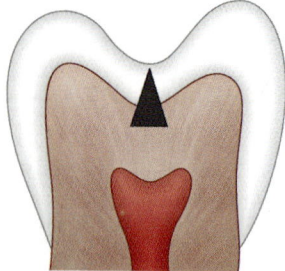 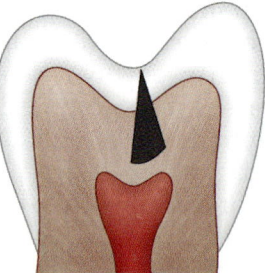

Incipient occlusal caries   Moderate occlusal caries   Severe occlusal caries

Fig. 38.3: Types of occlusal carious lesions

a. **Incipient lesions (Fig. 38.4):** Usually the early phase of lesion is difficult to locate on radiographs because it takes around 30–40% demineralization of the tissue to appear on the radiograph. Lesion appears as triangular shaped with its base towards the external tooth surface and its apex towards the dentin. Lesion is confined within the half of the thickness of the enamel, not extending beyond it. These lesions may also be seen as dots, bands or a thin line on the radiographs.

b. **Moderate lesions:** Lesions are extended beyond the inner half of enamel and confined to the outer half and not extending into the dentinoenamel junction. Shape of the lesion appears as a triangle on the radiograph, but may present as diffused radiolucency too (Fig. 38.5).

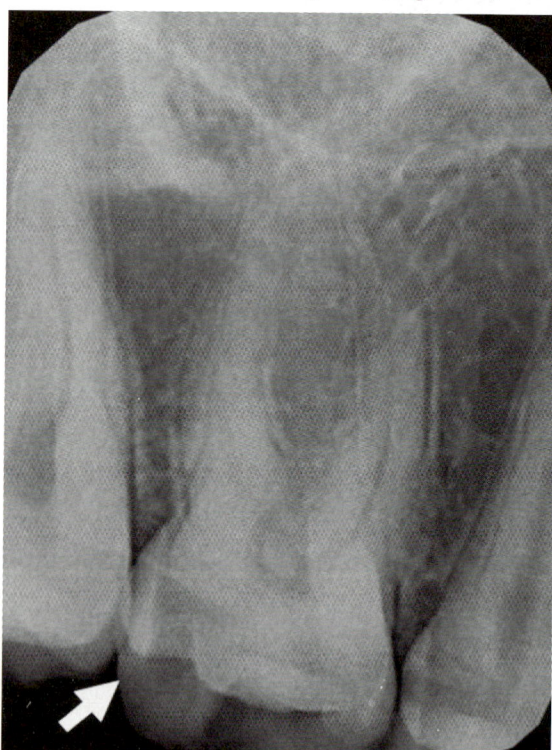

Fig. 38.5: Moderate proximal carious lesions

c. **Advanced lesions:** When lesions cross the dentinoenamel junction, it appears as second triangle-shaped lesion in dentin

Fig. 38.4: Incipient proximal carious lesions

with first triangle present in the enamel. The base of the lesion is located in the dentin and apex points towards the pulp space and it is confined to the inner half of the dentin. The second triangular shaped lesion is usually large in appearance and it spreads laterally along the direction of the dentinal tubules. As the lesion progresses, there is more amount of demineralization occurring, lesion may appear more diffused and irregular in shape (Fig. 38.6).

when compared to location of cervical burnouts (Figs 38.7 and 38.8).

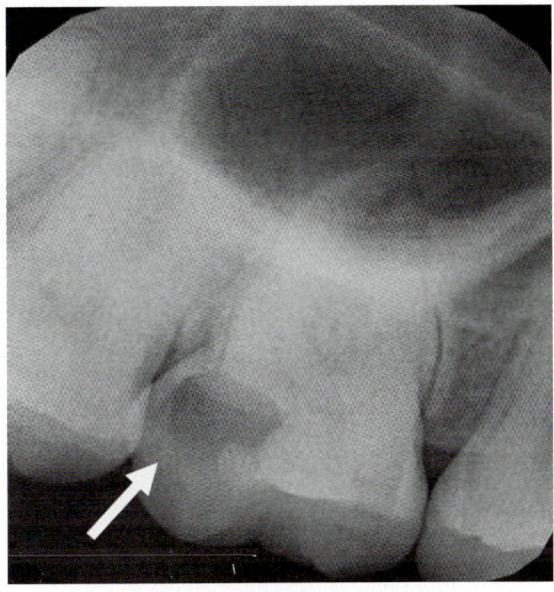

Fig. 38.7

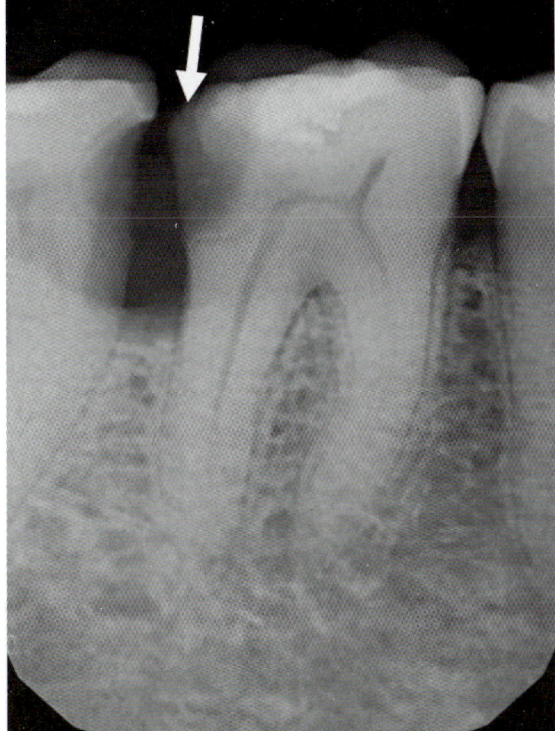

Fig. 38.6: Advanced proximal carious lesions

d. **Severe lesions:** These lesions extend beyond more than half of dentin and approaching the pulp chamber. These lesions appears as cavitations in the tooth when clinically examined.

Differential diagnosis: Proximal lesions are smooth surface lesions located typically at or below the tooth contact area and the free gingival margins. Lesion does not start below gingival margins, is a differentiating feature

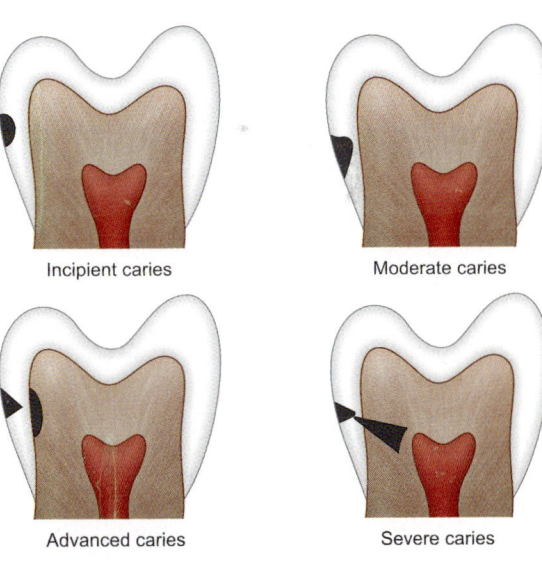

Fig. 38.8: Progression of proximal caries

Buccal and Lingual Surface Caries/ Cervical Caries (Fig. 38.9)

Buccal and lingual surfaces are involved with the carious process where enamel pits are affected by the carious process. These lesions are best detected on the clinical examination and difficult to diagnose on the radiographs due to superimposition of unaffected healthy surrounding enamel and dentinal tissues. Lesion appears as a small round-shaped radiolucency or shadow when present in the enamel, as the carious lesion progresses to dentin, it becomes more elliptical or semilunar. Also radiographically one distinct feature can be observed, the radiolucency is always surrounded by uniform spread of healthy unaffected enamel rods.

Root Surface Caries/Cemental Caries

Main etiological factor for the root caries is bacterial plaque accumulation over the cementum after gingival recession due to food lodgment, open contacts and tooth over eruptions. Lesions are rapidly spreading in nature due to physical properties of cementum, i.e. its softer nature leads to rapid destruction. Root caries associated with the posterior teeth can be visualized on the horizontal bitewing radiographs whereas the carious lesions on the anterior teeth are best visualized using periapical radiography. Radiographic appearance of root caries is described as ill defined notched, scooping out and saucer-like radiolucency present apical to the cementoenamel junction, but coronal to the bone height. Early lesions are difficult to be diagnosed radiographically. Mostly affecting molar and premolar teeth and is best detected clinically (Fig. 38.10).

Differential diagnosis: Cervical burnout may mimic root caries but a true carious lesion can be differentiated by the absence of an image of root edge and by the appearance of a diffused border where the tooth substance is lost.

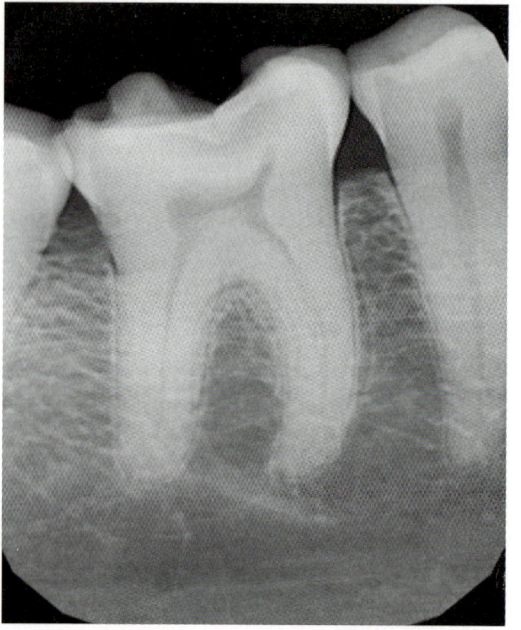

Fig. 38.9: Buccal carious lesions

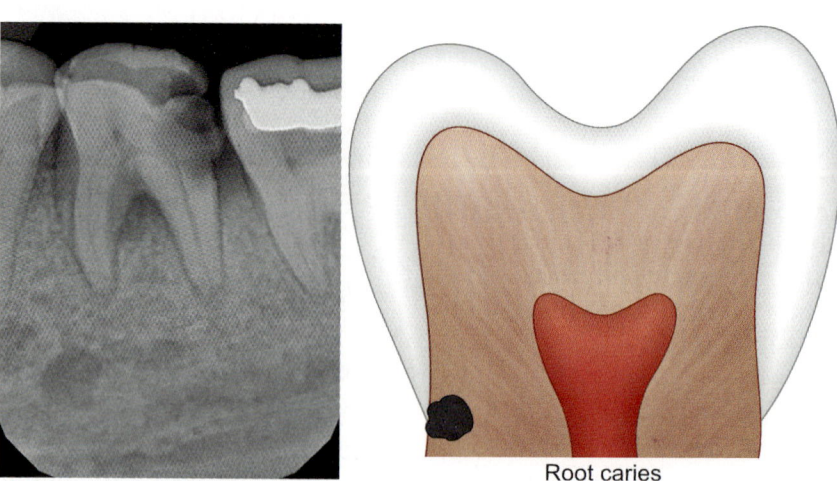

Root caries

Fig. 38.10: Root caries

Rampant Caries

Represents class of carious lesions which progress rapidly leading to severe destruction of the tooth tissue. Such lesions are associated with children presenting with poor dietary habits and oral hygiene status. Also such lesions can be seen in individuals with reduced salivary flow or xerostomia. Multiple teeth are involved and most of the lesions are at the advanced stages, i.e. approaching or invading the pulp. Radiographically large radiolucency can be seen suggesting severe tissue loss and pulp invasion.

Recurrent Caries/Secondary Caries (Fig. 38.11)

Development of lesion occurs at or under the pre-existing restorative margins that can be attributed to faulty cavity extensions, shaping or inadequate adaptation of restorative material. Radiographically, many factors are associated with the location and diagnosis of recurrent or secondary caries like visualization of lesion can be masked by the radiopacity of the overlying restorative material, location of carious lesion, i.e. caries beneath the interproximal margins can be located more easily than other locations and such lesions can be easily confused by radiolucent lining cement.

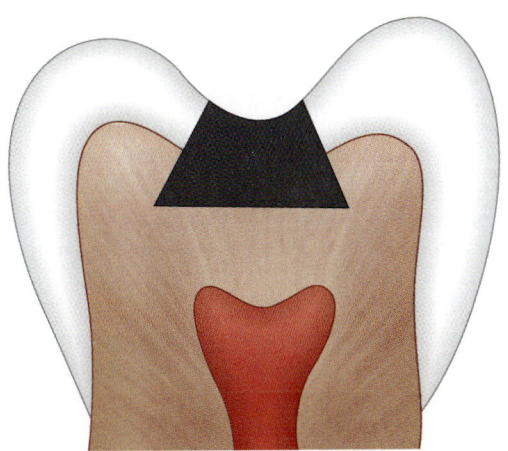

Fig. 38.11: Secondary caries

Differential diagnosis: Radiolucent cements or lining may be misdiagnosed as secondary caries. Differentiating features includes the fact that radiolucent cements present with sharp and well-defined outline reflecting the preparation and placement.

Cervical burnouts may also be misdiagnosed as secondary caries and can be distinguished on the condition that cervical burnout presents as triangle-shaped lesion which gets less apparent towards the center of tooth.

Appearance of secondary caries under amalgam restorations can be seen due to radiopaque ions released from the amalgam restorations, may cause area under restoration to appear radiolucent mimicking secondary caries.

Arrested Caries

Arrested caries lesions located on the occlusal pits and fissures are rarely detected on the radiographic imaging, but lesions on the proximal surface appear as vague or ill defined radiolucent notch. Usually the involved tooth surface with arrested caries lesions presents with no adjacent tooth contact.

Radiation Caries/Drug-related Caries

Patients undergoing radiation therapy of head and neck region leads to reduced salivary gland functions causing reduced salivary flow and change in oral microflora. All this if untreated leads to xerostomia in the oral cavity and xerostomia in-turn leads to progressive and severe, i.e. rampant tooth tissue destruction. Most frequent lesions can be seen as a radiolucent shadow commencing at the necks (cervical region) of teeth and spreads mesially and distally in patients with poor oral hygiene not using topical fluoride. Several adjacent teeth are often affected causing crowns to be lost with root fragments remaining. Radiographically lesion presents as radiolucent shadows around the neck of tooth with varying depth of destruction into enamel and dentin. These radiolucent appearances are diffused or non-uniform in shape. Many patients are taking drugs that produce xerostomia and that can result in a similar appearance of carious lesions.

Radiation caries can be classified as

- **Type I:** Represents the most common pattern which affects the cervical aspect of the teeth and extends along the cementoenamel junction. A circumferential carious lesion develops, it may lead to amputation of the coronal structure.
- **Type II:** Areas of dental surfaces demineralization occurs with generalized erosions and worn occlusal and incisal surfaces.
- **Type III:** Represents the least common pattern with appearances of change in color in the dentin structure. The crown eventually becomes dark brown/black with occlusal and incisal wear.

Summary of Differential Diagnosis of Dental Caries

a. **Cervical burnout:** Located at the neck of the teeth, triangular in shape, gradually becoming less apparent towards the center of the tooth, follows anatomical contour and the peripheral border appears intact. Many teeth in the same arch on the radiograph will appear to be affected.

b. **Internal resorption:** Enlarged pulp chamber. The margins are sharp and smooth.

c. **External resorption:** Seen at apices of teeth, blunt apex, smooth outline altering shape of root.

d. **Erosion cavity:** Saucer-shaped radiolucency with well-defined or diffuse borders.

e. **Non-opaque filling:** It will have sharpness and uniformity of the margins.

f. **Hypoplasia of enamel:** Several small dark spots are seen in multiple teeth. Irregular attrition or abrasion can also be included as DD of caries.

FREQUENTLY ASKED QUESTIONS

1. Write about various radiographic appearances of carious lesions.
2. Discuss radiographic differential diagnosis of caries.

BIBLIOGRAPHY

1. Shafer WG, et al. A Textbook of Oral Pathology. Philadelphia:WB Saunders;1983.p86.
2. Petersen PE, Bourgeois D, Ogawa H, Estupinan-Day S, Ndiaye C. The global burden of oral diseases and risks to oral health. Bull World Health Organ. 2005;83:661–9.
3. Peterson PE. The World Oral Health Report. Publication No. WHO/ NMH/ NPH/ORH/03.2. Geneva: World Health Organization; 2003.
4. Marcenes W, Kassebaum NJ, Bernabé E, Flaxman A, Naghavi M, Lopez A, et al. Global burden of oral conditions in 1990–2010: A systematic analysis. J Dent Res. 2013;92:592–7.
5. Hobdell M, Petersen PE, Clarkson J, Johnson N. Global goals for oral health 2020. Int Dent J 2003;53:285–8.
6. Mann J, Pettigrew JC, Revach A, Arwas JR, Kochavi D. Assessment of the DMF-S index with the use of bitewing radiographs. Oral Surg Oral Med Oral Pathol. 1989;68:661–5.
7. Creanor SL, Russell JI, Strang DM, Stephen KW, Burchell CK. The prevalence of clinically undetected occlusal dentine caries in Scottish adolescents. Br Dent J. 1990;169:126–9.
8. de Vries HCB, Juiken HMHM, Konig KG, vant Hof MA. Radiographic versus clinical diagnosis of approximal carious lesions. Caries Res. 1990;24:364–70.
9. Kidd EAM, Naylor MN, Wilson RF. Prevalence of clinically undetected and untreated molar occlusal dentine caries in adolescents on the Isle of Wight. Caries Res. 1992;26:397–401.
10. Rugg-Gunn AJ. Dental Caries. In: Welbury RR, editor. Paediatric Dentistry. Oxford: Oxford University Press; 1997.
11. Diniz MB, Rodrigues JA, Neuhaus KW, Cordeiro RCL, Lussi A. Influence of examiner's clinical experience on the reproducibility and accuracy of radiographic examination in detecting occlusal caries. Clinical Oral Investigations. 2010;14(5):515–23.

12. Hellen-Halme K, Lith A. Effect of ambient light level at the monitor surface on digital radiographic evaluation of approximal carious lesions, an in vitro study. Dentomaxillofacial Radiology. 2012;41:192–6.

13. Eric Whaites and Nicholas Drage. Essentials of Dental Radiography and Radiology. 5th ed. Churchill Livingstone;2013:Chapter 21:Dental caries and the assessment of restorations; Pp. 251–64.

14. De Araujo FB, Rosito DB, Toigo E, dos Santos CK. Diagnosis of approximal caries: radiographic versus clinical examination using tooth separation. Am J Dent. 1992 Oct;5(5):245–8.

15. Mejàre I. Bitewing examination to detect caries in children and adolescents—when and how often? Dent Update. 2005 Dec;32(10):588–90, 593–4, 596–7.

16. Mejàre I, Stenlund H, Zelezny-Holmlund C. Caries incidence and lesion progression from adolescence to young adulthood: a prospective 15-year cohort study in Sweden. Caries Res. 2004 Mar-Apr;38(2):130–41.

17. Mjör IA, Toffenetti F. Secondary caries: a literature review with case reports. Quintessence Int. 2000 Mar;31(3):165–79.

18. White, Stuart C, and Pharoah MJ. Oral Radiology: Principles and Interpretation. 6th ed. St. Louis, Mo: Mosby/Elsevier, 2009; Chapter no. 17: Dental caries; p270–81.

19. Vissink A, Jansma J, Spijkervet, FK, Burlage FR, Coppes RP. Oral sequelae of head and neck radiotherapy. Crit Rev Oral Biol Med. 2003; 14:199–212.

20. Jham BC, da Silva Freire AR. Oral complications of radiotherapy in the head and neck. Rev Bras Otorrinolaringol (Engl Ed). 2006; 72:704–8.

21. Kielbassa AM, Hinkelbein W, Hellwig E, Meyer-Lückel H. Radiation-related damage to dentition. Lancet Oncol. 2006; 7:326–35.

Radiologic Considerations in Periodontal Diseases

Radiography plays an important role in the diagnosis, study and treatment of periodontal disease. Radiographs can provide critical information for diagnosis and treatment planning and can also serve as baseline information for the assessment of treatment outcomes. However the radiographs are the adjunct to the clinical examinations and not a substitute for it.

A conventional or advanced radiographic method helps to assess the destruction of alveolar bone associated with periodontitis. It can be used to evaluate bone loss—horizontal or angular patterns (infra bony) defects, root morphologies/topographies, furcation, radiolucencies, endodontic lesions, endodontic mishaps, developmental anomalies and, root length and shape remaining in bone.

Limitations of Conventional Radiography

- Provide 2D view of 3D structures, therefore, fails to disclose the osseous destruction confined to buccal or lingual surfaces.
- Typically show less severe bone destruction, approximately 30% less than actually present.
- Measure bone level from CEJ is not valid when there is overeruption or severe attrition with passive eruption.
- Do not demonstrate soft tissue to hard tissue relation. (But if radiopaque material like gutta-percha inserted, base of the pocket can usually be recorded).

Classification for Periodontal and Peri-implant Disease and Conditions

(A new classification scheme for periodontal and peri-implant diseases and conditions—introduction and key changes from the 1999 classification)

I. Periodontal Health and Gingival Disease or Conditions

1. **Periodontal health and gingival health**
   a. Clinical gingival health on an intact periodontium
   b. Clinical gingival health on a reduced periodontium
2. **Gingivitis:** Dental biofilm induced
   a. Associated with dental biofilm alone
   b. Mediated by systemic or local risk factors
   c. Drug-influenced gingival enlargement
3. **Gingival disease:** Non-dental biofilm induced
   a. Genetic and developmental disorders
   b. Specific infections
   c. Inflammatory and immune conditions
   d. Reactive processes
   e. Neoplasms
   f. Endocrine, nutritional and metabolic diseases

g. Traumatic lesions

h. Gingival pigmentation

II. Forms of Periodontitis

1. Necrotizing periodontal disease
   a. Necrotizing gingivitis
   b. Necrotizing periodontitis
   c. Necrotizing stomatitis
2. Periodontitis as a manifestation of systemic diseases
   a. Stages
   b. Extent and Distribution
   c. Grade

III. Periodontal Manifestation of Systemic Diseases and Developmental and Acquired Conditions

1. Systemic diseases/conditions affecting the periodontal supporting tissue
2. Other periodontal conditions
   a. Periodontal abscess
   b. Endodontic-periodontal lesions
3. Mucogingival deformities and conditions around teeth
   a. Gingival phenotype
   b. Gingival/soft tissue recession
   c. Lack of gingiva
   d. Decreased vestibular depth
   e. Aberrant frenum and muscle position
   f. Gingival excess
   g. Abnormal color
   h. Conditions of exposed root surface
4. Traumatic occlusal force
   a. Primary occlusal trauma
   b. Secondary occlusal trauma
   c. Orthodontic forces
5. Prosthesis and tooth-related factors that modify
   a. Localized tooth-related factors
   b. Localized dental prosthesis-related factors

IV. Peri-implant Disease and Conditions

1. Peri-implant health
2. Peri-implant mucositis
3. Peri-implantitis
4. Peri-implant soft and hard tisuue deficiencies

RADIOGRAPHIC FINDINGS OF HEALTHY PERIODONTAL STRUCTURES

Before understanding the periodontal pathologies, assessment of healthy periodontium is important.

In health,

- Lamina dura around the root of the teeth appears as dense radiopaque line.
- Alveolar crest is located approximately 1.5–2 mm apical to the cementoenamel junctions (CEJ) of adjacent teeth.
- In the anterior region, the alveolar crest appears sharp.
- In the posterior region, the alveolar crest appears smooth and flat.
- Alveolar crests, when flat, meet with the lamina dura at the necks of the teeth, forming well-defined right angles.
- The normal periodontal ligament space appears as a continuous thin radiolucent line on the mesial and distal aspects of the teeth between the roots and the lamina dura and is of uniform thickness.

1. **Early radiographic changes in periodontitis:** Chronic periodontitis shows early bony changes as
   - Crestal irregularities, triangulation and interseptal bone changes
   - Interruption in the continuity of the lamina dura seen along the mesial or distal aspect of the interdental alveolar crest
   - Finger-like radiolucent projections extending from the crestal bone into the interdental alveolar bone. These projections are result of a deeper extension of the inflammation from the connective tissue of the gingiva.

2. **Evaluation of bone loss**
   - The radiograph actually indicates the amount of bone loss measured as the difference between the physiological bone and the remaining bone.

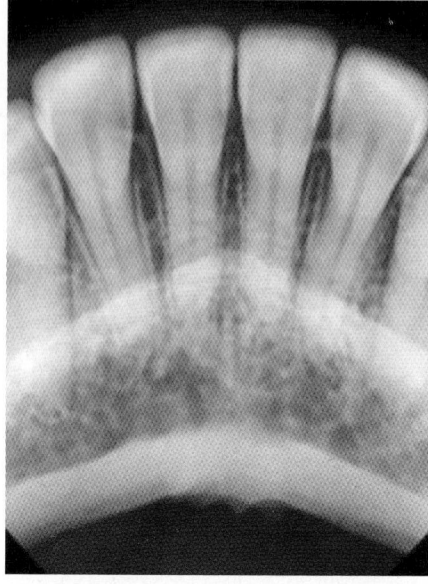

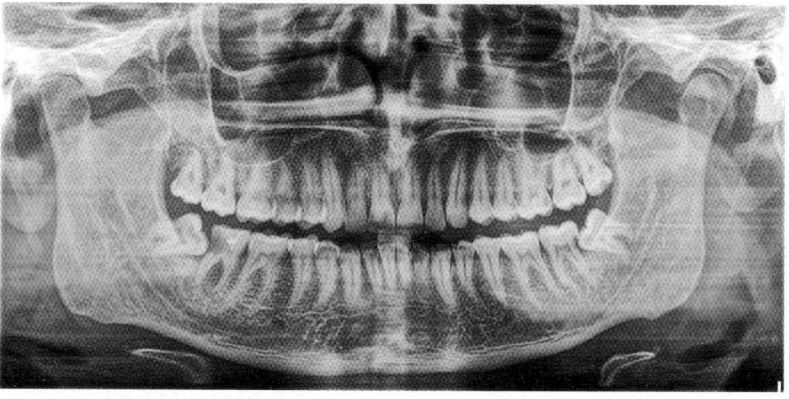

Fig. 39.1: Normal periodontium

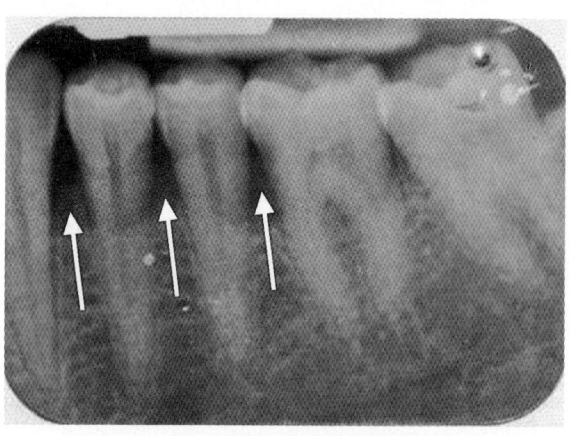

Fig. 39.2: Interdental bone loss

- Bone loss can be determined in terms of distribution, pattern and severity.
- When the bone loss occurs in less than 30% of the sites—localized bone loss.
- When the bone loss is greater than 30%— generalized bone loss
- When the bone loss occurs on a plane that is parallel to a line drawn from CEJ of a tooth to that of an adjacent tooth, it is called horizontal bone loss.
- When the bone loss occurs on a plane that is at an angle to a line drawn from CEJ of a tooth to that of an adjacent

tooth, it is called vertical or angular bone loss.

* Bone loss viewed on a dental radiograph can be defined as slight bone loss (1 to 2 mm), moderate bone loss (3 or 4 mm) and severe bone loss (5 mm or greater)

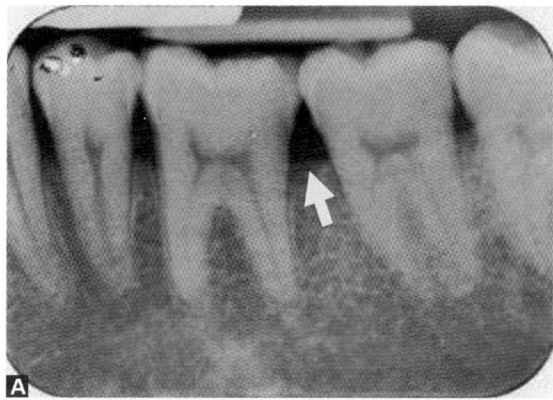

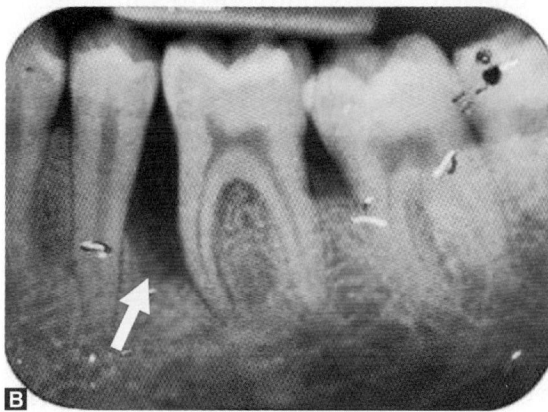

Fig. 39.3: (A) Horizontal bone loss. (B) Vertical bone loss

3. **Evaluation of furcation involvement**
   * Extension of the periodontal pocket between the roots of multirooted teeth is called furcation involvement.
   * Radiographs can be helpful in locating furcation involvement; however, the furcation involvement will not be seen unless the bone resorption extends apically beyond the furcation.
   * Mandibular molar furcation is much more sharply defined than the maxillary molar furcation.

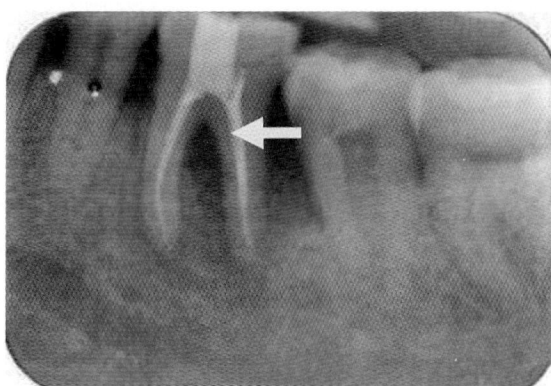

Fig. 39.4: Radiolucency in furcation area suggestive of furcation involvement

4. **Evaluation of crown root ratio**
   * Tooth stability is influenced by the amount of leverage placed on the periodontium.
   * An increase in length of the clinical crown produces unfavorable leverage on the periodontium.

5. **Hypercementosis**
   * Hypercementosis is seen occasionally on teeth with bone loss.
   * It may be a response to inflammation or to the increased occlusal loading on a tooth.

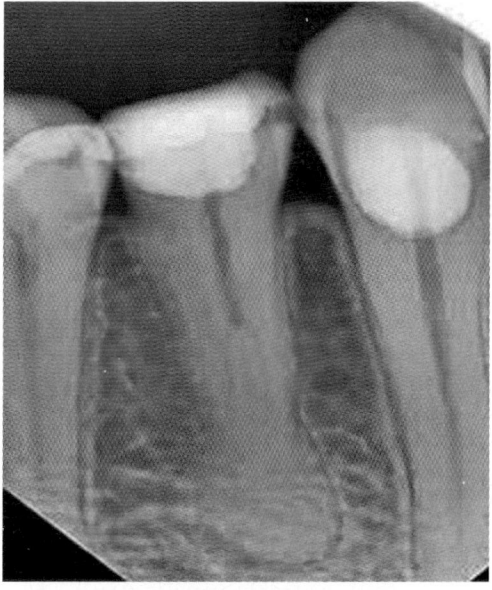

Fig. 39.5: Hypercementosis

RADIOGRAPHIC ASSESSMENT OF VARIOUS PERIODONTAL DISEASES

I. Periodontitis

A. Localized/generalized; Grade A, Grade B Periodontitis

Clinical features
- Supragingival and subgingival plaque and calculus
- Gingival swelling, redness and loss of gingival stippling
- Altered gingival margins
- Pocket formation
- Bleeding on probing
- Attachment loss
- Bone loss
- Furcation involvement
- Tooth mobility
- Pathologic migration
- Tooth loss

Radiographic features
After clinical examination, radiographic bone loss whether horizontal or angular gives the diagnosis of periodontitis.

B. Molar incisor relationship; Grade C Periodontitis

Primary features
- Rapid loss of attachment
- The subject is otherwise healthy
- Presence of familial aggregation

Secondary features
- Inconsistency of the low amount of present etiological factors.
- Strong colonization by *Aggregatibacter actinomycetemcomitans* and some population of *P. gingivalis*.
- Hyperresponsive macrophages and abnormal neutrophil function
- Self-limiting disease

Radiographic features
- Bone loss in maxillary and mandibular incisor and/or first molars usually bilaterally resulting in vertical arc-like destructive pattern (mirror images) in localized form of disease.

- With progression of the disease, there is generalized bone loss, less pronounced in premolars.

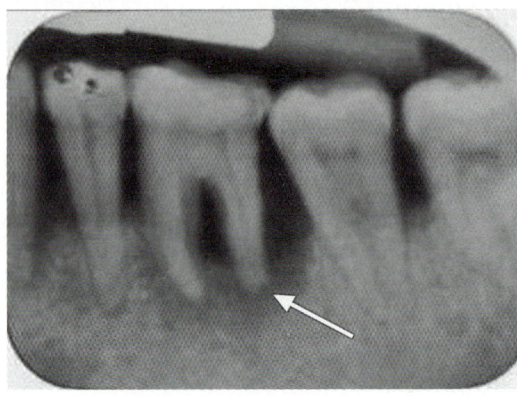

Fig. 39.6: Arc-shaped bone loss

Treatment
- Conventional periodontal therapy
- Antimicrobial therapy
- Surgical intervention
- Full mouth disinfection
- Host modulation therapy
- Restoration and rehabilitation of the lost teeth.

II. Periodontal Manifestation of Systemic Diseases and Developmental and Acquired Conditions

A. Other Periodontal Conditions

▶ **Periodontal Abscess**

Clinical features
1. *Acute periodontal abscess*
   - Mild-to-severe discomfort
   - Localized swelling
   - Periodontal pocket
   - Mobility
   - Elevation of teeth in socket
   - Tenderness to percussion or biting
   - Exudation
   - Elevated temperature
   - Regional lymphadenopathy
2. *Chronic periodontal abscess*
   - Dull pain
   - Slight tooth elevation

* Intermittent exudation
* Fistulous tract associated with deep pocket
* Usually without systemic involvement

Radiographic features
* Radiolucency on the lateral aspect of the root.
* Radiographic picture is not pathognomic for periodontal abscess because
  * Acute abscess gives no radiographic sign
  * Location of the abscess on the buccal and lingual/palatal aspect cannot be appreciated.
* Final diagnosis needs to be confirmed with the clinical findings.

Differential diagnosis
Pulpal abscess

Treatment options for periodontal abscess
* Drainage through pocket retraction or incision
* Scaling and root planing
* Periodontal surgery
* Systemic antibiotics
* Tooth removal

▶ Endodontic Periodontal Lesion

Clinical features
* Presence of inflammation, ulceration or sinus tracts
* Swelling or presence of abscess
* Tenderness on lateral percussion for periodontal inflammation

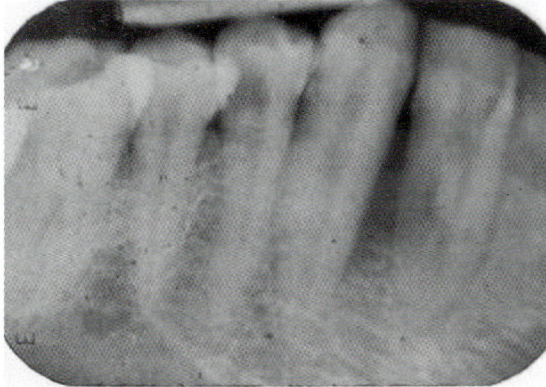

Fig. 39.7: IOPA showing bone loss around mandibular canine

* Tenderness on vertical percussion for apical periodontitis
* Mobility of teeth
* Non-vital teeth in case of endodontic involvement

Radiographic features
* If lesion is endodontic in origin: Periapical bone loss present
* If lesion is periodontal in origin: Varying degree of crestal bone loss present

Treatment
* *Primary endodontic lesion:* Root canal treatment
* *Primary periodontal lesion:* Periodontal therapy
* *Primary endodontic secondary periodontal lesion:* Root canal treatment followed by periodontal therapy

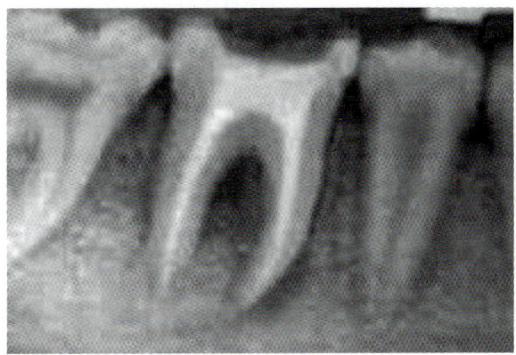

Fig. 39.8: Combined periodontal endodontic lesion

* *Primary periodontal secondary endodontic lesion:* Root canal treatment followed by periodontal therapy
* *Combined lesion:* Root canal treatment followed by periodontal treatment

B. Traumatic Occlusal Forces

▶ Trauma from occlusion

Clinical features
* Increased tooth mobility
* Attrition
* Positive fremitus test
* Tooth migration
* Sensitivity in teeth

Radiographic features
- Thickening of lamina dura
- Widening of the periodontal ligament space
- Advanced lesion have angular bone loss
- Root resorption from excessive forces on periodontium.

Treatment
Various treatment modalities include:
- Occlusal adjustments
- Management of parafunctional habits
- Splinting of teeth
- Orthodontic tooth movement
- Occlusal reconstruction
- Extraction of selected teeth.

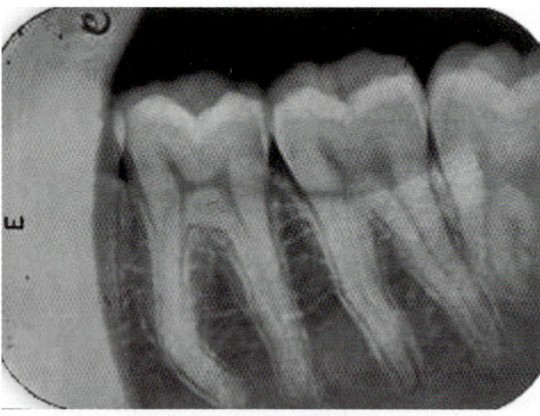

Fig. 39.9: Widening of periodontal ligament at the apex and thickening of the lamina dura

C. Prosthesis and Tooth Related Factors that modify or predispose to plaque-induced gingival diseases/periodontitis

i. Open contacts
Seen as open contacts clinically and radiographically results in food lodgement and subsequent bone loss.

Clinical features
- Open contacts
- Food lodgement
- Features of periodontitis

Radiographic features
- Crestal bone loss of varying degree
- Open contacts between the teeth

Treatment
- If required endodontic therapy
- Periodontal therapy
- Restoration of the contacts
- Interdental aid (Fig. 39.10)

ii. Iatrogenic factors
Clinical features
- Overcontoured restoration (Fig. 39.11)
- Symptoms and signs of periodontitis

Radiographic features
- Loss of the crestal alveolar bone
- Overhangs seen on the radiograph

Treatment
- Removal of the faulty restoration
- Periodontal therapy
- Re-restoration

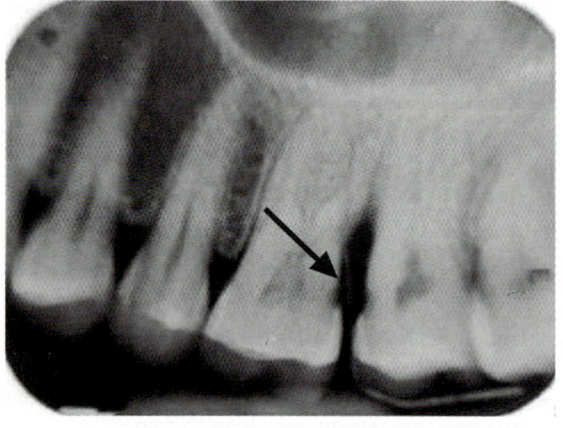

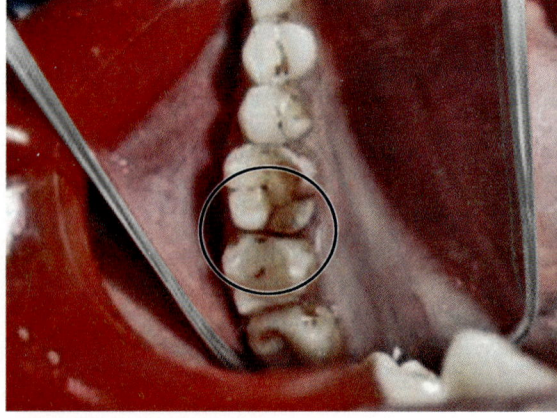

Fig. 39.10: Open contacts resulting in bone loss

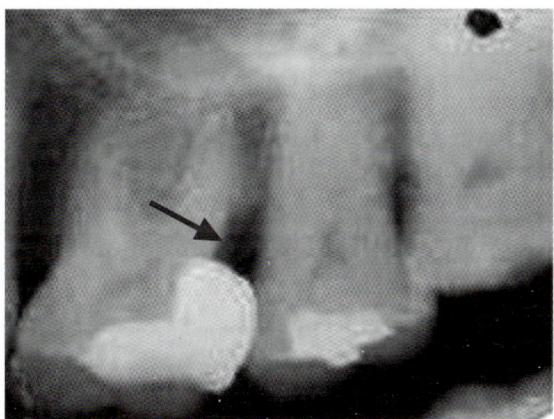

Fig. 39.11: Overhanging restoration with crestal bone loss

iii. Peri-implant disease and conditions

a. *Peri-implantitis*
   Clinical features
   × Increased peri-implant probing depth
   × Pain
   × Bleeding gums
   × Suppuration
   × Mobility of implant
   Radiographic feature
   Crestal bone loss around the implants.

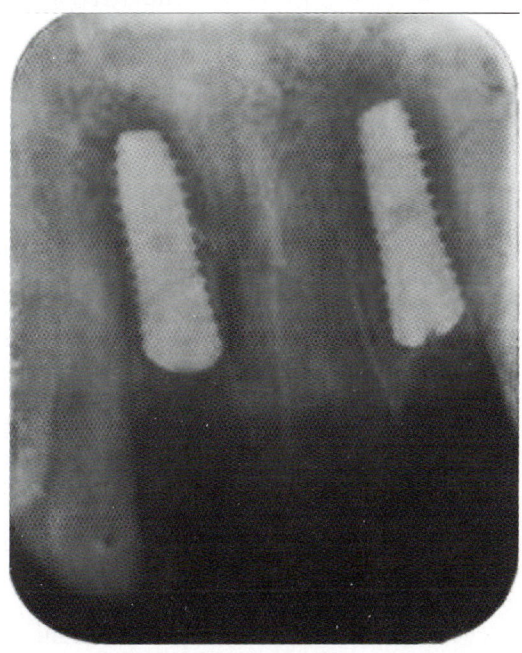

Fig. 39.12: Peri-implant bone loss

Treatment
AKUT protocol by Lang

Conventional Extraoral Panoramic Imaging (OPG)

Oral pantomography is used as substitute for full mouth IOPA. It can be used in follow-up treatment, progress of pathology, postoperative bony healing and prior to any surgical procedures (extraction of impacted teeth, enucleation of cyst). It is also used to view of the alveolar bone levels and evaluation of vertical height of alveolar bone before inserting osseo-integrated implants.

It has got a low exposure dose compared to full mouth IOPA. Broad anatomic region is imaged by this study. Anatomical structures are most identifiable and proper orientation of adjacent structures and generalized bone loss can be detected.

OPG has limitations of image distortion, lingual structures projection higher than buccal surfaces. Use of screen film combination results in less details than intraoral images. Overlapping of teeth and artifacts misinterpretation are its limitations.

Advanced Radiographic Techniques

Substantial advances in X-ray generator and X-ray technology have resulted in significant dose reduction and improved image quality. However, the basic information content of oral radiographic images has changed very little. Relatively few new technologies have emerged to address the critical needs in periodontal diagnosis. Digital imaging has been hailed as a panacea for many of the limitations associated with traditional film-based radiography. However, most of these limitations are associated with X-ray transmission and image interpretation and not with the choice of image receptor. Various advances include

× Radiovisiography (RVG)
× Computer-assisted densitometric image analysis system (CADIA)
× Digital subtraction radiograph

* Computer-based thermal imaging
* Computed tomography (CT)
* Helical computed tomography
* Cone beam computed tomography
* Magnetic resonance imaging (MRI)
* Bone scanning or radionuclide imaging

Conclusion

Dental radiographs play an integral role in assessment of periodontal disease. Periodontal examination is incomplete without accurate radiographs. The adoption of advances in the radiographic modality of the future, when based on sound scientific evidence, has the potential to transform the way we visualize the periodontal tissues. Digital image standardization, subtraction radiography, 3D imaging and quantitative image analysis are already a reality.

FREQUENTLY ASKED QUESTIONS

1. Write a short note on radiographic appearance of chronic periodontitis.
2. Enumerate radiologic appearances of periodontal conditions.

BIBLIOGRAPHY

1. Newman MG, Takei H, Klokkevold PR, Carranza FA. Carranza's Clinical Periodontology. Elsevier Health Sciences. 2011 Feb 14.
2. Caton JG, Armitage G, Berglundh T, Chapple IL, Jepsen S, Kornman KS, Mealey BL, Papapanou PN, Sanz M, Tonetti MS. A new classification scheme for periodontal and peri-implant diseases and conditions– Introduction and key changes from the 1999 classification. Journal of periodontology. 2018 Jun; 89:S1–8.
3. Lang NP, Lindhe J, editors. Clinical Periodontology and Implant Dentistry. 2nd Volume Set. John Wiley and Sons; 2015 Mar 25.
4. White SC, Pharoah MJ. Oral radiology-E-Book: Principles and interpretation. Elsevier Health Sciences; 2014 May 1.
5. AlJehani YA. Diagnostic applications of cone-beam CT for periodontal diseases. International journal of dentistry. 2014; 2014.
6. Misch KA, Erica SY, Sarment DP. Accuracy of cone beam computed tomography for periodontal defect measurements. Journal of periodontology. 2006 Jul 1;77(7):1261–6.
7. Walter C, Schmidt JC, Dula K, Sculean A. Cone beam computed tomography (CBCT) for diagnosis and treatment planning in periodontology: A systematic review. Quintessence Int. 2016 Jan 1;47(1):25–37.
8. Corbet EF, Ho DK, Lai SM. Radiographs in periodontal disease diagnosis and management. Australian Dental Journal. 2009 Sep;54:S27–43.
9. Vijay G, Raghavan V. Radiology in periodontics. Journal of Indian Academy of Oral Medicine and Radiology. 2013;25(1):24.
10. Lang NP, Berglundh T, Heitz-Mayfield LJ, Pjetursson BE, Salvi GE, Sanz M. Consensus statements and recommended clinical procedures regarding implant survival and complications. Int J Oral Maxillofac Implants. 2004;19(Suppl):150–4.
11. Jernberg GR, Bakdash MB, Keenan KM. Relationship between proximal tooth open contacts and periodontal disease. Journal of periodontology. 1983 Sep 1;54(9):529–33.
12. Brunsvold MA, Lane JJ. The prevalence of overhanging dental restorations and their relationship to periodontal disease. Journal of clinical periodontology. 1990 Feb;17(2):67–72.
13. Walto RE. Periodontal endodontic consideration, Principles and Practice of Endodontics. 3rd edition. 2002.

Diseases of Pulp and Periradicular Region

INTRODUCTION

Clinically and radiographically, disease free periapical area presents with intact lamina dura, uniform periodontal ligament space and absence of tenderness on percussion. Existence of interconnectivity between pulp and the periradicular tissues leads to reflection of pathologic process of one tissue or another in terms of inflammation and development of pathologies. Pulpal inflammation even before complete necrosis can cause the inflammatory response in the periradicular tissue. Bacteria, bacterial toxins, tissue debris, products of tissue necrosis and various immunological components from degrading pulpal tissue reaches the periradicular area leading to inflammation and destruction of otherwise healthy periradicular components. These inflammatory reactions range from widening of the periodontal ligament space to formation of periradicular abscess or granuloma, also the advanced sequel includes formation of cysts or osteomyelitis. Apart from the pulpal origin trauma, periodontal pathologies, neoplastic diseases and developmental disorders can be etiological factors for development of periradicular diseases. Mostly, the pulpal and periapical diseases are classified on the basis of clinical and radiographic features and the duration of lesion. Acute and chronic lesions can be categorized based on duration, i.e. disease

Box 40.1: Classification of pulpal diseases

Inflammatory diseases of the dental pulp

a. Reversible pulpitis

b. Irreversible pulpitis

   i. Symptomatic irreversible pulpitis (previously known as acute irreversible pulpitis)

   ii. Asymptomatic irreversible pulpitis (previously known as chronic irreversible pulpitis)

   iii. Chronic hyperplastic pulpitis

   iv. Internal resorption

Pulp degeneration

a. Calcific degeneration (radiographic diagnosis)

b. Atrophic degeneration (histopathologic diagnosis)

c. Fibrous degeneration

Pulp necrosis

process extending up to 7 to 10 days is considered as acute, whereas beyond this it is considered as a chronic lesion.

Symptomatic Apical Periodontitis/ Acute Apical Periodontitis

Painful inflammatory condition of periradicular tissues (Fig. 40.1) due to trauma, infection or irritation via root canal system regardless of the vitality status of tooth is acute apical periodontitis. The inflammation

TABLE 40.1: Clinical and radiographic features of pulpal diseases

Features of diseases	Reversible pulpitis	Acute irreversible pulpitis (symptomatic)	Chronic irreversible pulpitis (asymptomatic)	Chronic hyperplastic pulpitis (pulp polyp)	Pulp necrosis
1. Clinical	⚹ Pain (sensitivity) is short and sharp in nature which lasts for a moment ⚹ As the noxious stimulus is removed the pain is instantly relieved ⚹ More often pain is initiated by cold than hot food stimulus	⚹ Spontaneous pain that is usually caused by a hot or cold stimulus, and persists for several minutes to hours after stimulus removal ⚹ Pain is sharp, piercing and severe ⚹ Postural pain on change of position ⚹ Referred pain to adjacent teeth ⚹ Nocturnal pain	⚹ Asymptomatic in nature	⚹ Symptomless condition, Except during mastication when discomfort can be felt ⚹ Large, open cavity with direct approach to pulp chamber	⚹ Asymptomatic
2. Radiographic	⚹ No changes in periapical tissue	⚹ No changes in periapical tissue	⚹ No changes in periapical tissue	⚹ Large radiolucency involving crown and no changes in periapical tissue	⚹ No changes in periapical tissue

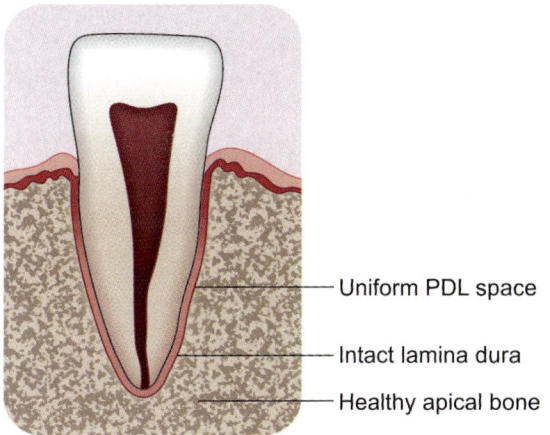

Fig. 40.1: Normal periradicular or periapical tissue

Uniform PDL space

Intact lamina dura

Healthy apical bone

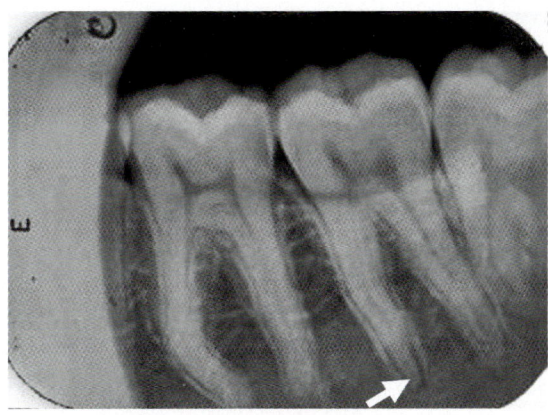

Fig. 40.2: Apical periodontitis—space widening of PDL

Box 40.2: Classification of periradicular diseases

1. Symptomatic periradicular diseases
   a. Symptomatic apical periodontitis (previously known as acute apical periodontitis)
      i. Vital tooth
      ii. Non-vital tooth
   b. Acute alveolar abscess
   c. Acute exacerbation of asymptomatic apical periodontitis (phoenix abscess)

2. Asymptomatic periradicular diseases
   a. Asymptomatic apical periodontitis (previously known as chronic apical periodontitis)
   b. Chronic alveolar abscess
   c. Radicular cyst
   d. Condensing osteitis

3. External root resorption

4. Persistent apical periodontitis

5. Diseases of the periradicular tissues of non-endodontic origin

is localized and restricted to the periodontal ligament (PDL) space due to rapid dilution of noxious bacterial content (Fig. 40.2).

Clinical Features

Patient can experience moderate to spontaneous discomfort due to increased inflammatory reactions in the pulp and the periapical tissues. Usually patient experiences pain, i.e. tenderness during mastication or closure of jaw. Tooth soreness and extrusion out of alveolar socket may also be present. Classical diagnostic characteristic of acute apical periodontium is pain on percussion or slight pressure.

Clinical presentation does not vary according to vitality status of tooth. Only vitality testing can establish a definitive diagnosis (Table 40.1).

Investigations

× **Vitality testing:** In cases of vital tooth, response can be recorded by means of vitality testings, i.e. cold, heat and electric, whereas in non-vital cases no response will be observed.

× **Radiographic assessment:** Infection and inflammation in the apical area forces the tooth slightly from the socket creating an increasing periodontal ligament space (widening) around the entire root which is apparent on the radiograph.

Treatment

Treatment depends upon vitality status of tooth and underlying etiology (Fig. 40.3). Re-establishing the occlusal harmony in cases of hyperocclusion and removal of irritant may lead to resolution of clinical signs and symptoms with associated vital tooth and in

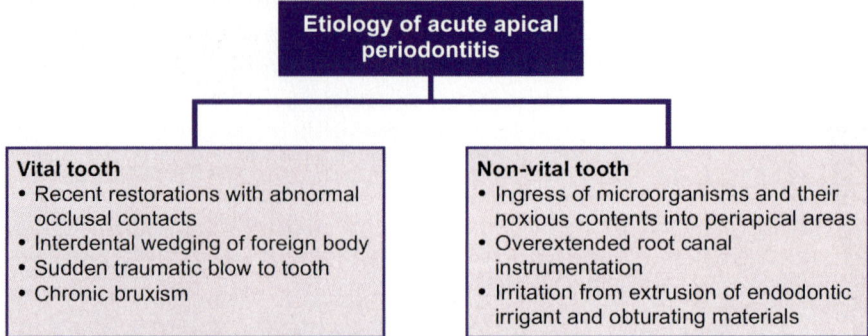

Fig. 40.3: Etiology of acute apical periodontitis

cases of non-vital tooth root canal therapy is indicated.

Acute Dentoalveolar Abscess (Periapical abscess/Periradicular Abscess)

It is localized collection of pus at the periapex of tooth after the pulpal necrosis, where the destructive infectious process is extended beyond the confines of tooth to the periradicular region via apical foramen.

Marked by rapid onset, spontaneous pain, and tenderness of the tooth to pressure, pus formation, and eventual swelling.

Etiology

- Trauma to pulp leading to necrosis.
- Chemical and mechanical irritation to pulp leading to necrosis.
- Bacterial invasion of necrotic pulp.

The primary symptom to be observed is presence of tenderness on percussion of the affected tooth. In later stages of disease progression, the patient presents with severe, throbbing pain and swelling of the overlying soft tissue. Swelling becomes more pronounced and extends beyond the original site and tooth becomes more painful, extruded and mobile. Systemically, patient reports with loss of sleep due to discomfort, slight-to-moderate rise in temperature, lymphadenopathy, chills, headache and foul smell in oral cavity. In the early stages of the disease, location of the involved tooth may be difficult due to the absence of clinical signs and symptoms but once the diseases process is established in the periodontium, it is easily located (Fig. 40.4).

Investigations

- **Vitality testing:** Clinical diagnosis can be made using electric pulp test or thermal tests as necrotic pulp does not respond any of these stimuli.
- **Radiographic assessment:** Radiographically, cavity, defective restoration, or

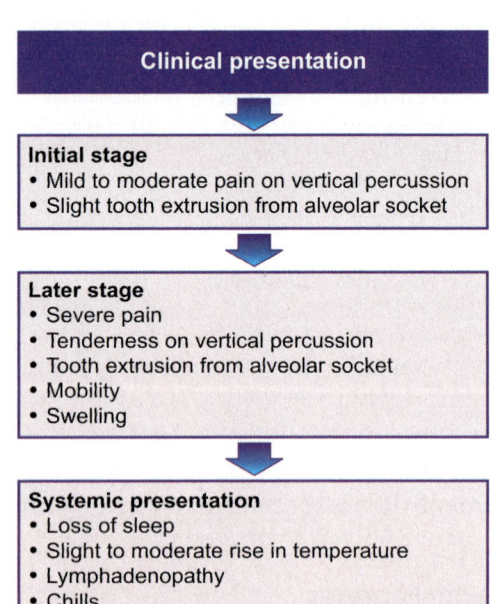

Fig. 40.4: Clinical presentation of acute dentoalveolar abscess

slight widening of the apical periodontal ligament space may be seen. Bone defects may not be seen in acute stages of infection as the infection is confined to medullary bone only, but in later stages slight unsharpness of the trabeculae may be seen at root apex.

TABLE 40.2: Clinical differentiation between acute apical periodontitis and abscess		
Clinical condition	Acute apical periodontitis	Periodontal abscess
Pain	Severe pain	Mild pain
Vitality status	Vital or non-vital	Tooth is mostly vital
Swelling	Absent	Present towards midsection of root and gingival border
Pockets	Absent	Present

Treatment

Immediate establishment of drainage either through root canal or through the incision and drainage is indicated as emergency choice of treatment followed by continuation of root canal treatment. Management of systemic complications and associated conditions includes prescription of antibiotics and analgesics.

Cellulitis

It is an infectious process which occurs as sequel following the acute inflammatory conditions. This is a rapidly spreading infection, where lesion may progress from bone to surrounding soft tissues and connective tissue planes. Symptoms include swelling, redness, pain and tenderness. On palpation of the tissues, they appear to be firm, indurate and grossly edematous. Infections can spread to the adjacent tissues depending upon the location of lesions, i.e. to adjacent areas including nose, maxillary sinus, floor of mouth, temporal fossa, facial spaces and face. Choice of treatment includes surgical incision and drainage under antibiotic coverage.

Dentoalveolar abscesses are subdivided as follows, depending on their radiographic appearance:

1. **Primary or neoteric abscess:** They are pulpoinflammatory or infectious conditions associated with teeth that have that have not developed apparent periapical radiographic changes.
2. **Secondary or recrudescent abscesses:** Which develop on a previously existing periapical radiolucent lesion that is granuloma cyst or scar.

Asymptomatic Apical Periodontitis/ Chronic Apical Periodontitis/ Periapical Granuloma

A long standing asymptomatic apical lesion presenting with growth of granulation tissue continues with periodontal ligament membrane, due to extension of infection from necrosis of pulp.

Etiology

Necrosis of pulp due to noxious stimulus followed by a continuous mild infection or irritation of the periradicular tissue leading to a productive cellular reaction and development of pathology.

Clinical Presentation

Usually asymptomatic. Apical periodontitis does not present with any subjective reaction which is clinically noticeable, except in rare cases when the lesion breaks down and undergoes suppuration. Patient presents history of pain which had subsided in due course of time.

Investigations

- **Vitality testings:** On thermal and electric vitality testing no response for tooth is observed.
- **Radiographic assessment:** Affected tooth presents with extensive caries, restoration, fracture or narrow canals. A well-defined

periapical radiolucent lesion with loss of lamina dura and size less than 2 cm without radiopaque border (hyper-osteotic border / sclerotic) is observed (Fig. 40.5).

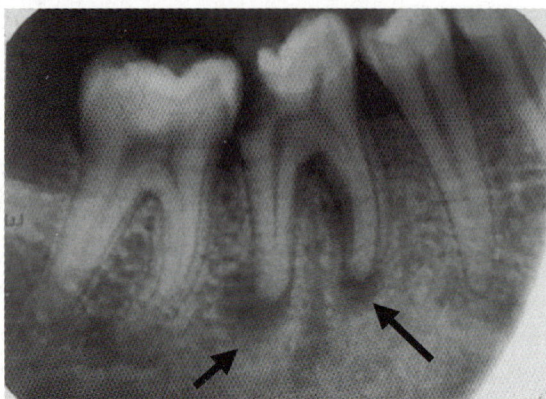

Fig. 40.5: Well-defined radiolucency without hyper-osteotic borders

Treatment

Treatment comprises root canal treatment of infected tooth, eliminating the focus of infection followed by repair of periradicular tissues.

Chronic Alveolar Abscess/Chronic Periapical Abscess

It is a long standing low grade inflammatory reaction of the periradicular tissues to the infection that occurs after the necrosis of pulpal tissue, with little or no discomfort to the patient. It is also associated with discharge of pus from sinus tract and presence of parulis which is made up of inflamed granulation tissue. Opening of parulis depends on the host resistance, i.e. it is open during active stage of lesion.

Etiology

Spread and extension of infection from infected root canal to periradicular tissues or pre-existing acute abscess conditions.

Clinical Presentation

Associated tooth is usually asymptomatic or mild painful response with history of trauma leading to tooth discoloration or presence of large open cavity in tooth leading to drainage via root canal system. Condition is discovered either on routine radiographic examination or presence of sinus tract. Usually, sinus tract is formed in the area of least resistance, i.e. buccal or facial cortical plates.

Investigations

a. **Vitality testing:** No response; suggestive of non-vitality.
b. **Radiographic assessment:** Signs of osseous breakdown can be observed with ill defined radiolucent area with loss of lamina dura. Area of diffused demineralization of the periapical bone can also be seen radiographically. Tracing of sinus tract can be done if in active state, using gutta percha cones which will indicate the offending tooth in radiograph (Fig. 40.6).

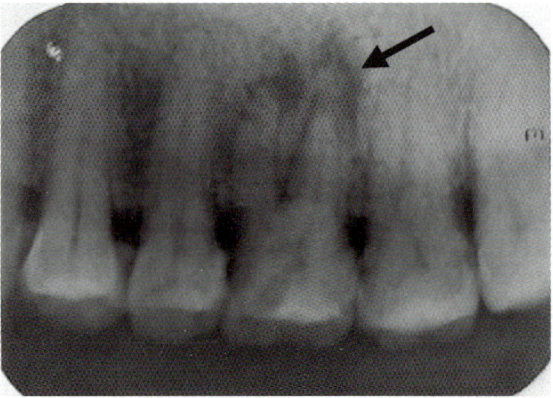

Fig. 40.6: Chronic periapical abscess showing ill-defined radiolucent lesion with loss of lamina dura

Acute Exacerbation of Chronic Periapical Abscess/Asymptomatic Apical Periodontitis (Phoenix Abscess)

Development of phoenix abscess is a classic example of disturbance of equilibrium between host defense and virulence factors. As the host defense fails to counteract the virulence of superimposed infection on chronic apical periodontitis lesion development is seen. Pulp vitality testing presents with no response and false positive response with electric pulp testing is associated with necrotic fluids present within root canal system. Well-defined radiolucency can be seen with associated root apex (Fig. 40.7).

Treatment

Treatment comprises root canal treatment of infected tooth, eliminating the focus of infection followed by repair of periradicular tissues.

Radicular Cyst

Cyst is defined as a pathologic cavity lined by epithelium and usually containing fluid or semisolid material. Radicular cyst is the most commonly associated cyst with the oral cavity, having strong male predilection and maxillary anterior region predominance (Fig. 40.8).

Clinical Presentation

Most of the radicular cysts are asymptomatic in nature during their developmental stages unless secondarily infected leading to discharge and pain. Large growing cystic lesion may present as swelling and mobility of tooth due to bone resorption. Due to accumulation of fluids in cyst cavity, there is gradual increase in size of developing cystic lesion causing drifting of teeth and leading to misalignment. The most confirmatory diagnosis is obtained from histopathology of the lesion.

Investigations

× **Vitality testings:** In most of the cases, the vitality testing gives negative response suggesting non-vital status of tooth. Only radiographic presentation of the lesion is positive.
× **Radiographic assessment:** Radiographically, a well-defined radiolucent lesion with size more than 2 cm² with thick hyperosteotic borders and periapical loss of lamina dura. Sometimes sclerotic border is discontinued due to secondary infections. The lesion appears round or pear-shaped usually associated with non-vital tooth with the epicenter of the lesion located at apex of involved tooth. Location of the cystic lesion may vary from the apical region to the lateral, when associated with lateral or accessory canal

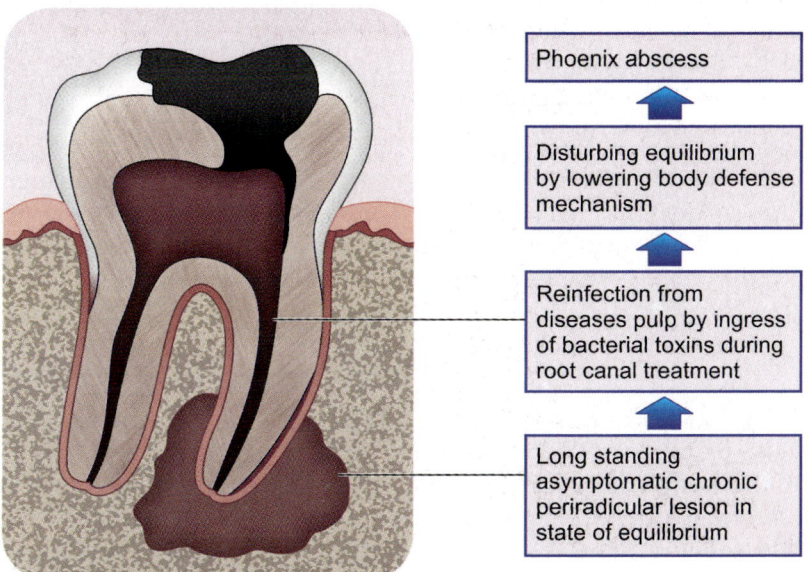

Phoenix abscess

⬆

Disturbing equilibrium by lowering body defense mechanism

⬆

Reinfection from diseases pulp by ingress of bacterial toxins during root canal treatment

⬆

Long standing asymptomatic chronic periradicular lesion in state of equilibrium

Fig. 40.7: Schematic presentation of development of phoenix abscess

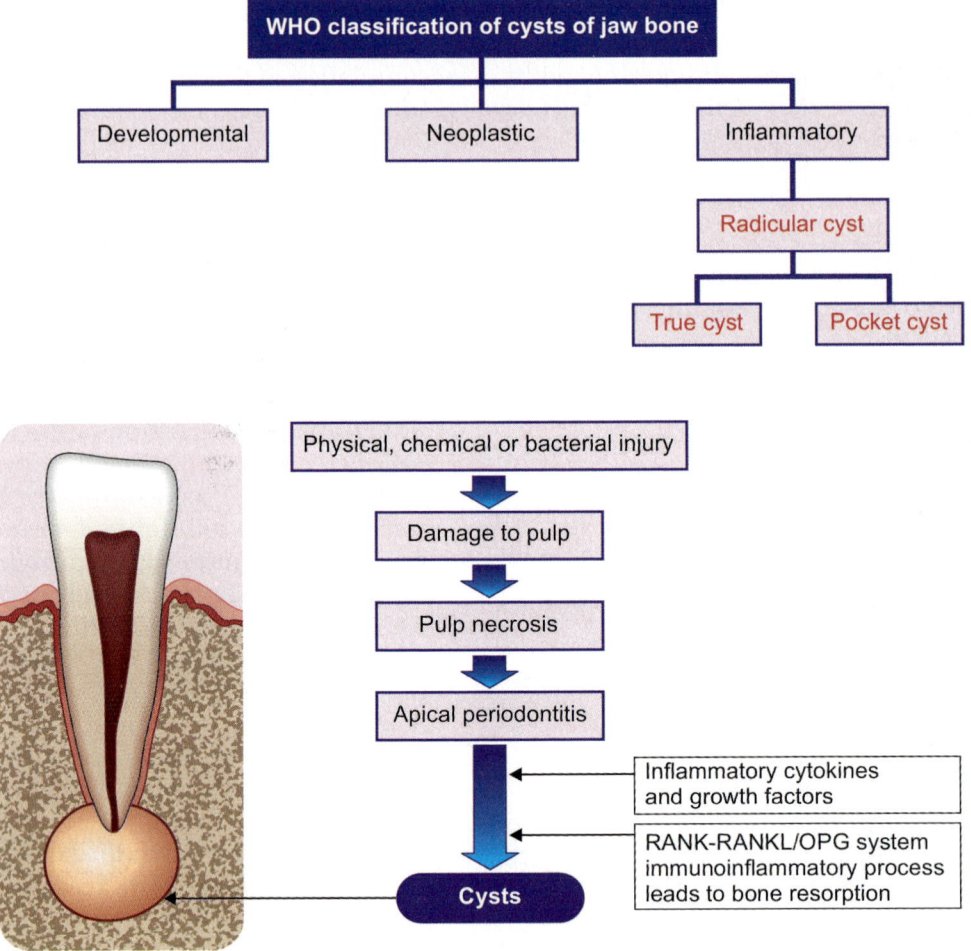

Fig. 40.8: Pathogenesis of radicular cyst

or deep periodontal pocket. If the lesion is associated with expansion, it mostly grows towards palatal cortical plate in maxillary and buccal cortical plate in mandibular bone or sometimes may perforate cortical bone (Fig. 40.9).

Treatment

In most of the cases radicular cysts are inflammatory in origin and nature and they can be treated with non-surgical root canal therapy successfully. Decompression procedures followed by non-surgical root canal therapy, have also been recommended to manage large radicular cysts, especially

those lesions are very close to vital structures such as maxillary sinus, mental foramen, or mandibular canal. However, failure of non-surgical management or presence of true radicular cysts might have to be treated surgically.

Condensing Osteitis

It is chronic inflammatory response of periradicular tissue towards mild low grade irritation from root canal system. Mandibular molars are frequently affected teeth in the dentition. Occurrence of this condition is due to constant mild irritation of periradicular tissues leading to increased osteoblastic

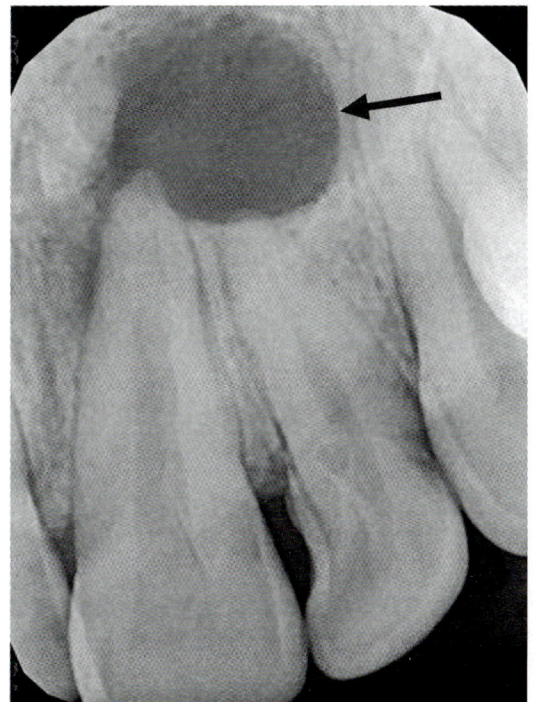

Fig. 40.9: Perforation of cortical bone

activity in alveolar bone. Condition is completely asymptomatic in nature with presence of positive response towards pulp vitality testing and treatment includes removal of irritant and if sign and symptom of irreversible pulpitis are observed then root canal treatment is indicated.

Rarefying Osteitis

This condition is also a reaction of periradicular tissue towards mild low grade irritation from root canal system leading to trabecular loss of alveolar bone and cannot be typically differentiated on a radiograph. Condition can only be identified histopathologically. Radiographically, lesion is found at the apex of non-vital tooth and can also be located on the lateral aspect of root when associated with a lateral canal. Edges of the radiolucency can be round to ovoid in shape with loss of lamina dura. Choice of treatment depends on the underlying etiology.

Periapical Scar

It represents a well circumscribed area of radiolucency associated with tooth previously treated endodontically. The exact etiological factors associated with the lesion includes apical curettage or root resection procedures. Structural and histological composition of the periapical scar tissue comprises fibrous connective tissue and may represent the end point of healing cycle.

Radiographic differential diagnosis of such lesion includes periapical abscess, cyst or granuloma. The involved tooth is usually asymptomatic and needs no therapeutic intervention.

Surgical Defect

Theses defects represent areas of failed bone deposition with osseous tissues after the surgical process. Usually condition is associated with otherwise clinically asymptomatic endodontically treated tooth and discovered on routine radiographic examination. Radiographically the lesions appear to be rounded, well defined and smoothly contoured not more than 1 cm in diameter. Shadows on the radiographs caused by the surgical defects usually reduces in size over the period of time and needs periodic evaluations.

Osteomyelitis (OML)

Definition: An inflammatory condition of the bone that begins as an infection of the medullary cavity, rapidly involves the harversian system and periosteum of that area.

Etiology

a. Spread of infection from the odontogenic infections
b. Trauma like untreated compound fractures
c. Infections extending from gingival ulcerations, lymph nodes, lacerations and hematogenic in origin.

Common Types

a. Acute suppurative osteomyelitis
b. Chronic suppurative osteomyelitis
c. Garre's osteomyelitis
d. Radiation osteomyelitis

▶ Acute Suppurative Osteomyelitis

Clinical presentation: Deep intense jaw pain with history of recent infection or extraction. Presence of abscess, diffused swelling, pus discharge, trismus, paraesthesia or anesthesia of lip (classic symptom) and systemically high intermittent fever.

Radiographic features: The most common location is the posterior body of mandible, whereas occurrence in maxilla is rare. The first radiographic evidence of acute form of osteomyelitis is decrease in the density of involved bone with loss of sharpness of existing trabeculae with blurred or fuzzy outline. Gradually, solitary or multiple radiolucent areas may be seen on radiograph, representing enlarged trabecular spaces due to foci of necrosis and frank bone destruction. In some cases, saucer-shaped area of destruction with irregular margins with teeth and some supporting bone is seen. There is loss of continuity of lamina dura around the involved teeth.

▶ Chronic Suppurative Osteomyelitis

Clinical presentation: Clinical features as similar to those present in acute cases but in milder form. Development of acute exacerbations can occur periodically.

Radiographic features: Similar to acute phase of osteomyelitis, the most common site is the posterior mandible. The periphery of lesion may be better defined than in acute phase. When the disease is active and is spreading through bone, the periphery may be more radiolucent and have poorly defined borders. Multiple radiolucencies of variable size with irregular outline and poorly defined borders are seen. In early stage, there is widening of marrow spaces and enlargement

of Volkmann's canal, so imparting 'mottled appearance'. The granulation tissue between living and dead bone produces irregular lines and zones radiolucency. It results in characteristic 'moth-eaten appearance' of established OML. Chronic osteomyelitis often stimulates the formation of periosteal new bone, which is seen radiographically as a single radiopaque line or a series of radiopaque lines (similar to onion-skin) parallel to surface of cortical bone. The roots of teeth may undergo external resorption and lamina dura may become less apparent, as it blends with surrounding granular sclerotic bone. In patients with extensive chronic osteomyelitis, the disease may slowly spread to mandibular condyle and into joint, resulting in a septic arthritis. Further, it may spread to inner ear and mastoid air cells. Chronic lesions may develop a draining fistula, which may appear as a well-defined break in the outer cortex or in the periosteal new bone (Fig. 40.10).

▶ Garre's Osteomyelitis

Clinical presentation: Most commonly seen in children and young adults with more prevalence in mandible than maxilla. Patient presents with chief complaint of toothache or pain in jaw and bony hard swelling on the outer surface of jaw.

Radiographic features: An intraoral periapical radiograph will show a carious tooth opposite the hard bony mass. Shadow of a thin convex shell of bone over the cortex, with radiolucent space between the two is seen. As infection persists, the cortex thickens and becomes laminated with alternating radiopaque and radiolucent layers (onion-skin appearance). As the lesion develops into a more chronic phase, cyclic and periodic acute exacerbations may produce more inflammatory exudate, which again lifts the periosteum from bone surface and stimulates the periosteum to form a second layer of bone. This is detected radiographically as a second radiopaque line almost parallel to

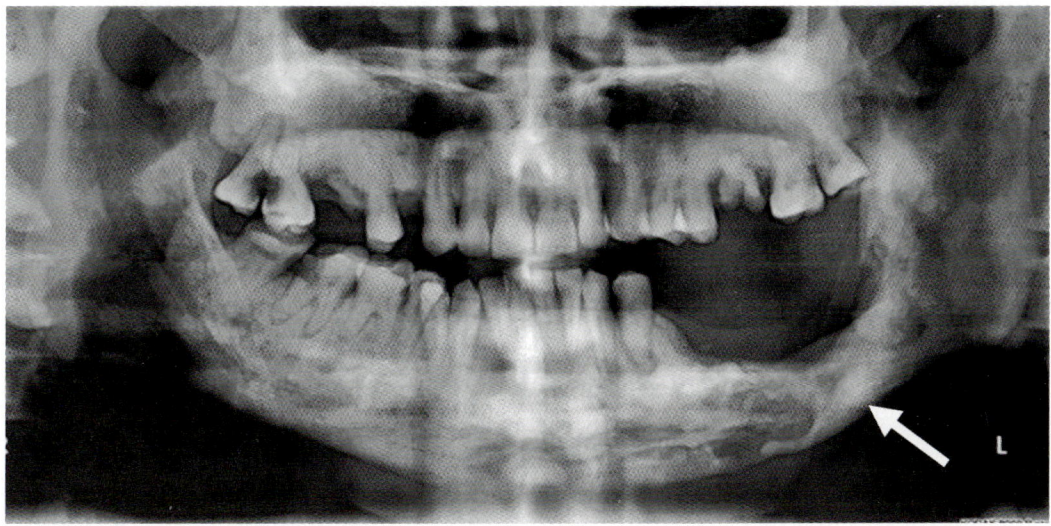

Fig. 40.10: Radiographic presentation of chronic superative osteomyelitis (Moth-eaten appearence)

first and separated from it by radiolucent band. This process may continue and result in several lines (onion-skin appearance), and eventually, a massive amount of new bone may be formed. This is refered to as proliferative periostitis and is seen more often in children.

▶ **Radiation Osteomyelitis**

Clinical presentation and radiographic features: Lesion is present in the mandible, especially the posterior mandible, is the most common location for osteoradionecrosis. An early characteristic change is a well-defined area of bone resorption within the outer cortical plate of mandible. Later changes are quite variable and may be predominantly lytic or sclerotic or a mixture. The periphery is ill-defined and similar to that in osteomyelitis. If the lesion reaches the inferior border of mandible, irregular resorption of this bony cortex often occurs. Radiation exposure may also stimulate the resorption of bone, especially in the maxilla, which may be similar in appearance to bone destruction caused by malignant neoplasm. There may be irregular widening of periodontal membrane space

similar to that seen in malignant neoplasia or it may stimulate periapical rarefying osteitis. There may be bone resorption, very similar to periodontal disease.

Radiographic consideration for the diagnosis of periapical lesions

- **Bone destruction:** Generally, 30–60% of regional bone destruction must have occurred for a change to be detected on the radiographs. Size of active growing lesion is usually larger than it appears on the radiograph.

- **Lamina dura:** Intact, widened or loss of lamina dura can be seen in the periapical radiographs. Its variation and presentation depends upon the stage of the active lesion in the periapical area.

- **Root resorption:** Root resorption can be a common feature of periapical inflammation or infection. Radiographically, the resorptive defects due to periapical inflammation usually presents with ragged margins of root surface while lesions like tumor can be linear.

Differential diagnosis for periapical radiolucent lesions:

TABLE 40.3: Common features of periodical pathologies

Features	Chronic alveolar abscess and phoenix abscess	Asymptomatic apical periodontitis/periapical granuloma	Radicular cyst	Periapical scar	Surgical defect
1. Type of pain	Asymptomatic	Asymptomatic	Asymptomatic	Asymptomatic	Asymptomatic
2. Swelling	⋆ Absent—marked by drainage via sinus tract or swelling in case of acute exacerbations	⋆ Absent	⋆ Absent in initial stages but later stages with expansion of cyst may be present	⋆ Absent	⋆ Absent
3. Vitality testing	⋆ Negative response	⋆ Negative response	⋆ Negative response	⋆ Negative response	⋆ Negative response
4. Pdl changes					
5. Lamina dura	⋆ Loss in apical area	⋆ Loss in apical area	⋆ Loss in apical area		
6. Shape of radiolucency	⋆ Ill defined	⋆ Well defined—round shaped without sclerotic borders	⋆ Well defined—round or pear shaped with sclerotic borders	⋆ Well defined	⋆ Well defined
7. Size of radiolucency		⋆ Thin radiopaque, less than 2 cm^2	⋆ Thick radiopaque, Larger than 2 cm^2	⋆ Surrounded by bone, depends on size of early defect and as healing progresses its size reduces	⋆ Surrounded by bone, depends on size of early defect and as healing progresses its size reduces, associated with histroy of apicectomy or surgery

Note: Hyperplasia of sinus mucosa, osteomyelitis and periapical cemento-osseous dysplasia are also considered as differential diagnosis but appearance of these lesions varies depending on the stage or chronicity of the lesion or stage.

FREQUENTLY ASKED QUESTIONS

1. Discuss radiographic differentiating features of chronic periapical abscess granuloma cyst.
2. Discuss differential diagnosis of periodical radiolucencies.

BIBLIOGRAPHY

1. Gutmann JL, Baumgartner JC, Gluskin AH, Hartwell GR, Walton RE. Identify and define all diagnostic terms for periapical/ periradicular health and disease states. J Endod. 2009;35:1658.
2. B. Suresh Chandra, V. Gopikrishna . Grossman's Endodontic Practice. 13th ed. India:Wolters Kluwer Health; 2014. Chapter 6: Diseases of the Periradicular Tissues; pp 112–145.
3. B. Suresh Chandra, V. Gopikrishna. Grossman's Endodontic Practice. 13th ed. India:Wolters Kluwer Health; 2014. Box 5.3: Clinical classification of the diseases of the pulp;p 97.
4. B. Suresh Chandra, V. Gopikrishna. Grossman's Endodontic Practice. 13th ed. India: Wolters Kluwer Health; 2014. Box 6.3: Clinical Classification of Diseases of Periradicular Tissues; p 113.
5. Abbott PV. Classification, diagnosis and clinical manifestations of apical periodontitis. Endodontic Topics. 2004;8:36–54.
6. Razavi SM, Kiani S, Khalesi S. Periapical lesions: a review of clinical, radiographic, and histopathologic features. Avicenna J Dent Res. 2014;6:e19435.
7. Lalonde ER. A new rationale for the management of periapical granulomas and cysts: an evaluation of histopathological and radiographic findings. J Am Dent Assoc. 1970;80(5):1056–9.
8. Natkin E, Oswald RJ, Carnes LI. The relationship of lesion size to diagnosis, incidence, and treatment of periapical cysts and granulomas. Oral Surg Oral Med Oral Pathol. 1984;57(1):82–94.
9. Weber AL. Imaging of cysts and odontogenic tumors of the jaw. Definition and classification. Radiol Clin North Am. 1993;31(1):101–20.
10. Scholl RJ, Kellett HM, Neumann DP, Lurie AG. Cysts and cystic lesions of the mandible: clinical and radiologic-histopathologic review. Radiographics. 1999;19(5):1107–24.
11. Patel S, Kanagasingam S, Pitt Ford T. External cervical resorption: a review. J Endod. 2009; 35(5):616–25.
12. Heithersay GS. Management of tooth resorption. Aust Dent J. 2007;52:S105–21.
13. Fernandes M, de Ataide I, Wagle R.Tooth resorption part I—pathogenesis and case series of internal resorption. J Conserv Dent. 2013 Jan;16(1):4–8.
14. Karjodkar F. Textbook of Dental and Maxillofacial Radiology. 2nd ed. India: Jaypee Brothers Medical Publishers (P) Ltd.; 2009.
15. Lin LM, Ricucci D, Lin J, Rosenberg PA. Non-surgical root canal therapy of large cyst-like inflammatory periapical lesions and inflammatory apical cysts. J Endod. 2009; 35: 607–15.
16. Nair PN. New perspectives on radicular cysts: do they heal? Int Endod J. 1998; 31: 155–160.
17. Martin SA. Conventional endodontic therapy of upper central incisor combined with cyst decompression: a case report. J Endod. 2007; 33:753–757.
18. Tandri SB. Management of infected radicular cyst by surgical decompression. J Conserv Dent. 2010; 13: 159–61.

Cyst of the Orofacial Regions

The word CYST (SIST) is derived from the Greek word cysts meaning a bladder. Kramer (1974) has defined a cyst as "a pathological cavity having fluid, semifluid or gaseous contents and which is not created by the accumulation of pus". Most cysts, but not all, are lined by epithelium. The higher frequency of cysts of the orofacial region can be attributed to the complex embryology and development of teeth with the presence of the numerous rests of odontogenic epithelium that remain after tooth formation.

The cystic content is secreted by either the cells lining the cavity or is derived from the adjacent tissue fluid. Based on accumulation of fluid within the cyst, it has a round or spherical shape. When the cyst is within the maxillary sinus, it enlarges in a concentric fashion resulting in a spherical shape, but when it grows within bone; its shape is influenced by the resistance of neighboring hard tissue.

Cysts of the oral and maxillofacial tissues that are not lined by epithelium are the mucous extravasation cyst of the salivary glands, the aneurysmal bone cyst and the solitary bone cyst.

CLASSIFICATION OF CYSTS

The cysts included here are those that are most common in the jaws and adjacent soft tissues (Table 17.1).

Odontogenic Cysts

Radicular Cyst

It is an epithelial-lined cyst of inflammatory origin; commonly called dental cyst or periapical cyst.

Radicular cyst most likely results from the cell rests of Malassez in the periodontal ligament. It is most commonly associated with periapical region of the non-vital tooth.

Clinical features: It occurs most frequently in the third to sixth decades and shows a slight male predominance. It is the most common type of cyst in the jaws and often produces no symptoms unless secondarily infected. When it becomes large, it may cause bony hard swelling on palpation, if the cortex is intact. There is crepitus, as the bone thins and becomes rubbery and fluctuant, if the outer cortex is perforated.

Radiographic features (Fig. 41.1): It is mostly associated with maxillary central incisor, which are most commonly affected by trauma; followed by mandibular first molar. It may affect deciduous molars. Teeth with a dens in dente have a higher incidence of pulp death and formation of radicular cyst. The cyst takes the periapical location of the involved tooth. It may appear on the mesial or distal surface of a tooth root at the opening of an accessory canal or infrequently in a deep periodontal pocket.

TABLE 41.1: Classification of cysts

I. Cysts of the jaws	II. Cysts associated with the maxillary antrum	III. Cysts of the soft tissues of the mouth, face and neck

A. Epithelial-lined cysts
 	
1. **Developmental origin**
a. Odontogenic
  i. Gingival cyst of infants
  ii. Odontogenic keratocyst
  iii. Dentigerous cyst
  iv. Eruption cyst
  v. Gingival cyst of adults
  vi. Developmental lateral perio-dontal cyst
  vii. Botryoid odontogenic cyst
  viii. Glandular odontogenic cyst
  ix. Calcifying odontogenic cyst
b. Non-odontogenic
  i. Midpalatal raphé cyst of infants
  ii. Nasopalatine duct cyst
  iii. Nasolabial cyst
2. **Inflammatory origin**
  i. Radicular cyst, apical and lateral
  ii. Residual cyst
  iii. Paradental cyst and juvenile paradental cyst
  iv. Inflammatory collateral cyst
B. Non-epithelial lined cysts
1. Solitary bone cyst
2. Aneurysmal bone cyst
	1. Mucocele
	2. Retention cyst
	3. Pseudocyst
	4. Postoperative maxillary cyst
		1. Dermoid and epidermoid cysts
		2. Lymphoepithelial (branchial) cyst
		3. Thyroglossal duct cyst
		4. Anterior median lingual cyst (intralingual cyst of foregut origin)
		5. Oral cysts with gastric or intestinal epithelium (oral alimentary tract cyst)
		6. Cystic hygroma
		7. Nasopharyngeal cyst
		8. Thymic cyst
		9. Cysts of the salivary glands: Mucous extravasation cyst; mucous retention cyst; ranula; polycystic (dysgenetic) disease of the parotid
		10. Parasitic cysts: Hydatid cyst; cysticercus cellulosae; trichinosis

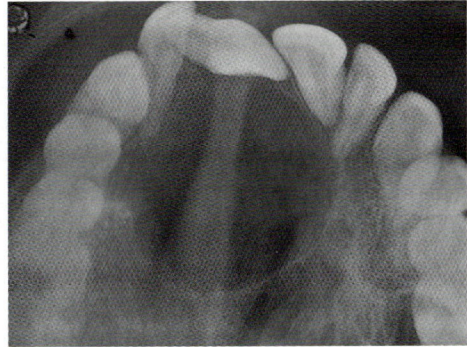

Fig. 41.1: Maxillary occlusal radiograph showing a large radicular cyst

It is round or oval in shape and has well-defined corticated borders unless secondarily infected and completely radiolucent. Loss of apical portion of the lamina dura is the most evident feature. It causes less or no effects on surrounding structures, when it is small. If a radicular cyst is large, there is displacement and resorption of the roots of adjacent teeth. The cyst may invaginate the sinus, the outer cortical plates of the maxilla or mandible may expand and may cause perforation of the buccal or lingual cortical plate or depress the inferior alveolar nerve canal.

Differential Diagnosis

Apical granuloma	0.5 × 0.5 cm, no aspirant
Lateral periodontal cyst	Offending tooth is vital
Periapical osseous dysplasia	Multiple teeth, mandibular incisors, tooth vital, initially radiolucent then mixed, lacks sclerotic border
Apical scar or a surgical defect	History of prior treatment

Management

Endodontic therapy followed by apicectomy
Enucleation
Surgical removal or marsupialization
Periodic radiographic follow-up, new bone forming first at the periphery and grows toward the center
Recurrence is rare

Residual Cyst

A cyst that remains after incomplete removal of the original cyst (a radicular, lateral, dentigerous, or another cyst) is called residual cyst. It is an epithelial-lined cyst of inflammatory origin.

It has been hypothesized that low-grade inflammation of the original cyst might predispose it to the formation of residual cysts.

Clinical features: The highest incidence is over 20 years of age. The male to female ratio is 3:2, and the maxilla is more favored than the mandible. It is asymptomatic and often is revealed incidentally on radiographs taken for evaluation of an edentulous area. There may be some expansion of the jaw or pain when the cyst is secondarily infected.

Radiographic features: Alveolar process and body of the jaw bones in edentulous areas is the preferred location. It may occur in both jaws, although it is found slightly more often in the mandible and is always above the inferior alveolar nerve canal. It is round or oval in shape, completely radiolucent and has well-defined corticated borders unless secondarily infected. The corticated borders may show some discontinuity at alveolar process giving rise to 'brandy wine glass' or 'flask-shaped' appearance.

A large residual cyst can cause displacement or resorption of adjacent teeth, or it may cause expansion of the outer cortical plates. The cyst may invaginate into the maxillary antrum. As the cyst is located in the odontogenic area, it may displace the mandibular alveolar nerve canal in an inferior direction.

Differential Diagnosis

Cyst-like anatomic patterns	History, previous and periodic radiograph
Odontogenic keratocyts	Thick cheesy aspirant
Stafne cyst	Located below the mandibular canal
Apical scar or a surgical defect	History of prior treatment

Management: It is treated by surgical enucleation or marsupialization, or both, if the cyst is large.

Dentigerous Cyst

The dentigerous cyst is the most common odontogenic cyst after the radicular cyst.

It is an epithelial-lined cyst of developmental origin. It forms around the crown of an unerupted or developing tooth. It initiates when fluid buildup in the layers of reduced enamel epithelium and the crown of the unerupted tooth. An eruption cyst is the soft tissue counterpart of a dentigerous cyst.

Clinical features: The peak incidence occurs during the second and third decades of life. The clinical examination shows a missing tooth or teeth and a hard swelling resulting in facial asymmetry. The patient typically has no pain or discomfort. If multiple dentigerous cysts are found, the patient should be evaluated for cleidocranial dysplasia. In this condition, there are multiple impacted supernumerary teeth and hence there is increased possibility of formation of dentigerous cyst. It has been estimated that dentigerous cystic changes occur in 0.81% of impacted third molars.

Radiographic features

Cyst appears as a pericoronal radiolucency
Well-defined cortex with a curved or circular outline

The teeth most frequently affected in order are the mandibular third molars, the maxillary canines, the mandibular premolars, and the maxillary third molars

Dentigerous cysts around supernumerary teeth account for about 5% of all dentigerous cysts, most developing around a mesiodens in the anterior maxilla

This cyst attaches at the cemento-enamel junction

May show central, lateral or circumferential location to the crown of impacted tooth (Fig. 41.2A)

Cysts related to maxillary third molars often grow into the maxillary antrum and may become quite large before they are discovered

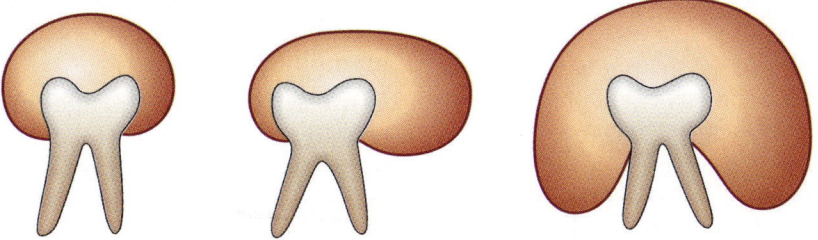

Fig. 41.2A: Central, lateral or circumferential location of cyst to the crown of impacted tooth

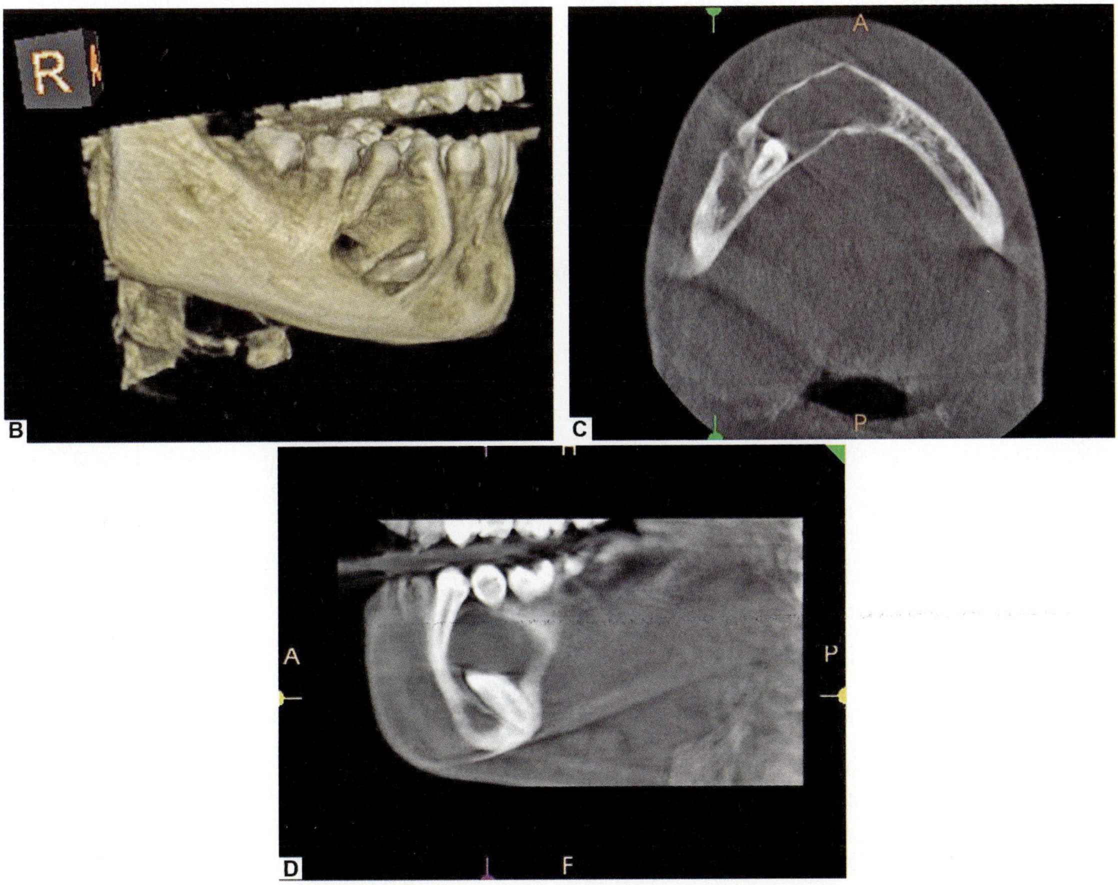

Fig. 41.2B: 3D image showing dentigerous cyst; **C.** Axial section of CBCT showing cystic lesion; **D.** Sagittal section of CBCT showing imapcted tooth with cystic lesion

As the cyst invaginates the antrum, the floor of the maxillary antrum may be displaced

May displace the associated tooth in an apical direction such that the maxillary third molars or canines may be pushed to the floor of the orbit

In mandible, the cysts may extend a considerable distance into the ramus and mandibular third molars may be displaced to the condylar or coronoid regions or to the inferior border of the mandible

A cyst may displace the inferior alveolar nerve canal in an inferior direction and often expands the outer cortex of the involved jaw

In cleidocranial dysplasia there are multiple impacted supernumerary teeth which may further develop multiple dentigerous cysts around them

Differential diagnosis: Table 41.2

Management: Dentigerous cysts are treated by surgical removal, along with impacted tooth. Large cysts may be treated by marsupialization before removal.

Complications: Mural ameloblastoma, squamous cell carcinoma and mucoepidermoid carcinoma have been reported to occur from the cyst lining of chronically infected cysts.

Buccal Bifurcation Cyst

It is also called mandibular infected buccal cyst, paradental cyst, and inflammatory paradental cyst. It is an epithelial-lined cyst of developmental origin. It may derive from the epithelial cell rests in the periodontal membrane of the buccal bifurcation of mandibular molars.

Clinical features: The age of occurrence is within the first two decades and involved teeth are vital. The common complaint is delay or lack of eruption of a mandibular first or second molar. The lingual cusp tips may be unusually projecting through the mucosa, elevated than the location of the buccal cusps. A hard swelling may occur buccal to the involved molar, and the patient has pain, if it is secondarily infected.

Radiographic features

The first molar is involved more frequently than the second molar

TABLE 41.2: Differential diagnosis				
Hyperplastic follicle	× OKC	× Small ameloblastic fibroma or cystic ameloblastoma	× Adenomatoid odontogenic tumors and calcified odontogenic cysts	× Radicular × cyst at the apex of a primary tooth
Size of normal follicular space is 2.5 × 2.5 mm	× A OKC does not expand the bone to the same degree as a dentigerous cyst	× It may be impossible to differentiate a small ameloblastic fibroma or cystic ameloblastoma from a dentigerous cyst if there is no internal structure	× Evidence of a radiopaque internal structure is sometimes found in these two lesions	× Surrounds the crown of the developing permanent tooth positioned apical to it, giving the false impression of a dentigerous cyst associated with the permanent tooth
Periodic recall	× May attach further apically on the root instead of at the cementoenamel junction	× Histologic examination	× Histologic examination	× Look for extensive caries or large restorations in a primary tooth
OKC, Odontogenic keratocyst				

Occasionally bilateral

Positioned in the buccal furcation of the affected molar.

The location is little distal to the furcation of the involved tooth

It has a circular shape with a well-defined cortical border

The internal structure is radiolucent

Most remarkable diagnostic characteristic is the tipping of the involved molar so that the lingual cusp tips being positioned higher than the buccal tips

Best diagnostic view is the mandibular occlusal cross-sectional (standard) projection, which demonstrates the abnormal position of the tooth roots

If the cyst is large enough, it may displace, resorb the adjacent teeth and cause an expansion of the buccal cortical plate

Periosteal new bone formation is seen on the buccal cortex adjacent to the involved tooth, if the cyst is infected secondarily

Differential diagnosis: Buccal bifurcation cyst is the only cyst that tilts the lingual cusp tips higher than the buccal and starts near the bifurcation region of the tooth.

Management: As the cyst does not recur, it is usually removed by conservative curettage because it and the involved molar should not be removed.

Odontogenic Keratocyst (OKC)

It is an epithelial-lined cyst of developmental origin. The epithelium in an odontogenic keratocyst has innate growth potential. Occasionally, bud-like proliferations of epithelium grow from the basal layer into the adjacent connective tissue wall and may give rise to satellite microcysts. The cystic lining is thin and fragile. Therefore, the recurrence rate is high. On aspiration, a yellowish viscous or cheesy material derived from the epithelial lining is retrieved.

Clinical features: OKC mostly develop during the second and third decades and has a slight male predominance. The cysts sometimes form around an unerupted tooth. It is usually free of symptoms until reaches a large size and clinically observable expansion of bone is very late. It grows along internal aspects in anteroposterior direction of jaws. The aspirate is thick yellow cheesy material.

Depending on location, various types of odontogenic keratocyst can be replacemental, envelopmental, extraneous and collateral (Fig. 41.3).

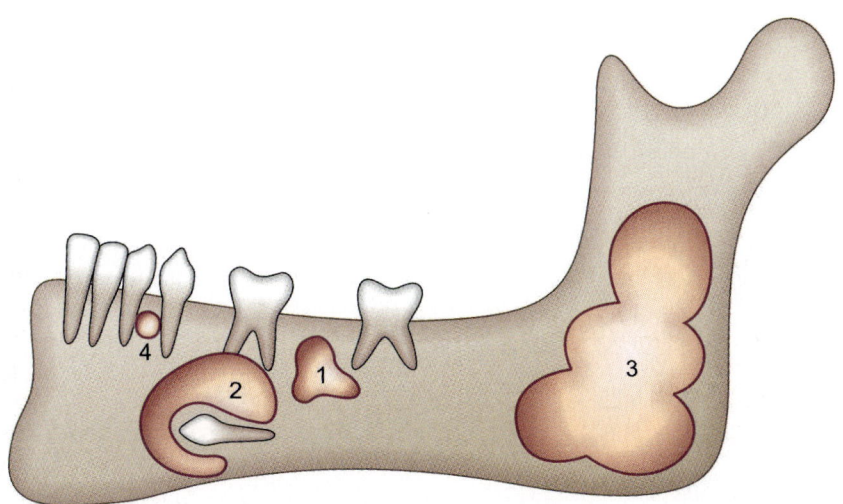

Fig. 41.3: 1—replacemental, 2—envelopmental, 3—extraneous and 4—collateral variety of OKC

Radiographic features: Ninety percent OKCs most commonly involve the posterior body of the mandible and more than 50% ramus. This cyst can be unilocular, multilocular and may have pericoronal position and is indistinguishable from a dentigerous cyst. The epicenter is located superior to the inferior alveolar nerve canal. OKC has a well-defined cortical border, unless they have become secondarily infected and smooth, round or oval shape or it may have a scalloped outline. It grows along internal aspects of the medullary bone in antero-posterior direction of jaws (Fig. 41.4) and minimal expansion occurs throughout the body of mandible except for the upper ramus and coronoid process. As the cyst invaginates the antrum, the floor of the maxillary antrum may be displaced, or a cyst may displace the inferior alveolar nerve canal in an inferior direction (Fig. 41.4A and B).

Differential diagnosis

OKC with solitary radiolucency	✗ Unicystic ameloblastoma ✗ Residual cyst ✗ Lateral periodontal cyst
OKC with pericoronal radiolucency	✗ Dentigerous cyst
OKC with multilocular radiolucency	✗ Odontogenic myxoma ✗ Simple bone cyst ✗ Mural ameloblastoma

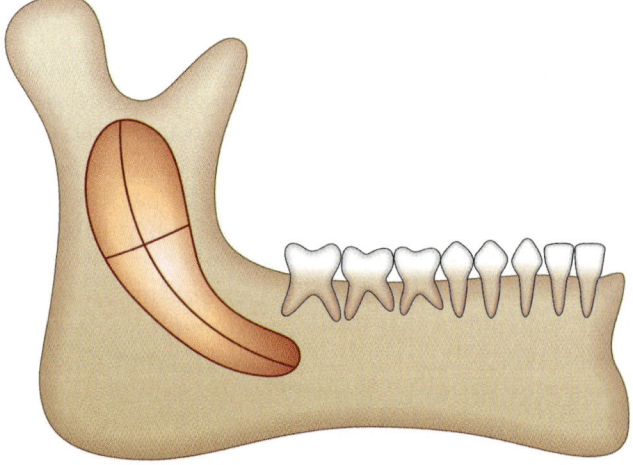

Fig. 41.4A: OKC grows along internal aspects of the medullary bone in anteroposterior direction of jaws

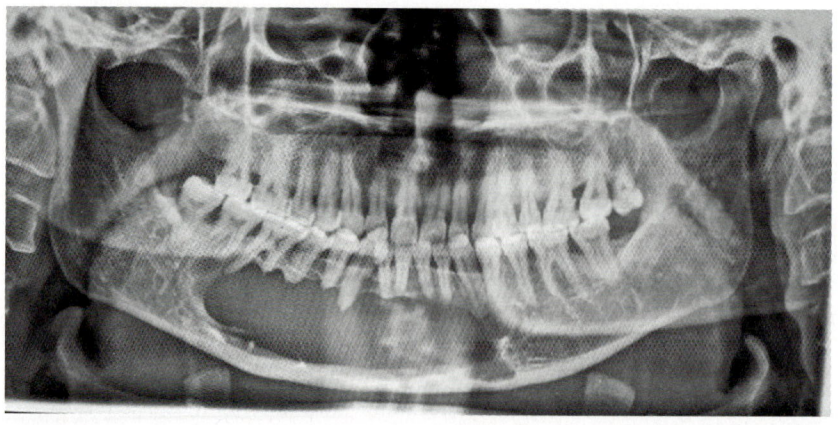

Fig. 41.4B: Multilocular radiolucency in anterior part of mandible extending on posterior aspect of right side

Management: OKC has a propensity to recur, complete surgical removal with stringent follow-up is necessary, a precise determination of the extent and location of any cortical perforations with soft tissue extension is best attained with computed tomography. In the case of multiple cysts and the possibility of basal cell nevus syndrome, a thorough radiologic examination allows accurate determination of the number of cysts and other osseous characteristics that confirm the diagnosis.

Basal Cell Nevus Syndrome

It is also called Gorlin Goltz syndrome. It is inherited as hereditary, autosomal dominant trait with variable expressivity. In this syndrome males and females are equally affected.

Clinical features: The age ranges in between 5–30 years. It involves three types of manifestations, viz cutaneous abnormalities, skeletal abnormalities, ectopic calcifications. The cutaneous abnormalities include multiple nevoid basal cell carcinomas of the skin, skeletal abnormalities may include bifid rib, mild mandibular prognathism, kyphoscoliosis, bifid ribs, synostosis of ribs, shortening of the metacarpals frontal and temporoparietal bossing, mild hypertelorism, polydactyly, syndactyly and vertebral fusion. Ectopic calcifications may show calcifications in falx cerebri, other parts of dura and in jaw cysts. The calcifications in the skin called calcinosis cutis. Typically, multiple OKCs appear in multiple quadrants earlier in life than solitary OKCs. The recurrence rate of OKCs is higher than the solitary variety.

Radiographic features: A thorough radiologic examination including CT imaging is required to detect all the jaw lesions. Multiple OKCs may develop bilaterally and can vary in size from 1 mm to several centimeters in diameter. A radiopaque line of the calcified falx cerebri may be prominent on the posteroanterior skull projection.

Differential diagnosis

✖ Multiple myeloma	✖ Cherubism	✖ Multiple dentigerous cysts
Generalized rarefaction of bone	Bilateral multilocular lesions but usually has significant jaw expansion	Lesion is more expansile
Punched out radiolucencies skull radiograph	Pushes posterior teeth in an anterior direction	Pericoronal radiolucencies attached to CEJ of impacted tooth

Management: OKCs are treated more aggressively than other solitary OKCs because there is greater propensity for recurrence. Follow-up the patient yearly for recurrence and new cyst formation. Apart from panoramic radiograph, CT imaging and genetic counseling is necessary.

Lateral Periodontal Cyst

Lateral periodontal cyst is assumed to arise from epithelial rests in periodontium lateral to the root of the tooth. It is an epithelial-lined cyst of developmental origin. In most of the cases, it is primarily diagnosed as an incidental radiographic finding as well-defined round or tears drop-shaped radiolucency. It may be seen as a cluster of small cysts, and referred to as botryoid odontogenic cysts. It represent as 0.8–2% of all odontogenic cyst.

Clinical features: The lateral periodontal cyst is equally seen in both the sexes and the age of occurrence ranges from the II to IX decades with the mean age is about 50 years. The lesion is less than 1 cm in diameter and, therefore, is usually asymptomatic. It mimics a lateral periodontal abscess, if it becomes secondarily infected. Due to its location, it can be misdiagnosed as a lesion of endodontic origin.

Radiographic features: The lateral periodontal cysts develop in the mandible, frequently in a region extending from the lateral incisor to the second premolar. It can appear in the maxilla, particularly between the lateral incisor and the cuspid.

It appears as a well-defined round or oval-shaped radiolucency. The botryoid variety may have a multilocular appearance (Fig. 41.5). Large cysts can displace adjacent teeth and small cyst may efface the lamina dura of the adjacent root.

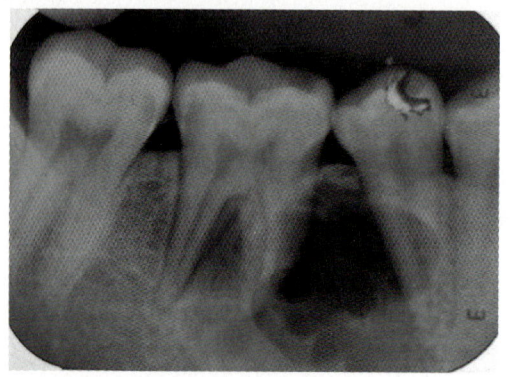

Fig. 41.5: IOPA showing botryoid variety showing a multilocular appearance

Differential diagnosis: Table 41.3

Management: Lateral periodontal cyst can be treated by simple enucleation.

Calcifying Epithelial Odontogenic Cyst

The calcifying odontogenic cyst was first described by Gorlin, et al. in 1962. It is an epithelial-lined cyst of developmental origin. It is comparatively uncommon in occurrence, constituting about 0.37—2.1% of all odontogenic tumors. It is a slow-growing, benign lesion and may manufacture calcified tissue identified as dysplastic dentin.

Clinical features: In calcifying epithelial odontogenic cyst, age ranges from 10 to 19 years of age, with a mean age of 36 years. It usually appears as a slow-growing, painless swelling of the jaw. The expanding lesion may perforate the cortical plate and extends into the soft tissue making it palpable.

Radiographic features: Most common location of calcifying epithelial odontogenic cyst is canines and incisors, i.e. anterior to the first molar. Both the jaws are almost equally involved. It manifests as a well defined and corticated cyst like radiolucency. Initially it is completely radiolucent and subsequently there is evidence of small foci of calcified white flecks. When it is associated with the impacted tooth, there is periapical radiolucency hindering its eruption. Displacement of teeth and resorption of roots may occur. As the lesion enlarges perforation of the cortical plate may be seen (Fig. 41.6).

Differential diagnosis: When the lesion has a pericoronal position with no internal calcifications dentigerous cyst, can be considered in differential diagnosis. If the lesion has internal calcifications, an adenomatoid odontogenic tumor, ameloblastic fibro-odontoma, and calcifying epithelial odontogenic tumor may be considered.

Management: Calcifying epithelial odontogenic cyst can be treated with enucleation and curettage.

TABLE 41.3: Differential diagnosis of lateral periodontal at cyst			
✗ Small OKC	✗ Mental foramen	✗ Radicular cyst at accessory canal	✗ Small ameloblastoma
Particularly collateral type mimics lateral periodontal cyst	Round well-defined radiolucency which changes its position on repeating the radiographs by giving different angulations	Round/oval well-defined radiolucency similar to lateral periodontal cyst but the offending tooth is non-vital	Botryoid variety may have a multilocular appearance. Aspiration is usually negative in ameloblastoma

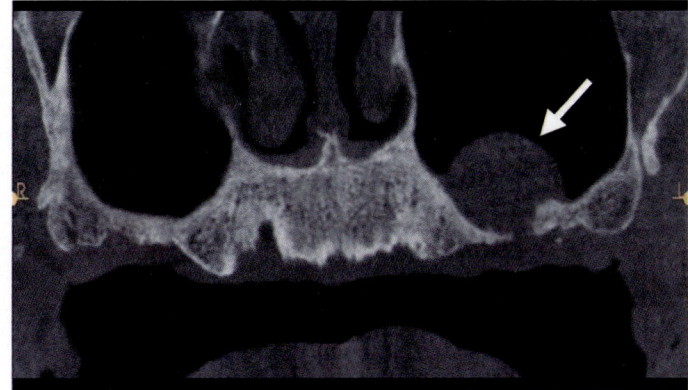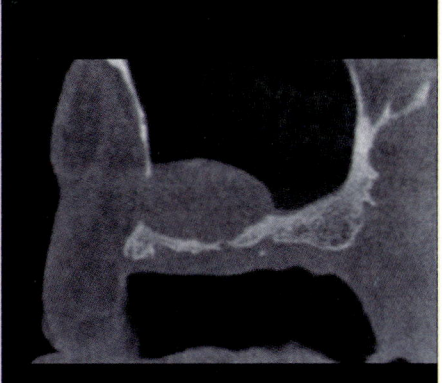

Fig. 41.6: Coronal and sagittal section shows cystic growth breaching cortex

NON-ODONTOGENIC CYSTS

Cyst of the Incisive Papilla

Cyst of the incisive papilla is the soft-tissue counterpart of a nasopalatine duct cyst, also known as the incisive canal cyst. It is a common non-odontogenic cyst that occurs in the midline in anterior maxilla, posterior to the central incisors.

Nasopalatine Duct Cyst

The nasopalatine duct cyst is also called nasopalatine canal cyst, incisive canal cyst, nasopalatine cyst, and median palatine cyst. It is a non-odotontogenic cyst of developmental origin.

It forms when the embryonic epithelial remnants of the nasopalatine duct, nasopalatine vessels and nerves undergo proliferation and cystic degeneration.

Clinical features: Nasopalatine duct cyst accounts for about 10% of jaw cysts. The age ranges from fourth to sixth decades. The male to female ratio is 3:1. It manifests as a small, well-defined fluctuant swelling just posterior to the palatine papilla. If the cyst is near the surface it is bluish in color and the deeper cyst shows normal appearing mucosa. The expanding cyst may penetrate the labial cortical plate and produce a swelling below the maxillary labial frenum or to one side. The cyst may bulge into the nasal cavity and can cause obstruction, flaring of the alae may cause distortion of the nasal septum. There may be a burning sensation or numbness over the palatal mucosa due to pressure from the cyst on the adjacent nasopalatine nerves. Sometimes, patient may report a salty taste.

Radiographic features: Most nasopalatine duct cysts are found in the nasopalatine foramen or canal. When this cyst extends posteriorly to involve the hard palate it is called a median palatal cyst. This cyst may not always be positioned symmetrically. The periphery is usually well defined and corticated and has a circular or oval shape. When the shadow of the nasal spine is superimposed on the cyst, it gives a heart shape. It is totally radiolucent. This cyst causes the roots of the central incisors to diverge, and sometimes root resorption occurs. The cyst may expand the labial and the palatal cortex. The floor of the nasal fossa may be displaced in a superior direction (Fig. 41.7).

Differential diagnosis

Large incisive foramen	Radicular cyst or granuloma
Asymptomatic	Absence of the lamina dura and enlargement of the periodontal ligament space around the apex of the central incisor

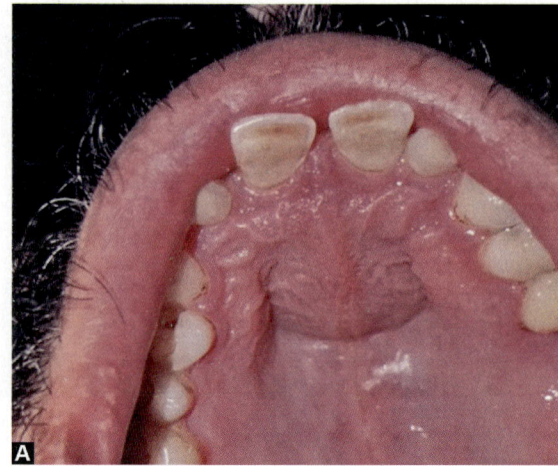

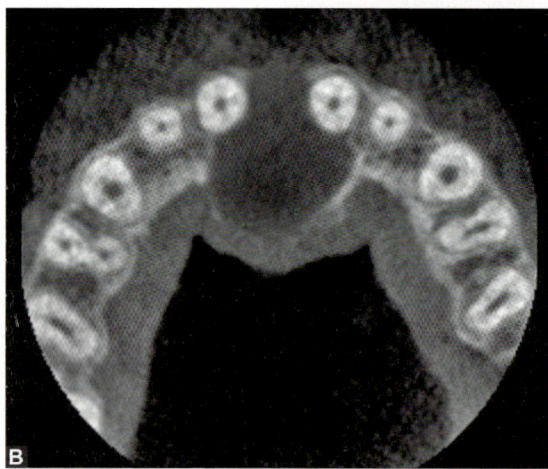
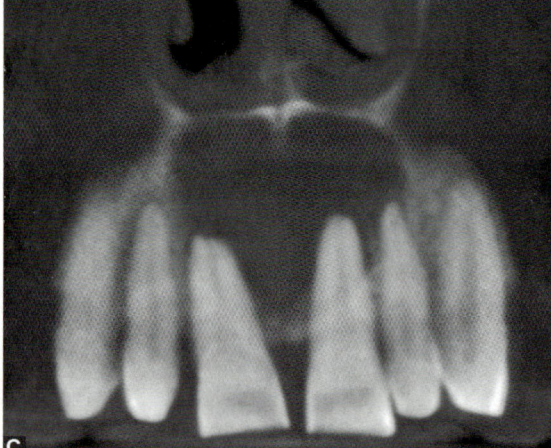

Fig. 41.7: A. Clinical presentation of cyst. **B. and C.** Axial and coronal sections of CBCT showing osteolytic cystic lesion

Management: The nasopalatine cyst is treated with enucleation in case of small cyst and with marsupialization, when it is large in size.

Nasolabial Cyst

It is also called nasoalveolar cyst. The exact origin of nasolabial cyst is unknown. It is a non-odontogenic cyst of developmental origin. It is said to be fissural cyst originating from the epithelial rests in fusion lines of the globular, lateral nasal, and maxillary processes.

Clinical features: Nasolabial cyst can occur in patients with the age range from 12 to 75 years, with a mean age of 44 years. About 75% of these lesions occur in females. There is a slight, unilateral swelling causing the obliteration of nasolabial fold, and the patient may complain of pain or discomfort. When large, it may bulge into the floor of the nasal cavity; distorts the nostrils and causes fullness of the upper lip. Infected cyst may drain into the nasal cavity.

Radiographic features: Nasolabial cyst is primarily soft tissue lesion seen adjacent to the alveolar process above the apices of the incisors. Conventional radiographs may not show any detectable changes, as this is a soft tissue lesion. CT or MRI can give an image of soft tissues.

Axial CT images with soft tissue window along with contrast may reveal a circular or oval lesion with slight soft tissue enhancement of the periphery. The internal structure appears homogeneous and relatively radiolucent compared with the surrounding soft tissues. Sometimes, it causes erosion of the underlying bone showing an increased radiolucency of the alveolar process under the cyst and apical to the incisors.

Differential diagnosis: Nasolabial cyst may simulate an acute dentoalveolar abscess and mucocele. The vitality test of the adjacent teeth should be carried out.

Management: Excision through an intraoral approach is indicated in the nasolabial cyst. This cyst is less likely to recur.

CYSTS ORIGINATING IN SOFT TISSUES OF THE MOUTH, FACE AND NECK

The cysts originating in soft tissues are thyroglossal duct cyst, branchial cleft cyst, lymphoepithelial cyst of parotid gland and dermoid cyst.

Thyroglossal Duct Cyst

Thyroglossal duct cyst is the most common congenital cyst and midline mass of the head and neck. It develops from epithelial remnants of the thyroglossal duct. It is the congenital cyst of soft tissue which appears as midline mass in the head and neck region.

Clinical features: Most of the thyroglossal duct cysts are detected in the first two decades of life. It usually occurs at the level of or below the hyoid bone in the midline of the neck. It is a slow-growing, painless mass, unless secondarily infected.

Radiographic features: The thyroglossal duct can occur anterior, posterior, superior, or inferior to the hyoid bone. The periphery of this cyst is usually well defined and has a curved outline. The internal structure on CT images is homogeneous and low attenuation lesion equivalent to fluid.

Branchial Cleft Cyst

The branchial cleft cyst is related to remnants of the first to fourth branchial arches. It is the most common congenital cyst of soft tissues. The cyst wall is usually composed of stratified squamous cell lining with some lymphoid tissue elements.

Clinical features: The branchial cleft cyst occurs in the second and third decades of life. It occurs anterior to sternocleidomastoid muscle in the lateral aspect of neck. It may have a preauricular position inferior to and behind the angle of the mandible if it is related to the first branchial arch, and sometimes related to the parotid gland. It manifests as a slow-growing, painless fluctuant swelling.

Radiographic features: The shape and internal image density of the branchial cleft cyst is cystlike. It has a lateral position which differentiates it from a thyroglossal cyst. It may be difficult to differentiate from a lymphoepithelial cyst, when associated with the parotid gland.

Lymphoepithelial Cyst of Parotid Gland

Lymphoepithelial cyst of parotid gland, is usually positioned within the parotid gland, the histologic appearance is very similar to a branchial cleft cyst. It is congenital cyst of soft tissues.

Clinical features: The mean age of occurrence is the fifth decade. It has a slight female predilection. It commonly manifests as a slow-growing enlargement in the parotid gland region. Few cysts may be related to HIV infections.

Radiographic features: Lymphoepithelial cyst has a circular cystic shape with an internal density of fluid, and it is typically located within the parotid gland.

Dermoid Cyst

Dermoid cyst is contemplated to be derived from trapped embryonic cells that are totipotential. It is lined with epidermis and cutaneous appendages and filled with keratin or sebaceous material and in rare cases with bone, teeth, muscle, or hair, and may be called a teratoma.

Clinical features: The age range of dermoid cyst is between 12 and 25 years and usually manifests as a slow, painless swelling. Only 1–2% develop in the oral cavity. Of these, about 25% occur in the floor of the mouth and on the tongue. About 10% or less arise in the head and neck with the orbital region most common. When located in the neck or floor of the mouth, these cysts may interfere with breathing, speaking, and eating. On palpation, cysts may be fluctuant or doughy, according to their contents (Fig. 41.8).

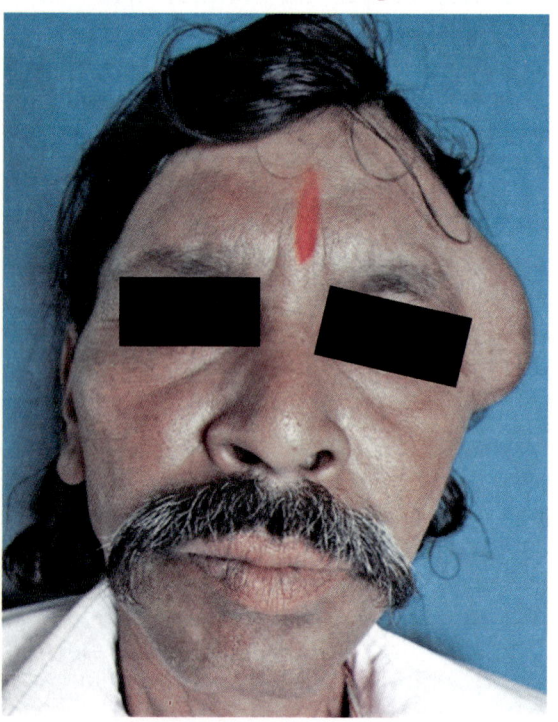

Fig. 41.8: Frontal view showing well-defined soft tissue lesion

Radiographic features: Dermoid cyst is well defined with a cystic shape. Occasionally, the internal aspect may be uniformly low attenuation equivalent to fluid or may have a soft tissue multilocular appearance. The radiopaque images, with characteristic shapes and densities, are apparent if teeth or bone form in the cyst.

Differential diagnosis: Includes ranula, thyroglossal duct cysts, cystic hygromas, and branchial cleft cysts.

CYSTLIKE LESIONS

Simple Bone Cyst (SBC)/Traumatic Bone Cyst

Simple bone cyst is also called traumatic bone cyst (Fig. 41.9). It is not a true cyst as the cyst represents as a cavity within bone that is lined by connective tissue. It may be empty, or it may contain fluid. Its etiology is unknown, although they may be a localized aberration in normal bone remodeling or metabolism.

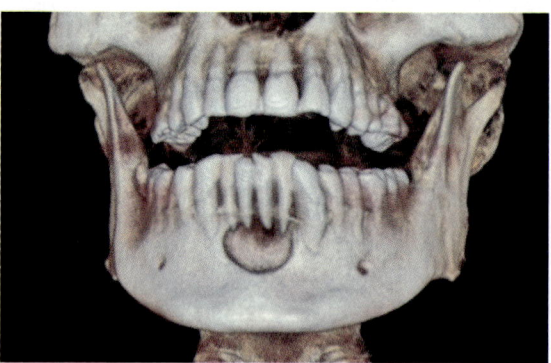

Fig. 41.9: 3D view with SBC involving mandibular anterior region

Clinical features: Simple bone cyst occurs in the first 2 decades of life, with a mean age of 17 years, and a male predominance of approximately 2:1. Multiple simple bone cysts can develop in osseous dysplasia which is seen in an older population. It is asymptomatic in most cases, pain or tenderness is rare. The teeth in vicinity are usually vital. They are discovered incidentally during radiographic examinations hence can become quite large. Aspiration usually produces only a few milliliters of straw-colored or sero-sanguineous fluid.

Radiographic features: Almost all SBCs can occur anywhere in the mandible but is seen most frequently in the ramus and posterior mandible in older patients. SBCs also frequently occur with cemento-osseous and fibrous dysplasia.

The periphery may vary from a well-defined, delicate cortex to an ill-defined border without a cortex that blends into the surrounding bone. The shape most often is smooth and curved, the superior border scallops between the roots of the teeth. The internal structure is unilocular or multilocular, even if the lesion does not usually contain true septa.

Differential diagnosis: SBCs may have an appearance similar to that of a true cyst, especially an OKC. It shows very little expansion and often have scalloped borders similar to those of an SBC. The diagnosis depends on surgical observations because the histopathologic features are not characteristic.

Management: The curettage of the cavity lining may be required; which begins bleeding and subsequent healing.

Aneurysmal Bone Cyst (ABC)

An aneurysmal bone cyst is considered to be a reactive lesion of bone. There is a proliferation of vascular spaces; fibroblasts; osteoclast-like cells; and reactive, poorly calcified woven bone. Aneurysmal bone cyst may be associated with fibrous dysplasia, central hemangioma, giant cell granuloma, and osteosarcoma.

Clinical features: In more than 90% of cases it occurs in younger than 30 years of age with predilection for females. It manifests as rapid bony swelling and the involved area may be tender on palpation.

Radiographic features: The mandible to maxilla ratio is of 3:2 with the predilection for the molar and ramus regions. The periphery usually is well defined, and the shape is circular and may show ballooning expansion.

It has a multilocular appearance. The septa are wispy, illdefined as seen in giant cell granulomas. In CT soft tissue window appearances may represent large vascular spaces. It may show extreme expansion of the outer cortical plates, can displace and resorb teeth. A CT scan is also recommended to determine the extent of the lesion better (Fig. 41.10).

Differential diagnosis: Table 41.4.

Management: Surgical curettage and partial resection along with follow-up may be required with the recurrence rate of 19–50% after curettage, and approximately 11% thereafter, respectively.

Stafne Bone Cyst

It was first described by Stafne in 1942. The etiology is unknown, but the condition is a developmental anomaly that develops in patients with age ranging in from 11 to 30 years.

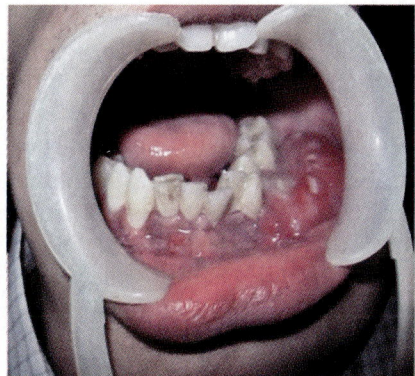
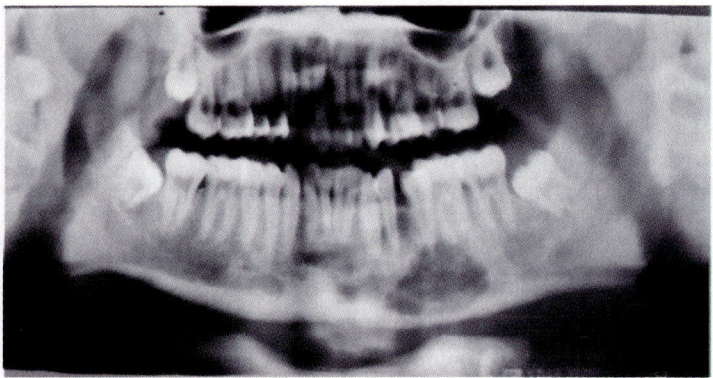

Fig. 41.10: Clinical and radiographic presentation of ABC

TABLE 41.4: Differential diagnosis

Giant cell granulomas	Ameloblastoma	Cherubism
Comparatively less expansion while aneurysmal bone cysts expand to a greater degree, and commonly involve the posterior parts of the mandible	Occurs in an older age group	Bilateral posterior involvement and both jaws

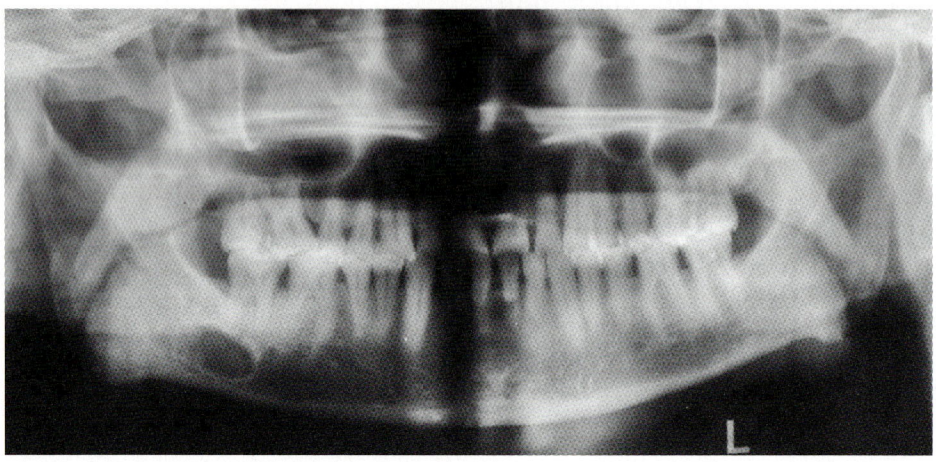

Fig. 41.11: OPG showing a well-defined ovoid radiolucency, inferior to mandibular canal on right side

It is not true cysts because no epithelial lining is present. The most common site is within the submandibular gland fossa, inferior to mandibular canal frequently close to the inferior border of the mandible (Fig. 41.10). Stafne bone cyst is thought to be linked with growth of the salivary gland adjacent to the lingual surface of the mandible.

Clinical features: Males are affected more than females; with a peak incidence in the fifth and sixth decades have been reported.

Radiographic features: It is a well-defined round, ovoid, radiolucency and diameter ranges from 1 to 3 cm. The most common location is inferior to mandibular canal frequently close to the inferior border of the mandible (Fig. 41.10). The borders are well defined with a dense sclerotic radiopaque margin which is thicker on the superior aspect. This appearance is the result of the X-rays passing tangentially through the relatively thick walls of the depression.

Differential diagnosis: The appearance and location of the Stafne cyst is characteristic and can be easily differentiated from odontogenic cysts and tumors as the odontogenic lesions are located above the inferior alveolar canal.

Management: Recognition of the lesion is important because this lesion doesn't require any treatment.

Cyst of the Maxillary Antrum/Mucocele/Pseudocyst

The mucosal cyst of the maxillary antrum, are mucocele or mucous retention cysts, The mucosal cyst is characterized by the absence of symptoms in most cases and are usually discovered on routine radiological examination. It appears as **dome-shaped** radiopacities with smooth and uniform outline present on the floor of the sinus.

They vary in size from minute to very large and may occupy the entire maxillary sinus. The smooth curved borders are well-defined but not corticated. There is no resorption of adjacent bone and typically thin radio-opaque line of the antral cortex is intact.

BIBLIOGRAPHY

1. Mervyn Shear, Paul Speight Cysts of the Oral and Maxillofacial Regions 2007. 4th edition. Blackwell, Munksgaard, Blackwell Publishing Ltd, 9600 Garsington Road, Oxford OX4 2DQ, UK.
2. White and Pharoah: Textbook of Oral Radiology, Principles and Interpretation. 5th edition.
3. Wood NK and Goaz PW. Differential diagnosis of oral and maxillofacial lesions. 5th edition. Harcourt Brace and Company Asia PTE Ltd. 1998.
4. Shear M. The Aggressive Nature of the Odontogenic Keratocyst; Is It a Benign Cystic Neoplasm? Part 1. Clinical and Early Experimental Evidence of Aggressive Behavior. Part 2. Proliferation and Genetic Studies. Part 3. Immunocytochemistry of Cytokeratin and Other Epithelial Cell Markers. Oral Oncology. 2002; 38, 219–226, 323–331, 407–15.
5. Shear M. Developmental odontogenic cysts. An update. J Oral Pathol Med. 1994 Jan;23(1):1–11. Review.[Medline: 8138974] [doi: 10.1111/j.1600–0714.1994.tb00246.x]
6. Iida S, Fukuda Y, Ueda T, Aikawa T, Arizpe JE, Okura M. Calcifying odontogenic cyst: Radiologic findings in 11 cases. Oral Surg Oral Med Oral Pathol Oral Radiol Endod. 2006;101:356–62.
7. Praetorius F, Ledesma-Montes C. Calcifying cystic odontogenic tumor. World Health Organization Classification of Tumors—Pathology and Genectics: Head and Neck Tumors. IARC Press, Lyon, 2005, p 313.

Diseases of Bones Manifested in the Jaws

The chapter focuses on the disorders of bones that involves the jaw bones also and can not be classified under other categories of diseases like cysts, tumors, etc.

OSTEOGENESIS IMPERFECTA
(BRITTLE BONE DISEASE)

Osteogenesis imperfecta (OI) is a heterogenous group of genetic disorders characterized by fragile and weak bones that break easily.

It is a rare clinical disease, occurring in 6–7 cases per lakh of population.

Etiopathogenesis

OI is a hereditary disease caused by mutations of the genes coding the chains of collagen type 1 gene. More than 90% cases are autosomal dominant. Other rare autosomal recessive forms of OI are due to defects in protein involved in cross-linking, hydroxylation, and mineralization of type 1 collagen, which leads to low tensile strength of collagen fibrils and hence brittle bones. Role of cartilage-associated protein (CRTAP), proly-13-hydroxylase-1 (P3H1/LEPRE1) and cyclophilin B (CyPB/PPIB) has also been postulated in the pathogenesis of OI.

Classification

David Sillence in 1979 gave the first classification of the disease based upon the clinical signs. Later on, other varities were added. Now, OI is classified into 15 subtypes based on the involved genes. However, for simplicity, the following classification has been recommended by the International Society of Skeletal Dysplasias.

Osteogenesis Imperfecta	Inheritance	Genes
Non-deforming OI (type I)	AD X-linked	COL1A/COL1A2 PLS3
Perinatal lethal (type II)	AD, AR	COL1A1/ COL1A2, CRTAP, LEPRE1, PPIB, BMP1
Progressive deforming (type III)	AD, AR	COL1A1/ COL1A2, CRTAP, LEPRE1, PPIB, FKBP10, SERPINH1, SERPINF1, WNT1
Moderate (type IV)	AD, AR	COL1A1/ COL1A2, CRTAP, FKBP10, SP7, SERPINF1, WNT1, TMEM38B
With calcification of the interossesous membrane and/or hypertropic callus (type V)	AD	IFITM5

Clinical Presentation

OI presents with variable clinical features based upon the severity of disease and the mutations. Disease characterization into mild, moderate and severe is generally based upon the number of bone fractures, degree of spine deformity and growth impairment. The major clinical manifestation is skeletal fragility. Other manifestations seen are skeletal deformity, joint laxity and bony sclerosis. Extra-skeletal manifestations include hearing loss, dentinogenesis imperfecta, blue/gray sclera, advancing deafness, beading of the ribs, hypercalciuria, aortic root dilatation, vascular, pulmonary complications and neurologic conditions such as macrocephaly, hydrocephalus, and basilar invagination. Type I, the mildest form of OI, is characterized by multiple fractures, blue sclera, brittle teeth, and hearing loss. Fractures are common in neonatal period, but rare after puberty. Type II is the most severe type, frequently causes death at birth or shortly after because of respiratory problems due to multiple rib fractures and small thorax.

Oral Manifestations

Craniofacial features include
* Wormian bones
* Blue sclera
* Triangular facies

* Frontal bossing
* Relative macrocephaly
* Flattened vertex and skull base
* Prominent occiput
* Maxillary hypoplasia with or without mandibular hyperplasia leading to Class III malocclusion
* Crossbite and open bite (Fig. 42.1A)

Dental alterations: Dental findings are more commonly associated with type III and IV OI. The appearance of teeth is similar to 'dentinogenesis imperfecta', however, the genetic mutations involved in both the diseases is different. Hence, the term 'opalecscent teeth' is used for dental features associated with OI.

* Blue, yellow or brown translucent teeth, more prominent in deciduous dentition
* Dentinal defects
* Severe attrition.
* Loss of vertical dimension
* Predisposition to development of periodontitis
* Delayed wound healing
* Increased incidence of impacted first and second molars (Fig. 42.1B)

Radiographic presentation
* Increased radiodensity of jaw bones
* Premature pulpal obliteration
* Shell teeth
* Thread like roots
* Narrow and corncob-shaped roots (Fig. 42.1C)

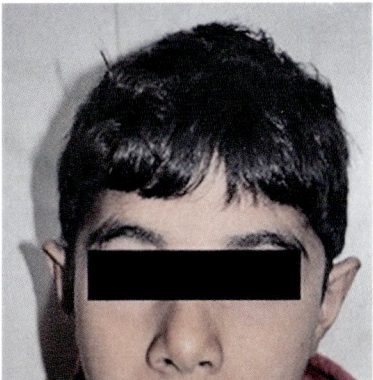 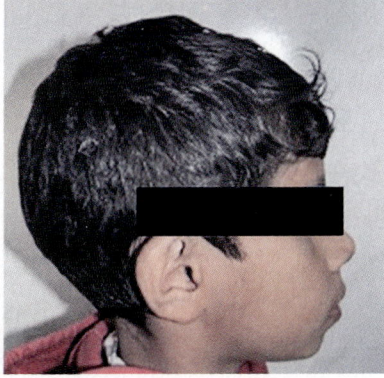 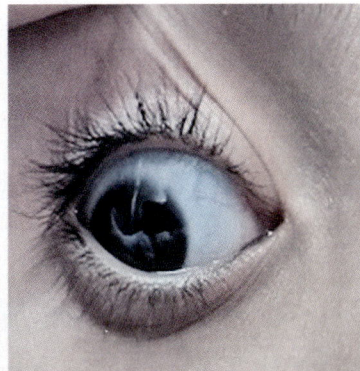

Fig. 42.1A: A case of osteogenesis imperfecta showing hypertelorism, frontal bossing, flattened vertex, prominent occiput and blue sclera.

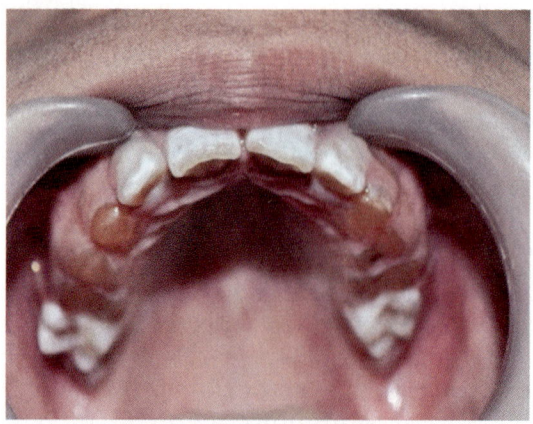

Fig. 42.1B: Intraoral photograph of a case of osteogenesis imperfecta and dentinogenesis imperfecta showing loss of enamel on deciduous teeth and discoloration

Diagnosis: Genetic testing is the most accurate investigation. Diagnosis requires correlation of clinical and radiographic features. Prenatal ultrasonography may be helpful for *in utero* diagnosis of disease. Bone biopsy is reserved for select cases. Serum alkaline phosphatase may be raised occasionally. Bone mineral density is far below the normal levels in majority of the cases.

Treatment: There is not yet a cure for OI. Treatment is individualized and depends on the severity of the disease and the age of the patient. Treatment is directed towards preventing or controlling the symptoms, maximizing independent mobility, and developing optimal bone mass and muscle

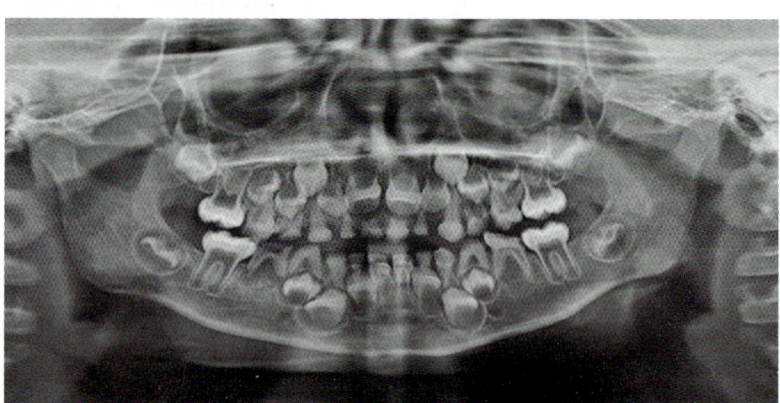

Fig. 42.1C: OPG of a patient with osteogenesis imperfecta and dentinogenesis imperfecta showing loss of enamel caps on deciduous teeth. Notice the cervical constriction and prominent pulp chambers in the permanent teeth. Also, the radiodensity of cortices is decreased

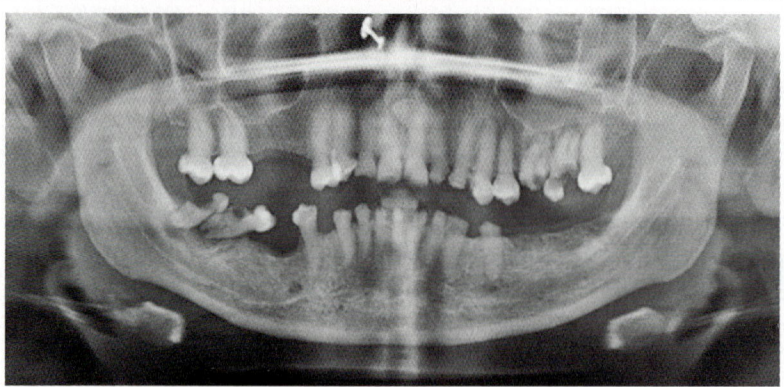

Fig. 42.1D: OPG of a patient with osteogenesis imperfecta and dentinogenesis imperfecta showing receded pulp chambers and loss of enamel caps on all the teeth

strength. Management of bone fractures and deformities may be difficult. Mainstay treatment is physiotherapy, rehabilitation and orthopedic surgery. Bisphosphonates are used in moderate-to-severe cases.

Dental treatment is very similar to dentinogenesis imperfecta. Full mouth rehabilitation may be required in some cases. Patients with significant malocclusion may require orthognathic or orthodontic corrections. Presurgical considerations include bleeding tendency, cardiac malformations, hyperthermia and difficult intubation.

Osteopetrosis (Albers-Schönberg's Disease or Marble Bone Disease)

Osteopetrosis is a group of rare hereditary skeletal disorders characterized by a marked increase in bone density. There is overgrowth and sclerosis of the bone, causing thickening of the cortices and narrowing of the marrow spaces. The prevalence of this disorder is estimated to be 1 in 100,000 to 1 in 500,000 persons.

Etiopathogenesis: The disease results from the failure of normal osteoclastic activity or differentiation, leading to a defect in remodeling of bone. Almost 30% cases have associated genetic abnormality. The genetic mutation seen in osteopetrosis causes defect in the proteins needed for osteoclastic activity. In some cases, the genes encoding the receptor RANK (receptor activator of nuclear factor-kappa B) interfere with formation of osteoclasts.

Clinical presentation: The disease may present clinically in a variety of subtypes. However, the three major clinical presentations are:
* The infantile form (autosomal recessive, malignant form)
* Intermediate form (autosomal recessive)
* The adult form (autosomal dominant, benign form) (Table 42.1).

Differential diagnosis: Endosteal hyperostosis, sclerosteosis, Van Bucham disease, infantile cortical hyperostosis, pyknodysostosis, craniometaphyseal dysplasia, diaphyseal dysplasia, melorheostosis, osteopathia striata, fluoride toxicity and secondary hyperparathyroidism.

Management: No specific treatment is required, other than management of complications. Prognosis of infantile form of the disease is poor with most patients dying within first decade. Bone marrow transplantation may be indicated in certain subtypes of the disease. If the osteomyelitis develops, it requires immediate attention to minimize osseous destruction. Managemnt typically includes drainage and surgical debridement with prolonged antibiotic therapy. Hyperbaric oxygen may be helpful in recalcitrant cases. Other alternative therapies such as interferon gamma 1b and calcitriol are still under research.

Paget Disease (Osteitis Deformans)

Paget disease of bone was first described by Sir James Paget in 1877, who described the clinical features and course of the disease in five patients and named the condition as 'osteitis deformans'. It is a metabolic disease characterized by increased and disorganized bone turnover affecting one or more skeletal sites. The disease initiates with an intense osteoclastic activity, with resorption of normal bone. After a period of time, vigorous osteoblastic activity leads to woven bone formation. It is the second most common metabolic disorder of bones after osteoporosis. The highest prevalence of the disease is found in the United Kingdom, followed by Spain, Italy, France, North America, Australia and New Zealand where the prevalence is 1–2% of the elderly population. It is rare in the Indian subcontinent and Southeast Asia. But, in recent years, due to unknown reasons, the decline in the incidence and severity of the disease has been observed in the high incidence countries.

Etiopathogenesis: Studies have identified several genes and loci involved in the

TABLE 42.1: Features of osteopetrosis

	Infantile form	Intermediate form	Adult form
Time of diagnosis	✗ At birth or early infancy	✗ Usually in first decade	✗ Most common form, discovered in adolescence
Clinical features	✗ Diffuse sclerosis of bones, failure of bone marrow, frequent fractures, growth impairment and cranial nerve compression leading to loss of hearing, blindness and facial palsy, susceptibility to infections	✗ Diffuse sclerosis of bones, short stature	✗ Less severe, mainly affects axial skeleton, cranial nerve or compression of recurrant fractures may occur
Laboratory investigations	✗ Normocytic anemia initially with hepatosplenomegaly ✗ Granulocytopenia	✗ Mild-to-moderate anemia, but rarely bone marrow failure	✗ Mostly asymptomatic
Craniofacial findings	✗ Broad face, hypertelorism, snub nose, frontal bossing	✗ Mandibular prognathism	
Oral considerations	✗ Osteomyelitis develops commonly after extraction of teeth, more commonly affecting the mandible. Delayed eruption of teeth, early tooth loss, poorly calcified teeth may be present	✗ Osteomyelitis may develop, dense bone of jaws	✗ Osteomyelitis may develop secondary to tooth extraction
Radiographic features	✗ Increased density of bones, defects in metaphyseal remodeling, loss of cortical differentiation, failure of tooth eruption, image of the roots are obliterated due to increased density	✗ Increased density of bones, unerupted teeth	

pathways that regulate osteoclast activity, responsible for Paget disease. The *CSF1, TNFRSF11A* and *TNFRSF11B, TM7SF4* genes, which promote differentiation of stem cells to osteoclasts, regulate osteoclastic differentiation and activity and formation of mature osteoclasts have been implicated in its pathogenesis. It has been estimated almost 40% of patients with a family history and 10% of patients with 'sporadic' disease carry a mutation in *SQSTM1* (p62) gene. The patients with the mutation of this particular gene have more severe disease.

Environmental factors like viral infection, dietary calcium deficiency during childhood, vitamin D deficiency and childhood rickets, excessive mechanical loading of the skeleton and environmental pollutants, have also been postulated to play a role in the pathogenesis of Paget disease.

Clinical presentation: The disease mainly affects the older patients with a male predilection. The most frequently affected bones are the pelvis (70% of cases), femur (55%), lumbar spine (53%), skull (42%) and tibia (32%). The affected bone is enlarged and weakened. Involvement of weight bearing bones may lead to 'simian stance'. Skull enlargement may cause increase in head circumference and 'tightening of hats'.

Bone pain is the commonest symptom of Paget disease. The pain is more severe at night, not worsened by exercise and not alleviated with rest. Other secondary presentations include bone deformity, fractures and neurologic complications such as headache, hearing loss, nerve compression syndromes and spinal stenosis. Cardiovascular complications may also be present in some patients.

The patients with Paget disease are at a substantially increased risk of osteosarcoma (<0.5% of patients). Secondary osteoarthritis may also develop due to abnormal biomechanical loading of joints and osteosclerosis affecting subchondral bone.

Craniofacial features: Jaw bones may be involved in 17% of the cases, with a predilection for maxilla. The patients may present with spacing of teeth, separation or movement of teeth causing malocclusion. In edentulous patients, ill fitted or tightening of dentures may be the presenting complaint. Enlargement of middle third of face may lead to nasal obstruction, enlarged turbinates, obliterated sinuses and deviated septum. In extreme cases, 'leontiasis ossea' may occur.

Radiographic presentation: Jaws are infrequently involved. When the jaw is affected, the 'osteoporosis circumscripta' (large circumscribed radiolucencies or ground glass appearance) may be present in early stage of the disease in skull bones. In later stages, patchy areas of oseteosclerosis are seen, the typical 'cotton wool appearance'.

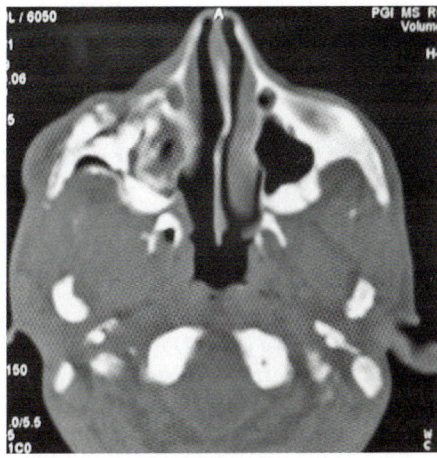

Fig. 42.2A: A patient suffering from osteopetrosis with multiple draining sinuses on face and bony deformity with respect to maxilla

Fig. 42.2C: CECT axial slice showing loss of architecture of right maxilla and soft tissue in the maxillary sinus

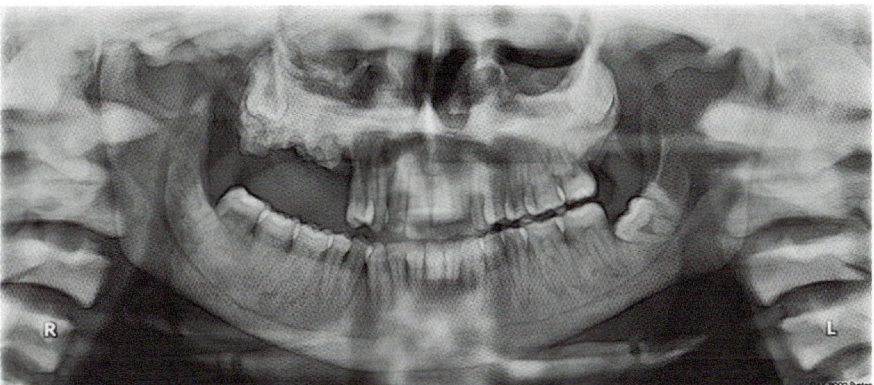

Fig. 42.2B: OPG of the same patient revealing dense sclerotic bone with loss of cortical differentiation, loss of lamina dura and thinning of inferior alveolar canal

These sclerotic patches tend to coalesce. The teeth may demonstrate generalized hypercementosis.

As the skull bones enlarges, 'pagetoid' appearance may be seen. The outer cortex may be thinnied but remains intact. When maxilla is involved, it may involve the sinus floor. The cortical boundries including sinus floor and lamina dura may become less evident.

Differential diagnosis
* Fibrous dysplasia (usually unilateral, seen in young age, encroach on antral space)
* Florid osseous dysplasia (centered over inferior alveolar canal, have a radiolucent capsule)
* Metabolic bone diseases (does not enlarge bones, alkaline phosphatase levels)

Diagnosis
* An increased serum alkaline phosphatase in patients who have otherwise normal liver function.
* Increased urine hydroxyproline levels
* In patients with limited disease extent, serum N-terminal propeptide of type 1 collagen or urinary N-terminal telopeptide of type 1 collagen may be helpful.
* Radiographic findings of osteosclerosis and osteolysis disrupting the normal trabecular pattern in affected bone, cortical thickening and bone expansion.
* Bone scintigraphy is helpful tool to evaluate the extent of disease.

Management: The management requires a multidisciplinary approach. Drugs that suppress bone turnover (antiresorptive treatments like bisphosphonates and calcitonin) can be helpful in treating pain that is due to increased metabolic activity, but most patients also require analgesics (NSAIDs, opiates, gabapentin and amitriptyline) and some require surgery to treat complications of the disease such as fractures and osteoarthritis. However, there is no evidence yet that bisphosphonates can decrease the associated complications or alter the natural history of the disease.

Points in case history to note:
* Any previous skeletal fractures or deformities.
* Familial history of similar disease
* Generalized pain in the bones
* Bony swellings or accompanying neural deficits

FIBRO-OSSEOUS LESIONS OF THE JAWS

Fibro-osseous lesions of the maxillofacial bones is a generic designation of a group of disorders characterized by the replacement of bone by a benign connective tissue matrix of spindle cells with varying amounts of woven bone. All these entities have overlapping histopathological features and are defined only by their growth pattern as apparent on radiographs.

Classification of Fibro-osseous Lesions

Numerous classifications have been proposed for fibro-osseous lesions and a wide diversity of lesions has been included under fibrosseous lesions such as developmental lesions, reactive lesions, and benign fibro-osseous neoplasms. But, most of these classification systems have been indulged in controversies and confusion regarding the terminology used.

The most acceptable classification that has gained wide recognition over the years was proposed by Waldron.

Waldron (1985):

I. **Fibrous dysplasia (FD)**
   A. Polyostotic
   B. Monostotic

II. **Fibro-osseous (cemental) lesions presumably arising in the periodontal ligament**
   A. Periapical cemental dysplasia
   B. Localized fibro-osseous-cemental lesion (probably reactive in nature)
   C. Florid cemento-osseous dysplasia (gigantiform cementoma)
   D. Ossifying and cementifying fibroma

III. **Fibro-osseous neoplasms of uncertain or debatable relationship to those arising in the periodontal ligament**
   A. Cementoblastoma, osteoblastoma and osteoid osteoma
   B. Juvenile active ossifying fibroma and other so-called aggressive, active ossifying/cementifying fibromas.

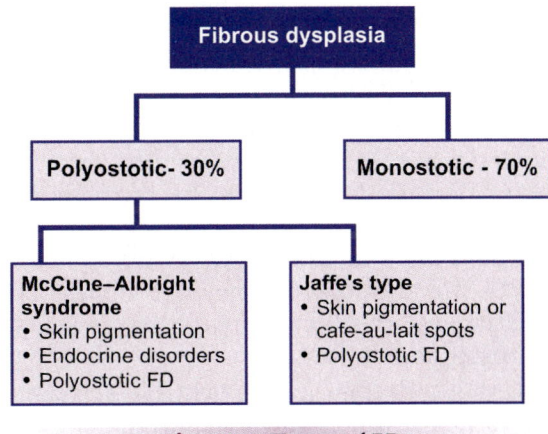

Fig. 42.3: Types of FD

This classification still remains the most valid classification.
   I. Fibrous dysplasia
   II. Cemento-osseous dysplasia
      A. Focal cemento-osseous dysplasia
      B. Periapical cemento-osseous dysplasia
      C. Florid cemento-osseous dysplasia
   III. Ossifying fibroma

I. Fibrous Dysplasia (FD)

Etiopathogenesis: FD is a benign fibro-osseous disease frequently affecting the jaw bones. It is believed to occur as a result of a developmental failure in the remodeling of primitive bone to mature lamellar bone or woven bone. This results in a mass of immature bony trabeculae enmeshed in dysplastic fibrous tissue. The affected bone undergoes a very slow (but never complete) remodeling process. Fibrous dysplasia is caused by a sporadic gene mutation of *GNAS 1a*. This is a somatic mutation, and therefore, lesions are not passed to successive generations. The lesion usually becomes static, once the skeletal growth stops, but proliferation may continue particularly in polyostotic form.

Types of FD

Figure 42.3.

Clinical Presentations

Site: Long bones are more commonly involved in the following frequency of occurrence, ribs> femur > tibia> maxilla > mandible.

Age : Polyostotic FD is usually seen in young patients below 10 years of age. Monostotic form occurs in slightly older age.

Gender: Monostotic form has no gender predilection, however, McCune-Albright syndrome almost exclusively affects the female patients.

Signs and symptoms: The disease is usually an incidental finding on radiography of facial bones, however, when the pathology is larger in size, the patient may present with unilateral facial swelling or enlarging alveolar process. Rarely, pain or neural deficit may be present (Fig. 42.4A).

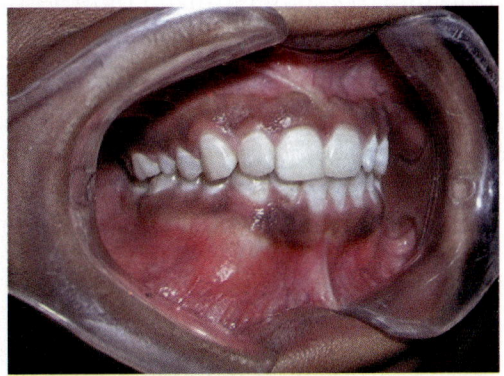

Fig. 42.4A: Fibrous dysplasia of mandible diagnosed incidentally on clinical radiographic examination. Expansion of buccal cortex can be appreciated from #43 to #47 region.

Radiographic Presentations

Location: Maxilla is twice more commonly affected as compared to mandible. The disease mostly occurs unilaterally and posterior part of jaws are frequently affected. Also, fibrous dysplasia is the most likely diagnosis when there are lesions elsewhere in the skeleton. Therefore, patients with FD of the craniofacial skeleton should be evaluated with a bone scan for the presence of postcranial lesions.

Periphery: Lesions often are ill defined with fuzzy transition zones. This occurs due to gradual blending of abnormal trabeculae in the surrounding bone. Rarely, the lesions may be well defined, especially in young patients.

Internal structure: Early lesions are radiolucent as the normal bone is replaced by dysplastic fibrous tissue. The early lesion characteristically is bounded by a distinct rim or shell of reactive bone. The lucent lesion with a thick sclerotic border is called the *rind sign*. As the remodeling of the fibrous tissue begins, woven bone is seen scattered throughout the radiolucency, giving the lesion a mixed appearance or *'peau d' orange appearance'*. The trabeculae formed are thin, short, irregular and abundant, imparting a texture of the *ground glass* or *swirling pattern* similar to fingerprint or *cotton wool* appearance. Sometimes, the mature lesions may be associated with simple bone cysts.

Effect on surrounding structures: The lesions may expand the bone to cause structural weakening and thinning of the cortices. The adjacent vital structures such as antral wall (especially anterolateral wall), inferior alveolar canal, erupting toothbuds may be displaced as the lesions expand. Lamina dura of the adjacent teeth disappears and periodontal ligament space is narrowed down. Rarely root resorption or hypercementosis may also be seen (Fig. 42.4B, C and D).

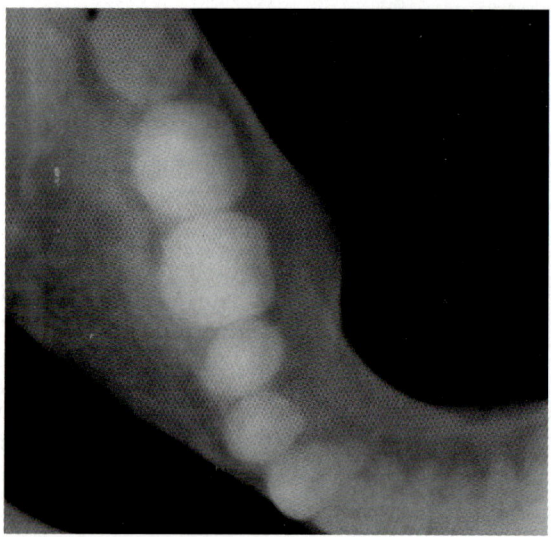

Fig. 42.4B: Mandibular occlusal radiograph showing fusiform enlargement. The typical ground glass appearance of fibrous dysplasia and indistinct margins of the pathology can be appreciated

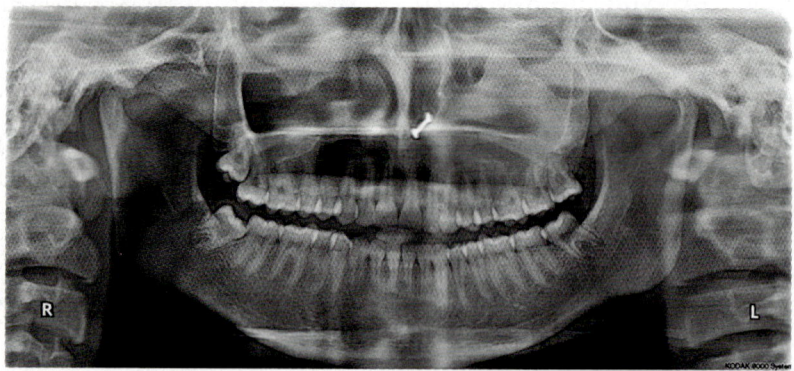

Fig. 42.4C: OPG of a patient with fibrous dysplasia showing ground glass appearance, loss of lamina dura and obliteration of left maxillary sinus

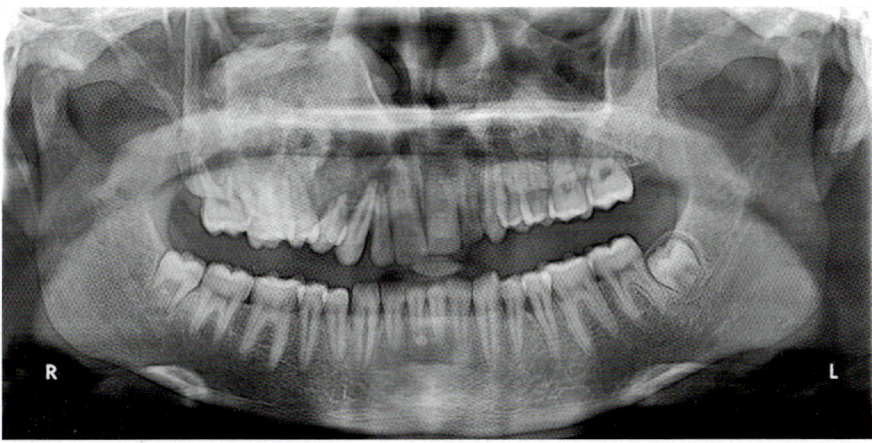

Fig. 42.4D: OPG reveals a well-defined radiopacity with a thin radiolucent capsule surrounding the opacity. The lesion shows a typical ground glass appearance and causes displacement of roots of the involved teeth

Investigations: Serum alkaline phosphatase levels are often elevated during active phases of this disease. Patients with the polyostotic form, must be evaluated to exclude hyperthyroidism, pituitary gigantism, or hypercortisolism. Polymerase chain reaction analysis with peptide nucleic acid may be used to study blood cells with the G protein gene (GNAS) mutation.

Management: The treatment is generally conservative. Surgery may be considered only if there is significant deformity, risk of pathological fracture, or symptomatic lesion.

Malignant transformation of FD occurs very infrequently, with reported prevalence ranging from 0.4% to 4%. Osteosarcoma makes up more than half of all the malignant, followed by fibrosarcoma and chondrosarcoma.

II. Osseous Dysplasia

Osseous dysplasias are the most common, yet least recognized form of benign fibro-osseous lesion. The distinction between the three subtypes is based solely on the clinical and radiographic manifestations with a little role of histopathology.

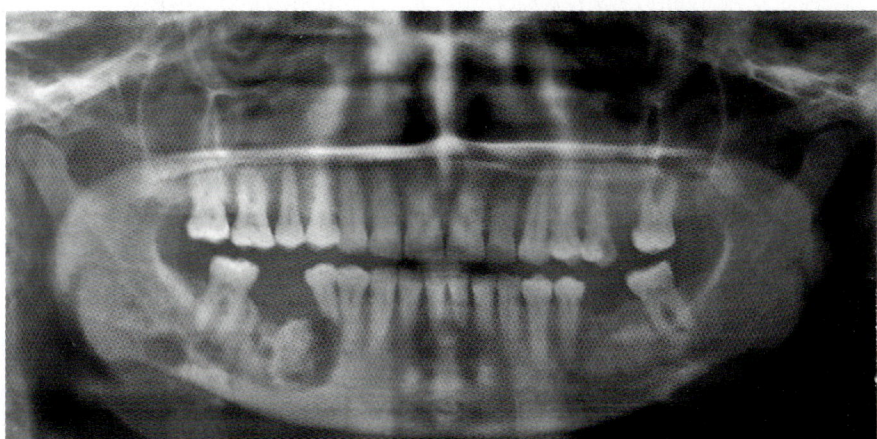

Fig. 42.5: OPG of a patient with florid osseous dysplasia showing an irregular radiopaque lesion with a radiolucent halo

Pathogenesis: These are reactive fibro-osseous lesions and are thought to arise from the periodontal ligament cells, where mature osteoblasts, cementoblasts and precursor cells reside.

The clinical radiographic features of the three varieties of osseous dysplasias are enumerated in Table 42.2.

Management: Management of these lesions usually depends on their size. Usually, multifocal or unifocal periapical osseous dysplasia needs no treatment. Larger forms of the disorder may require surgery to prevent further destruction.

Rarely, after extraction of the involved teeth, osseous dysplasias may become infected and develop features of osteomyelitis.

III. Ossifying Fibroma (Cementifying Fibroma; Cemento-ossifying fibroma)

Ossifying fibroma is classified and behaves as a benign bone neoplasm. Although, it is usually a benign, slow-growing, painless, and often asymptomatic tumor, a rapid growth pattern with a 'malignant' or aggressive behavior is sometimes noted, particularly, when the tumor is located outside the mandible. The neoplastic process is thought to originate from the elements of periodontal ligament. The lesion consists of highly cellular, fibrous tissue that contains varying amount of bone or cementum like tissue. The term for this juvenile ossifying fibroma (JOF) has been used for this lesion when patients are young.

Clinical Presentations

Site: Occurs almost exclusively in craniofacial region, with mandible being most commonly involved bone followed by ethmoid, frontal, and sphenoid sinuses, as well as the orbit, occiput, and temporal bone. Ossifying fibromas are characteristically monostotic. Less than 5% involve more than one bone.

Age: May occur in any age but, usually seen in young adults between second to fourth decades. The juvenile ossifying fibroma (JOF) occurs in first two decades of life.

Gender: Females are more commonly affected than males.

Signs and symptoms: The disease is usually asymptomatic and initially an incidental finding on radiography of facial bones, however, displacement of teeth may be an early clinical feature. JOF may result in deformity of the involved bone. When mid-face is involved, patients commonly have a painless swelling of the cheek, unilateral proptosis with diplopia, persistent nasal obstruction, rhinorrhea and epiphora, and recurrent epistaxis and hemoptysis.

Radiographic Presentations

Location: Occurs exclusively in facial bones and more common in mandible below the premolars and molars, above inferior alveolar canal. Maxillary lesions commonly involve canine fossa and zygomatic arch area.

Periphery: Lesions are typically well defined spherical lesions with smooth borders and a thin radiolucent halo, representing a capsule. Sometimes, the radiolucent halo may be surrounded by a sclerotic border.

Internal structure: Early lesions are unilocular radiolucent lesions. As they enlarge and mature, the internal structure becomes mixed radiolucent-radiopaque and then, completely radiopaque surrounded by a radiolucent rim. The density of internal structure depends upon the amount and pattern of calcification like whispy, flocculent pattern.

Effect on surrounding structures: The lesions expands the bone in a concentric pattern with equal growth in all the directions. The cortical plates maybe weakened and thinned out, but mostly remains intact. The lesion can grow into and occupy entire maxillary sinus. Inferior alveolar canal and adjacent teeth may be displaced as the lesions expand. Lamina dura of the adjacent teeth disappears and periodontal ligament space is obliterated. Resorption of teeth may occur.

TABLE 42.2: Features of various osseous dysplasias

Nomen-clature	Periapical osseous dysplasia (osseous dysplasia; cemental dysplasia; periapical cementoma; periapical FD; periapical ossifying fibroma)	Focal osseous dysplasia	Florid osseous dysplasia (florid cemento-osseous dysplasia; gigantiform cementoma; familial multiple cementomas)
Race and gender predilection	Usually seen in black females	Usually seen in black females	Usually seen in black females
Age	Almost exclusively after the age of 30 years	Usually during the 4th and 5th decades of life	Marked predilection for middle-aged to elderly
Site	Mandibular anterior periapical region, solitary or multiple, rarely exceed 1 cm in diameter.	Mostly, occurs in periapical region of mandibular posterior teeth in intimate association with the root apices or at the site of extraction	Usually widespread, extensive manifestation, may involve more than one quadrant. Both dentulous and edentulous areas are involved
Clinical presentations	Almost always asymptomatic, detected during a routine radiographic examination	Invariably asymptomatic	Invariably asymptomatic, large lesions may cause expansion of jaws.
Radiographic presentations	**Location:** Epicenter is in periapical area of mandibular incisors, usually involves multiple teeth	Periapical area of mandibular posterior teeth or extraction site, usually bilateral	Periapical area, usually involves multiple teeth in bilaterally symmetrical manner.
	Periphery: Round or oval, well defined lesions with a radiolucent halo of varying width. Serial radiographs have demonstrated that periapical osseous dysplasia initially manifests as multiple, well-circumscribed, non-corticate dradiolucent area at the apex of the tooth, that later coalesce to form larger irregular lesions	Usually, irregular lesions May be round or oval, well-defined lesions with a radiolucent halo of varying width	Irregular lesions with a radiolucent halo surrounded by a band of sclerotic bone.
	Internal structure: Initially, the lesions are predominantly radiolucent, but with time become mixed, then predominantly radiopaque	**Internal structure:** Initially, the lesions are predominantly radiolucent but with time become mixed, then predominantly radiopaque	**Internal structure:** Initially, the lesions are predominantly radiolucent but with time become mixed, then predominantly radiopaque.
	Effect on surrounding structures: loss of lamina dura, widened or thinner periodontal ligament space	**Effect on surrounding structures:** Loss of lamina dura, widened or thinner periodontal ligament space. Little or no expansion of jaws	**Effect on surrounding structures:** Loss of lamina dura, widened or thinner periodontal ligament space. Larger lesions may cause indulating expansion

Management: Surgical enucleation or resection is done. Recurrance is unlikely, even with large lesions due to presence of capsule.

Points in case history to note:

- First clinical feature is usually an asymptomatic swelling, causing facial deformity.
- The swellings are slow growing.
- Mostly, these lesions are incidentally diagnosed on radiographic examination of jaws.
- History of non-healing socket or persistent pain after extraction from the site of involved jaw.

FREQUENTLY ASKED QUESTIONS

1. Write classification of fibrosseous lesions.
2. Write clinical and radiographic features of fibrous dysplasia / ossifying fibroma.
3. Write a short note on Paget disease.
4. Write a short note on osteopetrosis.

BIBLIOGRAPHY

1. Neville BW, Damm DD, Allen CM, Chi A. Bone pathology. In: Oral and Maxillofacial Pathology. 4th ed. Elsevier.
2. Grace C. Petrikowski. Diseases of bone Manifested in Jaws. In: Oral Radiology Principles and Interpretation. 6th ed. Elsevier.
3. Alharbi SA. A Systematic Overview of Osteogenesis Imperfecta. Mol Biol. 2016, 5:1; DOI: 10.4172/2168–9547.1000150.
4. Gupta A, Khanna S, Gandhi P, Singh V. Maxillary Osteomyelitis Secondary to Osteopetrosis—A Rare Case Report. J Clin Diagn Res. 2010: 4(5), 3261–5.
5. Van Dijk FS, Sillence DO Osteogenesis Imperfecta: Clinical Diagnosis, Nomenclature and Severity Assessment. American journal of Medical genetics.
6. Fibro-osseous Lesions of the Oral and Maxillofacial Region: Retrospective Analysis for 20 Years. J Oral Maxillofac Pathol. 2013 Jan-Apr; 17(1): 36–40.
7. McCarthy Edward F. Fibro-Osseous Lesions of the Maxillofacial Bones. Head and Neck Pathol; 2013; 7:5–10.

Paranasal Sinus Diseases

INTRODUCTION

The paranasal sinuses are air-filled spaces located within the skull and facial bones. The four paired sets of paranasal sinuses are: maxillary, frontal, sphenoid, and ethmoidal. Various functions of the sinuses are lightening the weight of the skull, humidifying and heating inhaled air, increasing the resonance of voice, and providing a buffer against facial trauma. The maxillary sinuses are the largest of all paranasal sinuses.

DISEASES ASSOCIATED WITH THE PARANASAL SINUSES

The most important of all paranasal sinuses to the dentist are maxillary sinuses. The roots of maxillary posterior teeth are in proximity or in contact with the floor of maxillary sinuses. The maxillary sinus can pneumatize the maxillary alveolar and palatine bone to various extents (Fig. 43.1). Odontogenic pathologies can extend to the maxillary sinuses that can imitate sinus disease or vice versa. Hypoplasia of maxillary sinuses can

TABLE 43.1.	Development of paranasal sinuses		
Sinus	At birth	Growth	Beginning of radiological evidence
Maxillary	✗ Present at birth ✗ Starts at tenth intrauterine week	✗ Rapid growth from birth to 3 years of life and from 7–12 years of life. Pneumatization continues throughout adulthood	✗ Within 4–6 months after birth
Ethmoid	✗ Present at birth ✗ Starts at 3rd to 5th month of gestation	✗ Attains adult size by 12 years of age	✗ 1 year
Frontal	✗ Absent at birth ✗ Starts at the age of 2 years	✗ Continues to grow through puberty and stops at around 20 years of age	✗ 6 years
Sphenoid	✗ Starts at fourth fetal month ✗ Small or rudimentary at birth	✗ Reaches sella turcica: 7 years of age ✗ Dorsum sellae: Late teens ✗ Basisphenoid: Adult	✗ 4 years

occur unilaterally (Figs 43.2 and 43.3) or bilaterally and is often an incidental finding on radiographs.

This chapter focuses on the diseases associated with maxillary sinuses. These could be broadly divided into intrinsic and extrinsic categories. The intrinsic pathologies arise within the sinus and extrinsic pathologies originate outside the sinus and then either encroach on or infiltrate the sinus. Extrinsic diseases that can secondarily involve the sinus could be odontogenic inflammatory, cystic, benign neoplasm, malignant neoplasm, salivary gland related, systemic, traumatic, and/or syndromic.

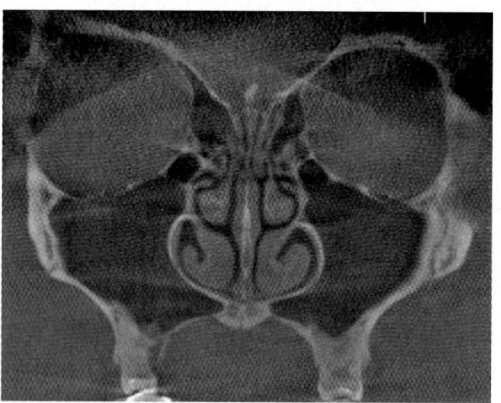

Fig. 43.1: Coronal CBCT section showing pneumatization of maxillary sinuses into alveolar and palatine processes of maxilla

General clinical features of sinus disease
* Percussion sensitivity of the teeth or cheek region
* Feeling of pressure
* Altered voice characteristics
* Pain on head movement
* Regional dysesthesia, paresthesia or anesthesia
* Swelling of the facial structures adjacent to the maxilla.
* Palatal swelling

Because of close proximity of the maxillary sinuses to the teeth and oral cavity, the signs and symptoms of sinus disease may first be reported to a dentist. A thorough investigation is necessary to determine if the disease is originating from within the sinus or outside the sinus, and to rule out any odontogenic causes. If it is difficult to reach to a diagnosis through conventional imaging modalities, evaluation through advanced imaging modalities should be considered.

Imaging Modalities (Table 43.2)

Intrinsic Diseases of Sinus

The intrinsic diseases of sinus are abnormalities that originate from tissues within the sinuses. This section explains the intrinsic diseases of the sinus.

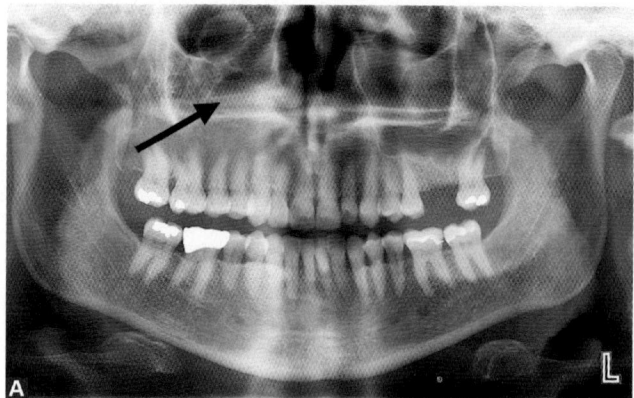
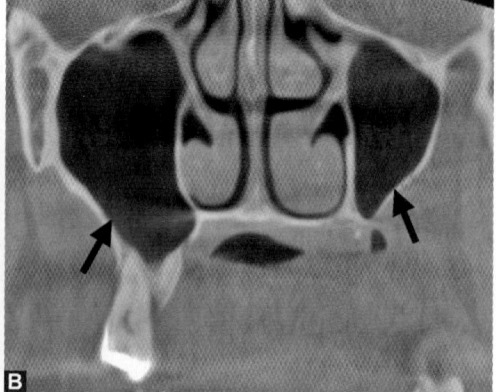

Fig. 43.2: (A) Panoramic radiograph showing hypoplastic right maxillary sinus. **(B)** Coronal CBCT section showing hypoplastic left maxillary sinus

Inflammatory Disease

Various infections either odontogenic or sinus origin, allergy, irritants (chemical or physical, like foreign bodies), or trauma can cause inflammation of the sinus mucosa. Radiographic images may show thickened sinus mucosa, air-fluid level, polyp, empyema, and/or retention cyst.

▶ 1. Mucositis

Localized thickening of the sinus mucosa is referred to as mucositis. The normal mucosal lining is usually 1 mm and not visible on radiographs. When sinus mucosa becomes inflamed due to infection, irritants or allergy, the sinus lining may increase 10–15 times of

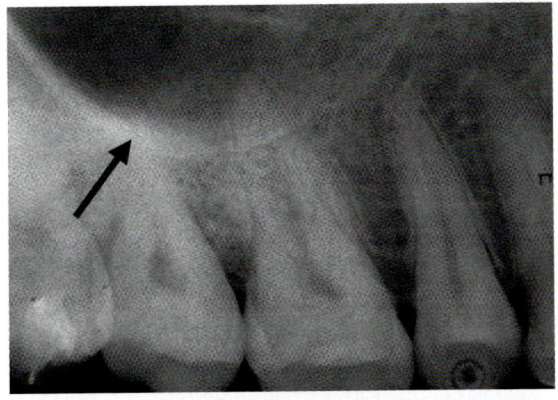

Fig. 43.3: Panoramic radiograph showing bilateral maxillary sinuses (solid arrow: Main sinus cavity (right side) and floor of the sinus (left side)) (dotted arrow: Posterior-lateral wall of maxillary sinus)

TABLE 43.2: Imaging modalities for diagnosing diseases of paranasal sinuses				
Imaging modality	Maxillary sinus	Frontal sinus	Ethmoidal sinus	Sphenoid sinus
Conventional radiography	✗ **Floor and relationship with maxillary posterior teeth:** Periapical radiograph, panoramic radiograph (Fig. 43.3), maxillary occlusal radiograph (Figs 43.4 and 43.5). ✗ **Posterior wall:** Panoramic radiograph (Fig. 43.3), lateral skull radiograph (Fig. 43.6a). ✗ **Main antral cavity (including lateral and medial wall, and roof:** Water's view (Fig. 43.6a) ✗ **Lateral and posterior borders:** Submentovertex view (Fig. 43.7a)	✗ Lateral skull projections (Fig. 43.6b), Water's view, (Fig. 43.6b). ✗ Caldwell view.	✗ Lateral skull projections (Fig. 43.5c), Submentovertex view (Fig. 43.7b), Caldwell view, Water's view.	Submentovertex view (Fig. 43.7c), Lateral skull projections, (Fig. 43.5d). Open mouth Water's view (limited view of sphenoid sinus).
CT/CBCT	✗ MDCT and CBCT provide superior images of ostiomeatal complex and sinus architecture in all three planes ✗ CBCT provides excellent air–mucosa–bone contrast ✗ CBCT showed 34% more pathologies than periapical radiographs and more expansion of lesions into the maxillary sinus, sinus membrane thickening			
MRI	✗ MRI gives superior images of soft tissues, particularly tumor extension and infiltration of the sinus ✗ It is also helpful to differentiate between soft tissue masses and retained fluid level in the sinuses			

Note: All the sinuses are visualized on lateral skull projections, but right and left sides are superimposed over each other

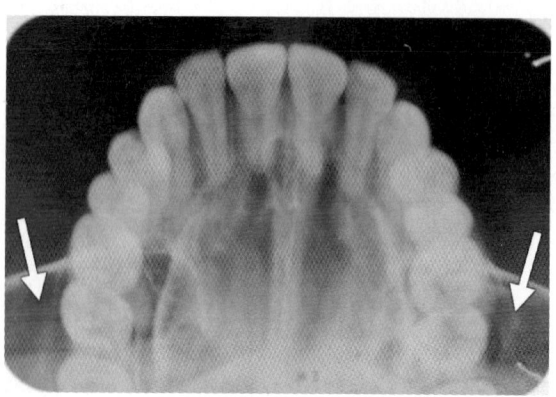

Fig. 43.4: True maxillary occlusal radiograph showing bilateral maxillary sinuses

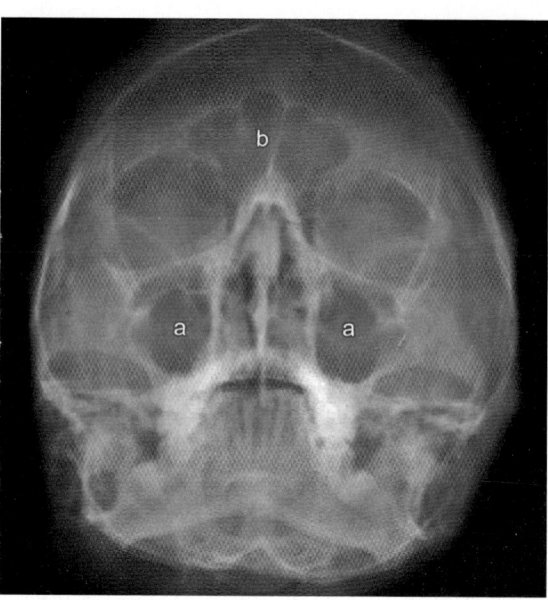

Fig. 43.6: Water's view showing (a) maxillary and (b) frontal sinuses

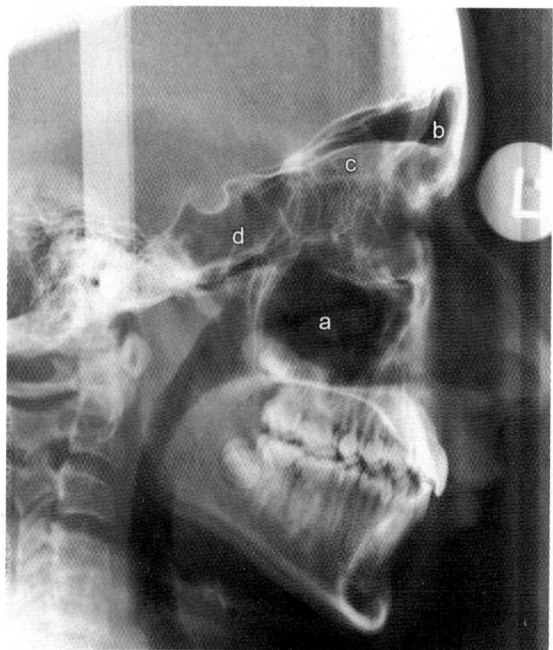

Fig. 43.5: Cropped lateral cephalometric radiographs showing (a) maxillary, (b) frontal, (c) ethmoid and (d) sphenoid sinuses

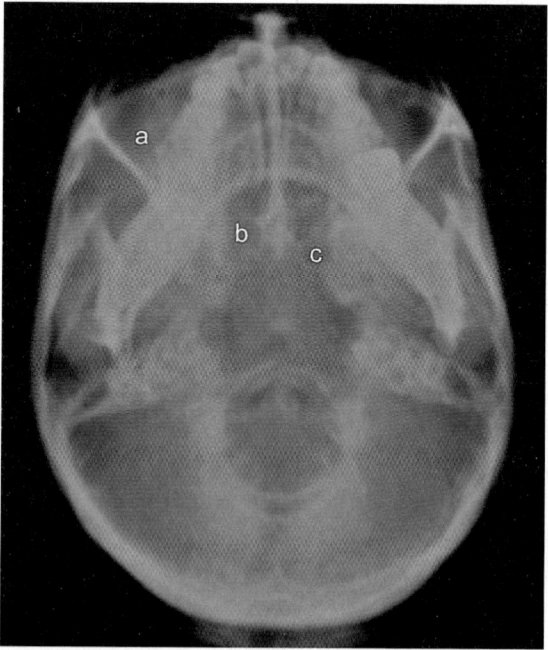

Fig. 43.7: Submentovertex view showing (a) maxillary, (b) ethmoidal and (c) sphenoid sinuses

normal thickness. Any mucosal thickening more than 3 mm is likely of pathological origin.

Clinical features: Usually patient does not have any symptoms. Mucositis is commonly discovered incidentally on the radiographs.

Imaging features: A well-defined, non-corticated soft tissue density band parallel to the sinus floor on conventional radiographs and CBCT images. (Fig. 43.9 and 43.10).

Management: Removal of the causative agent if symptomatic. Usually no treatment is necessary if asymptomatic.

▶ 2. Sinusitis

Generalized inflammation of the sinus mucosa caused due to bacteria, virus or allergen, when accompanied by clinical signs and symptoms, is called sinusitis. The sinuses are lined by respiratory epithelium and inflammation can cause ciliary dysfunction and retention of mucous secretion.

Retention of secretions sometimes can lead to blockage of ostiomeatal complex. The retained secretions in the sinus create a positive environment for bacterial growth. The most commonly affected sinus in children is ethmoid sinus and in adults is maxillary sinus. Possible reason for involvement of

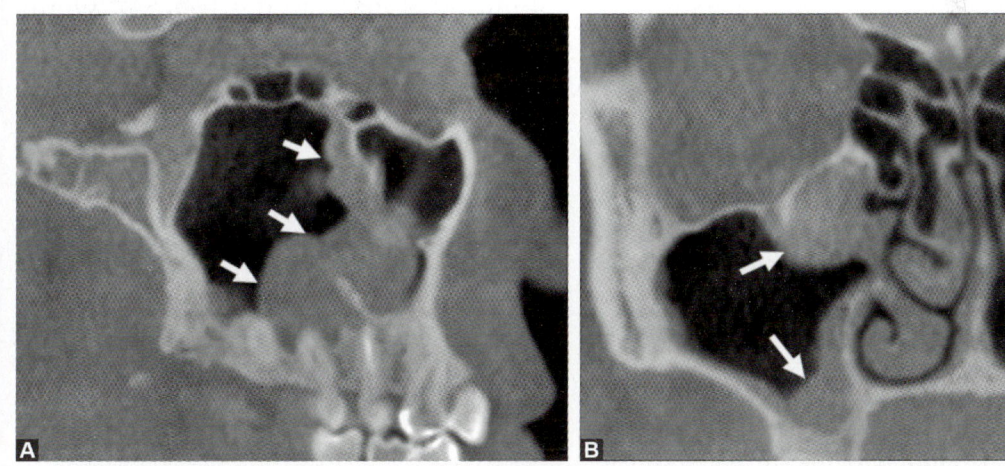

Figs 43.8A and B: A. Sagittal and **B.** coronal CBCT section showing mucositis

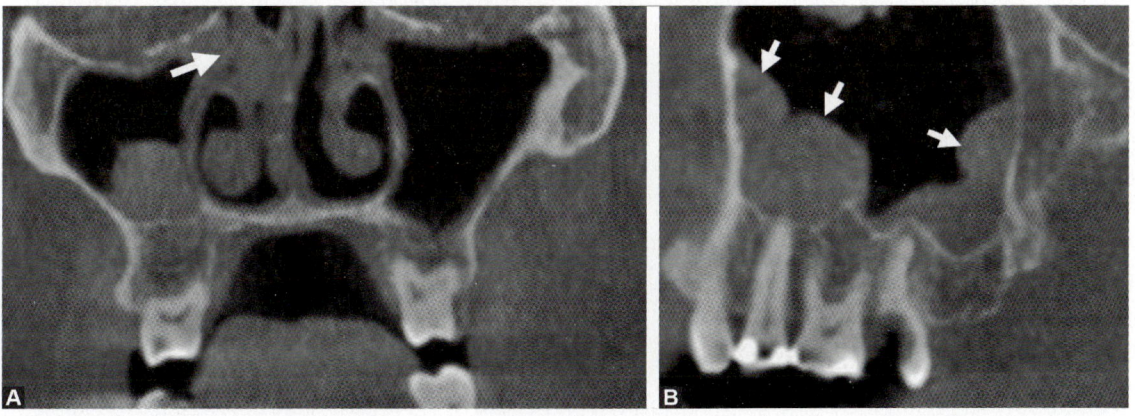

Fig. 43.9A and B: Polypoid mucosal thickening on the walls of maxillary sinuses on coronal and sagittal sections

ethmoid sinus in children is their position in the 'line of fire' as inspired particles impact and irritate the fragile ethmoid sinus lining.

When all the paranasal sinuses are affected, the condition is called pansinusitis. Pansinusitis in children could be related to a systemic condition called cystic fibrosis.

Sinusitis can be divided into five clinical categories.

- *Acute sinusitis:* Present for less than 2 weeks
- *Subacute sinusitis:* Present for 2 weeks to 3 months
- *Chronic sinusitis:* Present for more than 3 months
- Recurrent acute sinusitis
- Acute exacerbation of chronic sinusitis

Clinical Features

☞ Acute Maxillary Sinusitis

- It is commonly associated with common cold and occurs with nasal discharge or postnasal drip. If the acute infection persists, it can cause stuffiness or increased nasal discharge.
- The patient may feel pain, swelling, and tenderness on percussion over the involved sinus and headache.
- The maxillary sinusitis pain may refer to maxillary premolar or molar teeth of the affected side and teeth may become tender to percussion.

- Bacterial sinusitis may present with green or greenish yellow nasal discharge due to pigment-producing bacteria or due to antibacterial enzymes produced by white blood cells.
- Like any other sepsis in the body, acute infectious sinusitis can also cause fever, chills, malaise, and an increased leukocyte count.

Imaging features

On conventional radiographs

- Acute sinusitis shows mucosal thickening or opacification of the sinus. An air–fluid level can also be appreciated on the dependent area of the maxillary sinus.
- It is difficult to differentiate between air–fluid level and the mucosal thickening because both appear radiopaque.

On CBCT and CT

- Mucosal thickening or soft-tissue opacification of the sinus is noted.
- Air–fluid level, bubbly or frothy secretions are observed **(Fig. 43.10)**.
- Blockage of drainage pathways of ostiomeatal complex due to the inflamed mucosa may also be observed on CBCT or CT.

Resolving acute sinusitis shows a gradual increase in the radiolucency of the sinus. This increase in radiolucency indicates the sinus is gaining its normal air by shrinkage of thickened sinus mucosa and disappearance of fluid level.

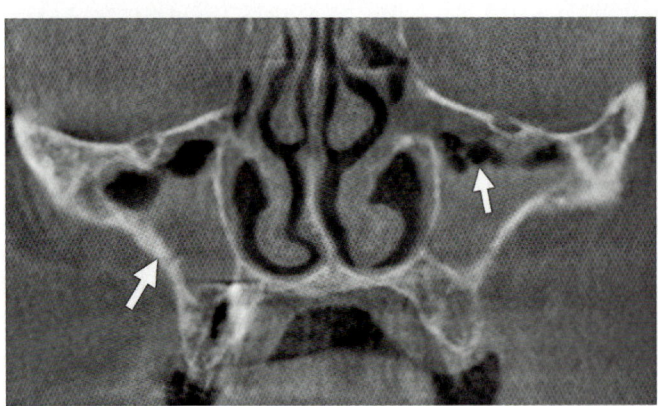
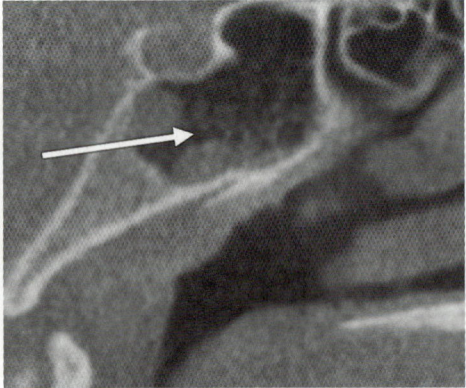

Fig. 43.10: Bilateral chronic sinusitis with acute exacerbation in left maxillary sinus and sphenoid sinus

Management

× Saline/steroid nasal spray.
× Decongestants, antihistamine, antibiotics (when necessary), and mucolytics.
× Surgical treatment (in rare cases) to prevent the development of complications.

☞ *Chronic Maxillary Sinusitis*

Clinical features

× When acute infection does not resolve by 3 months, it progresses to chronic sinusitis.
× Patients may experience chronic stuffiness and nasal or postnasal discharge. They may feel pain and discomfort during acute exacerbations.
× Several predisposing factors associated with chronic sinusitis are: Deviated nasal septum, presence of concha bullosa (pneumatization of the middle nasal concha), allergic rhinitis, dental infections (bacterial/fungal), asthma and cystic fibrosis.
× The order of involvement of sinuses in chronic sinusitis is ethmoid sinus > maxillary sinus > frontal and sphenoid sinuses.

Imaging features

× Mucosal thickening or soft tissue opacification with thickening and sclerosis of bony walls are the imaging findings of chronic sinusitis on both conventional and advanced imaging modalities (Fig. 43.11).
× The mucosal thickening may appear uniform or polypoid on radiographs. Infectious sinusitis shows smoother mucosal outline whereas allergic sinusitis shows more lobulated/polypoid appearance. The chronic sinusitis involving all the sinuses is called 'Pansinusitis' (Fig. 43.12).
× Occasional calcifications may also appear in the sinus.

Management

× Decongestants, antihistamine, antibiotics, antifungal, steroid nasal spray and mucolytics.
× Removal of predisposing factors is important for successful treatment.
× In case of recurrent or recalcitrant sinusitis, the surgical approach like functional endoscopic sinus surgery (FESS) is the treatment of choice.
× More extensive surgical procedure can be performed, if FESS fails.

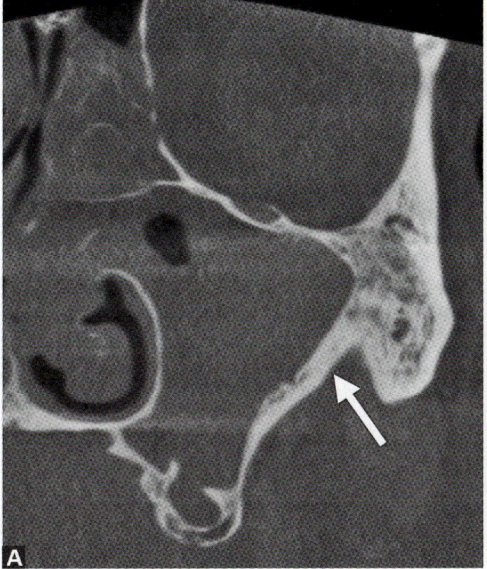 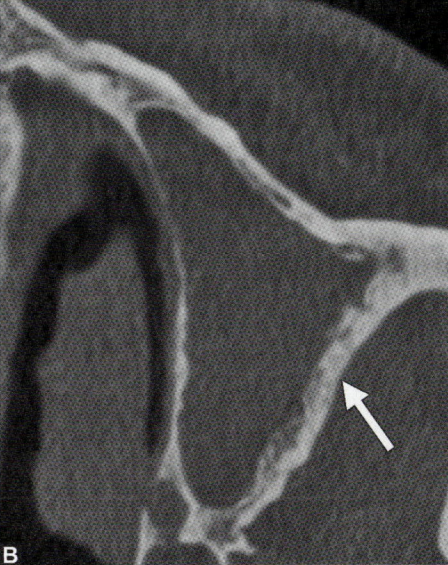

Fig. 43.11A and B: Chronic sinusitis: **A.** Coronal and **B.** axial sections of left maxillary sinus

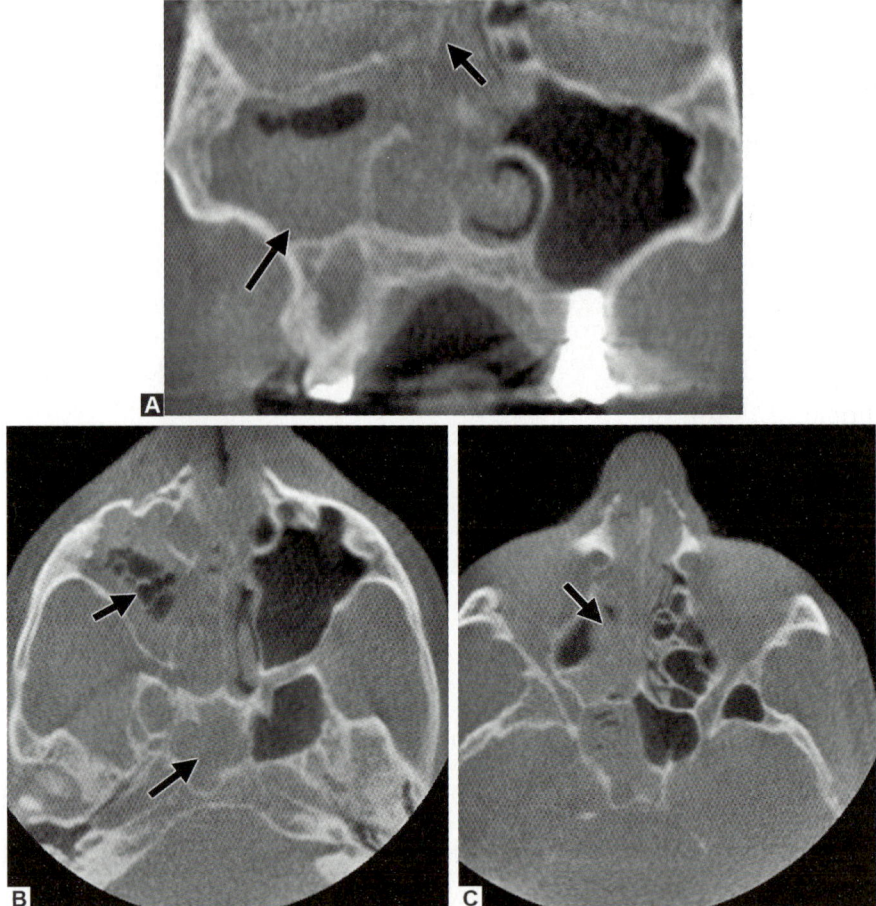

Fig. 43.12A to C: Pansinusitis

▶ 3. Retention Pseudocyst

Antral pseudocyst, mucous retention cyst, mucosal antral cyst, benign mucous cyst, benign mucosal cyst of the sinus pseudocyst, mesothelial cyst, interstitial cyst, lymphangiectatic cyst, false cyst, serous non-secretory intramural cyst.

Pathogenesis: Two suggested theories are:
1. When the secretory ducts of seromucous glands of sinus mucosa are blocked, the accumulation of pathologic secretions submucosally results in swelling of the tissue.
2. The degeneration of thickened inflamed sinus mucosa results in serous non-secretory retention cyst. This cyst

does not have an epithelium lining, hence it is called a 'pseudocyst'.

Clinical features
* Usually, it is an incidental finding on radiographs because the patient doesn't have any symptoms.
* Most commonly noticed in early spring or fall season which might be related to seasonal allergies or change in temperature.
* The pseudocyst may completely fill the sinus and cause pain and feeling of fullness and numbness.
* The pseudocyst may also extrude from the completely filled sinus and cause nasal obstruction and postnasal discharge.

- Sudden pressure changes due to sneezing or blowing of nose usually results in rupture of the pseudocyst.
- Sometimes, the pseudocyst continues to grow and herniate the nasal cavity and subsequently rupture. The rupture results in copious yellow discharge from the nose.
- It is most common in maxillary sinus followed by frontal and sphenoid sinus.

Imaging features

- Pseudocyst appears as a homogenous, well-defined, non-corticated, dome-shaped more radiopaque than the surrounding air with a broad base (Figs 43.13 and 43.14).

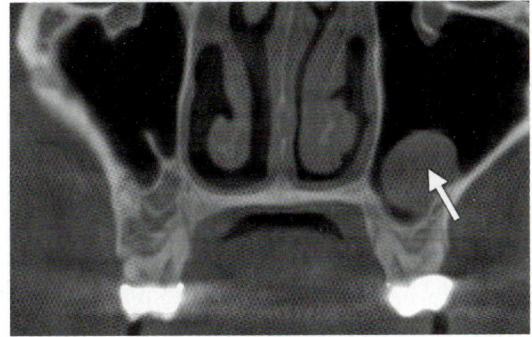

Fig. 43.13: Coronal CBCT section showing mucous retention pseudocyst

- It may occur unilaterally or bilaterally; there may be only one or multiple pseudocysts in one sinus.
- The size varies from as small as a fingertip or as large as completely filled sinus.
- The usual location of the pseudocyst is the floor of the sinus. It may also occur on the lateral wall or the roof of the sinus.
- The sinus floor remains intact.

Differential diagnosis

- **Odontogenic cyst:** When roots of maxillary posterior teeth are projected over a pseudocyst, the lamina dura remains intact with a normal width of periodontal ligament space. Radiographically, it is important to distinguish antral pseudocyst from an odontogenic cyst. The odontogenic cysts are rounded, or teardrop shape with corticated borders. There is a loss of lamina dura of the involved teeth. The floor of the

sinus is displaced superiorly and can be traced as a border of the cyst. Whereas, the pseudocyst is not lined by a corticated border and the sinus floor is not displaced.
- **Antral polyps of infectious or allergic origin:** Radiographically, antral polyps are multiple and have a narrower base than pseudocysts.
- **Neoplasm**
  - *Benign neoplasm:* Just like an odontogenic cyst, benign neoplasms (extrinsic to sinus) are separated from sinus by a radiopaque border and it is less likely dome-shaped.
  - *Malignant neoplasm:* Malignant neoplasm (extrinsic or intrinsic) destruct the cortical border of the sinus.

Management: No management required.

▶ 4. Polyps

The thickened mucous membrane of a chronically inflamed sinus frequently forms into irregular folds called polyps.

Clinical features

- It is most common in young patients.
- Because of the pressure effect, it may cause destruction.
- It is a severe condition, if it occurs in ethmoidal air cells. The medial wall of the orbit is a very thin bone called lamina papyracea (part of the ethmoid bone) and extension of the polyp from ethmoidal air cells into orbit through this thin medial wall can cause unilateral proptosis. It may originate from any part of the sinus wall.

Imaging features

- It appears as a homogenous polypoid-shaped soft tissue density on radiographs.
- It can block ostium and can cause bone destruction due to pressure effect (Fig. 43.15 and 43.16).

Differential diagnosis

- **Retention pseudocyst:** A polyp occurs in continuation with thickened mucous membrane lining, whereas adjacent mucous membrane is not apparent in pseudocyst. In the case of multiple

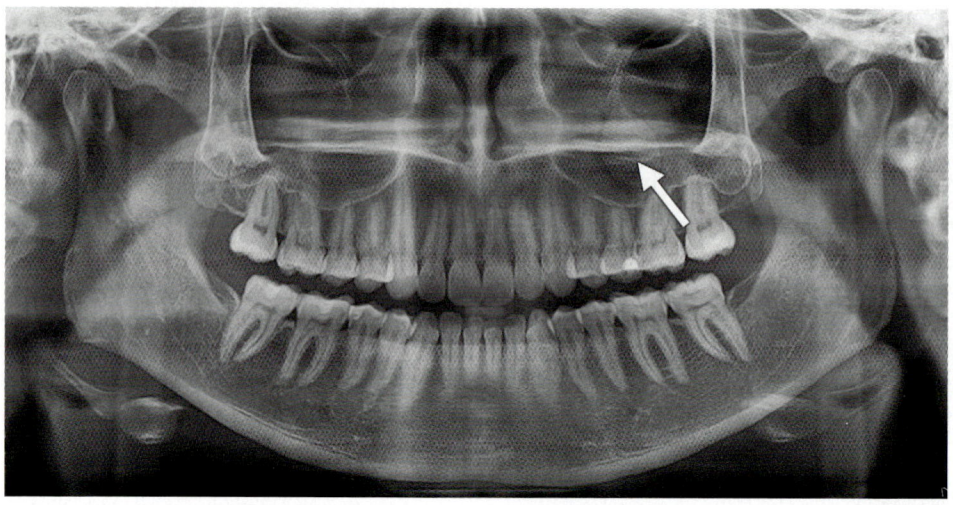

Fig. 43.14: Panoramic radiograph showing mucous retention pseudocyst

pseudocysts, polyposis should be given diagnostic preference.

- **Neoplasm:** It is difficult to distinguish between neoplasm and large polyp because both can cause the destruction of the adjacent bone. Just like a polyp, neoplasm can also be asymptomatic. In such cases, additional imaging and biopsy should be recommended (Figs 43.15 and 43.16).

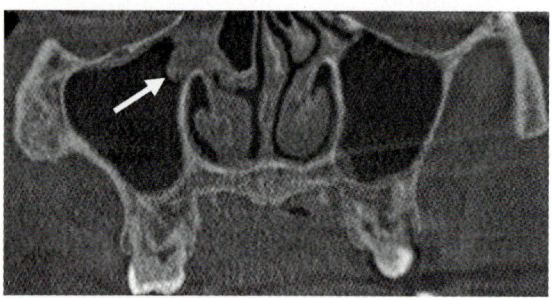

Fig. 43.15: Small polyp blocking ostium

▶ 5. Antrolith

Antroliths are calcified masses with a rough irregular surface formed by deposition of mineral salts around a nidus which may be endogenous such as inflamed mucosa, pus or clots or exogenous like tooth root, foreign body like dental material or food particle. The mineral salts are derived from antral secretions or inflammatory exudates.

Clinical features

- Smaller antroliths do not cause any discomfort to the patient and are incidentally discovered on radiographs.
- Large antroliths may cause pain, nasal obstruction, sinusitis or foul blood-stained discharge.

Imaging features

- Panoramic radiographs are not always the best modality to visualize antroliths because of the superimposition of the inferior nasal concha and zygomatic process over the sinuses.
- Panoramic radiographs should be supplemented with Water's projection.
- The exact location of the antroliths are best determined by CT or CBCT.
- Antrolith is a well-defined, round-to-ovoid shaped, smooth or irregular outlined lesion.
- It may appear as dense homogenous radiopacity or show a concentric ring of radiolucent and radiopaque material (Fig. 43.17).
- The size may vary from a few millimeters to a hazelnut.

Differential Diagnosis

- **Osteoma and exostosis:** These are continuous with the sinus walls, whereas antroliths are embedded in the sinus

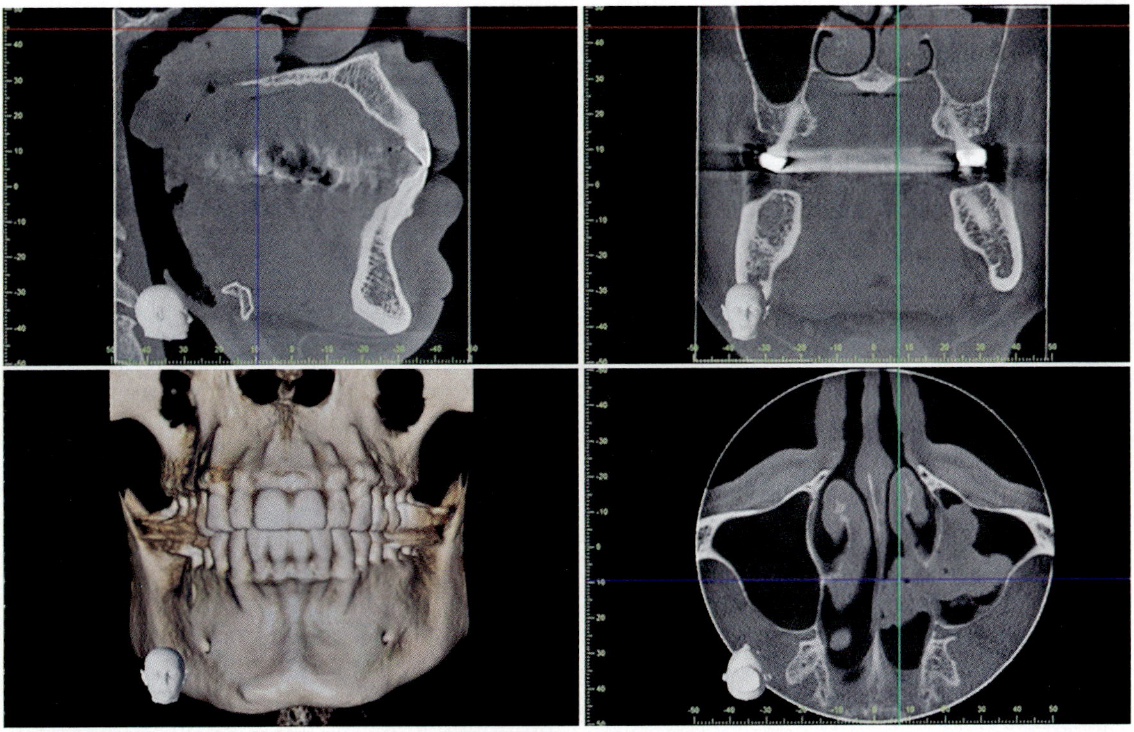

Fig. 43.16: Antrochoanal polyp in left maxillary sinus and nasal cavity extending into nasopharynx

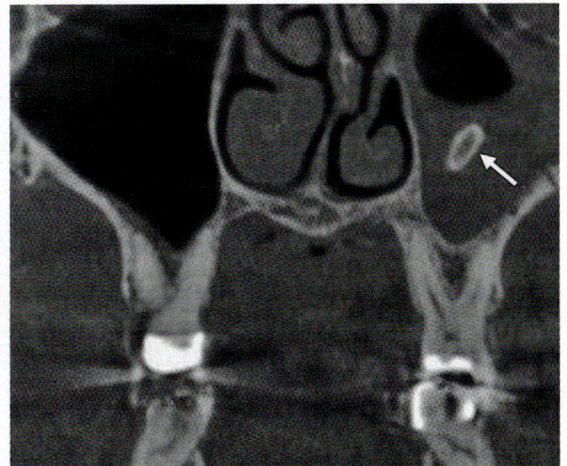

Fig. 43.17: Left maxillary sinus: Mucosal thickening with evidence of calcification suggesting an antrolith

mucosa and show no bony continuation with the sinus walls.

× **Root fragments:** Antrolith can be differentiated from root fragments by carefully examining the presence of root

canal and root canal anatomy. If the root fragment is displaced in the sinus, its position changes when the radiographs are taken with a different head position, unless it is stuck between bone and the sinus lining.

× **Mycolith:** It is seen in fungal sinusitis.

Management: An otolaryngologist consultation is recommended for large antrolith. Microscopic examination is required to differentiate it from low-grade maxillary sinus aspergillosis.

▶ 6. Mucocele (Pyocele)

A mucocele is a benign, epithelium-lined, expanding sac containing mucus, which usually develops when the sinus ostium becomes obstructed by chronic sinusitis, polyps or bone tumors. Expanding mucocele increases intra-antral pressure results in thinning, displacement, and destruction of the surrounding bone and can spread both intraorbitally and intracranially. When the cavity is filled with pus, it is termed an empyema, pyocele, or mucopyocele.

Clinical features: Frequency of occurrence: Frontal sinus (60–65%) > Ethmoid sinus (20–25%) > Maxillary sinus (10%) > Sphenoid sinus (1–2%).

☞ Frontal Sinus

- Recurrent frontal headache and swelling over the frontal sinus, are the key clinical features.
- Mucocele involving frontal sinus expands towards the least resistant wall. It tends to erode the thin superior orbital wall.
- When mucocele enters the orbit, it may cause decreased visual acuity, visual field abnormalities, diplopia, proptosis, ptosis, periorbital swelling, displacement of the globe, and restricted ocular movements.

☞ Ethmoidal Sinus

- Frontal headache or retro-orbital headache is one of the symptoms of ethmoidal sinus mucocele. If the mucocele extends from medial or posterior ethmoidal sinuses to orbital cavity through the thin medial wall (lamina papyracea) of the orbital cavity or through the apex of orbit, it may cause proptosis, exophthalmos, orbital displacement, and vision impairment.
- It may also extend to the nasal cavity and cause stuffiness of nose.
- Both frontal and ethmoid mucocele can extend into the cranial cavity with or without dural infiltrations.

☞ Maxillary Sinus

- When the mucocele expands and causes pressure over the superior alveolar nerve, causes radiating pain over the area supplied by the same nerve.
- The patient usually complains of fullness and swelling over the cheek.
- If the mucocele expands in the inferior direction, it may cause the destruction of the floor of the sinus and hence loosening of posterior teeth.

- If the lesion involves the medial wall, it may cause destruction/deformation of the lateral wall of nasal cavity.
- If the lesion extends superiorly, it may enter the orbit and may cause diplopia and/or proptosis.

☞ Sphenoid Sinus

- Headache is the most important symptom of sphenoid sinus mucocele. It should be differentiated from other causes of a headache.
- Expansion of sphenoid sinus may cause compression of the optic nerve and/or cavernous sinus. The compression of cavernous sinus can affect cranial nerves III, IV and VI. It may also cause ophthalmoplegia.

Imaging features: The overall shape of the sinus changes into more circular shape as the mucocele expands. Mucocele appears homogeneously radiopaque on radiographs. Bony walls of the sinus and intrasinus septae become severely thinned.

- When mucocele is associated with frontal sinus, the scalloped outline of the sinus may become smoothened by expanding mucocele. The superior orbital wall should be carefully examined on radiographs to look for any displacement or destruction.
- Ethmoidal sinus mucocele may cause displacement/destruction of lamina papyracea. Careful clinical examination and correlation with radiographs are mandatory to rule out any orbital extensions of the lesion (Fig. 43.18).
- Maxillary sinus mucocele may show displaced or resorbed tooth roots.
- Sphenoid sinus may displace sella turcica.
- Advanced imaging with CT/CBCT/MRI is recommended to know the exact extent of the lesion and effects on surrounding structures.

Differential diagnosis: Radiographically, it is difficult to distinguish between mucocele and cyst/neoplasm. A large odontogenic cyst may extend into maxillary antrum and may mimic mucocele.

Management: The prognosis of mucocele is excellent with surgical treatment. Maxillary antrum mucocele is treated by Caldwell-Luc procedure to excise the lesion. Mucocele involving frontal, ethmoidal or sphenoid sinus should be referred to an otolaryngologist for further evaluation.

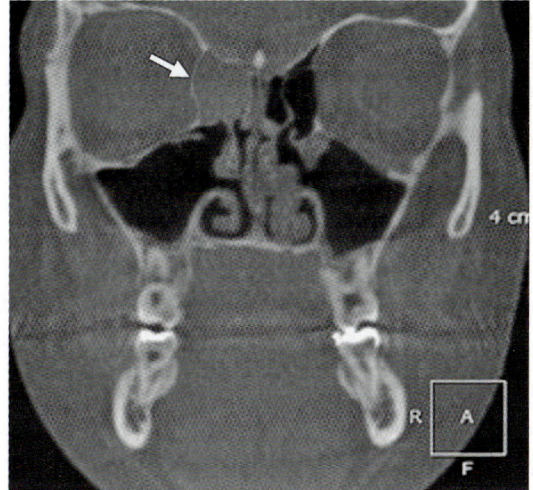

Fig. 43.18: Mucocele in ethmoid air cells

▶ 7. Neoplasm

Neoplasm of paranasal sinuses is most common in the maxillary sinus. Both benign and malignant neoplasms of sinus appear radiopaque like inflammatory lesions. The benign neoplasm usually causes displacement of sinus walls and malignant neoplasm causes destruction of sinus and adjacent structures. The common neoplasms of the maxillary sinus are squamous cell carcinoma and malignant salivary gland neoplasm.

☞ *I. Benign Neoplasms of the Paranasal Sinuses*

◆ *Osteoma*

Osteomas are benign, slow-growing, often asymptomatic mesenchymal neoplasm of the nose and paranasal sinuses.

Etiology: The controversial etiology of osteomas suggests embryonic, inflammatory, infectious, and traumatic origin.

Clinical features

- Frequency of occurrence: Frontal sinus (70–80%) > ethmoid sinus (20–25%) > maxillary sinus (5%) and sphenoid sinus (very rare).
- Paranasal sinus osteoma (PNSO) is the most common benign tumor of paranasal sinuses.
- The incidence rate ranges from 0.43% on conventional radiographs to 3% on CT/CBCT.
- Osteomas are twice more common in males than in females.
- Osteomas are most commonly diagnosed between the second to fourth decade of life.
- They are usually asymptomatic and diagnosed incidentally on radiographs. They may extend into nose, hard palate, orbit or intracranially.
- Symptoms are noted, if an osteoma causes obstruction of drainage pathway (ostium and/or infundibulum) or compresses or erodes adjacent structures. Headache is the most common symptom of frontal sinus osteoma.

Imaging features

- Osteomas are round to ovoid, homogeneously radiopaque structures (bone density) (Fig. 43.19).

Differential diagnosis:

- Antrolith
- Mycolith
- Tooth root
- Gardner syndrome (characterized by multiple osteomas, soft tissue tumors, and intestinal polyposis).

Management: The management depends on size, location, and age of the patient. Usually, no treatment is needed for asymptomatic small osteomas. Follow-up is recommended, especially for osteomas adjacent to the cranial walls. Surgery is recommended when lesion obliterates ostium and grows rapidly or show intracranial or intraorbital extension.

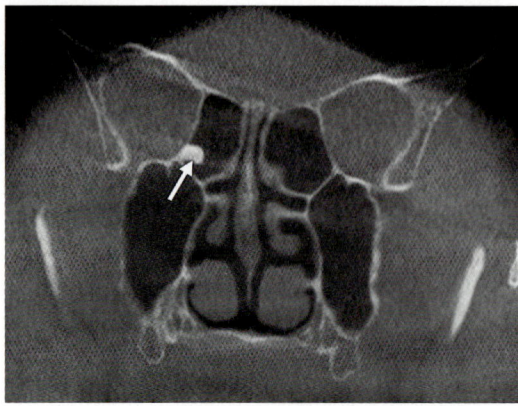

Fig. 43.19: Osteoma in right ethmoid air cell

☛ *Inverted Papilloma*

Inverted papilloma is a rare benign, locally aggressive neoplasm, arising from the ectodermal Schneiderian membrane. Inverted papilloma often erodes adjacent sinus bone similar to malignant neoplasm and it may extend to the nasal, oral, orbital and cranial cavity.

Clinical features
* It is most common in the fifth decade of life.
* Inverted papilloma is four to five times more common in men than women.

* The usual location is ethmoid or maxillary sinus.
* The initial symptoms are rhinorrhea, epistaxis, nasal obstruction, pain, headaches, hyposmia, and nasal masses.
* It is routinely diagnosed at a later stage after the onset of symptoms.
* The risk of malignant transformation ranges from 5–15%.

Imaging features
* Advanced imaging with CT and MRI will show a heterogeneous soft tissue density lesion occupying the sinus and often extending to nasal cavity. Due to the pressure effect, it may erode the adjacent bone and may mimic malignancy (Fig. 43.20A and B).
* *Note:* When a unilateral polyp is seen on radiographs, inverted papilloma and sinonasal tumor should always be considered in the differential diagnosis.

Management: The treatment varies from conservative removal to aggressive wide excision. Because of its locally aggressive nature and high recurrence rate, treatment should be planned carefully.

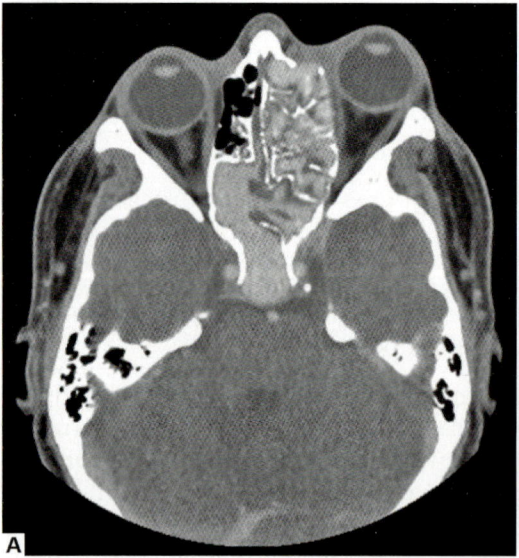
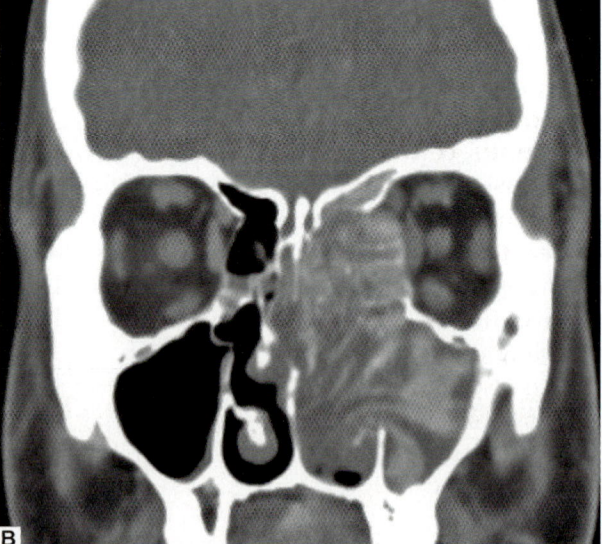

Fig. 43.20A and B: A. MDCT Axial section and **B.** coronal section showing involvement of left maxillary, ethmoid and sphenoid sinus by inverted papilloma (Image courtesy Dr M Noujeim)

II. Malignant Neoplasms of the Paranasal Sinuses

- Paranasal sinus neoplasms are rare and comprise 3% tumors of aerodigestive tract and only 1% tumors of the whole body.
- Squamous cell carcinoma is the most common (80–90%) malignant tumor of the paranasal sinuses.
- The clinical symptoms are similar to inflammatory sinusitis.
- The maxillary sinus (70%) is most commonly involved followed by ethmoid (20%), sphenoid (3%) and frontal sinuses (1%).
- It is difficult to determine the prognosis of these tumors because
    1. There are wide histological variants of paranasal sinuses tumors.
    2. These tumors are rare and there is no sufficient data to conduct studies.
    3. Unlike other tumors in the body, there are no universally accepted tumor staging system for the nose and paranasal sinuses tumors.
- When the lesion is near vital structures, the prognosis is poor.
- As patients usually seek treatment at an advanced stage, multimodality treatment is the mainstay of therapy.

Squamous Cell Carcinoma

Paranasal sinuses are lined by ciliated, pseudostratified columnar epithelium. Squamous cell carcinoma is the result of metaplastic changes in respiratory epithelium to squamous epithelium.

Clinical features

- It is most commonly noted in the sixth decade of life and is frequently seen in male patients (male:female ratio is 2:1).
- Patient with maxillary antrum carcinoma presents with a range of symptoms depending on the site of involvement.
- Lesion involving floor of the sinus can extend to alveolar process and may cause tooth pain, palatal or alveolar ridge swelling, mobility of teeth, and ill-fitting dentures.
- Lesion involving the medial wall of the sinus may extend to the nasal cavity and cause symptoms like nasal obstruction, epistaxis, mucosal discharge, and pain.
- Lesion extending into the lateral wall may cause swelling of the face and may extend inferiorly into the vestibule and may cause vestibular obliteration which in turn may cause pain in the maxillary posterior teeth.
- Superior and posterior involvement of maxillary sinus is prognostically important because of their proximity to orbit and ethmoid air cells superiorly and pterygoid plates and the pterygopalatine fossa posteriorly.
- Extension into orbit and/or ethmoidal air cell may cause intracranial spread.
- Posterior extension may cause invasion of muscles of mastication. Involvement of medial pterygoid muscles can lead to painful trismus.

Metastasis and Lymph Node Involvement

Lymph node metastases are relatively uncommon. Lymph node involvement indicates a poor prognosis. <10% cases present with distant metastasis and nodal metastases.

Imaging features

- Early malignant changes are non-specific radiographically. It is difficult to differentiate early changes from chronic sinusitis and polyps. It appears as homogeneously radiopaque mass of soft tissue density.
- As the lesion advances, it causes destruction of the sinus walls which can be noted on conventional radiographs including periapical and panoramic radiographs (Fig. 43.21). Involvement of alveolar bone show destruction around the teeth and irregular widening of the periodontal ligament space and can be appreciated on periapical radiographs.
- Medial wall destruction of the maxillary sinus is best noticed on Caldwell projection and lateral wall and floor destruction may be detected on a panoramic radiograph.

- MDCT / CBCT / MRI are preferred imaging modalities to know the exact extent of the neoplasm. MDCT is helpful to notice the soft tissue invasion of the neoplasm beyond the facial planes, extension into orbit, infratemporal fossa and cranial cavity. MRI is the best imaging modality to visualize soft tissue extension of the neoplasm and to differentiate mucus proliferation and soft tissue of neoplasm.

Management: Most of the paranasal sinus malignancies present at advanced stages. Surgical treatment along with postoperative radiation therapy is the preferred treatment modality.

III. Pseudotumor

(Invasive fungal sinusitis, inflammatory pseudotumor, fibroinflammatory pseudotumor, plasma cell granuloma, sinonasal fungal disease, mucormycosis, aspergillosis, zygomycosis of the paranasal sinuses, and *Rhizopus* sinusitis)

Inflammatory pseudotumor is a benign and rare process most commonly involving the lung and orbit but can be noted at any site in the body apparently related to diseases of fungal origin. The term 'inflammatory pseudotumor (IPT)' is used because clinically and radiographically it resembles malignant tumors.

Clinical features

- Clinical presentation depends on the site of the involvement and the symptoms are non-specific.
- The patient usually complains of recurrent infection.
- Pain is associated with nasal congestion, epistaxis, proptosis, dysphagia or cranial nerve involvement.
- These symptoms along with erythema, edema and fever may suggest inflammatory origin.
- In some patients, pseudotumor is associated with systemic diseases (Von Willebrand diseases, diabetes mellitus, or myelodysplasia) and immuno-compromised state.

Imaging features: The radiologic features of pseudotumor mimic malignant neoplasm. It usually causes erosion of the sinus walls. Soft tissue mass with sclerotic changes or calcifications can be noted (Fig. 43.22).

Differential diagnosis: The differential diagnosis of pseudotumor involves both benign and malignant neoplasm.

Managment

- Caldwell-Luc surgical technique
- Antrostomy
- Corticosteroid therapy, radiotherapy, chemotherapy, and surgery, all can be used, either alone or in combination.

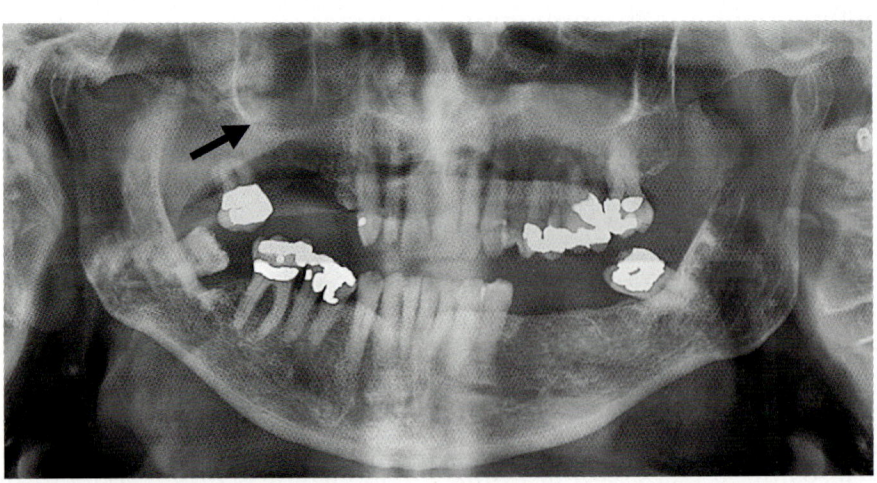

Fig. 43.21: Squamous cell carcinoma right maxillary sinus

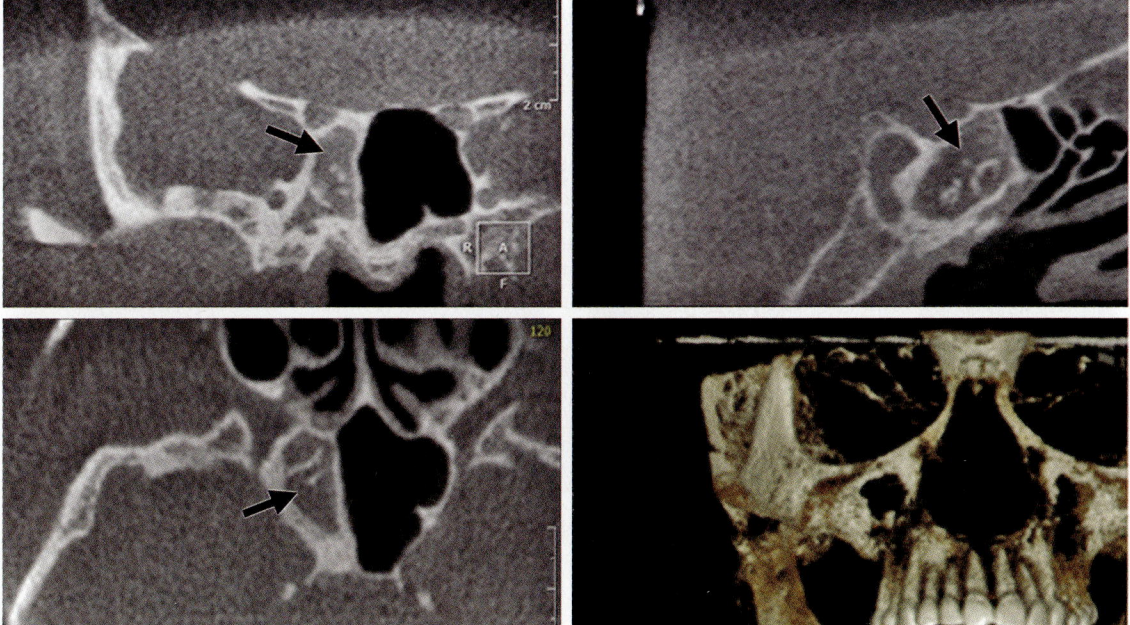

Fig. 43.22: CBCT sections showing opacification of right sphenoid sinus with calcifications suggesting fungal sinusitis

▶ 8. Extrinsic Diseases Involving the Paranasal Sinuses

☞ I. Inflammatory Diseases

◆ Maxillary Sinusitis of Dental Origin (MSDO)

- ✗ Pathological involvement of the maxillary sinus from dental diseases is a well-known entity in the literature. Maxillary sinusitis of dental origin is also known as odontogenic sinusitis, odontogenic rhinosinusitis, and odontogenic maxillary sinusitis.
- ✗ Different etiologic factors are periodontal disease, endodontic disease, root fractures, dental implants, dental extractions, oro-antral fistula, and iatrogenic causes such as extruded dental materials, displaced teeth, and foreign bodies.

Clinical features
- ✗ They range from no symptoms to sinonasal symptoms and/or endodontic symptoms. Sinonasal symptoms include congestion, rhinorrhea, retrorhinorrhea, facial pain, and foul odor.

- ✗ Absence of endodontic symptoms does not necessarily rule out endodontic etiology.

Imaging features
- ✗ Periapical radiographs often show superimposition of zygomatic process, maxillary sinus floor, and buccal cortical plate onto the dental roots, obscuring periradicular inflammatory changes.
- ✗ Limited field CBCT significantly improves the radiographic diagnosis.
- ✗ The unique imaging findings are periapical osteoperiostitis. The apical periodontitis leads to superior displacement of the sinus periosteum and subsequent deposition of a thin layer of new bone under the periosteum. This reactive bone formation is known as periapical osteoperiostitis (PAO). This reactive bone gives a thin, dome-shaped appearance on sinus floor and looks like a halo on radiographs (Fig. 43.23).

Treatment: The most important part of the treatment is to determine the etiology. The treatment options include non-invasive

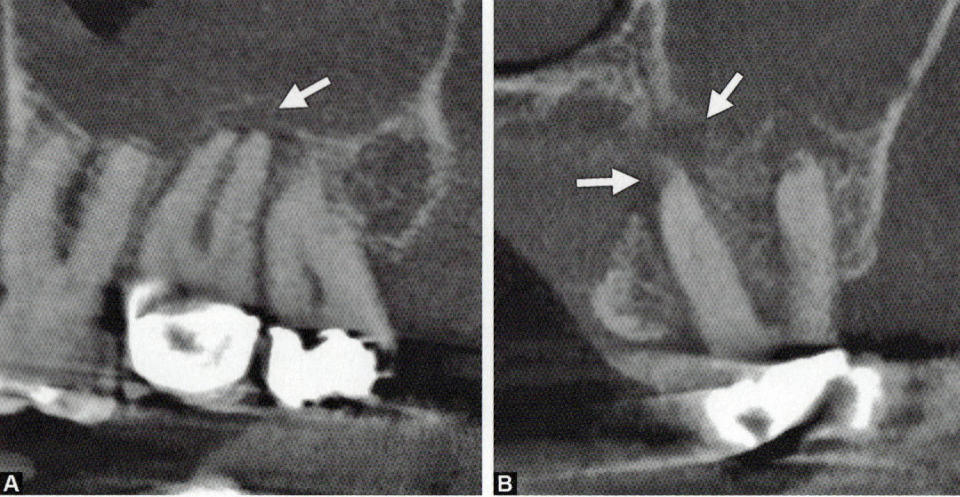

Fig. 43.23A and B: A. Sagittal and **B.** Coronal cross-sections of CBCT showing odontogenic sinusitis

endodontic treatment, periradicular surgery, and extraction of the offending tooth with or without antibiotics. In advanced cases of partially or completely obstructed sinus, surgical intervention may also be performed to establish drainage.

- ♦ *Displaced Dental Structures into the Sinus* (*Root/Foreign Bodies*)

Fractured tooth root as a result of trauma/iatrogenic causes or excess root canal filling material through the apices of the maxillary posterior teeth may extend into the maxillary sinus. Extension of dental structures into the sinus may cause maxillary sinusitis of dental origin (MSDO).

Clinical features

- ✗ Clinical features are non-specific and may resemble those of sinusitis later on.
- ✗ The dentist may notice a missing root fragment after extraction and unable to locate it into the socket.
- ✗ The dentist may ask the patient to hold the nose while attempting to breath (Valsalva maneuver). It may show bubbles within the fresh extraction socket. If the extracted tooth or any other foreign material is present for several days, it can cause mucosal thickening of the sinus lining.

Imaging features

- ✗ Displaced root fragment of maxillary posterior teeth/foreign material may be found anywhere in the sinus, but more commonly seen close to the floor of the sinus due to the gravity.
- ✗ On rare occasion, foreign material may be noticed submucosally between the sinus osseous walls and periosteum of the sinus.
- ✗ The foreign material typically appears as radiopaque on the radiographs (Fig. 43.24).
- ✗ A lateral maxillary occlusal view, Water's view or panoramic radiograph maybe helpful.
- ✗ The oroantral communication is difficult to be observed on these radiographs, if it is not involving, the mesial, distal or superior part of the alveolar process. Chronically displaced foreign material may also cause mucosal opacification of the sinus around causative agent and give rise to maxillary sinusitis of dental origin.

Differential diagnosis:

- ✗ Exostoses of the sinus wall
- ✗ Antrolith

Management

- ✗ Follow-up to observe eventual expulsion through the ostium by ciliary action of the sinus mucosa.
- ✗ Caldwell-Luc procedure

- Surgical intervention to treat advanced MSDO

II. Benign Odontogenic Cyst or Neoplasm

The odontogenic cyst or neoplasm affecting the maxillary sinus usually give similar appearance on the radiographs. The most common odontogenic cysts involving the maxillary sinus are the radicular cyst and dentigerous cyst. The most common odontogenic neoplasms involving the maxillary sinus are ameloblastoma and myxoma.

Clinical features

- Large cyst/neoplasm extending into sinus may cause facial deformity, nasal

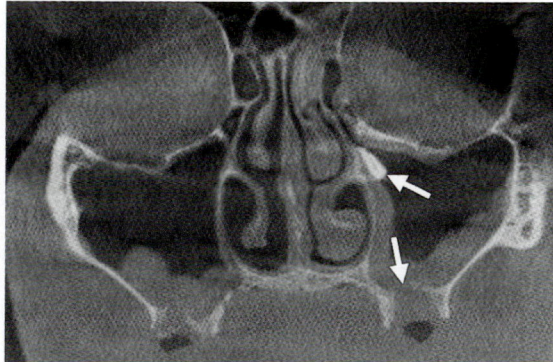

Fig. 43.24: CBCT coronal section showing root fragment in left maxillary sinus and oroantral communication

obstruction, palatal swelling, vestibular obliteration and displacement and/or loosening of the teeth.
- The borders of the growing lesion become indistinguishable from the sinus borders. As the lesion enlarges, it occupies sinus space and decreases the sinus volume.

Imaging features

- The lesion appears as ovoid, well-defined, corticated, homogenously radiopaque relative to the air-filled sinus cavity (Fig. 43.25).
- The cortication may be absent in aggressively growing lesions.
- The neoplasm may develop internal septation which mimic multilocular appearance.
- The neoplasm may stimulate dystrophic calcification depending upon the histologic nature of the neoplasm.
- Both cyst and neoplasms may displace the sinus floor and cause thinning of the cortex.
- Partially involved sinus gives the appearance of thin saddle over the cyst or neoplasm. The lesion may completely fill the sinus and may extend into adjacent structures.

Differential diagnosis

- Retention pseudocyst
- Antral loculation
- Maxillary sinusitis

Management: The management of the lesion depends on its extent and pathology.

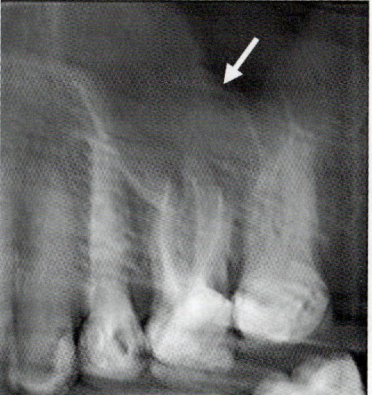
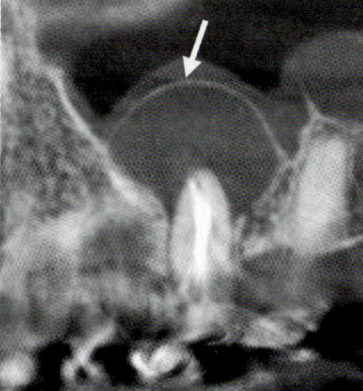
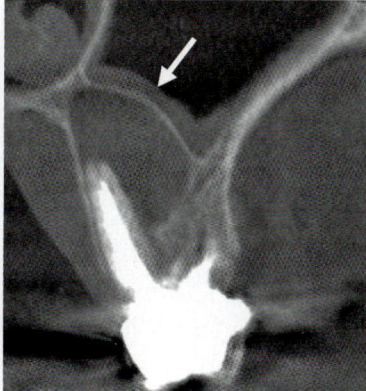

Fig. 43.25: CBCT sections showing radicular cyst with maxillary left first molar

Successful treatment may lead to healing of the area. It may cause 'collapse' of the sinus wall and irregular remodeling of the sinus floor with a radiolucent center projecting from the sinus floor.

☛ III. Malignant Neoplasms

The neoplasm originating from adjacent structures and extending to involve the paranasal sinuses include adenocarcinoma, soft and hard tissue sarcomas (**Figs 43.26A and B and 43.27A and B**), melanoma, meningioma (**Fig. 43.28**) and malignant lymphoma. Imaging features are often similar to malignancies arising within the sinus.

Synovial sarcoma of right masticator space involving maxillary sinus (images below).

☛ IV. Bone Dysplasia

Bone dysplasia may arise in any bone of the maxillofacial skeleton, causing expansion of the bone, displacement of the sinus borders and resulting in a smaller sinus on the involved side. Periapical or florid dysplasia occurring adjacent to maxillary posterior teeth behaves like a benign cyst or neoplasm.

Clinical features

× The sinus most frequently involved is sphenoid sinus, followed by the ethmoid and maxillary sinuses.

× Fibrous dysplasia is more common in children and young adults and the growth ceases at the skeletal maturity.

× The affected facial skeleton with fibrous dysplasia may result in facial asymmetry, sinus obliteration, proptosis, nasal obstruction, headaches or facial pain, recurrent sinusitis, and hyposmia, pituitary gland compression and impingement of the cranial nerves.

× The lesion may cause displacement of teeth.

Imaging features

× The most common radiographic feature of fibrous dysplasia is 'ground-glass' appearance with a thin cortex and without distinct borders which blends into the surrounding bone (**Fig. 43.29**).

× The sinus walls and floor are usually displaced but intact.

× The radiolucency of the sinus is partially or completely replaced by radiopacity of the lesion.

Differential diagnosis

× **Paget disease:** It usually spares the sinus and occurs in older patients.

× **Ossifying fibroma:** It has more tumoral expansion pattern than fibrous dysplasia and has a soft tissue capsule around it. However, it is difficult to distinguish

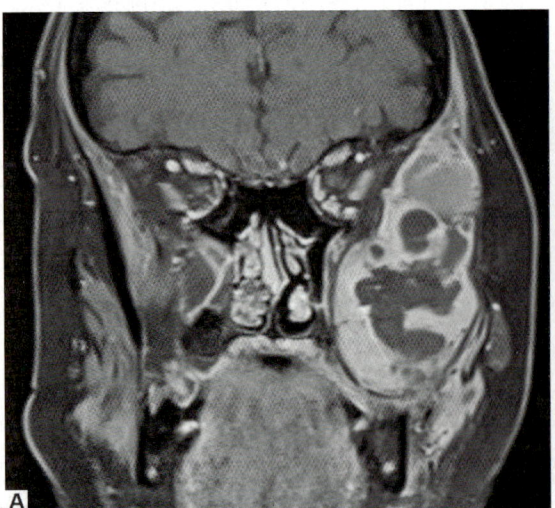

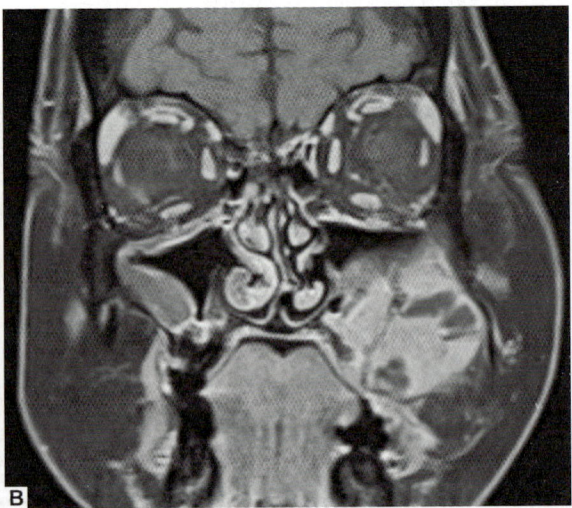

Fig. 43.26A and B: Coronal T1W fat saturated postcontrast MRI images

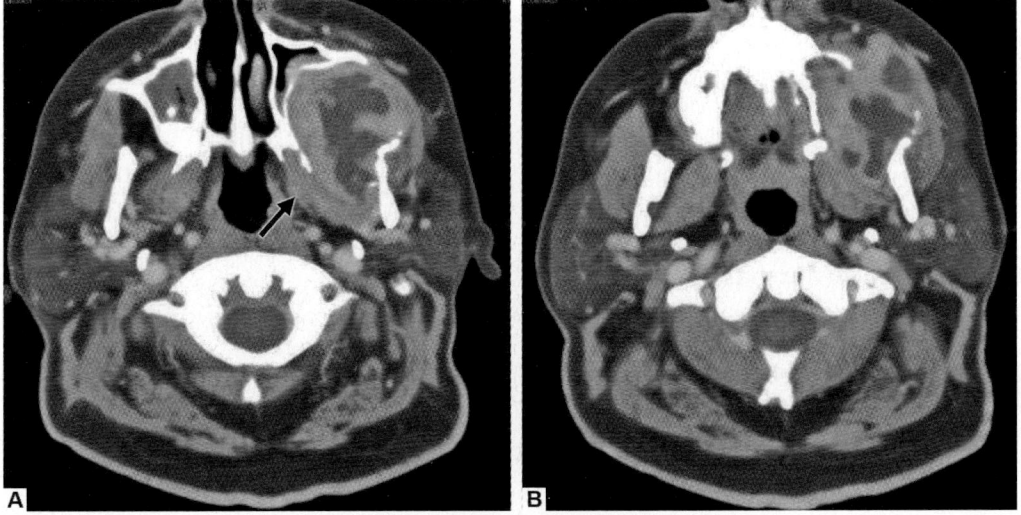

Fig. 43.27A and B: Axial CT soft tissue window postcontrast images

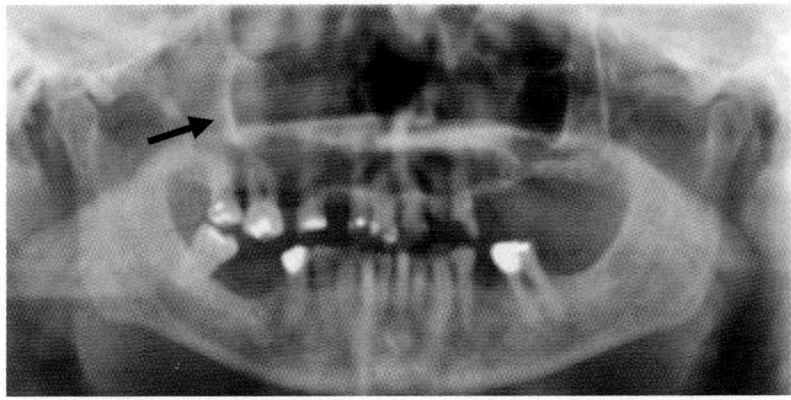

Fig. 43.28: Panoramic radiograph showing destruction of right maxillary sinus wall by metastatic lesion of meningioma

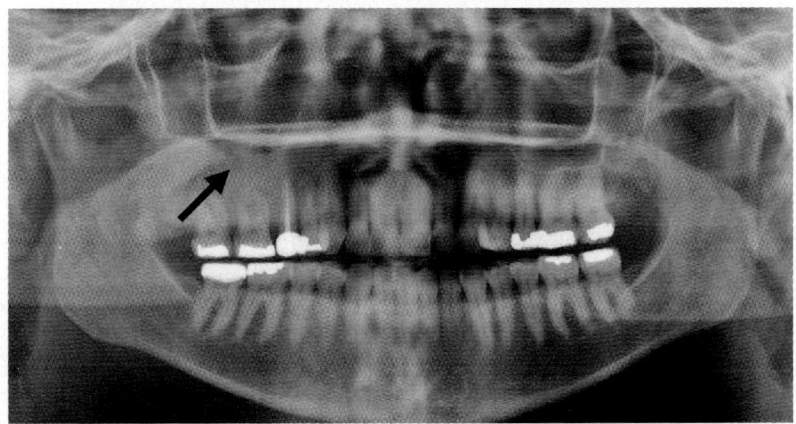

Fig. 43.29: Fibrous dysplasia in right maxilla displacing the floor of right maxillary sinus superiorly

both lesions radiographically. The most consistent radiographic feature is the shape of new bone encroaching on the sinus cavity is often parallel to the original shape of the sinus walls in fibrous dysplasia.

Management: Symptomatic treatment if needed in case of sinus infections. If Surgery is indicated, it is advisable to wait until late teenage to minimize the chances of regrowth and retreatment.

FREQUENTLY ASKED QUESTIONS

1. Write radiographic appearance of chronic sinusitis.
2. Write differential diagnosis of radio-pacities of maxillary sinus.
3. Classify diseases of sinus disorders and discuss radiographic appearances of them.

BIBLIOGRAPHY

1. Zachary J. Cappello, Arthur B. Dublin. Anatomy, Head, Sinuses, Paranasal. Treasure Island (FL): StatPearls Publishing; 2018 Jan.
2. Barry Berkovitz G. Holland Bernard Moxham. Oral Anatomy, Embryology, and Histology. 5th ed. Elsevier. 2017. Chapter 2. pp 9–10.
3. Stuart C. White, Michael J pharaoh. Oral Radiology Principles and Interpretation. 7th ed. Mosby Elsevier, Chapter 26. pp 472–91.
4. Karmody CS, Carter B, Vincent ME: Developmental anomalies of the maxillary sinus Trans Sect Otolaryngol, Am Acad Ophthalmol Otolaryngol. 84: 723–8, 1977.
5. Kaitlin Moore, Ann Ross. Frontal sinus development and juvenile age estimation. The anatomical record 300. 1600-17 (2017).
6. NesibeGu¨lYu¨kselAslier, Nuri Karabay, Gu¨ls¸ahZeybek, PembeKeskinog˘lu, Amac¸ Kiray, SemihSu¨tay, Mustafa Cenk Ecevit. The classification of frontal sinus pneumatization patterns by CT-based volumetry. Surgical and Radiologic Anatomy 38 (8), 923–30.
7. Loevner LA (2004) Paranasal Sinuses and Nose: Normal Anatomy and Pathologic Processes. In: von Schulthess G.K., Zollikofer C.L. (eds) Diseases of the Brain, Head and Neck, Spine. Springer, Milano.
8. Gray's anatomy. The Anatomical Basis of Clinical Practice. 39th Edition. Elsevier Churchill Livingstone 2005. Chapter 32.
9. Deepa V. Cherla, Senja Tomovic, James K. Liu, and Jean Anderson Eloy. The central Onodi cell: A previously unreported anatomic variation. Allergy Rhinol 4: e49 –e51, 2013; doi: 10.2500/ar.2013.4.0047.
10. Hodez C, Griffaton-Taillandier C, Bensimon I. Cone-beam imaging: applications in ENT. Eur Ann Otorhinolaryngol Head Neck Dis. 2011;128(2):65–78.
11. Low KM, Dula K, Burgin W, and von Arx, T. Comparison of periapical radiography and limited cone-beam tomography in posterior maxillary teeth referred for apical surgery. J Endod. 2008; 34:557–62.
12. David M Yousem. Imaging of sinonasal inflammatory disease. Radiology. 1993; 188:303–14.
13. Grace Petrikowski, Dania Tamimi, Lisa J. Koenig, and Susanne E. Perschbacher. Diagnostic Imaging: Oral and Maxillofacial. 2nd edition. Elsevier. Section 5. pp 857–954.
14. Eric Whaites, Nicholas Drage. Essentials of Dental Radiography and Radiology. 3rd edition. Elsevier Health Sciences. Chapter 27. pp 335–46.
15. Satish Nair, Emmanuel James, Angshuman Dutta, Sunil Goyal. Antrolith in the maxillary sinus: An unusual complication of endoscopic sinus surgery. Indian J Otolaryngol Head Neck Surg. 82 (January–March 2010) 62(1):81–3.
16. Langlais and Langland. Diagnostic Imaging of Jaw. (Williams and Willkins, 1995) Soft tissue calcification. Pp. 629–31.
17. CSH Tan, VKY Yong, LW Yip, S Amrith. An unusual presentation of a giant frontal sinus mucocele manifesting with a subcutaneous forehead mass. Ann Acad Med Singapore 2005; 34:397–8.
18. Claudio Ungari, Emiliano Riccardi, Gabriele Reale, Alessandro Agrillo, Claudio Rinna, Valeria Mitro, Fabio Filiaci. Management and treatment of sinonasal inverted papilloma. Annali di Stomatologia 2015; VI (3–4): 87–90.
19. Hasan Hu¨seyinArslan, HamdiTasli, Su¨leymanCebeci, Mustafa Gerek. The Management of the Paranasal Sinus Osteomas. The Journal of Craniofacial Surgery 2017 May;28(3):741–5.

20. Katzenmeyer K, Pou A. Neoplasms of the Nose and Paranasal Sinus. Dr. Quinn's Online Textbook of Otolaryngology. June 7, 2000.

21. Myers E, Suen J. Cancer of the Head and Neck, 3rd Edition: Neoplasms of the Nose and Paranasal Sinuses. WB Saunders Company. 1996.

22. Madhavi Patnana, Alexander B Sevrukov, Khaled M Elsayes, Chitra Viswanathan, Meghan Lubner, Christine O. Menias, Review. Inflammatory pseudotumor: The great mimicker. American Journal of Roentgenology. 2012;198: W217-W227. 10.2214/AJR.11.7299.

23. AAE Position Statement 2018. Maxillary Sinusitis of Endodontic Origin. P 1–7.

24. Lee J, FitzGibbon E, Chen Y, et al. Clinical guidelines for the management of craniofacial fibrous dysplasia. Orphanet Journal of Rare Diseases. 2012;7(Suppl 1): S2. doi:10.1186/1750–1172–7-S1-S2.

Soft Tissue Calcification and Ossification

Calcifications of various structures located in the head and neck regions are commonly found in patients seeking dental care. These are deposits of calcium salts, mostly calcium phosphate in the soft tissues.

The deposition of calcium salts in the skeleton is termed physiologic calcification. Whereas, deposition of calcium occurs in soft tissue in an unorganized fashion it is termed pathologic or heterotopic calcification.

Soft tissue calcifications in the head and neck region can be categorized as:

1. **Dystrophic calcifications**
   - Calcified lymph nodes
   - Dystrophic calcification in the tonsils
   - Cysticercosis
   - Arterial calcification
     - Monckeberg medial calcinosis/arteriosclerosis
     - Calcified atherosclerotic plaque
2. **Idiopathic calcifications**
   - Sialoliths
   - Phleboliths
   - Laryngeal cartilage calcifications
   - Rhinolith/Antrolith
3. **Metastatic calcifications**
   - Ossification of the styloid ligament
   - Osteoma cutis
   - Myositis ossificans

DYSTROPHIC CALCIFICATION

The deposition of calcium salts into primary sites of chronic inflammation or dead tissue.

This calcification usually is localized to the site of injury.

Dystrophic calcification may produce no signs or symptoms, although on enlargement a solid mass of calcium salts sometimes can be palpated.

Calcified Lymph Nodes

Dystrophic calcification occurs in chronically inflamed lymph nodes. The lymphoid tissue is replaced by hydroxyapatite like calcium salts. This condition may occur due to infections, granulomatous diseases, autoimmune disorders like rheumatoid arthritis, systemic sclerosis and metastases from distant calcifying neoplasms.

Clinical features: The most commonly involved lymph nodes are the submandibular, superficial and deep cervical nodes and sometimes, the submental and preauricular nodes. Calcified lymph nodes are generally asymptomatic. On palpation these nodes are single or multiple (series of lymph nodes chain); round or linear masses with variable mobility. They are often found incidentally on radiographic examinations.

Radiographic features: Calcified lymph nodes commonly observed at the submandibular region, near the angle of mandible or between the posterior border of the ramus and cervical spine. The image of the calcified node sometimes overlaps the

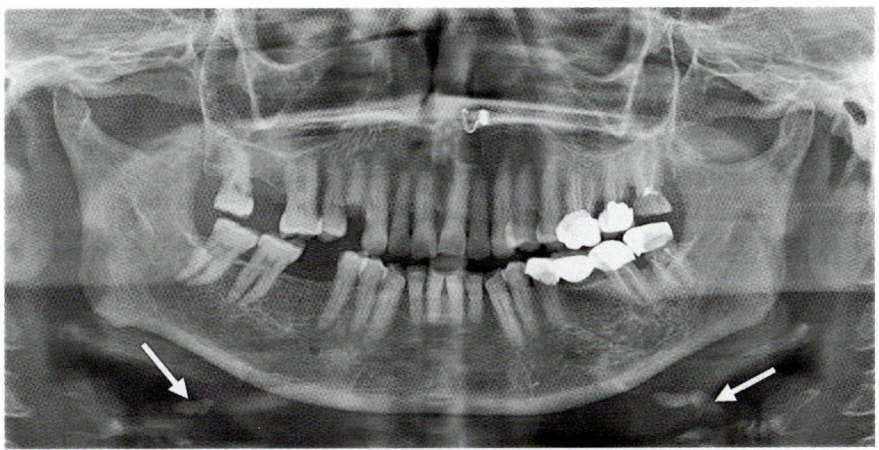

Fig. 44.1: Panoramic radiograph showing calcified lymph nodes (arrows)

inferior aspect of the ramus. The periphery is well defined and most often are irregular, lobulated with a cauliflower like appearance. The internal aspect may vary in the degree of radiopacity, giving the impression of a collection of spherical or irregular masses; multiple mottled radiopacities distributed along the course of a nodal chain and occasionally a laminated appearance or the radiopacity may appear only on the surface of the node (eggshell calcification). In absence of clinical symptoms, it is difficult to differentiate a calcified submandibular lymph node from a sialolith in submandibular gland, in such cases sialogram helps in differentiating these two entities (Fig. 44.1).

Dystrophic Calcification in the Tonsils
(Tonsillar Calculi, Tonsillar Stones, Tonsil Concretions and Tonsilloliths)

Tonsilloliths are rare concretions that are formed when repeated bouts of inflammation enlarge the tonsillar crypts. Incomplete resolution of organic debris (dead bacteria, pus, epithelial cells and food) can serve as the nidus for dystrophic calcification.

Clinical features: Tonsilloliths occur more frequently in adults than in children. It is hard in consistency; single or multiple; round, oval, cylindrical, irregular or pyramidal in shape;

and grayish-yellow, black, red-brown or dark gray in color, projecting from the tonsillar crypts, usually from the palatine tonsil. Small calcifications usually produce no clinical signs or symptoms. Giant tonsilloliths may cause stretching of lymphoid tissue and result in ulceration and extrusion.

Radiographic features: In the panoramic radiograph, tonsilloliths appear as single or multiple radiopacities that overlap the mid-portion of the mandibular ramus in the region where the image of the dorsal surface of the tongue crosses the ramus in the oropharyngeal airspaces. The most common appearance of tonsillolith is a cluster of multiple small, ill-defined radiopacities ranging from 0.5–14.5 cm in diameter. These calcifications appear slightly more radiopaque than cancellous bone and approximately the same as cortical bone (Fig. 44.2).

Cysticercosis

The name 'cysticercosis' derived from the Greek word 'Kystic' meaning bladder and 'Kercos' signifying tail. It is caused by the ingestion of the eggs of *Taenia solium* (pork tapeworm). Usually, when the larvae infect the intermediate host tissue (pig), it results in cysticercosis; and when ingested by the definitive host (human), these larvae

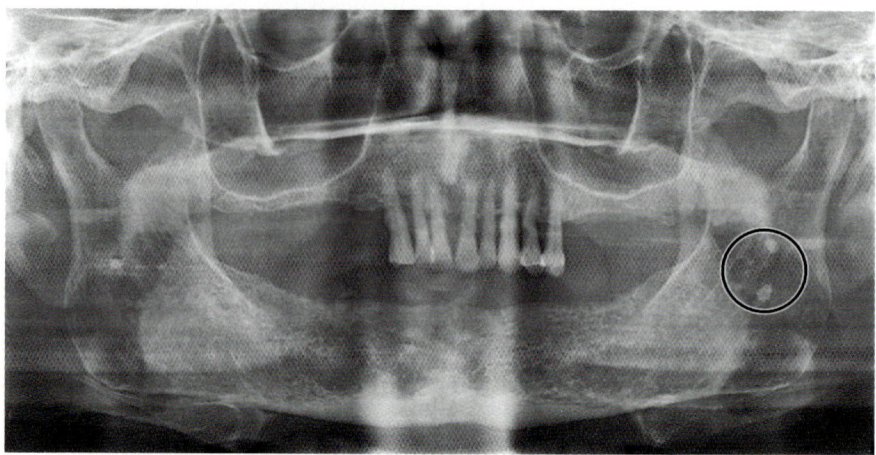

Fig. 44.2: Panoramic radiograph showing dystrophic calcification of tonsils (marked in circle)

complete their life cycle by developing into adult worms.

Clinical features: Any region of the oral cavity may be involved, but tongue (42.15%) is the most common site of predilection followed by labial (26.15%) and buccal mucosa (18.9%). Examination of the oral mucosa may disclose palpable, well-circumscribed soft fluctuant swellings, which resemble a mucocele or benign mesenchymal neoplasm. Multiple small nodules may be felt in the region of the masseter and suprahyoid muscles and in the tongue, buccal mucosa, or lip.

Radiographic features: Multiple well-defined elliptic radiopacities are viewed, resembling grains of rice with homogeneous and radiopaque internal aspect.

Arterial Calcification

Two distinct patterns of arterial calcification which can be identified both radiographically and histologically as—Monckeberg's medial calcinosis and calcified atherosclerotic plaque.

Monckeberg Medial Calcinosis/ Arteriosclerosis

Arteriosclerosis was first described by Monckeberg in 1903. The hallmark of arteriosclerosis is the fragmentation, degeneration and eventual loss of elastic fibers followed by the deposition of calcium within the medial coat of the vessel.

Clinical features: Most patients are asymptomatic initially, although later in the course of the disease cutaneous gangrene, peripheral vascular disease and myositis may occur as a result of vascular insufficiency. Patients with Sturge Weber syndrome also develop intracranial arterial calcifications.

Radiographic features: Medial calcinosis involving the facial artery or less commonly the carotid artery may be viewed on panoramic radiographs. From the side, the calcified vessel appears as a parallel pair of thin, radiopaque lines that may have a straight course or a tortuous path and is described as a 'pipe stem' or 'tram-track' appearance. In cross-section, involved vessels will display a circular or ring like pattern. There is no internal structure because the diffuse, finely divided calcium deposits occur solely in the medial wall of the vessels.

Calcified Atherosclerotic Plaque

Atheromas are calcified plaques composed of lipids and fibrous tissue, which are deposited on the walls of blood vessels and lead to atherosclerosis.

Radiographic features: These lesions may be visible in the panoramic radiograph in the soft tissues of the neck. It can be located superior or inferior to the greater cornu of the hyoid bone and adjacent to the cervical vertebrae C3, C4 or the intervertebral space between them. These soft tissue calcifications are multiple in number, irregularly shaped and differentiated from the surrounding soft tissues by their vertical linear distribution. These soft tissue calcifications are multiple in number, irregularly shaped and differentiated from the surrounding soft tissues by their vertical linear distribution. These soft tissue calcifications are usually multiple and irregular in shape and sharply defined from the surrounding soft tissues and they have a vertical linear distribution. The internal aspect is composed of a heterogeneous radiopacity with radiolucent voids (Fig. 44.3).

IDIOPATHIC CALCIFICATION

In idiopathic calcinosis, there is no identifiable cause and it appears to be multifactorial in origin.

Sialolith

Sialoliths are calcified deposits in the ducts of major and minor salivary glands or within the glands itself. Greater than 80% of the sialoliths occur in the submandibular gland or its duct followed by 6% in the parotid gland and 2%. In addition, the submandibular duct is longer, tortuous with a narrow orifice and the gland has an anti-gravity flow.

Clinical features: Sialoliths are round or ovoid in shape, rough or smooth in texture and yellowish in color. Usually, sialolith ranges from 1 mm to less than 1 cm in size. They usually occur singly but may be multiple, especially in the parotid gland. Patients with salivary stones may be asymptomatic, but they usually have a history of pain and swelling in the floor of the mouth and in the involved submandibular gland or in the cheek in case of parotid sialoliths. This discomfort may intensify at mealtimes.

Radiographic features: Sialoliths located in the duct of the submandibular gland usually are cylindrical and very smooth in their outlines. Some stones are homogeneously radiopaque and others show evidence of multiple layers of calcification (Fig. 44.4).

Phlebolith

Phleboliths are pathological, calcified vascular thrombi formed due to stasis of blood. Hemangiomas and developmental vascular malformations of the head and neck region are frequently associated with multiple phleboliths.

Clinical features: The involved soft tissue may be swollen, throbbing or discolored by the presence of veins or a hemangioma.

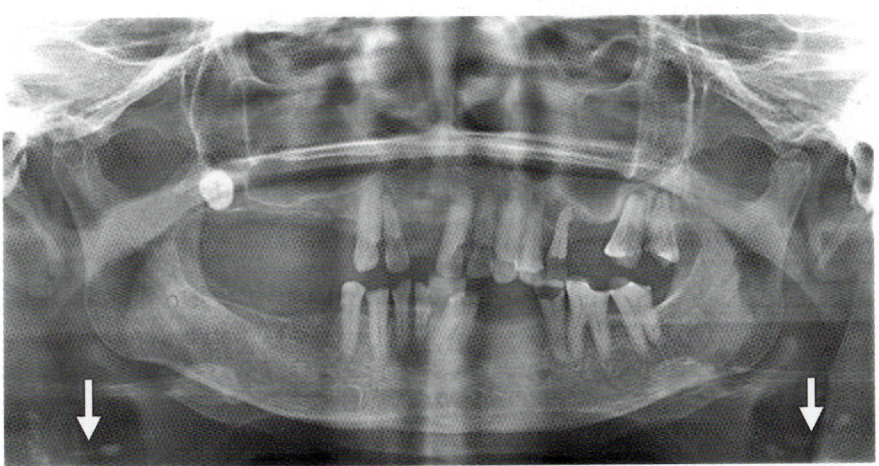

Fig. 44.3: Panoramic radiograph showing bilateral atheromas (arrows)

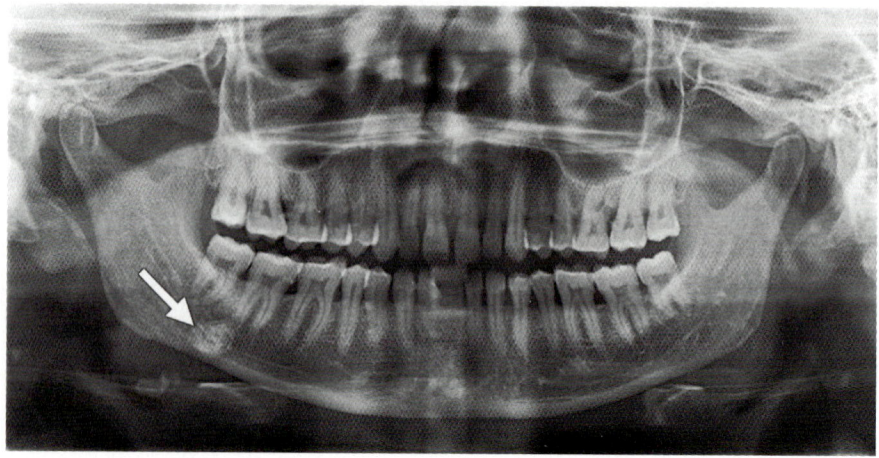

Fig. 44.4: Panoramic radiograph showing sialolith on the right side (arrow)

Applying pressure to the involved tissue should cause a blanching or change in color, if the lesion is vascular in nature. Auscultation may reveal a bruit in cases of cavernous hemangioma but not in the capillary type.

Radiographic features: The shape is round or oval in cross-section, up to 6 mm in diameter with a smooth periphery. If the involved blood vessel is viewed from the side, the phlebolith may resemble a straight or slightly curved sausage. The internal aspect may be homogeneously radiopaque but more commonly has the appearance of laminations, giving phleboliths a "bull's-eye or target appearance". The radiopaque center and concentric rings of calcification give an 'Onion skinning like' appearance.

Laryngeal Cartilage Calcifications

Both the thyroid and the triticeous (means grain of wheat) cartilages consist of hyaline cartilage, which has a tendency to calcify or ossify with advancing age. Calcification of tracheal cartilages is an incidental radiographic finding with no clinical features.

Radiographic features: The calcified triticeous cartilage is located on a lateral skull or panoramic radiograph within the soft tissues of the pharynx, inferior to the greater cornu of the hyoid bone and located adjacent to the superior border of C4. The superior cornu of a calcified thyroid cartilage is positioned medial to C4 and is superimposed on the prevertebral soft tissue. The size of triticeous cartilage ranges from 7 to 9 mm in length and 2 to 4 mm in width. The periphery is well defined and smooth and the geometry is exceedingly regular. Calcified tracheal cartilages generally present a homogeneous radiopacity but may occasionally demonstrate an outer cortex.

Rhinolith

Rhinolith is a Greek word where 'rhino' meaning nose and 'lithos' meaning stone. They are mineralized masses found within the nasal cavity. It originates from the deposition of magnesium, iron, calcium and phosphorus around a nidus, which can be endogenous or exogenous in origin.

Clinical features: Rhinoliths are generally seen in the floor of nose, about halfway between the anterior and posterior portions of the nasal cavity. They are present as grayish irregular masses and feel hard, bony and gritty on probing. Larger rhinoliths can lead to unilateral foul smelling nasal discharge, nasal obstruction, facial pain, headache, nasal bleeding, ear discharge, anosmia, palatal and septal perforation.

Radiographic features: Rhinoliths develop in the nose. These stones have a variety of shapes and sizes, depending on the nature of the nidus. They may present as homogeneous or heterogeneous radiopacities, depending on the nature of the nidus and may sometimes have laminations. Occasionally the density will exceed the surrounding bone.

Antrolith

Antroliths are calcified bodies that are formed as a result of mineral salt deposition around a nucleus within the antral cavity.

Clinical features: Stones are frequently covered by granulation tissue with a rich blood supply and its color may diverge from black to gray or white. These masses are usually asymptomatic, but they may be associated with dull pain mimicking sinusitis.

Radiographic features: Antroliths are observed as radiopaque masses of varying sizes and shapes with irregular borders and they are occasionally accompanied by antral mucosal swelling, fluid and polyps.

METASTATIC CALCIFICATION

The deposition of calcium salts in normal tissues is known as metastatic calcification and is almost always secondary to some derangement in calcium metabolism (hypercalcemia).

Ossification of the Stylohyoid Ligament

Ossification of the stylohyoid ligament usually extends downward from the base of the skull and commonly occurs bilaterally. However, in rare cases the ossification begins at the lesser horn of the hyoid or in the central area of the ligament. The associated conditions are Eagle syndrome, styloid syndrome and styloid chain ossification (Fig. 44.5).

Clinical features: The ossified ligament usually can be detected by palpation over the tonsil as a hard, pointed structure. Only a minority of patients have symptoms. Symptoms related to this ossified ligament are termed Eagle syndrome, which is expressed as one of two subtypes: Classic Eagle syndrome resulting from cranial nerve impingement, and the carotid artery syndrome, resulting from impingement on the carotid vessels.

Radiographic features: In a panoramic image the linear ossification extends forward from the region of the mastoid process and crosses the posteroinferior aspect of the ramus toward the hyoid bone. The styloid process appears as a long, tapering, thin, radiopaque process that is thicker at its base and projects downward and forward. It normally varies from about 0.5 to 2.5 cm in length. The ossified ligament has roughly a straight outline, but in some cases some irregularity may be seen in the outer surface. The farther the radiopaque ossified ligament extends

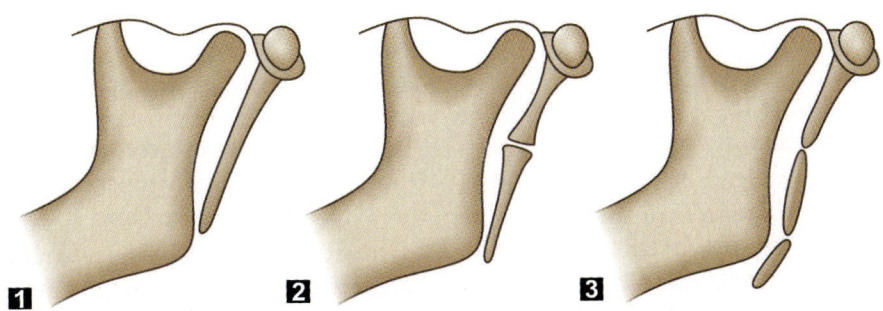

Fig. 44.5: The three types of radiographic appearances of styloid process (Type 1: Elongated; Type 2: Pseudoarticulated; Type 3: Segmented, respectively).

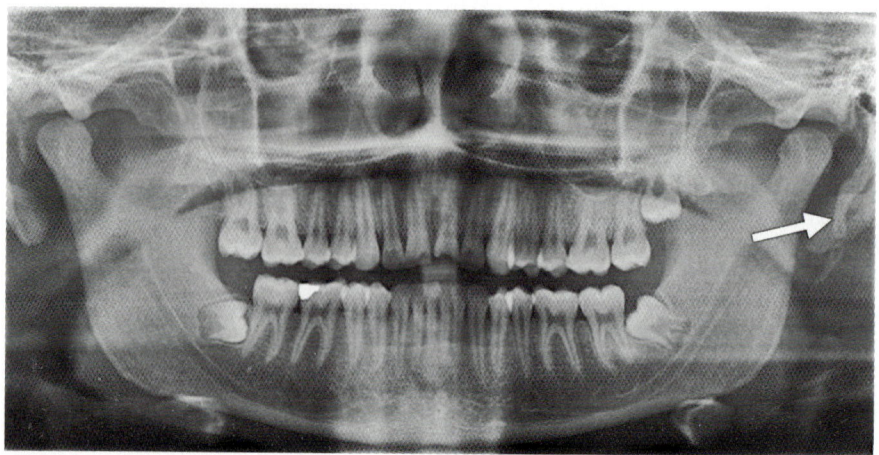

Fig. 44.6: Panoramic radiograph showing pseudoarticulated type of styloid process on the left side

toward the hyoid bone, the more likely it is that it will be interrupted by radiolucent, joint like junctions (pseudoarticulations). Small ossifications of the stylohyoid ligament appear homogeneously radiopaque. As the ossification increases in length and girth, the outer cortex of this bone becomes evident as a radiopaque band at the periphery (Fig. 44.6).

Osteoma Cutis

Osteoma cutis is a rare benign disorder where osseous nodules form in the reticular layer of normal skin. These nodules are formed by the deposition of lamellar bone and are characterized by osteocytes in the core and osteoclasts around the periphery.

Clinical features: Osteoma cutis can occur anywhere, but the face is the most common site. The tongue is the most common intraoral site. Osteoma cutis does not cause any visible change in the overlying skin other than an occasional color change that may appear yellowish white. If the lesion is large, the individual osteoma may be palpated.

Radiographic features: Radiographically, osteoma cutis most commonly appears in the cheek and lip regions. In this location the image can be superimposed over a tooth root or alveolar process, giving the appearance of an area of dense bone. Osteoma cutis appears as smoothly outlined, radiopaque, washer-shaped images. These single or multiple radiopacities usually are very small, ranging in size from 0.1 to 5 cm. The internal aspect may be homogeneously radiopaque but usually has a radiolucent center that represents normal fatty marrow, giving the lesion a doughnut appearance radiographically. Individual lesions of calcified cystic acne resemble a snowflake like radiopacity, which corresponds to the clinical location of the scar.

Myositis Ossificans

In myositis ossificans; fibrous tissue and heterotopic bone form within the interstitial tissue of muscle and associated tendons and ligaments. There are two principal forms: Localized and progressive.

Myositis Ossificans Traumatica

It is also called myositis ossificans circum-scripta, localized myositis ossificans or fibrodysplasia ossificans circumscripta. This condition results from acute or chronic trauma or from heavy muscular strain caused by certain occupations and sports.

Clinical features: The signs and symptoms of the MOT start immediately after the injury or up to 6 months later, but they may appear 20 years after trauma, as in some cases. The site of the precipitating trauma remains swollen, tender, and painful much longer than expected. The overlying skin may be red and inflamed, and when the lesion involves a muscle of mastication, opening the jaws may be difficult. After about 2 or 3 weeks, the area of ossification becomes apparent in the tissues; a firm intramuscular mass can be palpated. The localized lesion may enlarge slowly, but eventually it stops growing. The lesion may appear fixed, or it may be freely movable on palpation. The most commonly involved muscles of the head and neck are the masseter and sternocleidomastoid however, other muscles of mastication may be involved.

Radiographic features: The periphery of lesion commonly is more radiopaque than the internal structure. There is a variation in shape from irregular oval to linear streaks (pseudotrabeculae) running in the same direction as the normal muscle fibers. The internal structure varies with time from faintly homogeneous radiopacity to delicate lacy or feathery radiopaque internal structure.

Myositis Ossificans Progressiva

Myositis ossificans progressiva is also known as fibrodysplasia ossificans progressiva, Stone man disease or Muncher-Meyer disease. It is a rare hereditary disorder with autosomal dominant trait.

Clinical features: Mostly, the heterotopic ossification starts in the muscles of the neck and upper back region and then moves to the extremities. The disease commences with soft tissue swelling that is tender and painful and may show redness and heat, indicating the presence of inflammation. The acute symptoms subside, and a firm mass remains in the tissues. Stiffness and limitation of motion of the neck, chest, back, and extremities (especially the shoulders) gradually increase. In the advanced stages of the disease the 'petrified man' condition can be observed.

Radiographic features: The radiographic appearance of progressive myositis ossificans is similar to that described for the traumatic form. The heterotopic bone is more commonly aligned along the long axis of the involved muscle.

FREQUENTLY ASKED QUESTIONS

1. Discuss differential diagnosis of radiopacities at the angle of mandible.
2. Mention various causes of well-defined radiopacities which can detected in maxillomandibular region.

BIBLIOGRAPHY

1. Kirsch T. Determinants of pathological mineralization. Curr Opin Rheumatol. 2006;18(2):174–180.
2. Carter LC. Soft Tissue Calcification and Ossification. Oral Radiology Principles and Interpretations. 6th ed. St. Louis, Missouri: Mosby Elsevier; 2009. p. 526–540.
3. Karjodkar FR. Soft tissue calcifications and ossifications. Essentials of Oral and Maxillofacial Radiology. 1st ed. New Delhi: Jaypee Brothers Medical Publishers; 2014. P 503–515.
4. Mohan H. Cell Injury and Cellular Adaptations. Textbook of pathology. 6th ed. New Delhi: Jaypee Brothers Medical Publishers; 2010. p. 51–54.
5. Muto T, Michiya H, Kanazawa M, Sato K. Pathological calcification of the cervicofacial region. Br J Oral Maxillofac Surg. 1991; 29(2):120–122.
6. Bar T, Zagury A. Calcifications simulating sialolithiasis of the major salivary glands. Dentomaxillofac Radiol. 2007;36(1):59–62.
7. Neshat K, Penna KJ, Shah DH. Tonsillolith: A case report. J Oral Maxillofac Surg. 2001;59(6):692–693.
8. Hung CC, Lee JC, Kang BH, Lin YS. Giant tonsillolith. Otolaryngol Head Neck Surg. 2007;137(4):676–677.
9. Sezer B, Tugsel Z, Bilgen C. An unusual tonsillolith. Oral Surg Oral Med Oral Pathol Oral Radiol Endod. 2003;95(4):471–473.
10. Revel MP, Bely N, Laccourreye O. Giant tonsillolith. Ann Otol Rhinol Laryngol. 1998;107(3):262–263.

11. Castellano M, Marcolli G. A giant calculus of the tonsil, simulating a tumor. Minerva Med. 1966;57:1686–1688.

12. Gadgil RM. An unusual large tonsillolith. Oral Surg Oral Med Oral Pathol. 1984;58(2)237.

13. Pruet CW, Duplan DA. Tonsil concretions and tonsilloliths. Otolaryngol Clin North Am. 1987;20(2):305–309.

14. Hoffman H. Tonsillolith. Oral Surg Oral Med Oral Pathol. 1978;45(4):657–658.

15. Cox FE. History of human parasitology. Clin Microbiol Rev. 2002;15(4):595–612.

16. Prabhu SR. Oral Diseases in the Tropics. Lucknow: Oxford University Press; 1992. p. 126–129.

17. Nigam S, Singh T, Mishra A, Chaturvedi KU. Oral cysticercosis—report of six cases. Head Neck. 2001;23(6):497–499.

18. Krishnamoorthy B, Suma GN, Dhillon M, Srivastava S, Sharma ML, Malik SS. Encysted Tenia solium larva of the oral cavity: Case report with review of literature. Contemp Clin Dent. 2012;3(Suppl 2):S228–232.

19. Peacock M. Calcium metabolism in health and disease. Clin J Am Soc Nephrol. 2010;5(1):23–30.

20. Puvabanditsin S, Garrow E, Titapiwatanakun R, Getachew R, Patel JB. Severe calcinosis cutis in an infant. Pediatr Radiol. 2005;35(5):539–542.

21. Ogata Y, Okinaka Y, Takahashi M. Antrolith associated with aspergillosis of the maxillary sinus: report of a case. J Oral Maxillofac Surg. 1997;55(1):1339–1341.

22. Kumar V, Abbas AK, Aster JC. Cell Injury, Cell Death, and Adaptations. Robbins Basic Pathology. 9th ed. Philadelphia: Elsevier Saunders; 2013. p. 25–26.

23. Eagle WW. Elongated styloid process. Report of two cases. Arch Otolaryngol. 1937;25:584–587.

24. Fazeli P, Harvell J, Jacobs MB. Osteoma cutis (cutaneous ossification). West J Med. 1999;171(4):243–245.

25. Moritz DL, Elewski B. Pigmented post acne osteoma cutis in a patient treated with minocycline: Report and review of the literature. J Am Acad Dermatol. 1991; 24(5):851–853.

Trauma:
Teeth and Jaws

INTRODUCTION

Traumatic injuries to maxillofacial skeleton including dental structures have become prevalent in multiple trauma patients. Of all trauma patients, around 25% withstand a maxillofacial injury. Patients with only maxillofacial trauma have relatively less risk for life-threatening conditions; however, associated injuries like spinal cord injury can be dangerous for them if not diagnosed early. Accurate diagnosis is essential for the proper treatment of facial trauma to reduce postoperative morbidity for the victim. Understanding of the skeletal and soft tissue anatomy of the maxillofacial unit and proper clinical and radiographic evaluation are very important for the management of these victims.

Until recently, diagnostic imaging of facial trauma mostly comprised of standard facial and panoramic radiographs and, if the facility available, computed tomographic evaluation. In most cases, standard radiographic examination is sufficient and useful in evaluation of these injuries and their healing/repair. This chapter will discuss diagnostic imaging in the patient with maxillofacial trauma.

NORMAL ANATOMY

The facial skeleton is attached to the anterior cranial fossa and the sphenoidal bones.

Each of the facial bone can be identified on the frontal or lateral view of skull except hard palate and vomer (Fig. 45.1). Of the fourteen bones those form facial skeleton, two are single (vomer and mandible) and six are paired (maxillae, zygomatic, palatine, nasal and lacrimal bones; and inferior nasal conchae). While two maxillae are the largest immovable bones, other bones form the upper part of facial skeleton. The dentoalveolar portion of the maxilla forms a horizontal supporting structure for teeth and associated structures; and confines the hard palate.

Zygoma or malar bone forms the prominence of cheek and is located lateral to the zygomatic process of maxilla. The zygomatic process of temporal bone unites with the posterior slender extension of the zygoma to form the curved zygomatic arch. In the midline, the nasal septum is formed by the ethmoidal plate and the vomer. It provides a weak vertical support for the nasal bones and hard palate. The lacrimal bone lies in medial wall of the orbit and two nasal bones are fused form the bridge of nose. Both of these bones are thinnest and fragile bones of the face.

The largest and movable bone of the facial skeleton is mandible. Although, mandible is a single bone, it forms from two separate bones that unite in the midline by the end of first year of life and this part present in

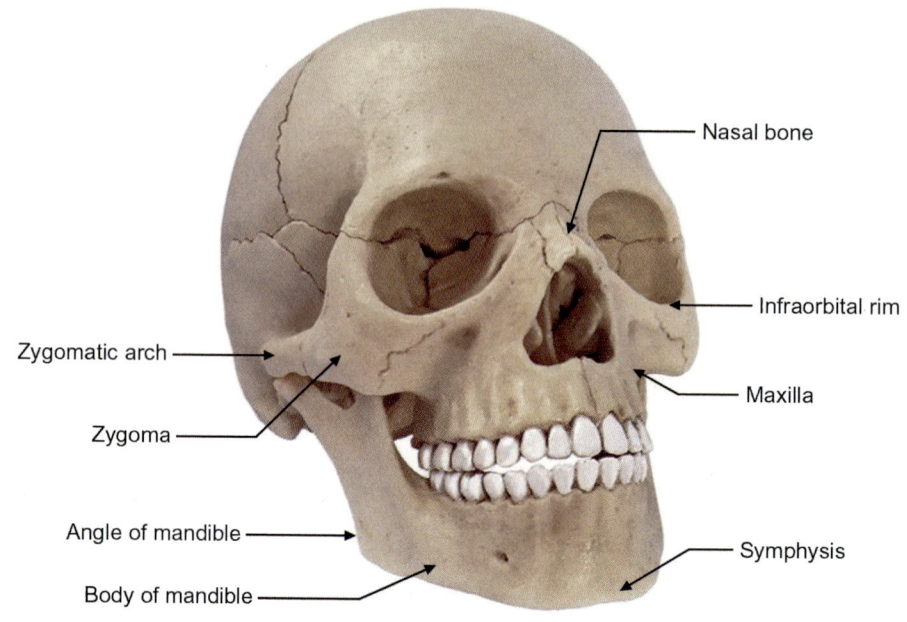

Fig. 45.1: Osteology of facial skeleton

the midline is termed symphysis. The angle of mandible divides the bone into two parts as body (anterior) and ramus (posterior). The ramus of mandible in superior portion is divided by mandibular or sigmoid notch into processes. The anterior process is coronoid process while posterior process is condyloid process. The latter contributes to the formation of temporomandibular joint along with glenoid fossa of temporal bone.

Etiology and Classification

The most common causes of facial injuries include vehicular accidents, assaults, falls, and sports-related injuries. The amount of force delivered by the impact to the facial skeleton plays an important role in the severity of the subsequent trauma. The injury level depends on the force and ranges from little comminution or displacement, or fracture displacement up to highly comminuted fractures along with alteration in facial skeletal structure. Hence, the cause of the injury is an important component in evaluation and assessment of the victim.

Maxillofacial trauma ranges from injuries to dental tissue (teeth and associated structures), simple fractures involving only one or two bony structures to complex injuries to osseous facial skeleton. Therefore, classification of facial trauma is important to outline diagnosis and develop a successful plan. Radiographic evaluation is a useful tool in classifying maxillofacial trauma and provides vital information for the initial diagnosis, treatment and follow-up.

Depending on the type of tissue or facial skeleton affected by trauma, injuries can be broadly divided into following categories:
1. Injuries to the teeth and their supporting structures
2. Fractures of the mandible
3. Fractures of the middle third of the facial skeleton
4. Other injuries involving skull bones, cranial base, cervical spine and intracranial tissue damage

Radiographic Examination

The radiographic examination should be planned after evaluation of signs and symptoms and clinical assessment. It should help to confirm the clinical diagnosis, identify fractures or foreign bodies, and obtain accurate information about severity of injury that may be obscured in clinical assessment. Need for multiple radiographs should also be considered to classify the fractures and plan best possible treatment for the patient. Further, limitations in radiographic examination should be evaluated depending on general state of the patient and the type and severity of other injuries. For example, patients with severe facial trauma are generally have intracranial damage and/or cervical spine injuries which need serious attention than any damage to orofacial structures. The radiographic investigation must, therefore, be weighed to each patient's needs.

For optimal treatment outcome, correct diagnosis of the severity of the injury is essential and must be achieved through a detailed history taking, clinical, and radiographic examination. Radiographs are important aid for differential diagnosis of traumatic dental and maxillofacial injuries. Intraoral radiographs are useful to identify the location, type, and severity of injuries of most dentoalveolar injuries.

Requirements

The ideal radiographic examination in facial injuries should include two radiographs at right angle, e.g. a periapical and an occlusal view. They should be reproducible and provide base-line assessment and subsequent follow-up. Additional chest and abdominal radiography to rule out suspected inhalation or swallowing of avulsed tooth should be planned. The radiographs should give information regarding type of injury, fracture site, degree of displacement of fractured fragments of tooth/alveolar bone. Follow-up radiographs should give information about healing response, complications like presence of root resorption and infection. In medicolegal aspect, they are considered a diagnostic measure of the first importance and also provide a visual record of the progress of the patient.

The expected radiographic features indicating a fractured site include a radiolucent line between the fragments, discontinuity in the outline shape of the affected bone.

Periapical Radiography

This is the most common radiographic examination, very easy to carry out and provides better resolution of the teeth and surrounding structures. Either paralleling or bisecting angle technique can be used. Paralleling technique is recommended as it provides accurate images with minimum distortion. Images obtained are reproducible and the response of the treatment can be evaluated in follow-up.

Bisecting angle technique is widely used as it does not require film holding device but the images are not reproducible. However in patients with limited mouth opening due to trauma, this technique is preferred.

A fracture of the crown of a tooth is easier to detect than a root fracture on radiograph. The fracture appears as a radiolucent line, or the missing part of the tooth is obvious. A root fracture also is seen as a radiolucent line, but is often difficult to reveal because of superimposition of trabeculae.

Techniques of object localization can also be employed for dentoalveolar fracture evaluation.

Occlusal Radiography

Occlusal radiography can be useful for both the jaws. This view can be used in combination with periapical radiography to rule out root fractures. Extrusion of anterior teeth can be evaluated on these radiographs. This view is very useful in patients with limited mouth opening and uncooperative children.

Panoramic Radiography

This view provides visualization of whole of maxilla and mandible including parts of zygomatic arches and condyles. Fractures of alveolar bone, body and symphysis of mandible can be easily visualized while fractures in anterior region may be obscured due to overlapping of cervical vertebrae. Evaluation of condylar and zygomatic arch fracture can also be done on panoramic view. Although fractures in walls of maxillary sinus, infraorbital margin can be suspected in panoramic view, additional extraoral views should be made to confirm them.

Assessment of Panoramic Radiograph

Sometimes, panoramic radiograph may not reveal a fracture. Therefore, it is crucial to correlate clinical findings during radiographic evaluation. In symphysis region, one should be careful to find out overlapping of fracture fragments. If there is any doubt, additional radiograph like PA skull should be recommended.

Important points to be considered during panoramic evaluation include the following:
1. Symmetry of mandible: Compare one side of mandible with other.
2. Half of the mandibular fractures are bilateral. Consider the mandible as a stiff ring of bone, as it is very common for a ring to have two fractures.
3. Evaluate angle and body areas for fractures.
4. Evaluate condylar areas for subtle fractures.
5. Check for the step deformity in the occlusal plane of teeth.
6. Always try to differentiate overlapping anatomic shadows of tongue space

and pharyngeal spaces that may mimic fracture lines.
7. Get familiar with routinely encountered artifacts on panoramic views.

Extraoral Radiography

Conventional film radiography is often used for the routine evaluation of maxillofacial trauma because of low cost, wide availability, and low radiation exposure. The extraoral views generally give an acceptable review of the facial bones and wherever there is suspicion about the extent of the injuries, they should be recommended. There is series of extraoral views and one can select one of more views as per the need of the victim. The various views include lateral oblique views of the mandible (body and ramus projections), posteroanterior views (skull, mandible and reverse Towne), occipitomental, submentovertex, and true lateral projections. Table 45.1 illustrates the site of facial injury and recommended projections.

The Water's view is obtained so that the petrous part of temporal bone lies entirely beneath the floor of the maxillary sinus, allowing clear visibility of the complete region. This view reveals the maxillary and ethmoidal air sinuses and anterior facial structures that include nasal bones, anterior orbital floors, zygomas, anterior lamina papyracea (the orbital lamina of ethmoid bone). This radiograph provides the outlines of the major segments of the midface buttresses.

The submentovertex view is obtained by using a vertex-submental beam or with the

TABLE 45.1: Extraoral radiographs in maxillofacial trauma

Trauma site	Projection	Region viewed
Mandible	✗ Lateral oblique ✗ PA mandible ✗ Reverse Towne	✗ Angle, body, and condyle ✗ Horizontal displacement at mandibular angles and condyles ✗ Condylar neck fractures
Maxilla and zygomatic region	✗ Occipitomental ✗ Submentovertex	✗ Orbital margins, malar buttress, maxillary sinus ✗ Zygomatic arch, supraorbital margin

patient upright with the neck hyperextended by using a submental-vertex X-ray beam. However, it is difficult to perform in the acutely traumatized patient and requires ruling out of any cervical spine injury. It is preferred to get mandibular symphysis superimposed on the frontal sinus. This view is useful in evaluating the medial and lateral walls of the maxillary sinus, the lateral wall of the orbit, and the sphenoidal margin of the temporal bone. The zygomatic arches can be seen if the projection is underexposed ('jug handle' view).

A reverse Towne projection is important for evaluation of the petrous ridges and mastoid air cells, mandibular condyles, and condylar necks. It helps in assessment of the subcondylar region and the inferior orbital fissure.

Advanced Imaging

Computed tomographic examination is most useful in complex maxillofacial trauma. This facility is now available in many hospitals and provides valuable information in head injury patients during early assessment. At the same time, the midfacial fractures can be diagnosed during scanning. Computed tomography is very important in the assessment of nasoethmoidal complex and orbital injuries. Computed reconstructions and 3D reconstruction can be mostly useful in multiple fractures (Fig. 45.2).

INJURIES TO THE TEETH AND THEIR SUPPORTING STRUCTURES

The different types of dental injuries include fractures and luxation of the teeth, fractures of the alveolar bone or combination of both. Tooth fracture may be coronal involving enamel, enamel and dentin or involving enamel, dentin and pulp. Root fractures may occur with or without coronal fractures.

Luxation injuries can be in the form of concussion, subluxation, extrusion, intrusion lateral displacement of avulsion of teeth. Fractures of the alveolar bone may involve socket, alveolar process or may involve the associated jaw. Traumatic injuries during mixed dentition period can cause displacement of developing tooth bud. When avulsion of tooth is found during clinical examination, swallowing or inhaling an avulsed tooth should be ruled out.

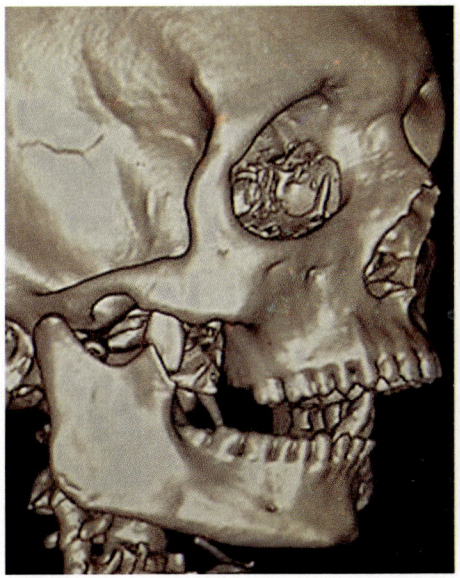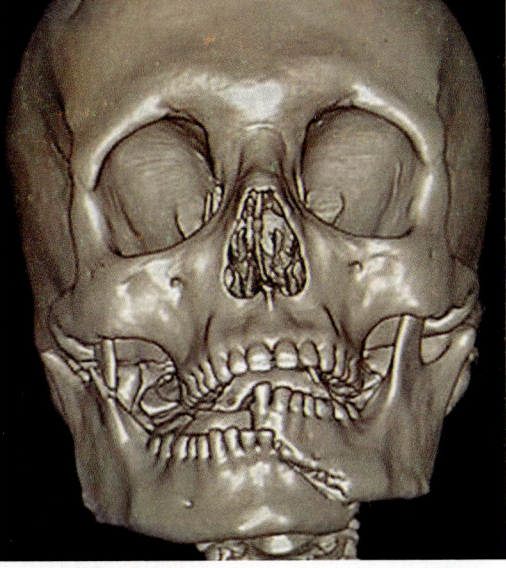

Fig. 45.2: 3D reconstruction image showing coronoid fracture and parasymphysial fracture. (Picture courtesy: Dr. Vijaykumar Girhe, Aurangabad)

Radiographic examination: Radiographic examination should be carried out for all traumatized dentoalveolar complex even though evident clinically to assess severity of damage caused by trauma. They also help in evaluation of healing process and postoperative complications.

The ideal radiographic examination should include two perpendicular views for example, periapical and occlusal views in anterior segment. A panoramic radiograph can be recommended to rule out jaw fractures. Chest and abdominal radiography should be performed if swallowing of avulsed tooth or foreign body is suspected. Soft tissue radiographs of lips or cheeks can be advised for evaluation of embedded foreign objects.

Radiographic interpretation: Radiographs should be evaluated for type of dental tissue injury, displacement of fractured tooth or root fragments. Careful observation of lamina dura and periodontal ligament space to check their discontinuity and widening respectively should be done. The trauma has affected the mixed dentition then stage of root formation, injury to the developing permanent tooth bud should be observed

carefully. If there is any radiolucent line in alveolar bone raising suspicion of alveolar fracture, panoramic radiographs can be made to evaluate further extension of fracture line.

Follow-up radiographs should be evaluated for signs of healing, development of secondary infection, crown or root resorption and condition of affected tooth bud.

Radiographs may pose difficulty in detection of root fractures due to overlapping of adjacent structures.

Fractures of the Mandible

Mandible is most commonly affected bone in facial traumatic injuries due to its shape and anatomic location. It can fracture at site of direct trauma and at other sites due to the impact of trauma. Various sites for fractures are shown in Fig. 45.3. Fractures of the mandible can be favorable or unfavorable depending on how the fracture line progresses and how the forces are exerted by muscles attached to the mandible. Direction of fracture line determines whether it is stable or unstable. Fractures running from posterior downward to anterior generally are

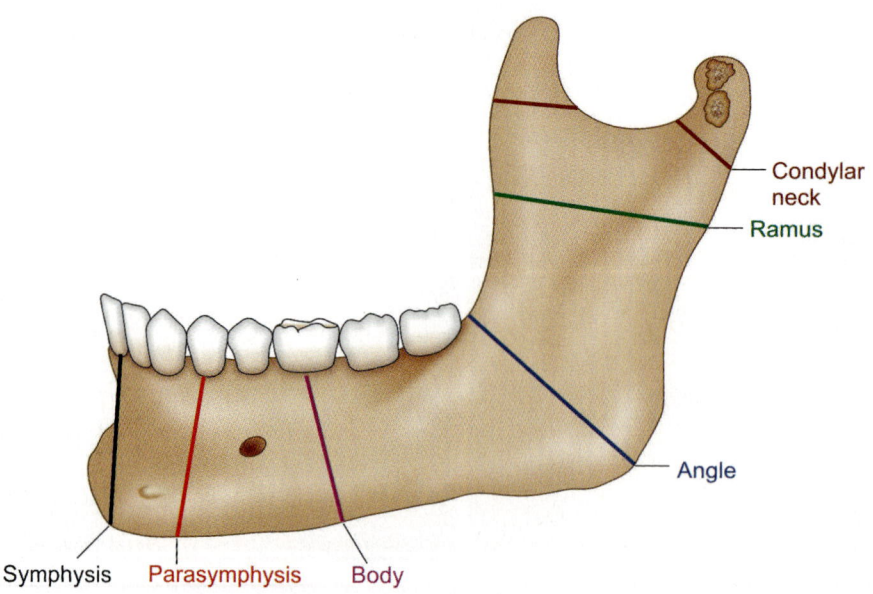

Fig. 45.3: Various fracture sites of mandible

favorable, because muscles pull the fractured fragments together.

Mandibular fractures are classified according to the anatomic region involved into: Symphyseal fractures, alveolar process fractures, fractures of the body or horizontal ramus, fractures of the angle, fractures of the ascending ramus, coronoid process fractures and fractures of the mandibular condyle.

Radiographic examination: The radiologic diagnosis of a suspected mandibular fracture initially depends on clnical examination of the victim. Whether the patient presents with an isolated injury or with multi-injury trauma is a determining factor. If one suspects only an isolated mandibular fracture, various radiographic views like posteroanterior (PA) view, Reverse Towne view, and bilateral oblique views are indicated. Availability of panoramic radiography can be the best adjuvant in diagnosis of mandibular fractures (Figs 45.4 and 45.5). One should plan to make two views atright angles to one another. If dentoalveolar complex is involved, intraoral views are recommended to evaluate teeth in the line of fracture.

Radiographic interpretation: Mandibular fractures are mainly diagnosed by radiolucent lines between the bony fragments. Displaced fracture fragments are easy to diagnose however fractures involving the buccal and lingual cortical plates may produce two radiolucent lines.

Presence of step deformity at inferior border of mandible is seen in displaced fracture segments. If the fracture fragments overlap on each other, a radiopaque line will be seen. As discussed earlier, forces of muscles attached and severity of impact force will determine the degree of displacement. Therefore, careful correlation of clinical findings with radiographic evaluation is vital for diagnosis and treatment plan.

Midfacial Fractures

Diagnosis of midfacial fracture is one of the most challenging areas in dental radiography. The factors like complex anatomy of facial skeleton, thin bones of orbital and nasal complex and maxillary sinuses play important role in their diagnosis and treatment plan. Therefore, sound knowledge of osteology and normal radiographic anatomy is essential. Additionally, understanding of direction of fracture lines, radiographic presentation of fracture site and prescription of correct radiographic projections are governing factors to reach the diagnosis.

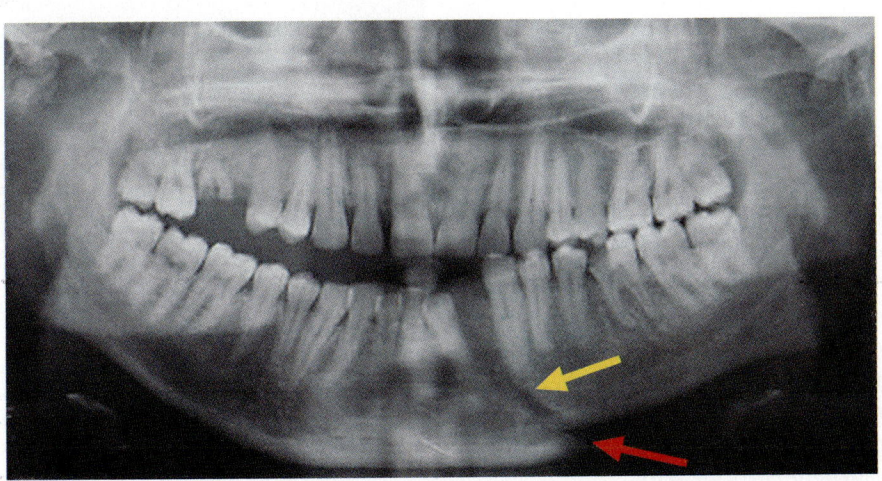

Fig. 45.4: Panoramic radiograph showing parasymphysial fracture (yellow arrow). Observe the step formation in inferior border (red arrow)

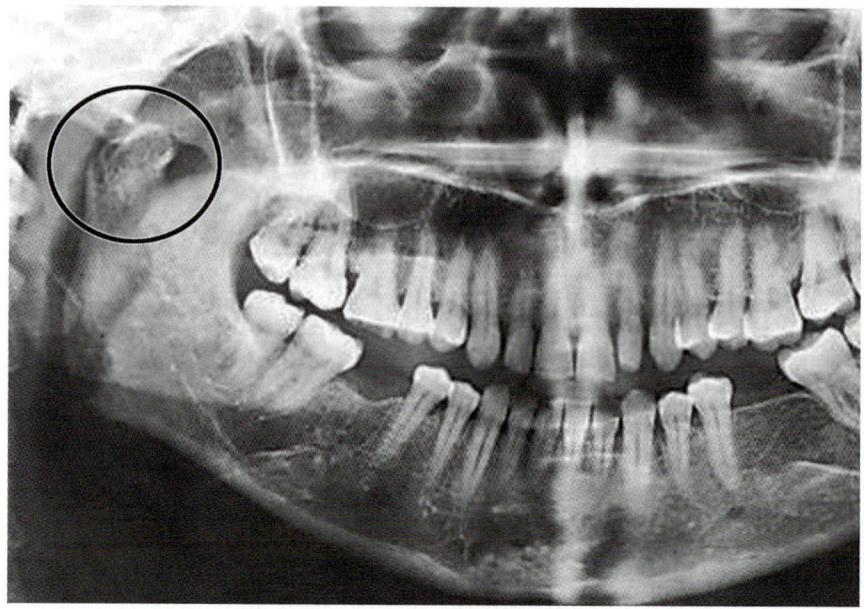

Fig. 45.5: Cropped panoramic radiograph showing condylar fracture

Classification

Most injuries to the middle third of the face are from the front, forcing part or parts of the facial skeleton downwards and backwards along the cranial base. The resulting lines of fracture follow the lines of weakness of the facial skeleton, as shown in Fig. 45.5. Thus fractures of the middle third of the face can be classified into following six categories:

1. Alveolar
2. Guerin's/Le Fort I
3. Pyramidal/Le Fort II
4. High transverse/Le Fort III
5. Naso-ethmoidal complex
6. Malar/zygomatic

1. **Alveolar fractures:** Alveolar fractures occur in the tooth bearing areas of the jaw. Dentoalveolar trauma may present in isolation, resulting from low-velocity blunt facial trauma to the anterior segment, or in combination with other facial fractures. Diagnosis and treatment planning for these patients can often be accomplished with the use of panoramic and periapical radiographs.

2. **Guerin's or Le Fort I fracture:** In this fracture, the palate and alveolus are

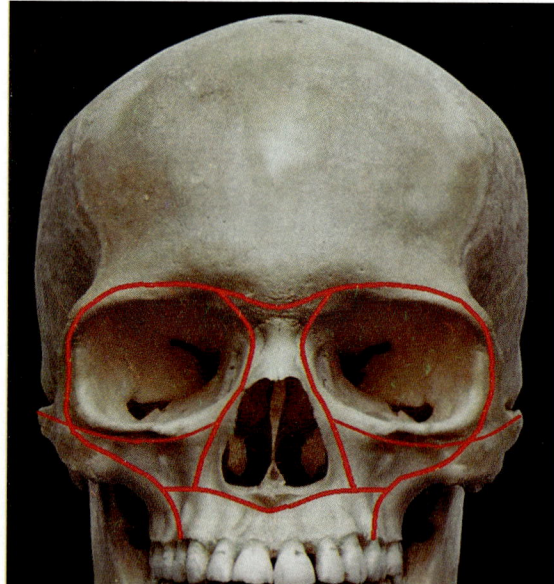

Fig. 45.6: Grid system of buttresses of maxillary complex

separated from the maxillary complex by a transverse fracture just above the floor of the nasal cavity, the maxillary sinuses and the vomer and the internal pterygoid plates.

3. **Le Fort II fracture:** Le Fort type II fracture is also called pyramidal fracture as the central portion of the face becomes separated from the skull as a pyramidal fragment. The fracture line runs across the nasal bridge, through lacrimal bones, the internal wall and floor of both orbits, obliquely across the anterior maxillary sinus, extending posteriorly to the lower pterygoid plates.

4. **Le Fort III fracture:** In this fracture, the maxillary complex is separated from the skull by a fracture line that crosses the lateral walls of both orbits and both orbital floors and crosses the midline at the root of the nose to involve the cribriform plate of the ethmoid bone. One must remember that all Le Fort III fractures are considered head injuries and should be treated as such. Further, as the anterior cranial fossa communicates with the nose through the fractured cribriform plate, there are high chances of ascending infection in this region.

5. **The nasal bone and nasoethmoidal complex fracture:** This may be involved separately or in combination with other fractures. Nasoethmoidal fractures can occur due to direct blow on the bridge of nose, and the nasal pyramid is displaced posteriorly, fracturing the nasal bones, frontal processes of the maxillae, lacrimal bones, ethmoid sinuses, cribriform plate, and nasal septum.

6. **Malar/zygomatic (tripod or trimalar) fracture:** These are the second most common isolated fractures of the face. Zygomatic bone may get fractured by a direct blow to the prominence of the cheek. The fracture line passes through the infraorbital margin, the anterior wall of the sinus, the malar buttress, the zygomatic arch and the frontal process of the zygomatic bone.

Radiographic examination: Radiographic examination of midfacial fractures is related to general condition, intracranial and spinal injuries and the severity of the facial trauma. Nevertheless, true lateral skull projection should be done in all cases to rule out fractures of the base of skull. This view reveals fluid level in the sphenoidal air sinus, a characteristic feature of fracture of base of skull. Minimum of two views at right angles should be carried out, although several views may be required. The occipitomental radiographs (Water's view) are the mainstay in midfacial fractures and should be evaluated from a distance for facial asymmetry. They delineates the nasal pyramid fractures and useful in finding the fractures in walls of maxillary and frontal sinuses, orbital rims and zygomatic tripod. During evaluation of occipitomental view, consider the malar bone as a seat of four-legged stool, wherein four legs include zygomatic arch, frontal process of zygomatic bone, infraorbital margin, and lateral wall of maxillary sinus **(Fig. 45.7A and B)**. These structures being weak are prone for fractures and need careful evaluation on occipitomental projection. Submentovetrex projections with reduced exposure should be made for fractures of zygomatic arches (Jug-handle view).

Panoramic radiography is particularly useful for fractures of the dentoalveolar area of the maxilla. When a fracture is suspected in a panoramic projection, especially in the maxillary sinuses or in the orbital rim, it is recommended that further radiographic projections should be taken for confirmation of fracture.

Radiographic interpretation: In anterior maxilla, fracture of the labial cortical plate may be seen on an occlusal radiograph. Sometimes, fracture of alveolar one may overlap the roots of teeth and can confuse the root fractures. Projection with different angulation can be useful in differentiation. The occipitomental (Water's) view provides a good image of the zygomatic bone and midface that will show the displaced fracture fragment **(Fig. 45.8)**.

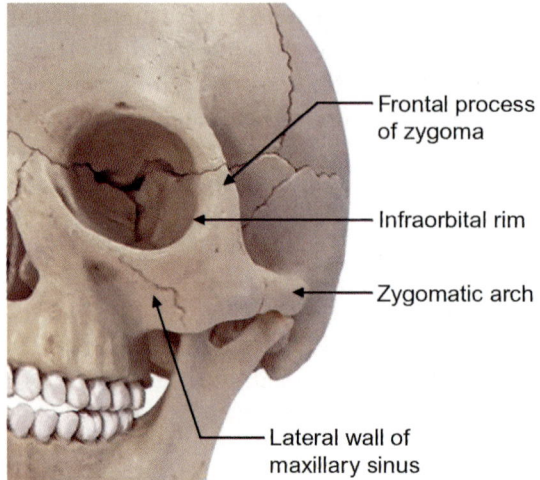

Fig. 45.7A: Zygomatic complex—note the four legs that should be evaluated on occipitomental view (Bony view)

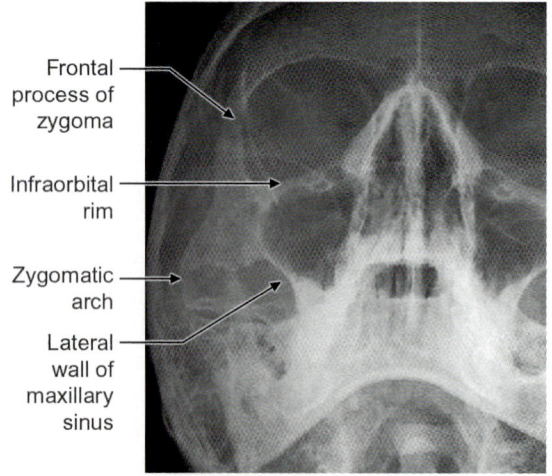

Fig. 45.7B: Zygomatic complex—note the four legs that should be evaluated on occipitomental view (radiographic view)

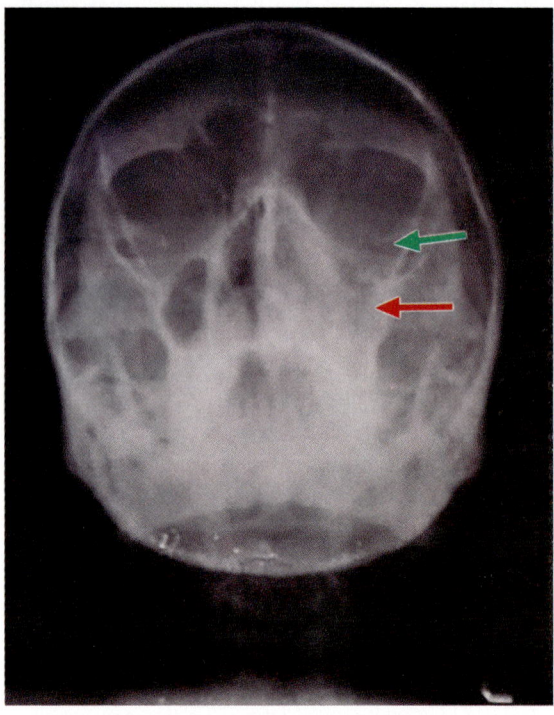

Fig. 45.8: Occipitomental view showing fractured left infraorbital rim (green arrow). Note the obscured left sinus (red arrow)

outweigh the need for management of facial trauma. Further, it is beyond the scope of this textbook to discuss these injuries in detail, but the most commonly used radiographic surveys, apart from conventional radiography, include computed tomography with 3D reconstruction. Intracranial injuries can be best evaluated with magnetic resonance imaging.

FREQUENTLY ASKED QUESTIONS

1. Correlate site of trauma and required radiographic investigation (scenario based).

OTHER FRACTURES AND INJURIES

Maxillofacial fractures may be associated with injury to skull vault, base of skull or cervical spines. The clinical assessment and severity of involvement of these structures in trauma mostly govern the need of the patient to receive emergency and life-supporting care. Most of the times, these situations

BIBLIOGRAPHY

1. White SC, Pharoah MJ. Oral Radiology: Principles and Interpretation. 6th edition. St. Louis, Mo: Mosby/Elsevier, 2009.
2. Whaites E. Essentials of Dental Radiography and Radiology. 5th edition. Edinburgh: Churchill Livingstone, 2007.

3. MacDonald D. Oral and Maxillofacial Radiology: A diagnostic Approach. John Wiley and Sons, 2011.
4. Moore UJ. Principles of Oral and Maxillofacial Surgery, 5th edition. Blackwell Science, 2001.
5. Roberts G, Longhurst P. Oral and Dental Trauma in Children and Adolescents. Oxford University Press, 1996.
6. Bali R, Sharma P, Garg A, Dhillon G. A comprehensive study on maxillofacial trauma conducted in Yamunanagar, India. J Inj Violence Res. 2013;5:108–16.
7. Kullman L, Al Sane M. Guidelines for dental radiography immediately after a dento-alveolar trauma, a systematic literature review. Dental Traumatology. 2012; 28: 193–9.
8. Naeem A, Gemal H, Reed D. Imaging in traumatic mandibular fractures. Quant Imaging Med Surg., 2017; 7: 469–79.
9. Tomich G, Baigorria P, Orlando N, Méjico M, Costamagna C, Villavicencio RL. Frequency and types of fractures in maxillofacial traumas. Assessment using multislice computed tomography with multiplanar and threedimensional reconstructions. Revista Argentina de Radiolog´ıa. 2011;75: 305–17.
10. Dolan KD, Jacoby CG, Smoker WR. The radiology of facial fractures. Radiographics. 1984; 4: 575–663.
11. Laine, JL, Conway, D, Laskin, DM. Radiology of maxillofacial trauma. Curr Probl Diagn Radiol. 1993; 22:145.
12. Moilanen A. Midfacial fractures in dental panoramic radiography. Oral Surg. Oral Med Oral Pathol. 1984;57:106–10
13. Shah S, Uppal SK, Mittal RK, Garg R, Saggar K, Dhawan R. Diagnostic tools in maxillofacial fractures: Is there really a need of three-dimensional computed tomography? Indian J Plast Surg. 2016; 49(2):225–33.

Index